Hair and its Disorders

Hair and its Disorders

Biology, Pathology and Management

Edited by

Francisco M Camacho MD
Head Professor and Chairman
Department of Dermatology
Surgical Dermatology and Venereology
Hospital Virgen Macarena
University of Seville
Seville
Spain

Valerie A Randall PhD
Department of Biomedical Studies
University of Bradford
Bradford
West Yorkshire
UK

Vera H Price MD, FRCP(C)
Professor of Clinical Dermatology
Department of Dermatology
University of California, San Francisco
San Francisco
USA

MARTIN ■ DUNITZ

© Martin Dunitz Ltd 2000

First published in the United Kingdom in 2000 by
Martin Dunitz Ltd
The Livery House
7–9 Pratt Street
London NW1 0AE

Tel: +44-(0)20-7482-2202
Fax: +44-(0)20-7267-0159
E-mail: **info@mdunitz.globalnet.co.uk**
Website: http://www.dunitz.co.uk

A CIP catalogue record for this book is available from the British Library

ISBN 1-85317-799-7

Distributed in the United States by:
Blackwell Science Inc.
Commerce Place, 350 Main Street
Malden MA 02148, USA
Tel: 1-800-215-1000

Distributed in Canada by:
Login Brothers Book Company
324 Salteaux Crescent
Winnipeg, Manitoba R3J 3T2
Canada
Tel: 1-204-224-4068

Distributed in Brazil by:
Ernesto Reichmann Distribuidora de Livros, Ltda
Rua Coronel Marques 335, Tatuape 03440-000
Sao Paulo,
Brazil

Composition by Wearset, Boldon, Tyne and Wear
Printed and bound in Italy by Printer Trento

Contents

Contributors

Howard P Baden MD
Professor of Dermatology
Harvard Medical School
Massachusetts General Hospital
Cutaneous Biology Research Center
Charlestown
MA 02129
USA

David de Berker MRCP
Consultant Dermatologist
Bristol Dermatology Centre
Bristol Royal Infirmary
Bristol
UK

Peter Bjerring MD PhD
Professor
Department of Dermatology
Marselisborg Hospital
University of Aarhus
8000 Aarhus C
Denmark

Ulrike Blume-Peytavi MD
Department of Dermatology
University Medical Centre Benjamin Franklin
The Free University of Berlin
12200 Berlin
Germany

Bernadette de Brouwer BSc
Skinterface sprl
Skin Study Center
Tournai 7500
Belgium

Jean Claude Bystryn MD
Professor of Dermatology
The Ronald O Perelman Department of
Dermatology
New York University School of Medicine
New York
NY 10016
USA

Francisco M Camacho MD
Head Professor and Chairman
Department of Dermatology, Surgical
Dermatology and Venereology
Hospital Virgen Macarena
University of Seville
Seville
Spain

Jérôme Castanet MD
Service de Dermatologie
Centre Hospitalier Universitaire de Nice
Hôpital Archet 2
06202 Nice
France

Cheng-Ming Chuong MD PhD
Professor
Department of Pathology
University of Southern California
Los Angeles
CA 90033
USA

George Cotsarelis MD
Department of Dermatology
University of Pennsylvania School of Medicine
Philadelphia
PA 19104
USA

Rodney P R Dawber MA, MB, ChB, FRCP
Consultant Dermatologist
Department of Dermatology
Churchill Hospital
Headington
Oxford
UK

D José Luis Díaz-Pérez MD, PhD
Professor of Dermatology
Department of Dermatology
University Hospital of Cruces
48903 – Baracaldo – Bilbao
Spain

Marna Ericson PhD
Senior Scientist
Department of Dermatology
University of Minnesota
Minneapolis
MN 55455
USA

Juan Ferrando MD
Associate Professor Dermatology
Department of Dermatology
Hospital Clínic
University of Barcelona
Barcelona
Spain

Bo Forslind MD PhD
Professor Medical Biophysics
Experimental Dermatology Research Group
Medical Biophysics MBB
Karolinska Insititute
Stockholm
Sweden

María-José García-Hernández MD
Assistant Professor
Department of Dermatology
University of Seville
Seville
Spain

Christoph C Geilen MD
Professor of Dermatology
Honorary Lecturer
University Medical Centre Benjamin Franklin
The Free University of Berlin
12200 Berlin
Germany

Sofia Georgala MD
Associate Professor Dermatology
Department of Dermatology
National University of Athens
A Sygros Hospital
Athens 16121
Greece

Ramon Grimalt MD
Department of Dermatology
Hospital Clínic
University of Barcelona
Barcelona
Spain

Rudolf Happle MD
Professor of Dermatology
Department of Dermatology
Philipp University of Marburg
35037 Marburg
Germany

María K Hordinsky MD
Professor
Department of Dermatology
University of Minnesota
Minneapolis
MN 55455
USA

Rolf Hoffmann MD
Professor of Dermatology
Department of Dermatology
University of Marburg
35033 Marburg
Germany

Koji Imamura MD
Wisconsin Regional Primate Research Center
and
Department of Human Oncology
University of Wisconsin
Madison
WI 537
USA

Kensei Katsuoka MD
Professor and Chairman
Department of Dermatology
Kitasato University School of Medicine
Sagamihara 228–8555
Japan

Nathalie Mandt MD
Department of Dermatology
University Medical Centre Benjamin Franklin
The Free University of Berlin
12200 Berlin
Germany

Andrew JG McDonagh FRCP
Department of Dermatology
Royal Hallamshire Hospital
Sheffield
UK

Ian McKay PhD
Senior Lecturer
Centre for Cutaneous Research
Queen Mary and Westfield College
University of London
London
UK

Andrew G Messenger MD
Consultant Dermatologist
Department of Dermatology
Royal Hallamshire Hospital
Sheffield
UK

Sven Müller-Röver MD
Centre for Cutaneous Research
Queen Mary and Westfield College
University of London
UK

Constantin E Orfanos MD
Professor
Department of Dermatology
University Medical Centre Benjamin Franklin
The Free University of Berlin
12200 Berlin
Germany

Jean-Paul Ortonne MD
Professor
Service de Dermatologie
Centre Hospitalier Universitaire de Nice
Hôpital Archet 2
06202 Nice
France

Huei-ju Pan
Wisconsin Regional Primate Research Center
and
Department of Human Oncology
University of Wisconsin
Madison
WI 537
USA

Ralf Paus MD
Professor of Dermatology
Department of Dermatology
University Hospital Eppendorf
University of Hamburg
Hamburg
Germany

Michael P Philpott DPhil
Centre for Cutaneous Research
Queen Mary and Westfield College
University of London
London
UK

Vera H Price MD, FRCP(C)
Professor of Clinical Dermatology
Department of Dermatology
School of Medicine
University of California, San Francisco
San Francisco
CA 94117
USA

Bianca Maria Piraccini MD
Department of Dermatology
University of Bologna
Bologna 40138
Italy

Valerie A Randall PhD
Department of Biomedical Studies
University of Bradford
Bradford
West Yorkshire
UK

Rachel Reynolds MD
Department of Dermatology
Cutaneous Biology Research Centre
Massachusetts General Hospital
Charlestown
MA 02129
USA

Dimitris G Rigopoulos MD
Assistant Professor of Dermatology
Department of Dermatology
University of Athens
A Sygros Hospital
Athens 16121
Greece

Marty E Sawaya MD PhD
Principal Investigator Clinical Research
ARATEC Clinical Trials
Ocala
FL 34478
and
Adjunct Professor
University of Miami School of Medicine
Miami
FL 33124
USA

Jerry Shapiro MD, FRCPC
Clinical Associate Professor
Director
University of British Columbia
Hair Research and Treatment Centre
Division of Dermatology
University of British Columbia
Vancouver
Canada

Rodney Sinclair MBBS, FACD
Senior Lecturer
Department of Dermatology
University of Melbourne
St Vincent's Hospital
and
Consultant Dermatologist
Skin and Cancer Foundtion
Melbourne
Australia

Desmond J Tobin BSc, PhD, CBiol, FIT
Lecturer in Biomedical Sciences
Department of Biomedical Sciences
University of Bradford
Bradford
UK

Antonella Tosti MD
Associate Professor of Dermatology
Department of Dermatology
University of Bologna
Bologna 40138
Italy

Hideo Uno MD
Wisconsin Regional Primate Research Center
and
Department of Human Oncology
University of Wisconsin
Madison
WI 537
USA

Dominique Van Neste MD PhD
Managing Director of Skinterface sprl
Skin Study Center
Tournai 7500
Belgium

David A Whiting MD FACP FRCP (Ed)
Clinical Professor of Dermatology and Pediatrics
University of Texas, Southwestern Medical
Center
and
Medical Director
Baylor Hair Research and Treatment Center
Dallas TX 75246
USA

Tobey Wu-Kuo
Department of Pathology
School of Medicine
University of Southern California
Los Angeles
CA 90033
USA

Hugh Zachariae MD PhD
Professor
Department of Dermatology
Marselisborg Hospital
University of Aarhus
8000 Aarhus C
Denmark

Preface

Hair is a mammalian characteristic which, in human beings, plays important roles in protection and social communication. This means that even common hair follicle disorders often cause marked psychological distress. Unfortunately, treatments have been hampered by the poor understanding of the complex system that is the hair follicle. Recently, the hair follicle has been the focus of much research and our knowledge of the basic biology of the follicle has been expanded dramatically with the advent of new cellular and molecular biological techniques. The location of stem cells in the bulge area, the identification of particular molecules involved in follicular development and hair cycling, and greater understanding of the mechanisms of androgen action in the hair follicle are just a few of the important developments. As a result of this research new and better therapeutic regimes have been introduced, particularly for androgen-dependent conditions.

This book contains sections on both the basic biology of the hair follicle and the various clinical conditions which occur. The up-to-date chapters have been contributed by basic scientists and clinicians who are internationally renowned for their exciting research on the normal and abnormal functioning of the hair follicle in health and disease. It contains the latest findings on the regulatory molecules involved including androgens and growth factors and the various model systems that have been established to investigate the follicle. The clinical sections cover hair disorders involving hair loss (androgenetic alopecia, alopecia areata), those associated with systemic disease, hair shaft abnormalities and disorders involving excessive hair growth (hypertrichosis and hirsutism). The current understanding of the aetiology, pathogenesis and forms of management of these disorders are discussed, including newly introduced therapy.

This book has been designed to be useful to everyone interested in the hair follicle from the basic scientist starting their research career investigating the exciting cell biological system of the hair follicle to an experienced clinician needing to be updated on the recent developments in understanding and therapy. Hopefully, it should not only update people in their fields and provide a long term reference book, but also encourage basic scientists to check details of specific disorders to confirm their ideas, and clinicians to tailor their patient management with greater knowledge of hair follicle biology.

We should like to thank all of the contributors who gave their time and thoughts to prepare the chapters. We should like to thank our families, friends and colleagues for their forbearance and support during the preparation of this book. In particular, Richard, Emily, Rosemary and Rosa Garrudo.

Happy reading

Francisco Camacho
Val Randall
Vera Price

Glossary

ACD	allergic contact dermatitis
ALA	amino levulinic acid
CA	cyproterme acetate
CHS	contact hypersensitivity
CTA	congenital triangular alopecia
CTS	connective tissue sheath
DP	dermal papilla
DHT	dihydrotestosterone
5α-DHT	5α-dihydrotestosterone
EE	ethinyl estradiol
FAGA	female androgenetic alopecia
HF	hair follicle
IRS	inner root sheath
LAHS	loose anagen hair syndrome
ORS	outer root sheath
SCM	S-carboxymethylated
SEM	scanning electron microscope
SL	spirolactone
SP	substance P

Section I

FOLLICLE BIOLOGY

1
Structure and function of the hair follicle

Bo Forslind

Introduction

The hair follicle is the structural unit responsible for the formation of a hair fibre. This is a highly important function as the production of appropriate hair is an important survival factor for many mammals. In humans hair plays important roles in social and sexual communication. The role of hair as an insulator for thermo-regulation and its importance for camouflage also mean that the type of hair formed by individual follicles at different times of the year must change. The dynamics of the follicle in the form of the alternating active and resting parts of the regular hair cycles enable different hairs to be produced in line with the season or with human sexual maturity. The hair cycle is discussed by Paus et al. in Chapter 6. The structure of the follicle determines the shape of the hair produced. From the organization of its components, the obvious function of the outer (ORS) and inner (IRS) root sheaths is to provide a mould, which determines the gross form of the hair fibre. The maturation of the different parts of the hair follicle follows a sequence through which the IRS is consolidated long before the corresponding maturation of the cortex occurs. Apparently the root sheath forms a rigid funnel-like structure through which the growth pressure of the newly formed cells of the hair bulb squeezes the cortex cells to obtain their elongated final form.

The growth rate of human scalp fibres is approximately 0.4 mm per day.[1,2] The complete keratinization process including cell division, protein synthesis and catabolic breakdown of nucleic acids, cell organelles, and so on that is, the differentiation of the cell into a completely keratinized cortical cell, occurs within 1 mm from the germinate area of the root.[3] Thus, it is inter-esting to note that it takes approximately 2.5 days for a cortex cell to pass from the stage of a newly 'born' cell through the highly metabolic phase of protein synthesis to reach the final state of a cell that is completely filled with fibrous and amorphous protein and partially deprived of water in the virgin hair fibre. Compare this with an epidermal cell, which, in about 6–10 days makes a corresponding journey to its end in the stratum corneum. This 'time-table' of hair cell differentiation explains why the hair is sensitive to metabolic interventions such as those caused by cytostatic drugs used in dermatological and cancer therapy.

The three-dimensional appearance of the follicle will determine the final form of the fibre— whether straight follicles as seen in Mongolians, slightly bent ones as seen in many Caucasians, and of helical form as seen in Africans—that will give rise to straight hairs, slightly wavy hairs and curly hairs respectively (Figure 1).[4] An additional function of the hair follicle as a unit is to serve as a sophisticated anchoring device for the hair fibre.

The function of human hair is generally regarded as ornamental in that essentially, we are naked with sparse distribution of hairs. The fact that men have pronounced body hair when sexually mature, such as that on the beard or chest, and part of the male population balds, sometimes at a comparatively young age, suggests that the primary function of human hair (or lack of it) is a sex-related signal. This is discussed further by Randall in Chapter 5. The hair fibre also operates as a sensory receptor, via the sensory nerve fibres, which inserts into the connective tissue sheath surrounding the follicle.

Aspects of the intimate relations between structure and function of the hair and its follicle

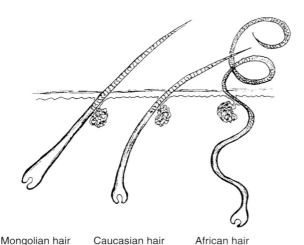

Mongolian hair   Caucasian hair   African hair

Figure 1

The hair follicle. The final form of a hair is determined directly by the shape of the hair follicle. A straight follicle (left) produces a straight hair with approximately round cross-section, a curved follicle a slightly curly hair (middle) and a helical form produces a tightly curled hair with an ellipsoidal cross-section.

will be highlighted in this review. Rather than merely dwelling on old facts, however, this review will also attempt to address several yet unanswered questions that, in the author's mind, appear to be crucial for the understanding of normal and pathological physiology of hair growth.

The topics addressed will be:

- During the differentiation of the cortex and cuticle cells is cysteine transported over the IRS and cuticles at levels above the bulb and, if this is the case, how?
- Compared with the cortex cells the cuticle cells appear inelastic. Is this expressed in the organization of the proteins in these cells?
- The cell envelope of the cuticle and cortex, respectively, is expected to have elastic properties but how is this material organized?
- What is the character of the intercellular cement between the cuticle of the cortex and cuticle of the IRS?

- How are the lipids in the intercellular spaces of the cuticle organized and what kind are they? Can the organization be that of crystalline domains surrounded by border zones in a fluid crystalline state? This would constitute an effective water trap and be a means to achieve control of the moisture in the hair fibre by allowing only very slow water evaporation.

General structure–function considerations surrounding the structure of the follicle

Looking in detail at the cellular entities of the hair follicle cross-section, it becomes clear that they differ to a notable degree in their final morphological look and their biochemical constituents. The differentiation process of *all* follicle cells has been termed 'keratinization' irrespective of whether the fibrous protein α-keratin is present in the cells or not. To avoid any inference that the biochemical components are the same in the different cell types that form the hair follicle, the use of the term *consolidation* in this text denotes the final stage of differentiation.

Light microscopy

The final form of a normal hair fibre is dependent directly on the shape of the hair follicle. A straight follicle produces a straight hair fibre with an approximately round cross-section, a curved follicle produces a slightly curly hair (see Figure 1). When the follicle adopts a helical form the resulting hair fibre will be tightly curled and the cross-section ellipsoidal to a greater or lesser extent.[4] To understand how disorders of the hair are expressed, it is important to understand how the process of keratinization is related to hair growth at a morphological level.[5] Our reference level will be in the mid-bulb where the hair follicle breaks when the fibre is pulled (Figure 2). This is the level of cell division for the hair fibre proper.[1,6] However, even this far down in the follicle the root sheaths are consolidated (or *keratinized* as some researchers have it), forming a rigid cylinder. Circular and longitudinal collagen fibres form an outside supportive reinforcement within the connective tissue sheath immediately adjacent to the structure called the external or outer root sheath (ORS) (see Figure 2). The rigidity of the root sheath is obviously paramount for the formation of a normal hair shaft. At the bottom of the hair follicle the invagination of the dermal papilla is a prominent feature (see Figure 2). The fact that the dermal papilla has a dome-like shape may have two functional reasons. Firstly, it provides an augmented matrix cell–dermal interface that can harbour the great number of dividing cells that produce the fast-growing (0.4 mm/day) fibre. Secondly the dome-shape supported from the dermal side by the connective-tissue gel provides a resistance against buckling of the basal lamina structure caused by the pressure of cell division, which therefore will be directed outwards, that is, along the fibre axis. (Think of the force exerted by dandelions sprouting through the asphalt of our roads.) The matrix cell region also harbours the melanocytes that contribute to the pigmentation of the hair fibre. In human hairs, the cuticle cells never contain pigment granules, which are found in the cortex and medulla cells.

The soft, initially non-keratinized cells of the cortex are forced to take on a longitudinal form, finally to get a length-to-width ratio of about 6:1, as they are pressed upwards in the funnel-like mould of the root sheath (Figure 3). In this process the newly synthesized keratin intermediate fibres (KIF)[7,8] are oriented along the longitudinal axis of the cell and also of the hair fibre itself.

This interpretation of fibre form origin is supported by findings in the spun glass hair condition (synonyms: cheveux incoiffable, pili canaliculi), which has completely normal keratin biochemistry and intracellular arrangement of the fibrous keratin, but weird and wiry fibres. This is caused by the lack of stability in the only partly consolidated root sheath cells, resulting in disorganized longitudinal grooves, which will cause hair fibre cross-section to have any form but a round or elliptical one.[9]

The hair fibres from the spun glass hair are interesting to compare with the normal contorted cross-section of hair fibres from apocrine gland regions of the integument, namely the axillae and the pubic region. Here the often 'T-bone steak'-like cross-section (Figure 4) serves to

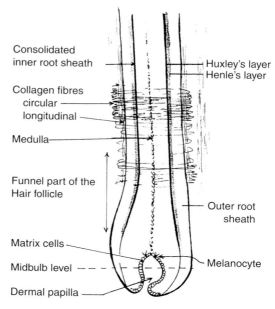

Figure 2

Schematic representation of the main components of the hair follicle. The connective tissue sheath is composed of collagen fibres that act like a 'corset', preventing sideways expansion of the follicle.

augment the surface area of the region by a factor of 5–10 for the benefit of a more effective odour release. (Remember that the classification of odours into pleasant or obnoxious is a matter of social preferences: the original utility of our

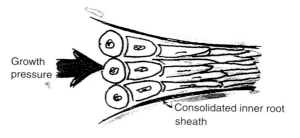

Figure 3

The ORS/IRS 'funnel' structure. This aligns the cortex and cuticle cells (cf. Figure 2 for location). ORS, outer root sheath; IRS, inner root sheath.

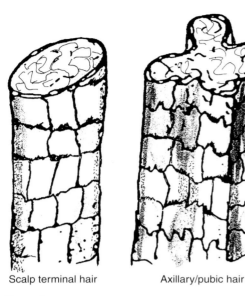

Scalp terminal hair   Axillary/pubic hair

Figure 4

A scalp or body hair cross-section is generally round or oval whereas the axillary and pubic fibres have a contorted cross-section. In the latter case, a large surface area is provided for apocrine secretion odour emission.

apocrine gland secretions is to attract the opposite sex.) Is the spun glass hair a breakthrough of a genetic information that should be contained just within areas of apocrine glands?

Transmission electron microscopy

Transmission electron microscopy (TEM) analysis of the hair follicle started with the pioneer publications of Birbeck and Mercer.[10] With few exceptions, works published since those days have been mainly qualitative, morphological descriptions, with few exceptions.[3] Over the years most of these publications have been reviewed in anthologies on hair, hair growth and hair disease.[6,11–17]

The connective tissue sheath

Externally to the hair follicle is a well-organized connective tissue sheath of collagen fibrils. The epithelial ORS cells of the follicle are separated from the connective tissue by a basal lamina, and adjacent to this are collagen fibrils orientated parallel to the follicle axis. Externally to these fibrils, are collagen fibrils in a circular arrangement at right angles to the former. Merkel cells have been observed attached to the basal lamina of the ORS.[18]

The root sheaths

The root sheath is formed by the ORS and the IRS (see Figure 2). The ORS has actually been shown to contain two different cells types: the most peripheral true ORS cells; and the so-called companion cells, which seem to adhere more closely to the Henle cells of the IRS than to the true ORS and which take on a flat, elongated form higher up in the follicle. The companion cells may play a role in the breakdown of the IRS.[18]

The ORS forms a non-keratinizing region at the periphery of the follicle and is continuous with the epidermis. In cross-section the ORS is generally of the same width but, in wool follicles, which are conspicuously deflected, the ORS is thicker on the deflected side.[18] The ORS cells contain many vacuoles, Golgi complexes, smooth and rough endoplasmic reticulum, mitochondria, and so on. The ORS also contains great amounts of glycogen[18,19] in the lower part of the follicle, suggesting the presence of an energy-consuming activity in these cells, for example, amino acid transport. Suggestions of such a transcellular route for cysteine have been proposed,[13,20] but this has not yet been substantiated by experimental evidence.

The structures that are the first to be consolidated in the hair follicle are the IRS cells; these obviously serve in union with the ORS and the connective tissue sheath as a mould for the emerging hair fibre. The main components of the IRS layer are the outer Henle layer and the inner Huxley layer. Both layers contain straight protein filaments (diameter ~8 nm) aligned along the axis of the follicle—an arrangement that is compatible with a structure not yielding on stress in the fibre axis direction (Figure 5). During the con-

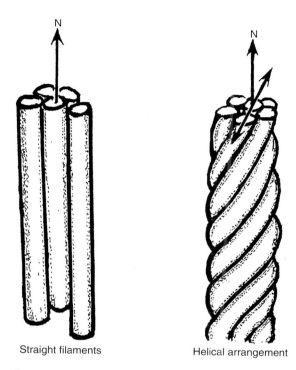

Straight filaments   Helical arrangement

Figure 5

Fibril arrangement. Stress is redistributed by a coil arrangement of fibrils in the cortex cells (right) leading to optimized yield properties compared with an aligned arrangement (left) as seen in the IRS cells.

solidation process, trichohyalin granules, which contain a morphous protein material, first emerge. Later these granules embed the filaments completely. Immediately adjacent to the Huxley layer is the cuticle of the IRS, the IRSC, which lacks fibrous proteins and which, in turn, is apposed to the fibre cuticle (FC).[18] In the final breakdown of the IRS, cellular components, ribosomes, nucleus and so on disappear in the differentiation process, which has many of the characteristics of apoptosis.

The consolidated IRS cells thus fulfil the requirement of forming a non-yielding cylindrical and funnel-like structure that will impose an elongated form onto the cortex and cuticle cells, when these cells are pressed through this rigid 'funnel' by the growth pressure exerted by the cell division process as discussed earlier. This is illustrated in Figure 3.

A functional hair fibre should have elastic properties and it is, therefore, a consequence of necessity that the IRS cells are cast off at the level of the sebaceous gland.

The cuticle

The innermost part of the IRS and the outermost part of the hair fibre proper sport cuticle cells that interdigitate to serve as an anchoring means for the hair fibre in the follicle (Figure 6). When the hair fibre emerges over the skin surface the cuticle cells adhere closely to the cortex and the free border of the cuticle cells has a slightly undulating profile (Figure 7). Only a few millimetres from the scalp the front edge of the cuticle cells is chipped off in small fragments, giving the

Growth direction

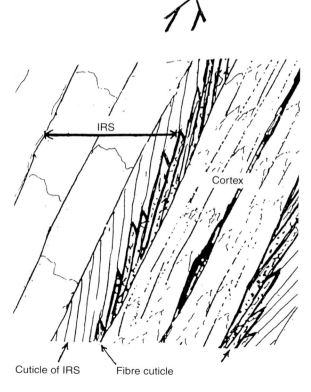

IRS

Cortex

Cuticle of IRS   Fibre cuticle

Figure 6

The 'Velcro' principle of the interdigitating cuticles of the cortex and the inner root sheath (IRS), respectively, serves as an anchoring means for the hair fibre in the follicle.

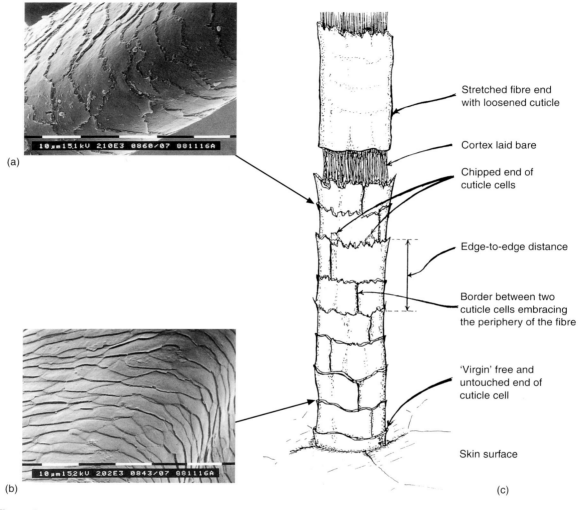

(a)

(b)

(c)

Stretched fibre end
with loosened cuticle

Cortex laid bare

Chipped end of
cuticle cells

Edge-to-edge distance

Border between two
cuticle cells embracing
the periphery of the fibre

'Virgin' free and
untouched end of
cuticle cell

Skin surface

Figure 7

The hair fibre surface structure. This alters with position on the protruding hair fibre. Scanning electron micrographs of the hair fibre cuticle substructures demonstrate the effect of physical and chemical agents causing destruction of the cuticle cell edges. The bottom micrograph (b) represents the untouched virgin segment; the top micrograph (a) depicts the weathered fibre, with chipped cuticle scales (Redrawn from Camacho-Montagna Aula Med, Trichology, 1997, Madrid).

free border a jagged appearance (see Figure 7). This chipping of the free edge suggests that the cuticle cells lack elasticity and are fragile. Their inferior elasticity compared with the cortex cells, which can be stretched to a great extent (100% in 100°C water vapour) has been demonstrated elegantly in tensile experiments using the scanning electron microscope (SEM) performed by Swift.[22]

The cuticle cells have approximately the same length as cortex cells, that is 120 μm (Figure 8) with a width of 20–80 μm. The morphology of the cuticle cells does not reveal any fibrous components under the transmission electron micro-

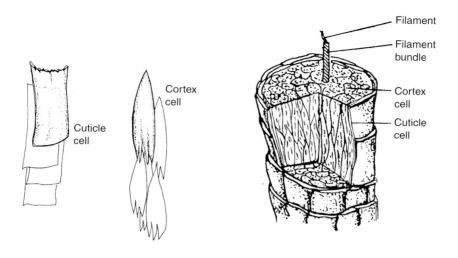

Figure 8

Schematic representation of hair fibre cross-section, cuticle and cortex cells. The width of a cuticle cell is 20–80 µm; while the width of a cortex cell is approximately 25 µm. (Adapted from ref. 13.)

scope.[21] Looking at the morphology of the cuticle of the cortex (i.e. the hair fibre) a dense, so-called A-layer resides inside the bounding surface membrane (Figure 9). This A-layer characteristically has a constant width and contains high amounts of sulphur.[22] The next two layers, the exocuticle and the endocuticle, vary in width. In conventional osmium preparations the exocuticle has dark-staining properties whereas the innermost part, the endocuticle contains low-contrast material, presumably nuclear and organelle debris. The cuticle membrane contains large amounts of ϵ-(γ-glutamyl-) lysine isopeptide cross-links, which render the cuticle membrane highly resistant to chemical treatments.[23,24] In spite of their low mechanical strength the cuticle cells nevertheless offer substantial protection to the cortex by being manifold overlayered like shingles. In cross-section, a human scalp hair will thus show more than five cuticle cells adhering closely to each other (cf. Figure 9).

When examining cuticle cell morphology in detail the endocuticle is found to have low chemical resistance compared to the outer exocuticle with the A-band and suffers the effects of chlorinated water and fungal invasion first.[25]

Approximately free access to this part of the cell is given at the chipped border of the free cuticle edge.

The hair fibre cuticle is not only a mechanical protection for the cortex cells, which form the bulk of the material in a hair fibre, but it also represents a structure that will control the water content of the fibre. During the development of the fibre cuticle, which includes the formation of the exocuticle, several transformation steps occur. Initially the fibre cuticle demonstrates a plasma membrane apposed to the IRS cuticle separated by an intercellular space. The original fibre cuticle plasma membrane is disrupted during a process that involves formation of the exocuticular resistant membrane (RM). On the fibre cuticle and IRS cuticle respectively, an intercellular lamina remains after cleavage along a previous central band. The emerging fibre will, therefore, expose a surface consisting of outer, paired lipid bilayers with a densely-stained underlying proteinaceous band, the exocuticle. Between the exocuticular-resistant membrane of two apposed fibre cuticles, there is, at the scale edge, an intercellular gap of 1–2 µm in length extending inwards from the scale edge. On the

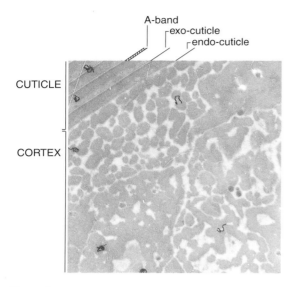

Figure 9

Fragment of an electron microscopic autoradiograph (^{35}S-cysteine) of a human hair fibre cross-section at a level approximately 250 μm above the mid-bulb region. Keratin synthesis is still in progress and the fibrous keratin is assembled in rounded bundles that tend to fuse into larger aggregates. Regions of a high sulphur content are the dense A-band and the exocuticle, as are the filament bundles of the cortex. Autoradiograph silver thread coils (black) denote the presence of radioactive label incorporation into A-band/exocuticle and filament bundles of cortex.

basis of the staining properties of the intercellular material between apposed fibre cuticles, Jones and co-workers[26] have suggested that the demonstrated unstained central band sandwiched between lightly-stained single laminae denotes a dual function of barrier and cellular adhesion.

In his thesis, Peet[27] demonstrated that about 90% of bound fatty acids were bound by thioester linkage to the cell membrane complex (CMC). The dominant bound fatty acid is a C_{21a} (18 methyleicosanoic acid), which is a branched type of fatty acid. There is a high degree of evolutionary conservation in the distribution of bound fatty acids in mammalian hair fibres, indicating a specific and important function. The biosynthesis of the C_{21a} lipids, which presumably derives from isoleucine, occurs well below the sebaceous gland. The high content of cysteine residues (12–18 mol % total cysteine) in epicuticle preparations, indicates that there are enough cysteine residues to create all necessary thioester bonds for fatty acids. Peet estimates that there are between five and ten fatty acid molecules per 100 amino acid residues for the surface of the cuticle membrane.

The fact the that C_{21a} fatty acids are branched means that their effective melting point is lower than that of corresponding straight-chain species, while remaining stable to oxidation, in contrast to unsaturated species. The function of the hydrophobic surface formed by these fatty acids is likely to be the spreading of sebum. In addition, short-chain branched fatty acids such as 14-methyleicosanoic acid have strong bacteriostatic properties for several Gram-positive organisms.

Jones et al.[26] have recently provided evidence for an asymmetrical distribution of this particular C_{21a} fatty acid. In maple syrup urine disease, a genetic disorder of abnormal carbohydrate metabolism, the membrane defect is found only at the upper surface of the fibre cuticle cell membrane. Largely the deficiency in C_{21a} is counterbalanced by an increase in C_{20} eicosanoic acid.

The ceramides found in wool were consistent with Type II cerebroside and Type III (ceramide from bovine brain) and were extractable with chloroform/methanol, in other words they were not found to be covalently bound to the protein.[25,28] It is notable that at low pH chlorine (Cl^-) releases bound fatty acids from keratin fibres, thus supporting the notion that there is a direct thioester attachment to cysteine residues.[25]

The membrane complex of the cuticle has been demonstrated to have other chemical properties than that of the cortex membrane complex. Using formic acid treatment, the cortex cell membrane complex yields ornithine and citrulline, amino acid derivatives not found in cortex membrane complexes.[23] A recent study demonstrated that CMCs from five distinct orders of Mammalia are remarkably consistent.[29] Lectin reactions proved the presence of glycoproteins and differences in lectin reactivity indicate differences in structures of the glycoproteins, the sugars mannose, galactose, N-acetylglucosamine, and N-acetylgalactosamine. The most abundant amino acids were serine, glutamic acid/glutamine and glycine.

The cortex

The size and organization of keratin filaments were investigated by transmission electron microscopy three decades ago. Special techniques involving the reduction of cysteine disulphide bonds were developed to visualize the low sulphur (high-molecular-weight) filament structures embedded in the random coil proteins of the sulphur-rich (low-molecular-weight) matrix.[10,30,31] The remarkable physical, tensile strength of hair fibres was later shown to be related to the filament organization and the cellular architecture of the cortex cells[8,13] (cf. Figures 5 and 8). Such information provides a background for the understanding of disorders involving changes in keratin formation and cellular adhesion.

With appropriate staining, cortex cells of a hair cross-section can be shown to contain an abundant mass of fibrils, mostly organized in coiled manners as denoted by the 'fingerprint whorl pattern' (Figure 10), which corresponds to an oblique, 'fish-bone'-like pattern in longitudinal thin sections.[3] The structural implication of such an arrangement is a gain in tensile strength by load distribution corresponding to that achieved when twining the parts of a wire or a rope. Mercer has suggested that the membranes of the cortex cells have rubber-like properties,[32] but this observation has not been validated by other researchers, although detailed biochemical analyses have been performed to identify the CMC protein(s) and sugars. In conclusion, it can be stated that the ultrastructural organization of the cortex cells thus allows them to be stretched extensively.

All methods used previously for the visualization of keratin filaments of the hair cortex have relied on a pre-treatment with chemicals, aimed at disrupting the disulphide bonds of the cysteine molecules that are characteristic of hair keratin. After such harsh treatment the sulphydryl groups are available to be easily reacted with osmium tetroxide (OsO_4) and a very high contrast is obtained for transmission electron microscopy. Conventional preparations seldom give a clearly defined 'keratin whorl pattern' of fibre cross-sections and several methods have been developed for the visualization of this pattern.[10,31] The risk of getting an artifactual picture of the keratin organization because of degradation of proteins in situ causing this contrast is obvious. An alternative method is to use uranyl acetate-stained sections of unfixed specimens.[33] When compared with specimens fixed in glutaraldehyde and OsO_4, this method yielded equal details in the keratin fine structure. The best contrast was obtained in relatively thick sections, or section areas thicker than the nominal 60 nm, where the filaments were depicted as 'rounded open spaces' in a stained, structureless matrix. A helical arrangement of filaments in the bundles is suggested by the 'fingerprint whorl patterns' seen in the cross-sections. Finally, this staining method allows the cellular envelopes ('membranes') to be well delineated (Figure 10). In contrast to what has been generally assumed, the fine details of hair and wool keratin organization in fibre cross-sections can thus be demonstrated without a previous chemical treatment aiming at disruption of disulphide bonds. The logical conclusion from these experiments is that the cross-linking induced by the glutaraldehyde fixation prevents the uranyl acetate from interacting with the proteins to any appreciable extent.[33]

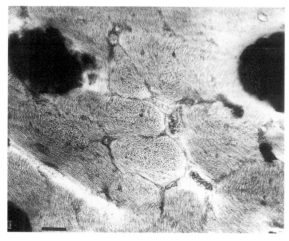

Figure 10

Electron micrograph demonstrating the 'finger print' whorl pattern arrangement of keratin filaments in hair fibre cross-section. (Reproduced with permission from *Acta Dermatol Venereol* 1991; **71:** 272.)

The medulla

In human scalp hairs, the medulla is often an inconspicuous part of the cross-section.[19] Frequently this entity is absent, interrupted or fragmented. In contrast to such findings in scalp hairs, the medulla is often unbroken and continuous along the length of the fibre in coarse-diameter hairs such as eyelashes, eyebrows and grey hair fibres. It is a well-known mechanical fact that a tubular structure is stiffer than a solid rod with the same mass per cross-section. Characteristically, and consequently, hair fibres with a continuous medulla are stiff, as demonstrated by the cilia of our eyelashes.

The medulla matrix cells are found at the top of the dermal papilla. It is unclear why they sometimes collapse to form the central cavity in medullated hair fibres. In sections of the fibre where the medullary space is not visible, medullary cells are still present. These cells contain scattered bundles of fibrillar material without any obvious orientation and are often vacuolated.[18] The periphery of the vacuoles is coated with amorphous protein material that appears as granules in the initial stages of differentiation. This protein has been shown to be almost completely devoid of cystine, but contains ε-(γ-glutamyl)lysine cross-links, which account for the very low solubility of the consolidated medulla.[24]

Sulphur content and the stabilization of keratin

The hallmark of keratins is that they have a characteristically high sulphur content, both in the high- and the low-sulphur fractions. In human hairs, the total sulphur content is close to 5% (cf. ref 21). The sulphur is mainly brought to the hair as part of the amino acid cysteine. It was an interesting finding that the bulk of sulphur incorporation occurs more than 200 μm above the level of cell division in the root.[3] This suggests that this rather large amino acid is transported by some unknown means over what, in the light and electron microscopes, are the apparently consolidated Henle and Huxley layers of the inner root sheath[20] (Figure 11). Support for such a transport mechanism can be found in the pres-

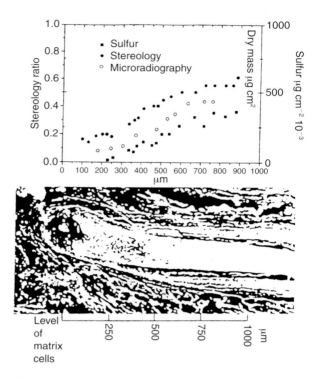

Figure 11

The active zone of growth is in the deepest part of the hair follicle. Morphometric data from development of keratinization and microradiographic data on mass increment and sulphur distribution in the hair follicle demonstrate that the cortex cells are fully keratinized within a distance less than 1 mm from the dermal papilla.

ence of glycogen in the ORS but it must be stressed that this notion has not yet found full experimental proof by repeated and unrelated observations. Interestingly Jones[34] has shown that the intermediate filament associated protein (the high-sulphur protein) synthesis occurs at a higher level of the presumptive hair shaft than the synthesis of the intermediate filament protein (the low-sulphur proteins).

The mass distribution given by quantitative microradiography shows a linear increase up to a level some 600–700 μm from the reference level.[35] Beyond this increase, there is a plateau in the mass distribution corresponding to a linear distance of 100–250 μm after which there is a second, rather small increase in the mass content (see Figure 11). Using stereological methods applied to electron micrographs of hair follicle cross-sections to estimate the content of keratin at different levels of the hair follicle, it has been demonstrated that this mass distribution accompanies the microradiographic mass curve like a twin.[3] When comparing the sulphur content of different levels in the hair follicle given by quantitative microradiography, this distribution adheres very closely to mass distribution curves (see Figure 11).

The interpretation of these quantitative data is straightforward. Keratin synthesis in the cortex cells increases in the metabolically active hair cells up to a level where the cells are completely filled with fibrous and amorphous keratin. The protein synthesis then comes to an end, as seen on the plateau region of the mass distribution curves when the nuclear and ribosomal material is decomposed. At the end of this degradation process of nucleic acids, the hair fibre is deprived of water. The fibre then attains its final diameter through a conspicuous contraction of the fibre resulting from loss of water (see Figure 11).

This differentiation process, in many respects, has the characteristics of apoptosis, namely programmed cell death. For example, the transformation of a lipid cell membrane into a protein envelope, the compacting, fragmentation and final loss of the nucleus and the loss of cytosolic nucleic acids are characteristics that are also found in the differentiation process of the epidermis and the nails. As yet, a precise knowledge of the details of how this cellular transformation comes about is lacking, although detailed information on the protein synthesis of the intracellular keratin and so on is available.

Often the reason for brittleness of hair fibres is a low sulphur content and this may be diagnostic for disease.[36–39] This aspect is dealt with further in Chapter 27.

Elements and trace elements of the hair follicle

The first subcellular maps of an element distribution ware made by a cytochemical technique developed by Swift.[22] Later a longitudinal distrib-

ution was given by a quantitative microradiographic assessment of sulphur.[35] It was not until the introduction of particle probes, however, that *simultaneous* recordings of elements and trace elements were possible, thus allowing actual quantitative relations between the content of particular elements to be assessed.[21,40–43] In his thesis, Bos[44] demonstrated that in longitudinal sections of human hair fibres, the elements and trace elements displayed varying distribution patterns, in other words that the bulb area had high iron and potassium levels, which fell rapidly to low levels during the consolidation process. In the bulb area, calcium measurements attained comparatively high values, which later decreased as the fibre was consolidated. In the emerging fibre, the calcium levels again reached high values owing to contamination.

The mineral content of the human hair fibre has been linked to the health status of the individual. It was recently shown, however, that contamination of the human hair fibre is often excessive and biologically relevant information can only be obtained from the virgin fibre, that is, the fibre of the follicle and the first few millimetres of the emerging fibre.[45] Bulk analysis of hair clippings consequently has no scientific support. Furthermore, correlated investigations into health status and concomitant analysis of single hair fibres and blood samples from the same individuals in a large population (preferably >100 individuals) is still lacking. This is a research area that still remains to be fully explored if elemental analysis is to provide support in clinical diagnosis in a wider context.

Conclusion

Although we understand much about the structure and function of the growing hair follicle and how it carefully produces the appropriate hair fibre, still much is unknown. Further understanding should enable the diagnosis and prevention of hair and possibly other health disorders.

Acknowledgements

This chapter is dedicated to the memory of Don Rivett, Australia and David Orwin, New Zealand, for their important contributions to keratin and hair fibre research.

References

1. Braun-Falco O: The histochemistry of the hair folli-cle. In: Montagna W, Ellis RA (eds.). *The Biology of Hair Growth*. New York, Academic Press, 1959: 65–90.
2. Braun-Falco O: Dynamik des normalen und pathol-ogischen Haarwachtums. *Archiv fur klinische und experimentelle Dermatologie* 1966; **227**: 419–452.
3. Forslind B, Swanbeck G: Keratin formation in the hair follicle. I. An ultrastructural investigation. *Exptl Cell Res* 1966; **43**: 191–209.
4. Lindelöf B, Forslind B, Hedblad M-A, Kaveus U: Human hair fibre form. Morphology revealed by light and scanning electron microscopy and com-puter aided three-dimensional reconstruction. *Arch Dermatol* 1988; **124**: 1359–1363.
5. Pinkus H: Embryology of hair. In: Montagna W, Ellis RA (eds.). *The Biology of Hair Growth*. New York, Academic Press, 1959: 1–32.
6. Montagna W: *Structure and Function of Skin*, 2nd edn. New York, Academic Press, 1962.
7. Fraser B, McRae T, Parry DAD, Suzuki E: Interme-diate filaments in α-keratins. *Proc Nat Acad Sci* 1985; **83**: 1179–1183.
8. Steinert PM: Structure, function, and dynamics of keratin intermediate filaments. *J Invest Dermatol* 1993; **100**: 729–734.
9. Stroud JD: Complementation of the inner root sheath of human hair. In: Brown AC, Crounse RG (eds.). *Hair, Trace Elements and Human Illness*. New York, Praeger, 1980: 163–168.
10. Birbeck MSC, Mercer EH: The electron microscopy of the human hair follicle. *J Biophys Biochem Cytol* 1957; **3**: 202–233.
11. Brown AC (ed.). *The First Human Hair Symposium*. New York, Medcom Press, 1974.
12. Brown AC: The integumentary system. In: GM Hodges, RC Hallowe (eds.). *Biomedical Research Applications of Scanning Electron Microscopy*. London, Academic Press, 1980; 65–125.
13. Forslind B: The growing anagen hair. In: Orfanos CE, Happle R (eds.). *Hair and Hair Diseases*. Berlin, Springer Verlag, 1990: 73–97.
14. Montagna W, Ellis RA: *The Biology of Hair Growth*. New York, Academic Press, 1959.
15. Orfanos C, Montagna W, Stuttgen R: *Hair Research*. Berlin, Springer Verlag, 1981.
16. Van Neste D, Lachapelle JM, Antoine JL: *Trends in Human Hair Growth and Alopecia Research*. Dor-drecht, Kluwer, 1989.
17. Wuepper KD, Norris DA, Messenger A (eds.): The fundamentals of hair biology. Cutaneous Biology Foundation 41st Symposium on the Biology of Skin, Snowmass July 25–29, 1992. *J Invest Derma-tol* 1993; **101**: 1S–152S.
18. Orwin DF: The cytology and cytochemistry of the wool follicle. *Int Rev Cytology* 1979; **60**: 331–374.
19. Parrakkal PF: The fine structure of the anagen hair follicle of the mouse. In: Montagna W, Dobson RL (eds.). *Hair Growth*. (Advances in Biology of Skin vol. 9). Oxford, Pergamon Press, 1969: 441–469.
20. Forslind B: Electron microscopic and autoradi-ographic study of S-35-L-cystine incorporation in mouse follicles. *Acta Derm Venereol (Stockh)* 1971; **51**: 9–15.
21. Forslind B, Li HK, Malmqvist KG, Wiegleb D: Ele-mental content of anagen hairs in a normal Cau-casian population studies with proton induced X-ray emission (PIXE). *Scanning Electron Microsc* 1986; **1**: 237–241.
22. Swift JA: The hair surface. In: Orfanos CE, Mon-tagna W, Stuttgen G (eds.). *Hair Research*. Berlin, Springer, 1981: 65–72.
23. Gillespie JM: The structural proteins of hair: Isola-tion, characterization and regulation of biosynthe-sis. Ch. 22. In: Goldsmith LA (ed.). *Physiology, Biochemistry and Molecular Biology of the Skin*. Oxford University Press, 1991: 625–659.
24. Harding HWJ, Rogers GE: Isolation of peptides containing citrulline and the cross-link, ∈(γ-glu-tamyl)lysine, from hair medulla protein. *Biochem Biophys Acta* 1976; **427**: 315–324.
25. Negri AP, Peet DJ, Wettenhall REH, Corneli HJ, Rivett DE: Covalently bound fatty acids and ceramides in wool. *J Text Indust* 1996; **87**: 608–611.
26. Jones LN, Horr TJ, Kaplin IJ: Formation of surface membranes in developing mammalian hair fibres. *Micron 1994;* **25**: 589–595.
27. Peet DJ: *Protein-bound Fatty Acids in Mammalian Hair Fibers*. Thesis, University of Melbourne.
28. Peet DJ, Wetenhall REH, Rivett DE: A comparative study of covalently bound fatty acids in keratinized tissues. *Comp Biochem Physiol* 1992; **102B**: 363–366.
29. Allen AK, Ellis J, Rivett DE: The presence of glyco-proteins in membrane complex of a variety of keratin fibers. *Biochem Biophys Acta* 1991; **1074**: 331–333.
30. Marshall RC: Characterization of proteins of human hair and nail by electrophoresis. *J Invest Dermatol* 1983; **80**: 519–524.

31. Rogers GE: Electron microscopy of wool. *J Ulstrastruct Res* 1959; **2**: 309–330.

32. Mercer EH: The contribution of the resistant cell membranes to the properties of keratinized tissues. *J Soc Cosmetic Chem* 1965; **16**: 507–514.

33. Forslind B, Andersson M: A new staining method for visualization of keratin filaments in hair fibre cross sections. *Acta Derm Venereol (Stockh)* 1990; **71**: 272–273.

34. Jones LN: Location and synthesis of hair structural proteins in human anagen follicles. *Br J Dermatol* 1996; **134**: 649–656.

35. Forslind B, Lindström B, Swanbeck G: Microradiographic and autoradiographic studies of keratin formation in the human hair. *Acta Dermat Venereol (Stockh)* 1971; **51**: 81–89.

36. Gummer CL, Dawber RPR, Price V: Trichothiodystrophy: an electron histochemical study of the hair shaft. *Br J Dermatol* 1984; **110**: 439–449.

37. Gummer CL, Dawber RPR: Trichothiodystrophy: an ultrastructural study of the hair follicle. *Br J Dermatol* 1985; **113**: 273–280.

38. Price VH: Structural anomalies of the hair shaft. In: Orfanos CE, Montagna W, Stuttgen G (eds.). *Hair Research. Status and Future Aspects.* Berlin, Springer, 1981: 363–422.

39. Venning VA, Dawber RPR, Ferguson DJP, Kanan MW: Weathering of hair in trichothiodystrophy. *Br J Dermatol* 1986; **114**: 591–595.

40. Forslind B: Clinical applications of scanning electron microscopy and energy dispersive X-ray analysis in dermatology—an update. *Scanning Microscopy* 1988; **2**: 959–976.

41. Forslind B, Kischner CW, Roomans GM (eds.): *The Integument.* Illinois, USA, Scanning Microscopy Inc, AMF O-Hare, 1985.

42. Forslind B, Wiren K, Malmqvist KG: Assessment of qualitative and quantitative data from pathological hairs—a critical evaluation of scanning electron microscopy and proton induced X-ray emission analysis. *Scanning Microscopy* 1987; **1**: 159–167.

43. Forslind B, Malmqvist KG, Wiren K: Genetic diseases, hair structure and elemental content. Ch. 19. In Rogers GE, Reis P, Ward KA, Marshall RC. (eds.). *The Biology of Wool and Hair*, London, Chapman & Hall 1988; 275–285.

44. Bos AJJ: *The Amsterdam Proton Microbeam. The Application of Micro-PIXE Measuring Trace Elements in Human Hair.* Thesis, Free University of Amsterdam, 1984.

45. Stocklassa B, Aransay-Vitores M, Nilsson G, Karlsson C, Wiegleb D, Forslind B: Evaluation of a new X-ray fluorescent analysis technique for the creation of a Nordic hair data base. Elemental distributions within the root and the virgin segment of hair fibers. [In press].

2

Developmental biology of hair follicles and other skin appendages

Tobey Wu-Kuo and Cheng-Ming Chuong

Introduction

Hair is the most prominent skin appendage in a human being. To understand its biology in development, one must take a step back to appreciate the commonality shared by hairs and other skin appendages. Skin forms the interface between organisms and their environment. The diversification of skin, with the formation of novel skin appendages during evolution, has provided animals with specialized structures and functions to interact with the environment and adapt to new niches. These diversifications include scales, feathers, hair follicles, claws, horns, hoofs, salivary glands, sebaceous glands, mammary glands, and so on (Figure 1).[1] Their functions vary from barrier and protection, to thermoregulation, communication, hunting, defense, flight, secretion, and so on. While Darwin's evolutionary theory provides a good basis as to why they exist, here we would like to explore how they form, from a developmental biology point of view. From a practical point of view, the understanding of the fundamental basic mechanism will also help us to manage diseases involving hair follicles as well as attempt to regenerate hair follicles from wounded skin or to engineer them from stem cells.

In this chapter, the morphogenetic processes, including skin appendage formation will first be described, including the principles and focussing on the specific examples of hair and feathers. The current understanding of the molecular basis of skin appendage morphogenesis will then be discussed, with an introduction of principles followed by specific categories of molecules. In terms of reference books, Sengel's Morphogenesis of skin[2] remains a classic, covering older literature, while Lucas and Stettenheim's Avian anatomy integument[3] is a good source of the biology of integument appendages, and Chuong's *Molecular Basis of Epithelial Appendage Morphogenesis*[4] includes chapters on different aspects of hair follicle and feather development and ectodermal dysplasia. For review papers, Hardy[5] and Chuong[6] have concise descriptions of hair and feather development respectively, and Oro and Scott[7] review the most recent molecular findings.

Morphogenetic processes of skin appendages

Different types of skin appendages are formed by variations of tissue interactions as adjuncts to a common theme.

Variations and convertibility of skin appendages

Skin appendages result from similar developmental processes. Skin appendages are topological transformations of originally flat epithelia into specialized structures that either protrude outward such as the hair, or invaginate inward as for a gland.[1,8] They then diverge into more complex skin appendages (Figure 1). Morphologically, however, they all begin by a thickening of the epidermis (formation of the epithelial placode). Treating hair follicles with retinoic acid at the time hair follicles are forming converts them into gland-like structures.[9,10] Treating chicken embryos with retinoic acid at the time

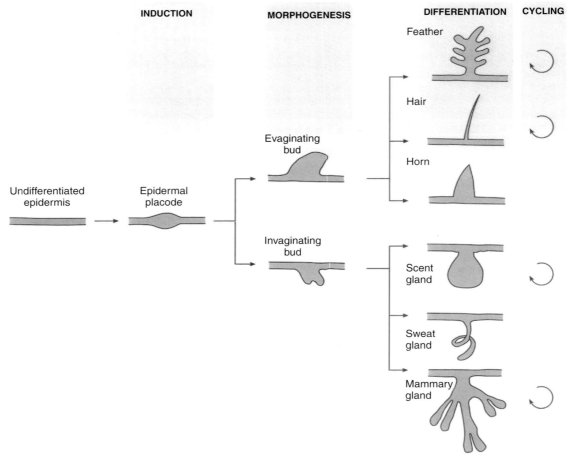

Figure 1

Prototypic processes of the formation of skin appendages. This figure demonstrates the different stages of development common to skin appendages—induction, morphogenesis, differentiation, and cycling. These four stages and their sub-stages are defined in the text. It also shows how the morphologically different skin appendages can arise from a common denominator. Skin appendages are products of epidermal–dermal interactions. For simplicity, only the epidermis is shown. The sweat gland itself does not cycle but the apocrine gland, a special kind of sweat gland, will regenerate after destroying itself during secretion.

scales are forming could transform the scales into feathers or vice versa.[11–13] These experiments have led to the recognition that skin appendages form in multiple stages,[11–12] share their earlier stages, and can be inter-converted between different skin appendage phenotypes at this time. Subsequently, it was shown that trans-genic mice over-expressing LEF-1, a β-catenin binding protein, grew hairs from the gum region.[14] Thus, perturbation in early stages of skin appendage formation can shift the balance and lead to morphological transformation, or the metaplasia of skin appendages.

Another clue to the common pathway of

epithelial appendages comes from the study of the human ectodermal dysplasia syndrome.[15,16] The ectodermal dysplasias are a clinically and genetically heterogeneous group of disorders identified by the absence of incomplete, or delayed, development of two or more cardinal signs: hair; nails; sweat glands; and teeth. The literal definition of 'ectodermal dysplasia' describes any developmental defect affecting the ectoderm, therefore, the spectrum of abnormalities may be significantly more broad than the cardinal signs, to include others such as the respiratory tract, heart, and so on. There are currently over 150 clinically recognized clinical phenotypes. Identifying the gene defects involved and proteins affected in these disorders would enable greater understanding of the fundamental mechanisms of skin appendage development and permit novel ways of managing diseases involving skin appendages to be devised.

Stages involved in skin appendage development

The stages outlined here are intended to provide a basic framework for the formation of different types of skin appendages (see Figure 1). This system is based on those described in Chuong and Widelitz[17] and can be used as a framework when the development of a new epithelial appendage is described. Examples of hairs, feathers and other appendages are described later. Comparisons among skin appendages are shown in Table 1.

1. **Induction stage:** forming skin appendage primordia.
   1A. Competence: both the epithelia and mesenchyma must be in a competent state for the formation of skin appendages.
   1B. Epithelial placode: local mesenchymal messages define a domain in the epithelial sheet to form an individual appendage.
   1C. Dermal condensation: further recruitment of dermal mesenchymal cells to consolidate and set the boundary (thus determining the size) of the primordia.

2. **Morphogenesis stage:** molding the primordia into a particular shape.
   2A. Antero-posterior (A–P) axis: endow an A–P axis to the radially symmetric primordia; this is important for functional elaboration.
   2B. Proximal-distal (P–D) axis: allow the primordia to elongate to a certain length (hair) or invaginate (glands).
   2C. Other morphogenetic events: such as branching (e.g. to produce feathers or glands).

3. **Differentiation stage:** the developing organ anlage differentiates into specific physical characteristics with specialized keratin (nail, hair, horn) or chemical (sweat gland, sebaceous gland) properties.

4. **Cycling:** opportunities for shedding and renewal of appendages particularly in the hair follicle and feather; these are modulated by physiological conditions (e.g. sex hormone levels); see Paus's Chapter (6) on cycling and Randall's on androgens (Chapter 5).
   4A. Anagen.
   4B. Catagen.
   4C. Telogen.

Architecture of skin appendages

The complex architecture of skin appendages results from successive molding of the epithelial sheet.

Hair follicle morphogenesis

The hair follicle is a complex organ composed of different types of epithelial and dermal tissues. (For a detailed description see Chapter 1 by Forslind.) How do hair follicles achieve this complexity?

Human hair follicle development has been described (see Figure 2 for the stages of the hair follicle modelled after Hardy[5]).[18–20] At approximately 75 days estimated gestational age, the induction of hair follicles becomes visible. The predated hair germ is a small accumulation of

Table 1 Comparison of the development of different skin appendages.

	Hair	Nail	Hoof	Horn	Feather	Scale
1. Induction stage	Epidermal placode Hair germ	Epidermal thickening over nail field, delineated by shallow grooves Matrix primordium forms at proximal groove	Groove in distal limb delineates the hoof field Epidermal thickening outlines the sole area	Epidermal thickening in the horn field Formation of many primary follicles in a spiral	Feather fields form over the tract region Epidermal placode thickening over each individual primordium	Scale field Individual scale placode
2. Morphogenesis stage	Dermal condensations proceed to form dermal papillae Down-growth of hair germ epithelia to wrap around dermal papillae and form hair fibers, inner and outer root sheath Note: Proliferation in matrix for continuous elongation	Dermal proximal nail fold formed by elongating matrix Elongation and expansion of matrix primordium Nail matrix, nail plate, nail bed, epo- and hypo-nychium form Note: Proliferation in matrix for continuous growth	Numerous dermal papilla in the coronary border Hoof 'wall' delinated by coronary border, develops primary and secondary epidermal lamellae The soft 'frog' regions form in the bottom of the sole	Numerous long dermal papillae Columns of medulla-like cells form at the papilar tips to collectively make the horn bud	Dermal condensations eventually invaginate to form dermal papillae Outward protrusion of epithelia to form feather buds; later invagination to form feather follicles Proliferation in feather collar epithelia for elongation of feather filaments; further branching formed by alternating zones of apoptosis	No dermal papilla formed Outward epidermal protrusion to form scale and hinge Do not elongate
3. Differentiation stage	Specialized hair keratins	Nail keratins	Tubular and intertubular keratins	Horn keratins	Feather β-keratins	α- and β-keratins
4. Cycling stage	Cycling	Continuous growth	Thickening	Continuous growth	Molting cycle	No cycling

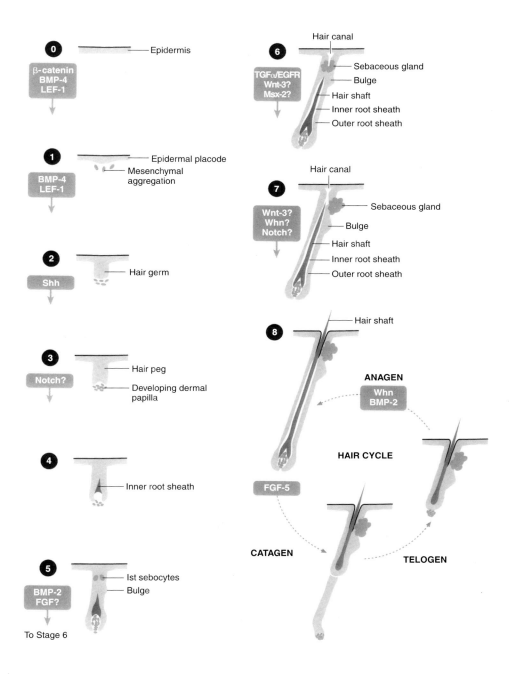

Figure 2

Hair follicle morphogenesis: stages and involved molecules. Hardy[5] developed a staging system for murine hair follicle morphogenesis: Stages 0–1 correspond to the induction phase here; Stages 2–4 correspond to the morphogenesis phase here; Stages 5–8 correspond to the differentiation phase here. This figure also shows the molecules that are shown or considered to be candidates to be involved in certain morphogenetic steps; namely; β-catenin,[33,137] BMP-2,[30] BMP-4,[79,137] FGF,[67] FGF-5,[73] LEF-1,[137] Msx ,[91] Noggin,[81] Notch,[124,138] Shh,[44,48] TGFa/EGFR,[60] Whn,[93,95] Wnt-3,[55] TGF-β2.[78]

mesenchymal cells spaced regularly below the dermal-epidermal junction. At approximately 80 days estimated gestational age, the hair germ becomes evident. This is a focus of basal epidermal cells that bud into the dermis and is surrounded by collections of aggregated mesenchymal cells. Soon a hair peg appears in which cells of the hair germ elongate deeper as cords of epithelial cells. The deepest portion of the fully elongated hair peg then flattens, forming a concave bulb-like structure to enclose the underlying mesenchymal cells, thus forming the follicular structure. The cells at the roof of the concavity become the matrix and will differentiate into the inner root sheath and hair fibers. The epithelial cells linking the matrix and interfollicular epidermis become the outer root sheath. The mesenchymal cells along the sides of the follicle become the follicle sheath, which is approximately two or three cell layers thick. At approximately 12–15 weeks estimated gestational age, several swellings appear on the side of the developing follicle during the formation of the bulbous hair peg. The uppermost swelling becomes the developing sebaceous gland and the lower one becomes the bulge, the site of attachment of the arrector pili muscles and the presumed site of follicle stem cells[21] (see also Chapter 3 by Cotsarelis). Some follicles will develop a third, smaller projection just proximal to the epidermis. These projections develop into apocrine sweat glands and ducts, which only complete development in certain regions such as in the axilla or groin, otherwise they become atrophic.

The epithelial matrix cells of the follicular bulb proliferate and differentiate to give rise to several concentric cones of cells. The innermost layers form the medulla, cortex and cuticle of the hair shaft. The outermost form the inner root sheath consisting of the cuticle and Huxley's and Henle's layers. Around 15 weeks, a hair canal is excavated. At this point, the inner root sheath, hair fiber and hair canal, begin to keratinize, and at 19 weeks, the first lanugo hair emerges.[20] The dermal components are the dermal papilla and the connective tissue sheath, which also have some inductive properties[22] (see Chapter 1 by Forslind for more detailed anatomy of hair follicles and for tissue interactions of follicle components).

In the final form of the follicle, the matrix epithelium overlies the dermal papilla, now a flame-shaped condensation of specialized dermal cells. The hair matrix is made up of undifferentiated epidermal cells, which proliferate and begin to differentiate as they move upward. The cells overlying the top and sides of the papilla keratinize, forming the three layers of the hair shaft. External to the hair shaft, are the three layers of the inner root sheath. The inner root sheath keratinizes low in the follicle, becoming a single functional unit at higher levels. The function of the inner root sheath is to coat and support the hair shaft up to the level of the isthmus (beginning at the bulge), at which point it desquamates. External to the inner root sheath, the outer root sheath does not keratinize below the isthmus. When the inner root sheath disintegrates at the isthmus, the outer root sheath then keratinizes. At the infundibulum, the outer root sheath begins to form a stratum granulosum and stratum corneum, becoming histologically indistinguishable from the surrounding epidermis.[23] Murine hair follicle morphogenesis basically follows the same architectural themes found in human development[5,24]; the difference is in the different gestational ages of mouse and human embryos.

Feather and other skin appendages

Similar to hair morphogenesis, the development of a feather goes through several stages defined by its morphologic characteristics and state of determination (see Figure 3). In the inductive stage, the placode is the first to become morphologically distinct, although some molecular events have occurred earlier. The dermal condensation is the accumulation of mesenchymal cells in the region of feather primordia. Short feather buds are first radially symmetric, but soon develop anterior–posterior asymmetry, slanting toward the posterior direction. At the long feather bud stage, the feather bud develops a proximal–distal axis and grows out of the body surface, in contrast to the hair pegs, which grow into the dermis. In the feather filament stage, a morphogenetic event unique to the bird takes place in which feather bud epithelia form barb and marginal plate epithelia, with distinct cellular

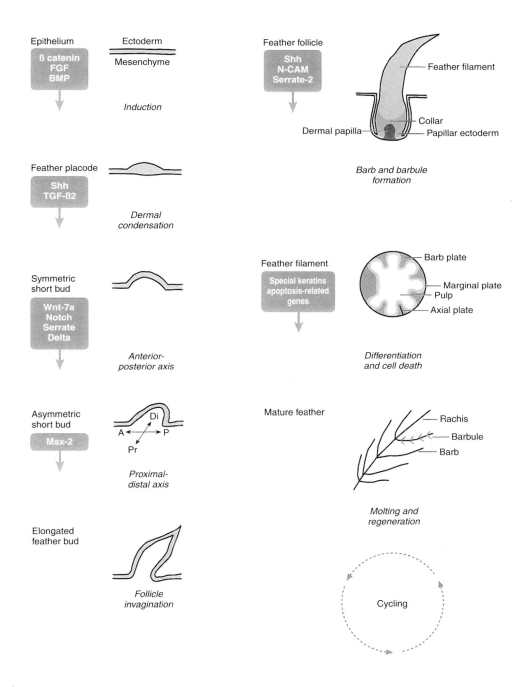

Figure 3

Feather Morphogenesis: Stages and involved molecules. Morphogenetic stages and phases are shown here. This figure also shows candidate molecules involved in certain morphogenetic steps; namely; β-catenin,[139] FGF,[140] BMP,[141] Shh,[142,143] TGF-β2,[144] Wnt-7a,[145] Notch,[126–128] Serrate,[126–128] Delta,[126–128] Msx-2,[89] N-CAM,[129] Serrate-2,[127]

fates of keratinization or death, thus forming barbs and the interbarb spaces between. More detailed reviews can be found in publications by Chuong et al,[25] Chuong and Widelitz,[17] Widelitz et al,[26] and Widelitz and Chuong.[27]

Nails, claws, hoofs, and horns are different skin appendages. Although their appearances are quite different, histological sections show that they are variations constructed using the same principles (see Figure 4). For instance, nails have a large nail matrix that is equivalent to the hair matrix, and nail papillary dermal papillae that are positive for neutral cell adhesion molecules (N-CAM) (our unpublished data), like the dermal papilla of the hair follicle.[28] They then form nail plate, eponychium and hyponychium, almost corresponding to the hairs and root sheaths. The claw has a similar structure, but has a terminal digit bony core between the claw plate and hyponychium, which makes it a good weapon. Hoof development starts with the formation of numerous dermal papillae in the coronary border, and also the sole area, which produces a thick hoof wall on the side, and a sole-and-frog region at the bottom. Horns are permanent structures made of keratin, in contrast to antlers that are made of bone and are shed annually. Horns are also formed by a large collection of well-aligned long dermal papillae that produce specialized horny keratins. In many cases, they also have a bony core. (Please see Figure 4 for a schematic drawing of nail/claw and horn formation). Further information on these skin appendages can be found in an article by Chapman.[29] A comparison of the development of different types of skin appendages can be seen in Table 1.

Molecular basis of skin appendage morphogenesis

Emerging principles

In recent years, many molecular pathways involved in skin development have been identified and their roles in skin appendages studied. Much new progress has been made since the production of transgenic and knock-out mice with skin abnormalities,[30] and the experimental approaches elucidating the different steps of feather morphogenesis.[31] Here, some emerging principles during the construction of skin appendages are outlined with reference to specific molecular pathways discussed below:

- Molecules involved in hair development are also involved in basal cell carcinoma or hair trichofolliculoma.[32,33] Therefore, skin appendages can be considered a regulated new growth, while tumors are a deregulated new growth. This is discussed below in the 'Sonic hedgehog and β-catenin' sections.

- The making of different skin appendages can be dissected into several morphogenetic steps (see Figure 1) where each step is controlled and mediated by many molecules (Figures 2 and 3). This must be taken into consideration when dealing with hair disorders. On the one hand, it reminds us that there is no single magical molecule that can do everything; on the other hand, it also explains the functional redundancy sometimes observed in knock-out mice.

- 'Competence' is the classical embryology term defined by the ability of the target tissue to respond to inducers and make a difference in cellular fates. The molecular basis of competence is the presence of receptors and other downstream signaling molecules to certain inductive signals. During development, competence states change spatially and temporally. This is an important area to study in order to evaluate the role of inducers and target tissues.

- Although molecules are important, cells may be treated as an integrative entity exhibiting the properties composed of the molecules unique to them. Dissociated cells show an amazing ability for self-organization in development[34–37] and self-renewal. The hair follicle of an adult mammal is unique in that it retains its morphogenetic signals, enabling it to regenerate itself.[38]

- In vivo, hair follicle stem cells are defined as self-renewing, pluripotential cells that form hair follicles. The isolation of hair follicle stem cells in vitro has been elusive because of this strict definition. From a developmental biology point of view, the term 'precursor' cells can be adopted to cover a wider category of epithelial cells at different developmental

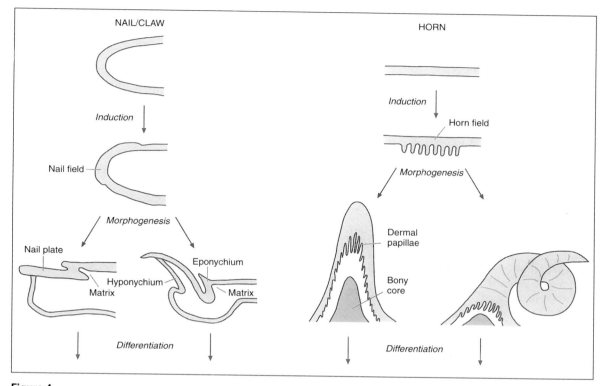

Figure 4

Schematic drawing of the formation of nails/claws and horns. Also see table 2 for description.
For nail/claw, after induction, a nail field is formed. The four phases of skin appendages development (induction, morphogensis, differentiation, and cycling), are highlighted. Depending on the way the epithelia in the nail field are folded, different shapes of nails (left) or claws (right) can form. *Wnt-7a* and *engrailed* have been shown to be involved in mouse claw formation.[146] *Msx 1, 2* are present in nail matrix.[147] For horns, clusters of elongated dermal papillae define a horn field. Different curvatures of horns may form due to differential cell proliferation. Left: horn of bull; right, horn of big horn sheep. It is possible *that Notch/serrate/delta* may be involved forming this curvature, similar to that in the slanting of feather buds.[126] Many signaling molecules used in other epithelial organogenesis may be shared by horns and nails. However, very few experimental data are available due to the impracticality of obtaining specimens.

stages along the pathway to becoming hair follicles.[39] Our job then becomes to identify markers and regulators of different stages of hair follicle precursor cells (see Chapter 3 by Cotsarelis for a more-detailed discussion on stem cells).

• The hair cycle shares many genes with hair follicle development, but is not completely similar. The hair cycle appears to be more sensitive to molecular changes. Several transgenic or knock-out mice do not show hair defects after birth but have problems entering the new anagen phase.

Major molecular pathways involved in skin appendage development

In the last decades, many molecules have been found to play important roles in the formation of skin appendages. Many of them are known growth factors,[40] while some more recent ones were originally identified as homologs to Drosophila *spp.*[41] The major molecular pathways involved in the development of skin appendages relevant to hair growth are listed below.

- Secreted signaling factors
    SHH pathway: Sonic hedgehog, Patched, Smoothened, Gli
    Wnt pathway: Wnt 3, Wnt 7a, frizzle, dishevelled
    EGF family: EGF, TGF-α
    FGF family: FGF-1,-2,-4,-7 (KGF)
    TGF-β family: TGF-β1,2,3, BMP-2,-4
    Others: IGF, PDGF, NGF, activins, etc.
- Nuclear factors
    Homeobox genes: Hox, Msx, Dlx
    Whn
    Hairless
    Tabby (EDA)
    Others: Id1-4, M-Twist, etc.
- Transmembrane molecules and extracellular matrix molecules
    Cadherins: P-, E-, N-
    Beta-catenin/LEF-1 pathway: β-catenin, LEF-1/TCF, APC
    Notch pathway: Notch, Delta, Serrate-1, Serrate-2
    Immunoglobulin family adhesion molecules: N-CAM, DCC, I-CAM
    Extracellular matrix proteins: tenascin, plasminogen activator and their inhibitors, collagen, fibronectin, laminin, proteoglycans, nexin
    Protease and modulators

Secreted signaling factors

Many morphogenes are secreted factors that have an effect on skin appendage morphogenesis. Some are discussed here; please also refer to Chapter 8 by Philpott for further discussion.

Sonic hedgehog pathway

Sonic hedgehog (Shh) is a secreted signaling molecule involved in many morphogenetic events and organ formation.[42] While both 'Patched' and 'Smoothened' are receptors for Shh, Patched functions as a repressor of Smoothened. Shh binds to and represses Patched, which then de-represses Smoothened[43,44] to lead to activation of the transcription factor Gli, thus altering gene expression.

The *Shh* gene is found in the feather placode, and ectopic *Shh* expression was shown to promote the formation of dermal condensations[45] and to require specific competent stages for effect.[46] In mice, it is expressed in the epithelium before the mesenchymal condensation, then in the epidermal placode, and expression continues into the hair bulb surrounding the dermal papilla.[47] In *Shh* null mice, the initiation of follicles is not affected, but the development of the follicles is arrested after Stage 2 (see Figure 2),[48,49] suggesting that *Shh* is essential for the progression from hair germ stage to hair peg stage.

The Gorlin syndrome[50] (also known as the basal cell nevus syndrome, BCNS) is a genetic human disease inherited in an autosomal dominant manner, that causes a diverse range of developmental abnormalities as well as a multitude of tumor types, the most common of which is basal cell carcinoma. Cloning showed that the mutation is in the *Patched* gene.[51] Subsequent studies showed that mutations in other molecules of the *Shh* pathway, for example Smoothened and Gli, are also involved in sporadic basal cell carcinomas.[52,53] On the experimental side, overexpressing *Shh* in the basal layer with a K14 promoter in transgenic mice led to the development of many features of the basal cell nevus syndrome, including the growth of invaginating hair follicles to form basal cell carcinoma-like tumors.[32] This is a good demonstration that basic molecular mechanisms are shared by development and cancer formation, with one being regulated and the other not.

The Wnt pathway

Wnt was originally found to be involved in tumor formation and development. It has many members; their receptors belong to the Frizzled family.[54] The *Wnt* pathway is involved in the control of hair growth and structure via its own signaling pathway. *Wnt-3* is expressed in developing and mature mouse hair follicles. Transgenic mice over-expressing *Wnt-3* in hair follicles and skin produced a short hair phenotype as a result of altered differentiation of hair shaft precursor cells.[55] This alteration also caused defects in hair shaft structure and composition resulting in cyclical balding of the transgenic mice.

In feather, *Wnt-7a* is found specifically in the posterior feather bud epithelium. Overexpression of *Wnt-7a* causes the whole bud to show posterior bud characteristics, and as a result, the buds do not elongate, suggesting the pivotal role played by the *Wnt* pathway in setting anterior–posterior and proximal–distal axes of skin appendages.[36]

Epidermal growth factor family

The epidermal growth factor family includes epidermal growth factor (EGF) and transforming growth factor-α (TGF-α) in relation to hair follicle morphogenesis. They both bind to the EGF receptor. Cohen[56] found that EGF stimulates the proliferation of epidermal and other epithelial tissues in animals. Keratinocyte growth is dependent on a combination of cell multiplication as well as cell migration.[57] They also noted that TGF-α is ten times more potent in inducing cell growth. For this reason, in this discussion the focus will be on TGF-α.

TGF-α is structurally related to EGF and binds to the EGF receptor. It is present in the normal neonatal and adult epidermal keratinocyte[58] and is even more potent than EGF in stimulating keratinocyte growth in vivo.[57] In fact, TGF-α overexpression is seen in skin diseases such as psoriasis, which is characterized by hyperproliferation.[59] TGF-α may play an important role in controlling follicular differentiation and keratinization.[40] While the EGF receptor is located on the outer root sheath, TGF-α is expressed in the inner root sheath. This suggests that hair growth is, in part, controlled by interactions between the EGF receptor and TGF-α, since the development and elongation of the hair shaft are believed to be dependent on the coordinated proliferation and migration of the inner and outer root sheaths.[60]

TGF-α deficient mice, or *waved-1*, show irregularly distributed and variably angled follicles.[61] This suggests that TGF-α may influence the proper positioning of follicles. The *waved-2* mutation, causing a phenotype similar to *waved-1*, was identified as a point mutation within the tyrosine kinase domain of the EGF/TGF-α receptor, which results in compromised receptor activation by its ligand.[60] EGF-receptor expression disruption is usually lethal; however, surviving mice show rudimentary whiskers with prematurely differentiated, thin, disoriented hair follicles, and separation of the hair shaft from the inner root sheath.[62–64]

Fibroblast growth factor family

The fibroblast growth factor (FGF) family has a wide range of biological activities.[65] The family consists of at least nine related proteins with remarkable mitogenic and morphogenetic effects on cells of ectodermal, mesodermal, and neuroectodermal origin. Different FGFs appear to be involved in different phases of skin appendage morphogenesis.

Several FGFs have been found to be involved in the development of skin appendages. Both FGF-1 and FGF-2 are distributed around the dermal-epidermal junction during follicle development, which implies that they may function in local tissue remodeling during follicle morphogenesis.[66] However, high concentrations seem to inhibit hair initiation. As the follicles mature, FGF-2 is associated with the outer root sheath at the interface between the bulb matrix and dermal papilla.[67] FGF-1 is found in the differentiating cells of the follicular bulb and is thought to participate in the formation of structural components of the follicle or fiber. In the feather, FGF-1, FGF-2, and FGF-4 can induce new feather buds from apteric regions of the embryo, and increase the size of feather buds through the merging of several buds.[68]

FGF-7 or keratinocyte growth factor (KGF) is a mitogen that is specific for epithelial cells. It is expressed specifically in the dermis, supporting the idea that KGF is important in the mesenchymal stimulation of epithelial cell growth.[69] In the follicle, KGF is located in the dermal papilla and its receptor is expressed in the epithelial compartment of the hair follicle. KGF accelerates the re-epithelialization and stimulates the proliferation and differentiation of early progenitor cells within hair follicles and sebaceous glands in wound beds and the adjacent dermis. In fact, both sebaceous glands and hair follicles were larger and more numerous in KGF stimulated areas.[70,71] Nevertheless, Guo and co-workers showed that ectopic expression of KGF at high levels in the basal cells of the epidermis inhibits the formation of primary hair follicles.[72]

FGF-5 is interesting in that it does not seem to influence hair development but prolongs the period of anagen.[73] In the normal follicle, FGF-5 is located in the lower third portion of the outer root sheath during late anagen. FGF-5-deficient mice had abnormally long hair and lengthened anagen. This suggests that FGF-5 may be involved in signaling the transition from anagen to catagen.

Transforming growth factor-beta/BMP family

The transforming growth factor-β (TGF-β) super-family is a multifunctional group of factors including growth, differentiation, and morphogenetic factors. These factors are seemingly involved in many processes of tissue development and repair.[74] The family members known to be involved in follicle development include TGF-β1 and 2 and the bone morphogenetic proteins, protein-2 and protein-4 (BMP-2 and BMP-4). The expression patterns of TGF-β isoforms suggest that they play key roles in hair development.[75] In vitro, the isoforms are expressed in the epidermis and are growth inhibitors of keratinocytes.[76] Overexpression of TGF-β1 in the epidermis results in a thinned interfollicular epidermis and drastically fewer hair follicles.[77] Conversely, squamous cell carcinomas are devoid of TGF-β.[76] Mice deficient in TGF-β2 but not TGF-β1 or TGF-β3, show a delay in hair follicle development and a reduction in the number of hair follicles.[78]

The bone morphogenetic proteins, protein-2 and protein-4 are expressed during hair follicle organogenesis.[79] BMP-4 is expressed transiently in the mesenchymal condensation just prior to hair follicle formation,[80] and may therefore be part of the initial dermal signals inducing follicular germ formation. BMP-2, however, is expressed in the epidermal placode, and in more advanced follicles, is found in the matrix and pre-cortex cells.[79] Transgenic mice overexpressing BMP-4 in the outer root sheath had a complete deficiency of hair growth after the first growth cycle and, therefore, progressive balding; however, the development phase appeared to be normal. It is believed that BMP-4 mimics the effects of BMP-2 on the outer root sheath cells rather than evoking any unrelated responses. This suggests that BMP-2 may regulate hair morphogenesis and hair cycling by negatively controlling the proliferative activity of follicular epithelial cells.[30]

Noggin is a known BMP antagonist. It has recently been shown to be present in the follicular mesenchyme of developing hair follicles in mice. In stage 1–3 hair follicles, noggin is seen in the mesenchymal condensation directly below the hair placode. In stages 4–6, it is present in the developing dermal papilla and proximal connective tissue sheath. Furthermore, it was shown that in noggin knockout mice, there is significant retardation in the induction and morphogenesis of hair follicles, while adminstration of noggin-soaked beads stimulated hair follicle induction in situ. Therefore, it suggested that noggin may prevent interactions between BMP's produced by the mesenchyme and placode with BMP receptor-1A. In support of this idea, it was shown that in embryonic skin organ culture, BMP-4 suppressed hair follicle induction with resulting reduction in epidermal thickness and proliferation. Noggin treatment then increases the number of hair placodes and accelerates hair follicle morphogenesis. The retardation of hair follicle induction and morphogenesis by BMP-4 is associated with an up-regulation in the number of TUNEL-positive cells in the hair placode. This is indicative of BMP-4 as an enhancer of apoptotic cell death.[81]

Other growth factors

There are many other growth factors involved in hair follicle morphogenesis that are not discussed here. These include the insulin-like growth factor family,[82] platelet-derived growth factor,[83,84] nerve growth factor, activins, and so on. Some of these are discussed in Chapter 9 by Dr Philpott.

Nuclear factors

Homeobox genes

Homeobox genes are a gene family that encodes transcription factors and therefore determines the developmental fate of a cell.[25,85] The major families include *Hox*, *Msx*, and *Dlx*. *Hox* genes are essential for the patterning and development of many segmental structures in vertebrates as well as invertebrates. In feather buds, *Hox* genes are found to form a body-position-dependent macrogradient and a feather-bud-position-dependent microgradient.[86] It was then suggested that *Hox* genes may play a role in the phenotypic determination of skin appendages via different combinations of *Hox* expression patterns.[25] The patterns of *Hox* genes in murine skin were found to vary temporally and spatially within the developing skin and hair follicles.[87] In the mouse embryonic skin, *Hox c8* was expressed in two graded patterns along the cephalocaudal and dorsal–ventral axis in the epithelial cells of the developing hair follicle, as well as the dermal papilla. *Hox d9* and *Hox d11* were expressed in the epithelial cells of the follicle during the formation of the hair bud. They both remained expressed in the fully developed hair but the expression was restricted to the differentiating matrix cells of the follicle bulb. *Hox d9* and *Hox d11* were switched off at the onset of catagen. *Hox d13* was expressed relatively late in hair follicle development and was restricted to the differentiating matrix cells of the follicle bulb.[87]

Hox expression in developing human skin was also studied and several *Hox* genes, including *HOXA4*, *HOXA5*, *HOXA7*, *HOXB4*, *HOXB7*, and *HOX C4*, exhibit spatial and temporal changes in developing epidermis, dermis, and hair follicles.[88] However, owing to difficulty in obtaining specimens, issues on regional specificity have not been addressed in detail.

Other homeobox genes associated with the development of skin appendages are *Msx-1* and *Msx-2*.[89] *Msx-1* and *Msx-2* are found in the feather placode and later in the proliferating matrix epithelia of follicles. The level of *Msx-2* may be important in regulating the appropriate length of skin appendages. Cyclic AMP, a reagent that inhibits skin-appendage growth, also suppresses the expression of *Msx-1* and *Msx-2*.[89] Mice with over-expression driven by cytomegalovirus (CMV) showed shrunken matrix epithelium and shortened hair.[90]

Winged helix nude

Mutations in the *winged helix nude* (*Whn*) gene result in the nude mouse and rat phenotypes.[92] The nude mouse may appear hairless but the dermis actually contains the same number of hair follicles as a wild-type mouse. The hair follicles, however, are aberrant and not completely developed.[93] The keratinization of the hair follicles is abnormal and characterized by short, bent hair shafts that rarely protrude from the follicles. The *Whn* gene codes for a transcription factor in the winged-helix domain family. This family of proteins developmentally regulates and directs tissue specific transcription and decisions regarding cell fate. It is also involved during anagen phase directing cells as they transform from proliferating to postmitotic differentiating cells.[94] *Whn* has been shown to be expressed specifically in epithelial cells of developing hair follicles and to function as a transcription factor that can suppress the expression of differentiation responsive genes. Over-expression of *whn*

led to the hyperproliferaton of keratinocytes, and hair follicles remained continuously in anagen.[95] Therefore, *Whn* appears to regulate the balance between epithelial cell growth and differentiation.[96] Most recently, a genetic defect in human *Whn* was found with phenotypes similar to nude mice.[97]

Hairless

Mutation of the *hairless* (*hr*) gene in mice results in complete baldness beginning with the first catagen phase, although these mice were born with seemingly normal hair follicles. These normal-appearing hair follicles disintegrate leaving behind utriculi and dermal cysts.[98,99] In the mouse hairless phenotype, the outer root sheath disintegrates except for two epithelial cell populations: the distal outer root sheath cells, which form the utriculi, and the remnants of the bulge, which may form epithelial outgrowths or dermal cysts. Recently, the recessively inherited human alopecia universalis was found to be defective in the *hairless* gene.[100]

Transmembrane molecules and extracellular matrix molecules

Cell adhesion molecules are known to mediate cell interactions in regulating cell migration, growth, and differentiation—events that are critical in the development of skin and its appendages.[101] The concept of 'topobiology', the investigation of place-dependent molecular interactions of cell surfaces or with substrates that result in changes in cell regulation,[102] was applied to analyse hair development.[103] This field emphasizes that different groups of cells can create differential surface tension forces to alter cell shape on the basis of their adhesion properties during the formation of hair follicles.

Tabby

The *tabby* mouse gene (*Ta*) is the murine homolog of human *anhydrotic ectodermal dysplasia* (*EDA*) gene.[104] The *tabby* phenotype shares the EDA features of hypoplastic hair, teeth and eccrine sweat glands.[105] It is important because it is the first gene characterized for EDA[106] and may be involved in the development of different kinds of skin appendages. The function of the tabby gene product has yet to be determined; it contains a single transmembrane domain and a collagenous domain, which shares similarities with other membrane-associated proteins.[107] It has been suggested that the *Ta* gene may be involved in a signal transduction pathway involving EGF. In tabby mice, there appears to be a reduction of EGF receptors.[108] Injections of EGF rescued the phenotype of delayed eyelid opening and incisor tooth eruption in the *tabby* mouse mutant[109] and induced the development of functional eccrine sweat glands.[110] Recently, the gene for mouse *downless* was cloned and shown to be a member of the tumor necrosis factor receptor family. The mutant phenotype and expression pattern suggests that downless is likely to be the receptor for tabby.[111]

Cadherins

The cadherins are a family of calcium-dependent cell-adhesion molecules that are important for sorting cells into tissues and for establishing cell polarity.[101] L-CAM, or E-cadherin, was found in the developing feather placode, and perturbation of L-CAM led to abnormal feather morphogenesis and patterning.[112]

The expression of E- and P-cadherins in hair follicle development was studied by Hardy and Vielkind.[113] They found that when the ectoderm gave rise to the periderm and epidermis, E-cadherin was present on all epithelial layers. However, it then decreased in expression in the placode and hair pegs, while maintaining expression in the periderm and epidermis. Later the elongating follicles were completely negative for E-cadherin in the presumptive hair matrix. In the follicle, there was positive staining in the outer root sheath cells, the elongating inner root sheath, and the outermost layer of the hair bulb (the outer root sheath precursor cells). P-cadherin was also present in the periderm and epidermis before follicle initiation. Later, however, P-cadherin was lost in the periderm and epidermis, but retained moderate staining in the basal epidermis; it was also prominent in the placodes, hair pegs, and the presumptive matrix of elongating follicles. Later, it was also found in the hair matrix and moderately in the outer root sheaths of differentiating hair follicles.

Using antibodies against E- and P-cadherin interferes with skin morphogenesis and hair follicle morphogenesis in vitro.[114] It has been suggested that E-cadherin may be required to maintain the integrity of epithelial tissues, while P-cadherin is essential for the segregation of basal layers from the upper layers.[115,116] The shift from E-cadherin to P-cadherin on placodal cells may be in response to instruction for the epidermis to make a skin appendage.[113]

β-catenin / LEF-1 pathway

Beta-catenin binds the cytoplasmic domain of cadherin, and also binds to several other proteins including cytoskeleton proteins, and other adenopolyposis coli (APC). Activation of the pathway leads to accumulation of β-catenin in the cytoplasm, allowing it to interact with LEF-1/TCF, thus generating a functional transcription factor complex.[117,118] Therefore, the β-catenin pathway provides a molecular mechanism to transmit extracellular signals to the nucleus.[117] This pathway is present in keratinocytes. Active β-catenin driven by K14 in mice caused de novo hair follicle morphogenesis.[33] In some interfollicular segments, however, the new 'hair germs' progressed into epitheliod cysts, which strongly resembled human trichofolliculomas. As the mutant mice aged, they developed visible tumors whose histology resembled pilomatricomas. Indeed, a high percentage of human pilomatricomas are also found to have a mutation in β-catenin.[119]

Lymphoid enhancer factor-1 (LEF-1) is a DNA-binding protein in the family of high mobility group (HMG) proteins.[120] It acts to induce a sharp bend in the DNA helix and is dependent on other enhancer-bound proteins to activate transcription.[121]

LEF-1 is expressed in the ectoderm even before the dermal condensations are formed. Overexpression of *LEF-1* leads to the formation of hairs in the gum region.[14] On the other hand, *LEF-1* null transgenic mice have scant hair, and markedly reduced pelage and vibrissae follicles.[38,122] These studies suggest the importance of the β-catenin/LEF-1 pathway in the new growth of skin, whether they are regulated or de-regulated.

Notch pathway

The Notch pathway is important in many developmental processes, particularly the specification of epithelial cell fate.[123] The ligands include Delta and Serrate/Jagged. This pathway is involved in hair follicle development. High levels of *Notch* are expressed in the epithelial compartment, and are expressed as different cell types become distinguishable in the developing follicles. The cells that express high levels of *Notch* are the matrix cells as they undergo transition from mitotic precursors to discrete, differentiating cell types.[124] In development, *Notch-1* is expressed in the ectodermal-derived cells of the hair follicle, the inner cells of the epidermal placode and follicle bulb, and the suprabasal cells in the mature outer root sheath. *Delta-1* is only expressed during development and is specifically located in the mesenchymal cells of the pre-papilla (below the placode). *Serrate-1* or *Serrate-2* seems to overlap with *Notch-1* at all stages of development.[125]

Recent work also suggests that the notch pathway is involved in the patterning of feather development. Chen et al[126] demonstrated specific spatial expression patterns of *chicken (C)-Notch-1, C-Delta-1,* and *C-Serrate-1* toward posterior feather buds. They conducted recombination experiments with rotation showing that the appearance of these mRNAs precedes the new polarity of feather buds, thus suggesting that the Notch pathway is involved in the establishment of the anterior–posterior axis of feather buds. The Notch pathway is involved in early feather pattern formation.[127,128] Mis-expressing Delta-1 has a dual role—promoting feather bud development and inhibiting lateral buds. In the scale area, new feather buds are induced by Delta-1. The data suggests that the Notch pathway is important in guiding the fate of epithelial cells.

Immunoglobulin family adhesion molecules
N-CAM is a calcium-independent neural cell-adhesion molecule. In feather development, it was found at low levels in all presumptive dermis before patterning, in the distal bud epithelium, and in the matrix epithelia above the dermal papilla. It is expressed at high levels in the dermal condensation, dermal papilla, and marginal plate epithelium.[129,130] Perturbation of N-CAM leads to uneven segregation of dermal condensations.[101]

In mouse skin, prior to placode formation, N-CAM is found in all mesenchymal cells but not in epithelia. In the hair peg stage, N-CAM is found in most epithelial cells, though asymmetrically, being brighter on the longer, posterior side. In the elongating follicle, the expression changes again to the interfollicular mesenchyme,

mesenchymal sheath, and the dermal papilla. N-CAM continues to stain positively in the dermal papilla and the mesenchymal sheath of the follicle in the differentiating follicle, but also in the caudal outer root sheath near the follicle neck. N-CAM may reinforce cell adhesion during morphogenetic movements in areas of decreased calcium levels.[113] In the hair cycle, N-CAM remains high in dermal papilla.[28]

Deleted in colorectal carcinoma (DCC), a gene originally identified as the gene deleted in colorectal carcinoma, is a transmembrane protein composed of immunoglobulin domains. It is mainly expressed in the epithelia and neural tissue. In epithelia, it is enriched in the basal layer of the epidermis and crypt region on intestinal villi.[131] In hair follicles, it is enriched in the bulge region.[28] Its location suggests its role in growth control of epithelial cells. However, in neural development, it is shown to be involved in regulating neurite migration.[132] These two categories of function may also be found to be linked, pending further research.

Extracellular matrix proteins
These matrix proteins play pivotal roles in epithelial–mesenchymal interactions during the development of many organs. For example, tenascin, fibronectin, proteoglyeans and other matrix proteins have been shown to be important for feather and hair development.[101,133,134] Morphogenesis of skin appendage follicles also involves active tissue remodeling and, therefore, another area that deserves more attention is the study of proteases and their regulators. Indeed, plasminogen activator inhibitors have been shown to be involved in the development of hair, nail and skin.[135,136] Although these topics have been discussed only briefly, these are important issues.

Summary and conclusions

Skin appendages include hairs, feathers, nails, glands, horns, and so on. They are the topological transformation of an epithelial sheet resulting from epithelial–mesenchymal interactions. A new staging system and morphogenetic pathways that are common to different skin appendages have been discussed, showing that they are variations of a common theme. The principles of these morphogenetic processes and their molecular basis, including signaling molecules and adhesion molecules, have also been described. Skin appendages represent regulated new growths whereas skin tumors represent deregulated new growths.

It is hoped that what is learned in the field of developmental biology of skin appendages can be applied to the study of epidermal precursor cells to influence morphogenesis and differentiation in tissue regeneration and engineering. In the next decade, we hope to understand how a complex skin appendage such as the hair follicle can be formed from a piece of epithelium during development. Knowledge may be gleaned from both signaling molecules and nuclear factors (the morphogenesis designers) and from cell adhesion molecules and extracellular matrix proteins (the morphogenesis mediators).

Another important direction is the characterization of epidermal precursor cells, including stem cells. These precursor cells can form complex epidermal organs during development. If these 'principles of development' can be learnt, this may aid the study and practice of wound healing and regeneration, the bioengineering of skin, and the management of skin tumors. With the human genome project approaching an end, many genes will be known, analogous to the words in a dictionary. Tissue engineering requires us to know the language of cells. Learning developmental biology is like learning the grammar of this language so we can try to use words, that is genes, to construct manuscripts, that is an organ such as a hair follicle.[8]

Acknowledgments

We are grateful for support from NIH (CMC), NSF (CMC), and USC medical student award from the Baxter Foundation (TWK). We thank Mr Roger Kuo for his help with computer graphics and Dr Widelitz for reviewing the manuscript.

References

1. Chuong CM: Morphogenesis of epithelial appendages: variations on top of a common theme and implications in regeneration, In: Chuong CM, (ed.). *Molecular Basis of Epithelial Appendage Morphogenesis*. Austin, Texas, RG Landes, 1998: 3–13.
2. Sengel P: Morphogenesis of skin. In: Abercombie M, Newith DR, Torrey JG (eds.). *Developmental and Cell Biology Series*. Cambridge, University Press, 1976: 1–277.
3. Lucas AM, Stettenheim PR: Avian anatomy: integument. In: *Agriculture Handbook 362*. Washington DC, Agricultural Research Services, US Department of Agriculture, 1972.
4. Chuong CM (ed.): *Molecular Basis of Epithelial Appendage Morphogenesis*. Austin, Texas, RG Landes, 1998.
5. Hardy MH: The secret life of the hair follicle. *Trends Genet* 1992; **8**: 55–61.
6. Chuong CM: The making of a feather: homeoproteins, retinoids and adhesion molecules. *BioEssays* 1993; **15**: 513–521.
7. Oro A, Scott MP: Splitting hairs: dissecting roles of signaling systems in epidermal development. *Cell* 1998; **95**: 575–578.
8. Chuong CM, Noveen A: Phenotypic determination of epithelial appendages: genes, developmental pathways, and evolution. *J Invest Dermatol* (In press).
9. Hardy MH: Glandular metaplasia of hair follicles and other responses to vitamin A excess in cultures of rodent skin. *J Embryol Exper Morphol* 1968; **19**: 157–180.
10. Viallet JP, Dhouailly D: Retinoic acid and mouse skin morphogenesis. II. Role of epidermal competence in hair glandular metaplasia. *Develop Biol* 1994; **166**: 277–288.
11. Dhouailly D, Hardy MH, Sengel P: Formation of feathers on chick foot scales: a stage dependent morphogenetic response to retinoic acid. *J Embryol Exper Morphol* 1980; **58**: 63–78.
12. Chuong CM, Ting SA, Widelitz RB, Lee YS: Mechanism of skin morphogenesis. II. Retinoic acid modulates axis orientation and phenotypes of skin appendages. *Development* 1992; **115**: 839–852.
13. Kanzler B, Prin F, Thelu J, Dhouailly D: CHOXC-8 and CHOXD-13 expression in embryonic chick skin and cutaneous appendage specification. *Devel Dynam* 1997; **210**: 274–287.
14. Zhou P, Byrne C, Jacobs J, Fuchs E: Lymphoid enhancer factor 1 directs hair follicle patterning and epithelial cell fate. *Genes Devel* 1995; **9**: 570–583.

15. Pinheiro M, Freire-Maia N: Ectodermal dysplasias: a clinical classification and a causal review. *Am J Med Genet* 1994; **53**: 153–162.

16. Slavkin HC, Shum L, Nuckolls GH: Ectodermal dysplasia: a synthesis between evolutionary, developmental, and molecular biology and human clinical genetics. In: Chuong CM (ed.). *Molecular Basis of Epithelial Appendage Morphogenesis*. Austin, Texas, RG Landes, 1998: 15–30.

17. Chuong CM, Widelitz RB: Feather morphogenesis: a model of the formation of epithelial appendages. In: Chuong CM (ed.). *Molecular Basis of Epithelial Appendage Morphogenesis*. Austin, Texas, RG Landes, 1998: 57–72.

18. Paus R, Cotsarelis G: The biology of hair follicles. *New Eng J Med* 1999; **341**: 491–497.

19. Serri F, Cerimele D: Embryology of the hair follicle. In: Orfanos CE, Happle R, (eds.). *Hair and hair diseases*. New York, Springer-Verlag, 1989: 1–17.

20. Holbrook KA, Minami SI: Hair follicle embryogenesis in the human. *Annals NY Acad Sciences* 1991; **642**: 167–196.

21. Cotsarelis G, Sun TT, Larker RM: Label retaining cells reside in the bulge area of pilosebaceous unit: implications for follicular stem cells, hair cycle, and skin carcinogenesis. *Cell* 1990; **61**: 1329–1337.

22. Reynolds AJ, Jahoda CA: Hair matrix germinative epidermal cells confer follicle-inducing capabilities on dermal sheath and high passage papilla cells. *Development* 1996; **122**: 3085–3094.

23. Sperling LC: Hair anatomy for the clinician. *J Am Acad Dermatol* 1991; **25**: 1–17.

24. Philpott M, Paus R: Principles of hair follicle morphogenesis. In: Chuong CM (ed.). *Molecular Basis of Epithelial Appendage Morphogenesis*. Austin Texas, RG Landes, 1998: 75–110.

25. Chuong CM, Widelitz RB, Jiang TX: Adhesion molecules and homeoproteins in the phenotypic determination of skin appendages. *J Invest Dermatol* 1993; **101**: 10S–15S.

26. Widelitz RB, Jiang TX, Noveen A, et al.: Molecular histology in skin appendage morphogenesis. *Microsc Res Tech* 1997; **38**: 452–465.

27. Widelitz RB, Chuong CM: Early events in skin appendage formation: induction of epithelial placodes and condensation of dermal mesenchymal cells (In press).

28. Combates NJ, Chuong CM, Stenn KS, Prouty SM: Expression of two Ig family adhesion molecules in the murine hair cycle: DCC in the bulge epithelia and NCAM in the follicular papilla. *J Invest Dermatol* 1997; **109**: 672–678.

29. Chapman RE. In: Bereiter-Hahn J, Matoltsy AG, Richards KS (eds.). *Biology of the Integument, 2.*

Vertebrates. Berlin, Springer-Verlag, 1986: 293–317.

30. Blessing M, Nanney LB, King LE, Jones CM, Hogan BLM: Transgenic mice as a model to study the role of TGF-β-related molecules in hair follicles. *Genes Devel* 1993; **7**: 204–215.

31. Chen CW, Chuong CM: Avian integument provides multiple possibilities to analyse different phases of skin appendage morphogenesis. *J Invest Dermatol* (In press).

32. Oro AE, Higgins KM, Hu Z, Bonifas JM, Epstein EH, Scott MP: Basal cell carcinomas in mice over-expressing sonic hedgehog. *Science* 1997; **276**: 817–821.

33. Gat U, DasGupta R, Degenstein L, Fuchs E: De novo hair follicle morphogenesis and hair tumors in mice expressing a truncated β-catenin in skin. *Cell* 1998; **95**: 605–614.

34. Garber B, Kollar EJ, Moscona AA: Aggregation in vivo of dissociated cells, 3. Effect of state of differentiation of cells on feather development in hybrid aggregates of embryonic mouse and chick skin cells. *J Exper Zool* 1968; **168**: 455–472.

35. Lichti U, Scandurro AB, Kartasova T, Rubin JS, LaRochelle W, Yuspa SH: Hair follicle development and hair growth from defined cell populations grafted onto nude mice. *J Invest Dermatol* 1995; **104**: 43S–44S.

36. Widelitz RB, Jiang TX, Chen CW, Stott NS, Chuong CM: Wnt-7a in feather morphogenesis: involvement of anterior–posterior asymmetry and proximal–distal elongation demonstrated with an in vitro reconstitution model. *Development* 1999; **126**: 2577–2587.

37. Jiang T-X, Jung H-S, Widelitz RB, Chuong C-M: Self organization of periodic patterns by dissociated feather mesenchymal cells and the regulation of size, number and spacing of primordia. *Development* (in press).

38. Stenn KS, Combates NJ, Eilertsen KJ, et al.: Hair follicle growth controls. *Dermatol Clinics* 1996; **14**: 543–558.

39. Chuong CM, Jung HS, Noden D, Widelitz RB: Lineage and pluripotentiality of epithelial precursor cells in developing chicken skin. *Biochem Cell Biol* 1998; **76**: 1069–1077.

40. Peus D, Pittelkow MR: Growth factors in hair organ development and the hair growth cycle. *Dermatol Clinics* 1996; **4**: 559–572.

41. Chuong CM, Widelitz RB, Ting-Berreth S, Jiang TX: Early events during avian skin appendage regeneration: dependence on epithelial-mesenchymal interaction and order of molecular reappearance. *J Invest Dermatol* 1996; **107**: 639–646.

42. Ingham PW: The *patched* gene in development and cancer. *Curr Opin Genet Devel* 1998; **8**: 88–94.

43. Marigo V, Davey RA, Zuo Y, Cunningham JM, Tabin CJ: Biochemical evidence that patched is the hedgehog receptor. *Nature* 1996; **384:** 176–179.

44. Stone DM, Hynes M, Armanini M, et al.: The tumour-suppressor gene *patched* encodes a candidate receptor for Sonic hedgehog. *Nature* 1996; **384:** 129–134.

45. Ting-Berreth SA, Chuong CM: *Sonic Hedgehog* in feather morphogenesis: induction of mesenchymal condensation and association with cell death. *Devel Dynamics* 1996; **207:** 157–170.

46. Morgan BA, Orkin RW, Noramly S, Perez A: Stage-specific effects of sonic hedgehog expression in the epidermis. *Devel Biol* 1998; **201:** 1–12.

47. Iseki S, Araga A, Ohuchi H, et al.: Sonic hedgehog is expressed in epithelial cells during development of whisker, hair and tooth. *Biochemical and Biophysical Res Comm* 1996; **218:** 688–693.

48. St-Jacques B, Dassule HR, Karavanova I, et al.: Sonic hedgehog signaling is essential for hair development. *Curr Biol* 1998; **8:** 1058–1068.

49. Chiang C, Swan RZ, Grachtchouk M, et al.: Essential role for Sonic hedgehog during hair follicle morphogenesis. *Devel Biol* 1999; **205:** 1–9.

50. Gorlin RJ: Nevoid basal cell carcinoma syndrome. *Dermatol Clin* 1995; **13:** 13–25.

51. Johnson RL, Rothman AL, Xie J, et al.: Human homolog of patched, a candidate gene for the basal cell nevus syndrome. *Science* 1996; **272:** 1668–1671.

52. Xie J, Murone M, Luoh SM, et al.: Activating smoothened mutations in sporadic basal-cell carcinoma. *Nature* 1998; **391:** 90–92.

53. Dahmane N, Lee J, Robins P, Heller P, Ruiz I, Altaba A: Activation of the transcription factor Gli1 and the Sonic hedgehog signaling pathway in skin tumours. *Nature* 1997; **389:** 876–881.

54. Saldanha J, Singh J, Mahadevan D: Identification of a Frizzled-like cysteine rich domain in the extracellular region of developmental receptor tyrosine kinases. *Protein Sci* 1998; **7:** 1632–1635.

55. Millar SE, Willert K, Salinas PC, et al.: WNT signaling in the control of hair growth and structure. *Devel Biol* 1999; **207:** 133–149.

56. Cohen S: The stimulation of epidermal proliferation by a specific protein (EGF). *Devel Biol* 1965; **12:** 394–407.

57. Barrandon Y, Green H: Cell migration is essential for sustained growth of keratinocyte colonies: the roles of transforming growth factor-α and epidermal growth factor. *Cell* 1987; **50:** 1131–1137.

58. Coffey RJ Jr., Derynck R, Wilcox JN, et al.: Production and autoinduction of transforming growth factor-α in human keratinocytes. *Nature* 1987; **328:** 817–823.

59. Elder JT, Fisher GJ, Lindquist PB, et al.: Overex- pression of transforming growth factor α in psoriatic epidermis. *Science* 1989; **243:** 811–814.

60. Luetteke NC, Phillips HK, Qiu TH, et al.: The mouse waved-2 phenotype results from a point mutation in the EGF receptor tyrosine kinase. *Genes Devel* 1994; **8:** 299–413.

61. Luetteke NC, Qiu TH, Peiffer RL, Oliver P, Smithies O, Lee DC: TGF-α deficiency results in hair follicle and eye abnormalities in targeted and waved-1 mice. *Cell* 1993; **73:** 263–278.

62. Hansen LA: Altered hair follicle morphogenesis in epidermal growth factor receptor deficient mice. *J Invest Dermatol* 1996; **820:** (Abstract).

63. Sibilia M, Wagner EF: Strain-dependent epithelial defects in mice lacking the EGF receptor. *Science* 1995; **269:** 234–238.

64. Threadgill DW, Dlugosz AA, Hansen LA, et al.: Targeted disruption of mouse EGF receptor: effect of genetic background on mutant phenotype. *Science* 1995; **269:** 230–234.

65. Ornitz DM, Xu J, Colvin JS, et al.: Receptor specificity of the fibroblast growth factor family. *J Biol Chem* 1996; **271:** 15292–15297.

66. Du Cros DL, Isaacs K, Moore GPM: Distribution of acidic and basic fibroblast growth factors in ovine skin during follicle morphogenesis. *J Cell Sci* 1993; **105:** 667–674.

67. Du Cros DL: Fibroblast growth factor and epidermal growth factor in hair development. *J Invest Dermatol* 1993; **101:** 106S–113S.

68. Widelitz RB, Jiang TX, Noveen A, Chen CW, Chuong CM: FGF induces new feather buds from developing avian skin. *J Invest Dermatol* 1996; **107:** 797–803.

69. Finch PW, Rubin JS, Miki T, Ron D, Aaronson SA: Human KGF is FGF-related with properties of a paracrine effector of epithelial cell growth. *Science* 1989; **24:** 752–755.

70. Pierce GF, Yanagihara D, Klopchin K, et al.: Stimulation of all epithelial elements during skin regeneration by keratinocyte growth factor. *J Exper Med* 1994; **179:** 831–840.

71. Danilenko DM, Ring BD, Yanagihara D, et al.: Keratinocyte growth factor is an important endogenous mediator of hair follicle growth, development, and differentiation. *Am J Pathol* 1995; **147:** 145–153.

72. Guo L, Yu QC, Fuchs E: Targeting expression of keratinocyte growth factor to keratinocytes elicits striking changes in epithelial differentiation in transgenic mice. *EMBO J* 1993; **12:** 973–986.

73. Hebert JM, Rosenquist T, Gotz J, Martin GR: FGF5 as a regulator of the hair growth cycle: evidence from targeted and spontaneous mutations. *Cell* 1994; **78:** 1017–1025.

74. Massague J: TGF-beta signal transduction. *Ann Rev Biochem* 1998; **67:** 753–791.

75. Paus R, Foitzik K, Welker P, Bulfone-Paus S, Eichmuller S: Transforming growth factor-β receptor type I and type II expression during murine hair follicle development and cycling. *J Invest Dermatol* 1997; **109:** 518–526.

76. Glick AV, Kulkarni AB, Tennenbaum T, et al.: Loss of expression of transforming growth factor β in skin and skin tumors is associated with hyperproliferation and a high risk for malignant conversion. *Proc Natl Acad Sci USA* 1993; **90:** 6076–6080.

77. Sellheyer K, Bickenbach JR, Rothnagel J, et al.: Inhibition of skin development by overexpression of transforming growth factor β 1 in the epidermis of transgenic mice. *Proc Natl Acad Sci USA* 1993; **90:** 5237–5241.

78. Foitzik K, Paus R, Doetschman T, Paolo DG: The TGF-beta 2 isoform is both a required and sufficient inducer of murine hair follicle morphogenesis. *Devel Biol* 1999; **212:** 278–289.

79. Lyons KM, Pelton RW, Hogan BLM: Organogenesis and pattern formation in the mouse: RNA distribution patterns suggest a role for bone morphogenetic protein-2A (BMP-2A). *Development* 1990; **109:** 833–844.

80. Jones CM, Lyons KM, Hogan BLM: Involvement of *bone morphogenetic protein-4* (BMP-4) and *VGR-1* in morphogenesis and neurogenesis in the mouse. *Development* 1991; **111:** 531–542.

81. Botchkarev VA, Botchkareva NV, Roth W, et al.: Noggin is a mesenchymally derived stimulator of hair-follicle induction. *Nature Cell Biology* 1999; **1:** 158–165.

82. Philpott MP, Sanders DA, Kealey T: Effects of insulin and insulin-like growth factors on cultured human hair follicles: IGF-I at physiologic concentrations is an important regulator of hair follicle growth *in vitro*. *J Invest Dermatol* 1994; **102:** 857–861.

83. Ross RR: Platelet-derived growth factor. *Ann Rev Med* 1987; **38:** 71–79.

84. Takakura N, Yoshida H, Kunisada T, Nishikawa S, Nishikawa SI: Involvement of platelet-derived growth factor receptor-α in hair canal formation. *J Invest Dermatol* 1996; **107:** 770–777.

85. Scott GA, Goldsmith LA: Homeobox genes and skin development: a review. *J Invest Dermatol* 1993; **101:** 3–8.

86. Chuong CM, Oliver G, Ting SA, Jegalian BG, Chen HM, De Robertis EM: Gradients of homeoproteins in developing feather buds. *Development* 1990; **110:** 1021–1030.

87. Kanzler B, Viallet JP, Le Mouellic H, Boncinelli E, Duboule D, Dhouailly D: Differential expression of two different homeobox gene families during mouse tegument morphogenesis. *Int J Dev Biol* 1994; **38:** 633–640.

88. Stelnicki EJ, Komuves LG, Kwong AO, et al.: HOX

89. Noveen A, Jiang TX, Ting-Berreth SA, Chuong CM: Homeobox genes Msx-1 and Msx-2 are associated with induction and growth of skin appendages. *J Invest Dermatol* 1995; **104:** 711–719.

90. Jiang TX, Liu YH, Widelitz RB, et al.: Epidermal dysplasia and abnormal hair follicles in transgenic mice over-expressing homeobox gene Msx-2. *J Invest Dermatol* 1999; **113:** 231–238.

91. Wang WP, Widelitz RB, Jiang TX, Chuong CM: Msx-2 and the regulation of organ size: epidermal thickness and hair length. Submitted to *J Invest Dermatol* as a syllabus for Tricontinental Hair Research Societies.

92. Nehls M, Pfeifer D, Schorpp M, Hedrich H, Boehm T: New member of the winged-helix protein family disrupted in mouse and rat nude mutations. *Nature* 1994; **3372:** 103–107.

93. Kopf-Maier P, Mbonko VF, Merker HJ: Nude mice are not hairless. A morphological study. *Acta Anat (Basel)* 1990; **139:** 178–190.

94. Lee D, Prowse DM, Brissette JL: Association between mouse nude gene expression and the initiation of epithelial terminal differentiation. *Devel Biol* 1999; **208:** 362–374.

95. Prowse DM, Lee D, Weiner L, et al: Ectopic expression of the nude gene induces hyperproliferation and defects in differentiation: implications for the self-renewal of cutaneous epithelia. *Devel Biol* 1999; **212:** 54–67.

96. Brissette JL, Li J, Kamimura J, Lee D, Dotto GP: The product of the mouse *nude* locus, *Whn*, regulates the balance between epithelial cell growth and differentiation. *Genes Devel* 1996; **10:** 2212–2221.

97. Frank J, Pignata C, Panteleyev AA, et al.: Exposing the human nude phenotype. *Nature* 1999; **398:** 473–474.

98. Mann SJ: Hair loss and cyst formation in hairless and rhino mutant mice. *Anat Rec* 1971; **170:** 485–500.

99. Panteleyev AA, van der Veen C, Rosenbach T, Muller-Rover S, Sokolov VE, Paus R: Towards defining the pathogenesis of the hairless phenotype. *J Invest Dermatol* 1998; **110:** 902–907.

100. Ahmad W, Faiyaz M, Haque F, et al.: Alopecia universalis associated with a mutation in the human *hairless* gene. *Science* 1988; **279:** 720–724.

101. Jiang TX, Chuong CM: Mechanism of skin morphogenesis. I. Analyses with antibodies to adhesion molecules tenascin, N-CAM, and integrin. *Devel Biol* 1992; **150:** 82–98.

102. Edelman GM: Morphoregulatory molecules. *Biochemistry* 1988; **27:** 3533–3543.

103. Müller-Röver S, Paus R: Topobiology of the hair

follicle: adhesion molecules as morphoregulatory signals during hair follicle morphogenesis. In: Chuong CM (ed.). *Molecular Basis of Epithelial Appendage Morphogenesis*. Austin Texas, RG Landes, 1998; 283–314.

104. Srivastava AK, Pispa J, Hartung AJ, et al.: The Tabby phenotype is caused by mutation in a mouse homologue of the EDA gene that reveals novel mouse and human exons and encodes a protein (ectodysplasin-A) with collagenous domains. *Proc Natl Acad Sci USA* 1997; **25**: 13069–13074.

105. Sundberg JP: The Tabby (Ta), Tabby-c (Tac), and Tabby-J (Taj) mutations, chromosome X. In: Sundberg JP (ed.). *Handbook of Mouse Mutations with Skin and Hair Abnormalities*. Boca Raton, Florida, CRC Press, 1994: 455–462.

106. Bayes M, Hartung AJ, Ezer S, et al.: The anhidrotic ectodermal dysplasia gene (EDA) undergoes alternative splicing and encodes ectodysplasin-A with deletion mutations in collagenous repeats. *Hum Molec Genet* 1998; **7**: 1661–1669.

107. Ferguson BM, Brockdorff N, Formstone E, Nguyen T, Kronmiller JE, Zonana J: Cloning of *Tabby*, the murine homolog of the human EDA gene: evidence for a membrane-associated protein with a short collagenous domain. *Hum Mol Genet* 1997; **6**: 1589–1594.

108. Vargas GA, Fantino E, George-Nascimento C, Gargus JJ, Haigler HT: Reduced epidermal growth factor receptor expression in hypohidrotic ectodermal dysplasia and Tabby mice. *J Clin Invest* 1996; **97**: 2426–2432.

109. Kapalanga J, Blecher SR: Effect of the X-linked gene Tabby (Ta) on eyelid opening and incisor eruption in neonatal mice is opposite to that of epidermal growth factor. *Development* 1990; **108**: 349–355.

110. Blecher SR, Kapalanga J, Lalonde D: Induction of sweat glands by epidermal growth factor in murine X-linked anhidrotic ectodermal dysplasia. *Nature* 1990; **345**: 542–544.

111. Headon DJ, Overbeek PA: Involvement of a novel Tnf receptors homologue in hair follicle induction. *Nat Genet* 1999; **22**: 370–374.

112. Gallin WJ, Chuong CM, Finkel LH, Edelman GM: Antibodies to liver cell adhesion molecule perturb inductive interactions and alter feather pattern and structure. *Proc Natl Acad Sci USA* 1986; **83**: 8235–8239.

113. Hardy MH, Vielkind U: Changing patterns of cell adhesion molecules during mouse pelage hair follicle development (I). *Acta Anatomica* 1996; **157**: 169–182.

114. Hirai Y, Nose A, Kobayashi S, Takeichi M: Expression and role of E- and P-cadherin adhesion molecules in embryonic histogenesis. II. Skin morphogenesis. *Development* 1989; **105**: 271–277.

115. Nose A, Takeichi M: A novel cadherin in cell adhesion molecule, its expression patterns associated with implantation and organogenesis of mouse embryos. *J Cell Biol* 1986; **103**: 2649–2658.

116. Fujita M, Furukawa F, Fujii K, Horiguchi Y, Takeichi M, Imamura S: Expression of cadherin cell adhesion molecules during human skin development: morphogenesis of epidermis, hair follicles, and eccrine sweat ducts. *Arch Dermatol Res* 1992; **284**: 159–166.

117. Behrens J, von Kries JP, Kuhl M, et al.: Functional interaction of β-catenin with the transcription factor LEF-1. *Nature* 1996; **382**: 638–642.

118. Van der Wetering M, Cavallo R, Dooijes D, et al.: Armadillo coactivates transcription driven by the product of the Drosophila segment polarity gene dTCF. *Cell* 1997; **88**: 789–799.

119. Chan EF, Gat U, McNiff JM, Fuchs E: A common human skin tumour is caused by activating mutations in beta-catenin. *Nat Genet* 1999; **21**: 410–413.

120. Travis A, Amsterdam A, Belanger C, Grosschedl R: LEF-1, a gene encoding a lymphoid-specific with protein, an HMG domain, regulates T-cell receptor a enhancer function. *Genes Devel* 1991; **5**: 880–894.

121. Giese K, Cox J, Grosschedl R: The HMG domain of lymphoid enhancer factor 1 bends DNA and facilitates assembly of function nucleoprotein structures. *Cell* 1992; **69**: 185–195.

122. Van Genderen C, Okamura RM, Farinas I, et al.: Development of several organs that require inductive epithelial-mesenchymal interactions is impaired in LEF-1 deficient mice. *Genes and Devel* 1994; **8**: 2691–2703.

123. Kopan R, Cagan R: Notch on the cutting edge. *Trends Genet* 1997; **13**: 465–467.

124. Kopan R, Weintraub H: Mouse notch: expression in hair follicles correlates with cell fate determination. *J Cell Biol* 1993; **121**: 631–641.

125. Powell BC, Passmore EA, Nesci A, Dunn SM: The notch signalling pathway in hair growth. *Mechan Devel* 1998; **78**: 189–192.

126. Chen CW, Jung HS, Jiang TX, Chuong CM: Asymmetric expression of notch/delta/serrate is associated with the anterior-posterior axis of feather buds. *Devel Biol* 1997; **188**: 181–187.

127. Crowe R, Henrique D, Ish-Horowicz D, Niswander L: A new role for Notch and Delta in cell fate decisions: patterning the feather array. *Development* 1998; **125**: 767–775.

128. Viallet JP, Prin F, Olivera-Martinez I, Hirsinger E, Pourquie O, Dhouailly D: Chick Delta-1 gene expression and the formation of the feather primordia. *Mechan Devel* 1998; **72**: 159–168.

129. Chuong CM, Edelman GM: Expression of cell-adhesion molecules in embryonic induction, I.

Morphogenesis of nestling feathers. *J Cell Biol* 1985a; **101**: 1009–1026.

130. Chuong CM, Edelman GM: Expression of cell-adhesion molecules in embryonic induction: II. Morphogenesis of adult feathers. *J Cell Biol* 1985b; **101**: 1027–1043.

131. Chuong CM, Jiang TX, Yin E, Widelitz RB: cDCC (chicken homologue to a gene deleted in colorectal carcinoma) is an epithelial adhesion molecule expressed in the basal cells and involved in epithelial-mesenchymal interaction. *Devel Biol* 1994; **164**: 383–397.

132. Fazeli A, Dickinson SL, Hermiston ML, et al.: Phenotype of mice lacking functional Deleted in colorectal cancer (Dcc) gene. *Nature* 1997; **386**: 796–804.

133. Kaplan EK, Holbrook KA: Dynamic expression patterns of tenascin, proteoglycans, and cell adhesion molecules during human hair follicle morphogenesis. *Devel Dynam* 1994; **199**: 141–155.

134. Couchman JR: Hair follicle proteoglycans. *J Invest Dermatol* 1993; **101**: 605–645.

135. Lavker RM, Risse B, Brown H, et al.: Localization of plasminogen activator inhibitor type 2 (PAI-2) in hair and nail: implications for terminal differentiation. *J Invest Dermatol* 1998; **110**: 917–922.

136. Lyons-Giordano B, Lazarus GS: Skin abnormalities in mice transgenic for plasminogen activator inhibitor 1: implications for the regulation of desquamation and follicular neogenesis by plasminogen activator enzymes. *Devel Biol* 1995; **170**: 289–298.

137. Kratochwil K, Dull M, Farinas I, Galceran J, Grosschedl R: LEF-I expression is activated by BMP-4 and regulates inductive tissue interactions in tooth and hair development, *Genes Dev* (1995) **9**: 570–583.

138. Weinmaster G, Roberts VJ, Lemke G: A homologue of *Drosophila* Notch expressed during mammalian development, *Development* 1991; **113**: 199–205.

139. Noramly S, Freeman A, Morgan BA: Beta-catenin signaling can initiate feather bud development. *Development* 1999; **126**: 3509–3521.

140. Widelitz RB, Jiang TX, Noveen A, Chen CWJ, Chuong CM: FGF induces new feather buds from developing avian skin. *J Invest Derm* 1996; **107**: 797–803.

141. Jung HS, Francis-West PH, Widelitz RB, et al.: Local inhibitory action of BMPs and their relationships with activators in feather formation: implications for periodic patterning. *Dev Biol* 1998; **196**: 11–23.

142. Morgan BA, Orkin RW, Noramly S, Perez A: Stage-specific effects of sonic hedgehog expression in the epidermis. *Dev Biol* 1998; **201**: 1–12.

143. Ting-Berreth SA, Chuong CM: Sonic Hedgehog in feather morphogensis: induction of mesenchymal condensation and association with cell death. *Dev Dyn* 1996; **207**: 157–170.

144. Ting-Berreth SA, Chuong CM: Local delivery of TGF-beta2 can substitute for placode epithelium to induce mesenchymal condensation during skin appendage morphogenesis. *Dev Biol* 1996; **179**: 347–359.

145. Widelitz RB, Jiang TC, Chen CWJ, Stott NS, Chuong CM: Wnt-7a in feather morphogenesis: involvement of anterior-posterior asymmetry and proximal-distal elongation demonstrated with an in vitro reconstruction model. *Development* 1999; **126**: 2577–2587.

146. Loomis CA, Harris E, Michaud J, Wurst W, Hanks M, Joyner AL: The mouse Engrailed-1 gene and ventral limb patterning. *Nature* 1996; **382**: 360–363.

147. Reginelli AD, Wang YQ, Sassoon D, Muneoka K: Digit tip regfeneration correlates with regions of Msx1 (Hox 7) expression in fetal and newborn mice. *Development* 1995; **121**: 1065–1076

3

Hair follicle stem cells: their location and roles

George Cotsarelis

Introduction

The stratum corneum and hair shaft are the functional end-products of epidermal and hair follicle proliferation and differentiation. Both the plate-like stratum corneum and the cylindrical hair shaft serve their biological roles at the surface of the skin. As these structures are sloughed and shed from the skin, they are constantly replenished through proliferation and terminal differentiation of keratinocytes in the proliferative pool of the epidermis and hair follicle. This proliferative pool of cells is ultimately regenerated by stem cells.

What is a stem cell?

A stem cell is a relatively undifferentiated, multipotent, generally quiescent cell with a high proliferative potential that gives rise to both other stem cells and more proliferative transient amplifying cells. Transient amplifying cells comprise the actively dividing cells within the proliferative pool; they are responsible for the immediate replenishment of cells that are lost to the environment after terminal differentiation. Other stem cell attributes include the ability to proliferate in response to wounding and hyperproliferative stimuli, high β_1 and α_6 integrin expression, a distinct biochemical profile, and a life-span that exceeds that of the organism (for reviews, see[1,2]).

Much evidence supports the concept that the epidermis is organized into a hierarchy of stem, transient amplifying and terminally differentiated cells.[3-6] Each stem cell in the epidermis is responsible for maintaining a column of cells. This arrangement, called an 'epidermal proliferative unit', suggests that one stem cell generates approximately nine transient amplifying cells

that give rise to the overlying cells.[4,6] In hair follicles, the organization is more complicated (see Figure 1 and later text), because the lower follicle must regenerate at the onset of anagen, and the relatively undifferentiated cells in the hair bulb

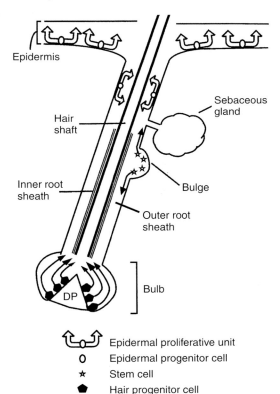

Figure 1

Epithelial stem cell system of the hair follicle and epidermis. Epithelial stem cells in the hair follicle bulge generate at least four progenitor cell types (one epidermal and three hair cell types). DP, dermal papilla. Modified with permission from Cotsarelis et al.[7]

Table 1 A comparison of the stem cell attributes shown by various follicular and epidermal epithelial cells (see Figure 1). EPU, epidermal proliferative unit; CFE, colony forming efficiency. Modified with permission from Cotsarelis et al.[7]

Stem cell attributes	Bulge cells		Hair matrix cells		Central cell of EPU	Interfollicular epidermal cells
	Rodent	Human	Rodent	Human	Rodent	Human
Slowly cycling	Yes [8]	Yes[9]	No[8]	No	Yes, but not as slow as bulge[10]	Likely[11,12]
High proliferative potential						
In vitro (CFE)	Yes[13]	?/not under current culture conditions[14]	No, not under current culture conditions[13]	No, not under current culture conditions[14]	?	Yes[15]
In vivo	?	?	No	Yes	?	Yes[4,16]
Long-lived	Yes[9,10]	?	No	No	No[17]	?
Multipotent	Likely[18]	Likely[14]	Likely[19]	Likely	No	No
Express high integrin levels	?	Yes[9]	?	No[9]	?	Yes[3]
Proliferate at anagen onset	Yes[20]	Yes[9]	No	No	NR	NR
Distinct keratin profile	Yes	Yes[9,21]	May not express keratin[19]	?	?	?
Proliferate in response to wounding	Yes	?	NR	NR	Yes	Likely

generate at least seven different cylindrical cell layers of the hair and follicle. Our hypothesis is that the bulge keratinocytes best satisfy the wide array of stem cell criteria (see Table 1), and these cells may serve as the ultimate reserve of both epidermal and hair follicle keratinocytes.

Why study stem cells?

The study of stem cells has yielded a better understanding of many organ systems. Although, originally, stem cells were thought to reside only in rapidly proliferating tissues, it is now clear that even tissues such as muscle and the central nervous system—both previously thought to be 'static' or non-proliferative—actually possess stem cells.[2] Tissues presumably are set up with this hierarchical nature because this allows for regeneration and repopulation after wounding, in the face of hyperproliferative stimuli or during normal cycling, as in the hair follicle.

The understanding and manipulation of stem cells has generated a wide range of clinical applications in many self-renewing tissues. For example, the localization of corneal epithelial stem cells to the limbus of the eye[22,23] led to the development of new techniques for corneal transplantation, and to cures for certain types of blindness.[24,25] Identification of hematopoietic stem cell markers resulted in the ability to perform autologous peripheral stem cell transplants and gene therapy.[26] Early work indicates that stem cells in muscle will be important for gene therapy.[27,28]

Epithelial stem cells may also be the site of origin for tumors. In the cornea, for example, most epithelial dysplasias and neoplasms arise in the limbal region, where stem cells are found.[29] Epidermal stem cells may give rise to cutaneous tumors. Several lines of evidence indicate that epidermal stem cells are the targets of chemical carcinogens, and these studies suggest that the slowly cycling nature of stem cells predisposes these cells to the accumulation of genetic alterations, which eventually may lead to tumor formation.

The hair follicle is an important source of skin

cancers.[1] In particular, based primarily on morphological and biochemical (keratin expression) data, certain types of tumors are thought to arise from the hair follicle bulge. Pinkus[30] noted that histologically the bulge may 'resemble very much the structure of trichoepithelioma'. Similar morphological observations have suggested that many basal cell carcinomas (BCCs) originate from the follicular outer root sheath, and possibly the bulge as well. Biochemically, both trichoepitheliomas and basal cell carcinomas express cytokeratin profiles found in normal follicular outer root sheath cells, and we showed that approximately one third of basal cell carcinomas and 13/13 trichoepitheliomas were positive for cytokeratin 15, a bulge cell marker[31] (see later text).

Location of hair follicle stem cells

In the skin, keratinocytes possessing the salient features of epithelial stem cells—namely their slowly cycling nature and high proliferative capacity—have been identified by in vitro and in vivo methodologies.

In vitro assessment of proliferative potential

Individual epidermal keratinocytes display varying abilities to form colonies in cell culture systems.[15] Colony forming efficiency, calculated as number of colonies/total number of plated cells, can be used as an indication of the number of stem cells in a particular region of the follicle. In rats, this type of analysis localizes stem cells to the hair follicle bulge.[13] Surprisingly, in human hair follicles, colony forming efficiency localizes stem cells to the lower outer root sheath, which is well outside of the bulge region.[14] This portion of the follicle undergoes degeneration during hair follicle regression (catagen), therefore, the exact location of human hair follicle stem cells, as determined by in vitro analysis is unclear.

In vivo detection of slowly cycling cells

Label–retaining cell analysis results in the in vivo detection of quiescent cells that are thought to be stem cells. Since stem cells are highly proliferative during development, they can be labeled with nucleoside analogs, such as tritiated thymidine (^{3}H-TdR) or bromodeoxyuridine (BrdU), which are administered to neonatal mice. After a chase period when no label is present, only slowly cycling cells remain labeled and are detected using autoradiography or immunohistology. These types of studies in mice clearly demonstrate that label–retaining cells are present in both the epidermis and hair follicle bulge.[8,10,32,33] However, recent studies utilizing very long chase periods for over 1 year show that the slowest cycling cells within the entire cutaneous epithelium reside in the bulge.[10] Given that the life-span of a mouse is roughly 2 years, it is likely that these cells persist throughout the mouse's lifetime.

By taking advantage of the human skin/scid mouse model, we studied the distribution of label-retaining cells within human hair follicles.[9] Hair follicles that retain a normal morphologic and functional appearance have been transplanted successfully to immunocompromised mice in the past.[34] These transplanted follicles produce a normal appearing hair shaft, and transit through the different phases of the hair follicle cycle.[9,35] Since hair is normally shed from grafts 2–4 weeks after grafting, in a similar type of effluvium that occurs following hair transplantation, we reasoned that hair follicle stem cells must be proliferating during the regeneration of the lower follicle at the transition from telogen to anagen prior to the onset of new hair shaft growth. To label these proliferating stem cells, we administered BrdU continuously for 2 weeks from 3–5 weeks after grafting. These stem cells were labeled for this prolonged period to increase the likelihood of 'capturing' stem cell proliferation, because these cells are thought to proliferate only briefly to produce transient amplifying cells that repopulate and regenerate the follicle.[8] The proliferative behavior of the hair follicle epithelium throughout the hair cycle is summarized in Table 2. In addition to cells within the hair follicle bulge, nearly every basal epidermal cell was labeled after 2 weeks of continuous labeling, as seen previously in mouse skin.[8,38]

To identify slowly cycling label-retaining cells, the grafts were chased for 4 months after the labeling period. During this time, rapidly proliferating transient amplifying cells of the lower follicle dilute their label, and only slowly cycling cells remain labeled (see Table 2). After the 4 month chase period, label-retaining cells were present in the bulge areas of hair follicles. No label-retaining cells were present in the bulb area or lower outer root sheath. Thus, in both mouse and human hair follicles, slowly cycling stem cells reside in the hair follicle bulge.

Defining the hair follicle bulge

The hair follicle bulge marks the lowermost portion of the 'permanent' hair follicle. Keratinocytes below the bulge degenerate during catagen. The bulge is a prominent structure in human fetal skin, however, in adult anagen hair follicles it is relatively inconspicuous. Investigators have, therefore, used the arrector pili muscle as a marker for the bulge, but the attachment site of the arrector pili muscle varies among different hair follicles and sometimes is located below the bulge.[39] Therefore, without a marker for the bulge cells, it has been difficult to draw conclusions about the precise location of human hair follicle stem cells, especially with respect to the bulge area.

In our experiments, we discovered that human bulge cells selectively express cytokeratin 15 (K15) throughout all stages of the hair cycle in different types of follicles, indicating that the bulge is composed of a biochemically distinct, permanent population of cells within the hair follicle outer root sheath.[9] K15 expression in the follicle is found in the basal cell layer of the outer root sheath of the lower isthmus and the secondary germ, the traditional site of follicular stem cells in telogen follicles.[40] Our operational definition of the bulge, therefore, is not simply limited to the morphologic bulges that attach to the arrector pili muscle, but also includes these other K15 positive areas.

Markers of epithelial stem cells

Epithelial stem cells have been localized to specific areas within tissues based on their biochemical properties. For example, the location of corneal epithelial stem cells in the limbus was initially inferred by keratin expression patterns.[22] The corneal epithelium expresses keratins 3 and 12 throughout the basal and suprabasal layers, while the limbal epithelium—peripheral to the corneal epithelium—expresses these keratins only in the suprabasal layer. This expression pattern suggested that the limbal basal epithelium contained biochemically more 'primitive' cells that differentiated into corneal epithelium. Subsequently, kinetic analyses demonstrated that slowly cycling label retaining cells were, indeed, concentrated in the limbus and absent in the central cornea.[23] Importantly, however, no marker specific for the stem-cell-rich limbus was identified, rather, the lack of differentiation markers implied that this area was less differentiated. The situation is similar in the hematopoietic system, in which stem cells are identified by their lack of specific differentiation markers.

Within the epidermis, β_1-integrin was shown to be a marker for keratinocyte stem cells. Keratinocytes with high colony-forming efficiency

Table 2 Proliferative activity within the hair follicle epithelium.[9,36,37,54] To identify hair follicle stem cells as label-retaining cells, the proliferative behavior of the hair follicle throughout the hair follicle cycle must be considered. The nucleoside analogue, BrdU, is infused during anagen onset (*) to label the stem cells as they proliferate. Stem cells in the bulge retain the label as they remain quiescent during the remainder of the hair cycle, while the proliferating matrix cells dilute out their label. Modified with permision from Lyle et al.[9] © Company of Biologists Ltd.

	Anagen	Catagen	Telogen	Anagen onset*	Anagen
Stem cells (bulge)	Quiescent	Quiescent	Quiescent	Proliferating	Quiescent
Matrix cells (bulb)	Proliferating	Degenerating	Absent	Regenerating	Proliferating

also possess high levels of β_1-integrin.[3] Within the epidermis, keratinocytes that express high levels of β_1-integrin on their surface (called β_1 bright cells) are located above rete ridges. In the follicle, β_1-bright cells are concentrated in the bulge area of the hair follicle.[9] α_6-integrin, another cell surface protein involved in adhesion, may be even more specific for epidermal stem cells, although its expression in the hair follicle has not been examined.[11] The high levels of integrins on stem cells may explain why they adhere quickly to substrates in vitro. This ability has been used to enrich for epidermal stem cells, and Bickenbach et al demonstrated that label-retaining cells can be enriched in this manner.[32] These findings indicate that isolation of stem cells in vitro is feasible and opens the door for ex vivo approaches to gene therapy.

In addition to integrins, cytokeratin expression also correlates with levels of differentiation within the skin. Within stratified squamous epithelia, such as the epidermis, hair follicle and cornea, cytokeratin expression generally defines populations of cells in similar states of differentiation.[41,42] For example, within the epidermis, the keratin pair 5/14 is expressed predominantly in the basal layer of the epidermis, which is composed of proliferating, relatively undifferentiated keratinocytes.[43] As keratinocytes leave the basal layer and become postmitotic and more differentiated, they cease production of K5/14, and begin to produce K1/K10.

Since cytokeratin 19 (K19) is thought to be a stem-cell marker,[21] we examined K19 expression in relation to K15 expression. Although K19 positive cells co-localized with K15-positive cells in the basal layer of the outer root sheath within the bulge area, K19-positive cells extended downward throughout the entire basal layer of the outer root sheath from the bulge to the bulb.[9] K15-positive cells, therefore, comprise a subset of K19-positive cells in the human hair follicle. These data suggest that both K15 and K19 are markers of relatively undifferentiated keratinocytes in the bulge, however, K15 appears restricted to the permanent portion of the follicle containing β_1-integrin bright cells and label-retaining cells, while K19 is present in more differentiated transient amplifying cells in the lower follicle as well. These findings agree with those of Jones et al[44] who suggested that only a subset of follicular K19-positive cells represent true stem cells. Based on our data, it is likely that the K15-positive keratinocytes comprise this subset. Our studies also support the notion that loss of K15 expression may be one of the earliest signs of the transition from stem to transient amplifying cell, and that the K15-negative/K19-positive phenotype may indicate that these cells are 'early' transient amplifying (TA$_1$) cells.

Interestingly, we also identified K15 cells clustered in the lower outer root sheath of approximately one-third of anagen follicles,[9] in an area where Rochat et al[14] and Moll[36] found the highest number of presumptive stem cells in vitro. Since these few discrete cells were also qualitatively integrin bright, they may represent very early transient amplifying cells or stem cells that have migrated down during anagen. Although the significance of this biochemical heterogeneity of the lower outer root sheath is unclear, perhaps the presence or absence of these K15-positive cells in the lower outer root sheath indicates the position of the follicle within the hair follicle cycle (e.g. early versus late anagen).

Bulge activation hypothesis

Based on the location of follicular stem cells in the bulge area, and the mesenchymal-epithelial interactions necessary for hair growth, we defined four important elements for hair follicle cycling: (i) bulge activation; (ii) dermal papilla activation; (iii) the limited proliferative potential of matrix keratinocytes: and (iv) the upward migration of the dermal papilla[8,9] (Figure 2). Defects in any of these steps could result in abnormal hair growth or hair loss.

It was demonstrated that bulge proliferation occurs preferentially at the onset of anagen,[9,20] when the lower follicle regenerates, including the hair matrix cells that subsequently generate the hair shaft and its surrounding inner root sheath. Experimentally, the bulge in the mouse hair follicle is responsive to hyperproliferative stimuli such as hair plucking, retinoic acid and phorbol esters.[20] These stimuli result in bulge proliferation and subsequent hair growth, but they can be blocked by corticosteroids.[45] The signals involved in bulge activation during the normal hair cycle are not well understood, but many candidate molecules are now known (see Chapter 6).

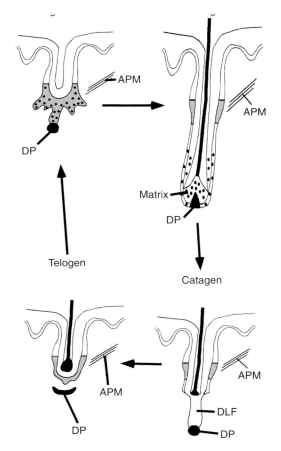

Figure 2

Stem cells and the hair follicle cycle. The shaded area represents slowly cycling bulge cells. Keratinocytes in the K15-positive bulge function as stem cells, which proliferate at anagen onset in response to a signal from the dermal papilla (DP). During anagen, bulge cells become quiescent and remain so throughout the remainder of the hair cycle. The duration of anagen may be determined by the finite proliferative potential of matrix keratinocytes. During catagen, the degenerating lower follicle (DLF) pulls up the DP, so that it comes to rest adjacent to the bulge during telogen. Proliferating cells are denoted by black dots. APM, arrector pili muscle. Modified with permission from Lyle et al.[9] © Company of Biologists Ltd.

Signals that activate the bulge are thought to arise from the adjacent dermal papilla.

The dermal papilla is a cluster of cells derived from the mesenchyme at the base of the follicle.[46] Cells within the dermal papilla proliferate in early to mid anagen (dermal papilla activation), possibly in response to angiogenic factors derived from matrix keratinocytes.[47] The dermal papilla has powerful inductive influences on immature and adult keratinocytes.[48] For example, dermal papilla cells from rat vibrissae (whisker follicle) transplanted to back skin in neonatal rats result in induction of vibrissa follicle formation.[49] Normally, however, the juxtaposition of the dermal papilla with the bulge cells at anagen onset is necessary for continued hair follicle cycling. If the dermal papilla does not ascend to the level of the bulge during catagen, a new hair will not form. This is illustrated vividly in mice and humans carrying the hairless mutation, in which the dermal papilla remains stranded in the subcutaneous fat during first catagen, and the subjects permanently lose their hair, presumably because the dermal papilla never activates the stem cells in the bulge.[8,50]

In contrast to bulge cells, matrix cells proliferate extremely rapidly. However, they eventually differentiate terminally, and therefore are analogous to transient amplifying cells. The number of cell divisions that matrix cells undergo can vary widely among different hair follicles with different anagen durations. It is possible that the inherent proliferative potential of the matrix cells determines the duration of anagen. Nevertheless, other factors, such as fibroblast growth factor 5 (FGF5), clearly influence matrix cell division.[51] FGF5 knockout mice (angora phenotype) have a prolonged anagen duration, and FGF5 is up-regulated at the end of anagen, suggesting that matrix cell division is controlled by FGF5. Notwithstanding, even angora mice eventually enter catagen, thus leaving open the possibility that the matrix cells possess an innate finite proliferative potential.

Hair follicle stem cells and alopecia

Alopecias can be classified into permanent and non-permanent types.[52] The localization of hair follicle stem cells to the bulge area may explain why some types of inflammatory alopecias are permanent or scarring (such as lichen planopilaris and discoid lupus erythematosis), while others (such as alopecia areata) are non-scarring or reversible. In scarring alopecias, inflammation surrounds the more superficial portion of the follicle, and involves the bulge area, suggesting that the stem cells necessary for follicle regeneration are damaged. In contrast, in alopecia areata—the prototypical non-scarring alopecia—the inflammatory infiltrate engulfs the bulb region of the hair follicle that is composed of more differentiated bulge cell progeny. Since this area is immediately responsible for hair shaft production, its destruction leads to hair loss. Nevertheless, the bulge area remains intact, and a new lower anagen follicle and subsequent hair shaft can potentially regenerate. Even patients with long-standing (e.g. decade-long) alopecia areata may regrow their hair either spontaneously or in response to immunomodulation.[53]

Jaworsky et al showed that, in patients with early androgenetic alopecia, the bulge appears to be a primary target for assault by an inflammatory infiltrate.[54] Over time, this damage could contribute to the irreversible nature of androgenetic alopecia as well. The bulge area also appears to be specifically attacked in early graft versus host disease that may result in alopecia.[55] By further characterizing the interaction of the immune system not only with bulge cells, but with the hair follicle in general, new strategies for treating inflammatory alopecias could be devised.

Future research

Further characterization of the bulge cells may lead to insights into not only the treatment of alopecia, but also of excess hair growth (e.g. hirsutism, hypertrichosis). By ablating bulge cells using exogenous agents (e.g. lasers, suicide genes), hair follicles could be destroyed selectively. Studies to determine the effect of bulge cell ablation on epidermal homeostasis are also necessary. Ultimately, given the accessibility of the follicle, cutaneous gene therapy targeting the bulge cells seems feasible.

References

1. Miller SJ, Sun TT, Lavker RM: Hair follicles, stem cells, and skin cancer. [Review]. *J Investig Dermatol* 1993; **100**: 288S–294S.
2. Morrison SJ, Shah NM, Anderson DJ: Regulatory mechanisms in stem cell biology. *Cell* 1997; **88**: 287–298.
3. Jones PH, Watt FM: Separation of human epidermal stem cells from transit amplifying cells on the basis of differences in integrin function and expression. *Cell* 1993; **73**: 713–724.
4. Kolodka TM, Garlick JA, Taichman LB: Evidence for keratinocyte stem cells in vitro: long-term engraftment and persistence of transgene expression from retrovirus-transduced keratinocytes. *Proc Natl Acad Sci* 1998; **95**: 4356–4361.
5. Morris R, Fischer S, Slaga T: Evidence that a slowly cycling subpopulation of adult murine epidermal cells retains carcinogen. *Cancer Res* 1986; **46**: 3061–3066.
6. Potten C, Morris R: Epithelial stem cells in vivo. *J Cell Sci (Suppl)* 1988; **10**: 45–62.
7. Cotsarelis, G, Kaur P, Dhouailly D, Hengge U, Bickenbach J: Epithelial stem cells in the skin: definition, markers, localization and functions. *Exper Dermatol* 1999; **8**: 80–88.
8. Cotsarelis G, Sun TT, Lavker RM: Label-retaining cells reside in the bulge area of pilosebaceous unit: implications for follicular stem cells, hair cycle, and skin carcinogenesis. *Cell* 1990; **61**: 1329–1337.
9. Lyle S, Christofidou-Solomidou M, Liu Y, Elder D, Albelda S, Cotsarelis G: The C8/144B monoclonal antibody recognizes cytokeratin 15 and defines the location of human hair follicle stem cells. *J Cell Sci* 1998; **111**: 3179–3188.
10. Morris R, Potten C: Highly persistent label-retaining cells in the hair follicles of mice and their fate following induction of anagen. *J Invest Dermatol* 1999; **112**: 470–475.
11. Li A, Simmons PJ, Kaur P: Identification and isolation of candidate human keratinocyte stem cells based on cell surface phenotype. *Proc Natl Acad Sci USA* 1998; **95**: 3902–3907.
12. Batacsorgo Z, Hammerberg C, Voorhees JJ, Cooper KD: Flow cytometric identification of proliferative subpopulations within normal human epidermis and the localization of the primary hyperproliferative population in psoriasis. *J Exper Med* 1993; **178**: 1271–1281.
13. Kobayashi K, Rochat A, Barrandon Y: Segregation of keratinocyte colony-forming cells in the bulge of the rat vibrissa. *Proc Natl Acad Sci USA* 1993; **90**: 7391–7395.
14. Rochat A, Kobayashi K, Barrandon Y: Location of

stem cells of human hair follicles by clonal analysis. *Cell* 1994; **76**: 1063–1073.

15. Barrandon Y, Green H: Three clonal types of keratinocyte with different capacities for multiplication. *Proc Natl Acad Sci USA* 1987; **84**: 2302–2306.

16. Compton CC, Gill JM, Bradford DA, Reganer S, Gallico GG, O'Connor NE: Skin regenerated from cultured epithelial autografts on full-thickness burn wounds from 6 days to 5 years after grafting. *Lab Invest* 1989; **60**: 600–612.

17. Morris RJ, Potten CS: Quantification of a highly persistent subpopulation of epidermal cells in the hair follicles of mice and their fate following plucking. *J Invest Dermatol* 1995; **104**: 578 [Abstract].

18. Kamimura J, Lee D, Baden HP, Brisette J, Dotto GP: Primary mouse keratinocyte cultures contain hair follicle progenitor cells with multiple differentiation potential. *J Invest Dermatol* 1997; **109**: 534–540.

19. Reynolds AJ, Jahoda CA: Hair matrix germinative epidermal cells confer follicle-inducing capabilities on dermal sheath and high passage papilla cells. *Development* 1996; **122**: 3085–3094.

20. Wilson C, Cotsarelis G, Wei ZG, et al.: Cells within the bulge region of mouse hair follicle transiently proliferate during early anagen: heterogeneity and functional differences of various hair cycles. *Differentiation* 1994; **55**: 127–136.

21. Michel M, Torok N, Godbout M-J, et al.: Keratin 19 as a biochemical marker of skin stem cells in vivo and in vitro: keratin 19 expressing cells are differentially localized in function of anatomic sites, and their number varies with donor age and culture stage. *J Cell Sci* 1996; **109**: 1017–1028.

22. Schermer A, Galvin S, Sun T-T: Differentiation-related expression of a major 64K corneal keratin in vivo and in culture suggests limbal location of corneal epithelial stem cells. *J Cell Biol* 1986; **103**: 49–62.

23. Cotsarelis G, Cheng SZ, Dong G, Sun TT, Lavker RM: Existence of slow-cycling limbal epithelial basal cells that can be preferentially stimulated to proliferate: implications on epithelial stem cells. *Cell* 1989; **57**: 201–209.

24. Hodson S: Cultivating a Cure for Blindness. *Nature* 1997; **387**: 449.

25. Tsubota K, Satake Y, Kaido M, et al.: Treatment of severe ocular-surface disorders with corneal epithelial stem-cell transplantation. *N Engl J Med* 1999; **340**: 1697–703.

26. Bernstein ID, Andrews RG, Rowley S: Isolation of human hematopoietic stem cells. *Blood Cells* 1994; **20**: 15–24.

27. Miller JB, Schaefer L, Dominov JA: Seeking muscle stem cells. *Curr Topics Develop Biology* 1999; **43**: 191–219.

28. Pavlath GK, Thaloor D, Rando TA, Cheong M, English AW, Zheng B: Heterogeneity among muscle precursor cells in adult skeletal muscles with differing regenerative capacities. *Develop Dynam* 1998; **212**: 495–508.

29. Waring GO, Roth AM, Ekins MB: Clinical and pathologic description of 17 cases of corneal intraepithelial neoplasia. *Am J Ophthalmol* 1984; **97**: 547–559.

30. Pinkus H: Multiple hairs. *J Invest Dermatol* 1951; **17**: 291.

31. Jih D, Lyle S, Elenitsas R, Elder D, Cotsarelis G: Cytokeratin 15 expression in trichoepitheliomas and a subset of basal cell carcinomas suggests they originate from hair follicle stem cells. *J Cutan Pathol* 1999; **26**: 113–118.

32. Bickenbach JR, Chism E: Selection and extended growth of murine epidermal stem cells in culture. *Exper Cell Res* 1998; **244**: 184–195.

33. Bickenbach J, Mackenzie I: Identification and localisation of label retaining cells in hamster epithelium. *J Invest Dermatol* 1984; **82**: 618–622.

34. Gilhar A, Pillar T, Etzioni A: The effect of topical cyclosporin on the immediate shedding of human scalp hair grafted onto nude mice. *Br J Dermatol* 1988; **119**: 767–770.

35. Van Neste D, de Brouwer B, Tetelin C, Bonfils A: Testosterone conditioned nude mice: an improved model for experimental monitoring of human hair production by androgen dependent balding scalp grafts. In: Van Neste D, Randall VA (eds.). *Hair Research for the Next Millennium*. New York, Elsevier Science, 1996: 319–326.

36. Moll I: Proliferative potential of different keratinocytes of plucked human hair follicles. *J Invest Dermatol* 1995; **105**: 14–21.

37. Commo S, Bernard BA: Immunohistochemical analysis of tissue remodelling during the anagen-catagen transition of the human hair follicle. *Br J Dermatol* 1997; **137**: 31–38.

38. Morris R, Fischer S, Slaga T: Evidence that the centrally and peripherally located cells in the murine epidermal proliferative unit are two distinct cell populations. *J Invest Dermatol* 1985; **84**: 277–281.

39. Pinkus H: Embryology of hair. In: Montagna W, Ellis RA (eds.). *The Biology of Hair Growth*. New York, Academic Press, 1958.

40. Silver AF, Chase HB: DNA synthesis in the adult hair germ during dormancy (telogen) and activation (early anagen). *Develop Biol* 1970; **21**: 440–451.

41. Lane EB, Wilson CA, Hughes BR, Leigh IM: Stem cells in hair follicles. Cytoskeletal studies. *Ann N Y Acad Sci* 1991; **642**: 197–213.

42. Schirren CG, Burgdorf WHC, Sander CA, Plewig G: Fetal and adult hair follicle: an immunohistochemical study of anticytokeratin antibodies

in formalin-fixed and paraffin-embedded tissue. *Am J Dermatopathol* 1997; **19**: 334–340.

43. Coulombe PA, Kopan R, Fuchs E: Expression of keratin K14 in the epidermis and hair follicle—insights into complex programs of differentiation. *J Cell Biol* 1989; **109**: 2295–2312.

44. Jones PH, Harper S, Watt FM: Stem cell patterning and fate in human epidermis. *Cell* 1995; **80**: 83–93.

45. Stenn KS, Paus R, Dutton T, Sarba B: Glucocorticoid effect on hair growth initiation: a reconsideration. *Skin Pharmacol* 1993; **6**: 125–134.

46. Reynolds AJ, Jahoda CA. Inductive properties of hair follicle cells. *Ann N Y Acad Sci* 1991; **642**: 226–41.

47. Stenn K, Pernandez L, Tirrell S: The angiogenic properties of the rat vibrissa hair follicle associated with the bulb. *J Invest Dermatol* 1988; **90**: 409–411.

48. Jahoda CA, Reynolds AJ: Dermal-epidermal interactions. Adult follicle-derived cell populations and hair growth. [Review] [53 refs]. *Dermatol Clin* 1996; **14**: 573–583.

49. Oliver RF: The experimental induction of whisker growth in the hooded rat by implantation of dermal papillae. *J Embryol Exper Morphol* 1967; **18**: 43–51.

50. Ahmad W, Faiyaz ul Haque M, Brancolini V, et al.: Alopecia universalis associated with a mutation in the human hairless gene. *Science* 1998; **279(5351)**: 720–724.

51. Hebert JM, Rosenquist T, Gotz J, Martin GR: FGF5 as a regulator of the hair growth cycle: evidence from targeted and spontaneous mutations. *Cell* 1994; **78**: 1017–1025.

52. Paus R, Cotsarelis G: The biology of hair follicles. *N Engl J Med* 1999; **341**: 491–497.

53. Olsen EA (ed.): *Disorders of Hair Growth: Diagnosis and Treatment*. New York, McGraw-Hill, 1994.

54. Jaworsky C, Kligman AM, Murphy GF: Characterization of inflammatory infiltrates in male pattern alopecia: implications for pathogenesis. *Br J Dermatol* 1992; **127**: 239–246.

55. Sale GE, Beauchamp MD, Akiyama M: Parafollicular bulges, but not hair bulb keratinocytes, are attacked in graft-versus-host disease of human skin. *Bone Marrow Transplant* 1994; **14**: 411–413.

4
Hair pigmentation

Jérôme Castanet and Jean-Paul Ortonne

Introduction

Melanocytes synthesize a cell-specific product, the pigment melanin, in highly organized organelles, the melanosomes. The melanosomes undergo a complex maturation process while being transferred to the tips of dendrites that ramify among neighbouring keratinocytes. Each epidermal melanocyte establishes contact with 30–40 keratinocytes, forming the so-called epidermal melanin unit, and transfers melanosomes and melanocytes to these keratinocytes.

Although the biology of follicular and of epidermal melanocytes seems similar in several aspects (in particular, the steps of melanogenesis), a striking feature of pigmented hair growth is that the activity of hair melanocytes located in the hair matrix, unlike that of those in the epidermis, is under cyclical control, and that melanogenesis and anagen are tightly coupled.[1]

Melanocyte biology

Embryogenesis

Melanoblasts, originating from the neural crest, reach all body regions. They invade the epidermis from the dermis and differentiate into active melanocytes. Both melanoblasts and active melanocytes migrate from the epidermis and become incorporated into the hair bulb. Thus, the proliferation, the migration and the differentiation of melanoblasts and melanocytes are key events in the embryogenesis of the pigment cell system of the skin. The presence, densities and distribution of melanocytes have been deter-mined.[2] Presumptive melanocytes, with a dendritic phenotype, are present in the human embryonic epidermis after 50 days estimated gestational age (EGA) and in the skin even earlier (40–50 days EGA) – that is, before the formation of primitive hair germs (ninth week EGA). Scattered melanocytes are present in hair pegs (90–105 days EGA). In the bullous hair pegs (>195 days EGA), these melanocytes are clustered specifically in the bulb, among the matrix cells that line the concavity proximal to the dermal papilla. Melanocytes in this position are large, melanized and typically 3–8 in number. Melanocytes were not obvious in the remainder of the follicle. In the 125-day fetal epidermis, the hair and the cells that give rise to the hair in the bulb are outlined by the density of melanin granules that they contain, demonstrating that the melanosomal transfer between melanocytes and keratinocytes has already occurred. The genetic control of the homing and route of migration of pigment cells into the epidermis and the factors that regulate the proliferation and differentiation of pigment cells still need to be better characterized in humans. Tyrosine kinase receptor, *c-kit*, activated by stem cell factor, seems important in transducing the signals to support melanoblast survival and migration towards the hair follicles in the embryo.[3] The signal transduction pathway between the *c-kit* receptor and the transcription factor microphthalmia (MITF) has also been discovered.[4]

Melanogenesis

Hair color is brought about by the various amounts of the different melanins that are synthesized under genetic controls.[5] Melanin synthesis is an enzymatic process that

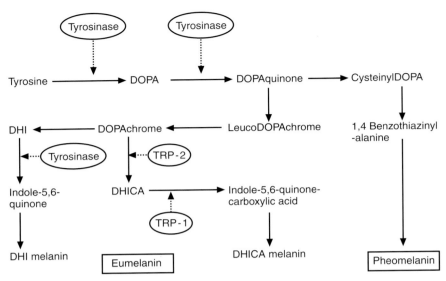

Figure 1

Genesis of eumelanin and pheomelanin

transforms tyrosine into eu- and pheomelanin (Figure 1). Several enzymes mediate this reaction, including tyrosinase, tyrosinase-related protein-1 (TRP-1), and tyrosinase-related protein-2 (TRP-2). Eumelanins are black to brown and are insoluble in all solvents, whereas pheomelanins are reddish-brown and alkali-soluble. From the amino-acid tyrosine to the various types of melanins, the metabolic pathway depends on the overall balance of a number of regulatory factors. The first two steps of melanogenesis are common for all melanins and are catalysed by tyrosinase. Tyrosinase, a copper-containing enzyme, is the main regulatory factor of the global level of melanogenesis; it maps to chromosome 11. The tyrosinase gene has been cloned and sequenced, and regulatory elements identified.[6,7] Tyrosinase catalyses the hydroxylation of tyrosine to 3-4-dihydroxyphenylalanine (DOPA) and the oxidation of DOPA to DOPAquinone. At that point the process of melanogenesis diverges.

Synthesis of eumelanins

The transformation of DOPAquinone into DOPAchrome occurs spontaneously, without the need for a catalytic enzyme activity. Spontaneously, DOPAchrome is transformed into 5,6-dihydroxyindole (DHI), in the absence of

the enzyme DOPAchrome tautomerase (DCT). In contrast, DCT catalyses the transformation of DOPAchrome into DHI-2 carboxylic acid (DHICA). DCT is identical to TRP-2. TRP-2, which maps to chromosome 13, determines the carboxyl content of melanins. Metal ions, such as Co^{2+}, Cu^{2+}, Ni^{2+}, may mimic DCT activity; however, the biological relevance of this observation is unknown. White hairs might contain less copper than black hairs.[8] Tyrosinase catalyses the oxidation of DHI to indolequinone, but peroxidase can also use DHI as a substrate. TRP-1, which maps to human chromosome 9, might generate the indole-quinone carboxylated derivative from DHICA; however, its precise catalytic function is still in dispute. TRP-1 might also interact with tyrosinase, stabilizing its catalytic function.[9] Finally, polymerization of indole-quinone leads to eumelanins. Eumelanins are heterogenous polymers of all the cyclized derivatives of DOPAquinone (mainly DHI and, to a lesser extent, DHICA). DHI-derived melanins are black and flocculent, whereas DHICA-derived melanins are yellowish and finely dispersed.[10]

Synthesis of pheomelanins

Pheomelanins arise by oxidative polymerization of cysteinylDOPAS and contain sulfur.[11] Pheomelanins are polymers or mixtures of polymers that contain a 1,4-benzothiazine unit, also found in the trichochromes. Such a biogenetic relationship between these two types of pigments explains why they are often found together in pheomelanin hair. They result from DOPAquinone and cysteine through formation and subsequent oxidation of 5-s-cysteinylDOPA and 2-s-cysteinylDOPA. The latter steps and the regulatory processes of the pheomelanin synthesis are much less characterized.

Switching mechanisms

Switching mechanisms, which are not fully understood, determine whether eumelanins or pheomelanins are produced by the follicular melanocytes. The key step in the switch is the transformation of DOPAquinone into cysteinylDOPAS rather than DOPAchrome. The addition of sulfur-containing amino acid, cysteine and/or glutathione, to quinone is a rapid event that occurs spontaneously, without a catalytic enzyme. Thus, the effective concentration of sulfydrils in melanocytes and their availability more specifically within the melanosomes are probably important factors in the switching mechanisms.[11] Their concentration might directly determinate the various proportions of pheo- and eumelanins arising from DOPAquinone. However, regulation of this biochemical pathway might arise at several levels. First, activity of the enzymes of the glutathione system, such as the glutathione reductase, peroxidase and transpeptidase, affects the tissues' sulfhydryl content and might regulate the metabolic fate of DOPAquinone. Such a view is supported by analysis of the levels of glutathione and related enzymatic activities in guinea pig skin of different colors. Second, it has been proposed that the role of cysteine/glutathione as regulatory factor in switching melanogenesis type is not tied to its absolute presence or absence, but rather to its effective concentration within the melanocyte at a given time.[12] Third, the melanosomal membrane may also play an important regulating role by controlling the uptake of melanogenesis substrates and sulfhydryls.

However, the clear-cut biochemical classification of melanins into two types probably does not reflect the entire complexity of the biological situation in the living human skin. First, a third group of melanins, oxymelanins, might arise by partial peroxidative cleavage of DHI.[13] They are of similar color to pheomelanins but devoid of sulfur. Second, a copolymerization process involving both eu- and pheomelanins may occur in vivo, leading to mixed-type melanins, which are mixtures of both types in various proportions.

Melanosome biology

Melanin biosynthesis takes place in melanosomes, highly organized, ellipsoidal, membrane-bound organelles.[14] Melanosomes are formed by the fusion of coated vesicles with immature melanosomes. Coated vesicles originate from the Golgi network and carry the enzyme machinery for melanogenesis and monomeric melanin precursors.[15] A non-enzymatic protein, the product of the silver locus, is present within the coated vesicles:[16] this protein seems to play a role in anchoring melanin polymers to the melanosome matrix.[17] Immature melanosomes originate from the smooth endoplasmic reticulum and contain lipid located in the outer surface, structural proteins assembled within the melanosomes and constituting the matrix core, and finally enzymatic proteins. In mice, a recessive gene at the pink-eye dilution locus (p-gene) results in pigmentary dilution of hair and eyes. Oculo-albinism type II is due to mutations in the human homolog of the murine p-gene. The pink-eyed dilution locus product (p-gene) is probably a component of premelanosomes that may be a tyrosine transporter or a link between the matrix and the membrane. Pink-eyed dilution mice melanocytes exhibit 50% of the amount of tyrosinase activity, compared to non-agouti black mice, and have slightly decreased levels of TRP-1 and TRP-2 catalytic activities but contain only 2% of the amount of eumelanin. This is consistent with the role of p protein as a substrate transporter.[18]

Melanin formation takes place only after the fusion of the two melanosomes components, leading to a progressive deposition of melanins on the internal matrix corresponding to several stages of melanosomes at the ultrastructural level.

Dendrite formation and melanosome transport

Dendrite formation by epidermal melanocytes may probably be promoted in vivo by ultraviolet

(UV) light, factors produced by keratinocytes, and direct keratinocyte–melanocyte contact.[19] Mature melanosomes are transferred from the perikaryon of the melanocytes to the tips of the dendrites through the motive action of cytoskeletal proteins, actin and microtubulin. Motor proteins, ATPases that transduce energy from ATP hydrolysis into direct movement along cytoskeletal elements, certainly play a major role in dendrite formation and melanosome transport.

In follicles, melanosomes are then transferred from the melanocytes to the keratinocytes in a manner similar to that described for the epidermis; there are currently four hypothese for the transfer: pinching-off of an inserted melanocyte dendrite tip; membrane fusion between the melanocyte and the keratinocyte; release of melanosome into the intercellular space; and direct inoculation.[20] The hair melanosomes are 2–4 times larger than the epidermal ones and are usually distributed singly. Next, melanin granules become embedded in keratin. A small number of melanosomes are found associated with the sponge-like keratin of the hair medulla; most are in the cortex, their long axis being parallel to the hair surface, while the cuticle cells, the inner root sheath, contain none or only a few melanosomes.[20]

Melanocyte attachment and motility

E-cadherin is assumed to be responsible for heterotypic interactions between keratinocytes and melanocytes.[21] Integrins are probably important for the interaction of melanocytes with the basement membrane and keratinocytes.[22] However, this aspect of melanocyte biology is probably of less importance in regard to hair color.

Follicular melanocytes

Distribution of melanocytes in active hair follicles

The total number of follicles in the scalp of an adult man has been estimated at about 100 000 (a significant loss of hair follicles occurs with advancing age). The bulb of each active follicle is formed by a thick cortex made up of keratinized cells cemented together. The cortex is surrounded by a cuticle, the inner root sheath, and the outer root sheath which is continuous with the superficial epithelium. The epithelium of each hair follicle encloses at its base a small stud of dermis known as the dermal papilla. The entire follicle is surrounded by a connective tissue sheath formed of collagenous fibers, a few elastic fibers and fibroblasts. Further details of the structure and function of the hair follicle are given in Chapter 1 by Forslind.

When considering the distribution of active and inactive melanocytes, the hair follicle can be divided into four parts.[23] Melanotic portions A and D are, respectively, the upper part of the follicle, with melanocytes in the wall of the pilary canal, and the upper part of the bulb in contact with the upper papilla. Portion B comprises the middle and lower follicle and possesses amelanotic melanocytes (DOPA-negative) along the outer root sheath (ORS). Portion C is the amelanotic ORS of the bulb. Hair-follicle melanocytes thus consist of two morphologically and functionally different types: pigmented and dendritic melanocytes, present in the infundibulum and bulb, and amelanotic and nondendritic melanocytes, present in the ORS of the middle and lower follicle.[24]

However, active, DOPA-positive melanocytes may be observed in the outer root sheath of the middle and lower part of the hair follicles in some circumstances, such as after X-ray irradiation, dermabrasion, exposure to UV rays and oral photochemotherapy. While human hair-follicle melanocytes are not yet routinely cultured, this has been performed.[25,26] Two subpopulations of cells were observed: small, bipolar, amelanotic melanocytes that proliferated well; and large, intensely pigmented melanocytes that did not. Further, hair follicle and epidermal melanocytes differed antigenically: hair follicle melanocytes expressed some antigens associated with alopecia areata, but not antigens associated with vitiligo, whereas the reverse was true for epidermal melanocytes.[26]

Melanocytes and the hair cycle

Hair follicles show intermittent activity. In the adult human scalp, the activity of each follicle is independent of its neighbours, a pattern known as mosaic. The duration of activity (anagen) varies greatly, usually ranging from 7–94 weeks, but may last as long as 3 years. Activity is followed by a short transitional phase (catagen) lasting about 2 weeks in the human scalp, and a resting phase (telogen) which lasts a few weeks. This is described in more detail in Chapter 6 by Paus et al. Hair bulb melanocytes are active only during a specific phase of hair production, namely anagen stages II through VI, whereas tyrosinase synthesis occurs during the early anagen stage.[27] Early anagen is also characterized by ultrastructural changes: an increase in volume of the cytoplasm, an increase in dendricity, the development of the Golgi complex and rough endoplasmic reticulum, and, finally, an increase in the size and number of melanosomes. No synthesis of tyrosinase occurs during catagen and telogen. During catagen and telogen, the melanocytes exhibit a scanty cytoplasm, a poorly developed Golgi complex and a nucleus with prominent heterochromatin patterns. They contain only a few small premelanosomes. These observations demonstrate that not only proliferation but also melanogenesis is linked to the hair cycle. At the end of anagen, scalp follicles show a gradual thinning and lightening of pigment at the base of the hair shaft. The melanocytes in the upper part of the bulb lose their dendrites and become amelanotic and indistinguishable from the matrix cells. From the onset of catagen, the connective tissue sheath thickens, with a characteristic corrugation in the epithelium, and the dermal papilla becomes released. Subsequently, the club hair moves towards the skin surface. Above the papilla, the epithelial strand is reduced to the secondary germ. When the next hair cycle starts, the secondary germ elongates, becomes invaginated by the papilla and gives rise to a new bulb with melanocytes.

The factors that control both hair growth and pigmentation are currently unknown, although apoptosis of hair bulb keratinocytes is responsible for catagen-associated tissue regression at the end of anagen.[28] Towards the end of anagen, retraction of dendrites and the suppression of melanogenesis are the earliest signs of imminent tissue regression, even before structural changes are apparent in the hair bulb. Subsequently, pigmented melanocytes disappear from the bulb.

The fate of bulb melanocytes during catagen, as well as the source of bulb melanocytes for successive hair generation, remains elusive. One hypothesis is that hair bulb melanocytes survive successive hair cycles. Studies of the mouse hair follicles during catagen and telogen suggest that melanocytes are scarce but persist in an undifferentiated state in the epithelial column.[29] They may be the survivors of the preceding population. Bulbar melanocytes might arise from the transfer of these undifferentiated cells during the early anagen phase, with also an increased number of pigment cells, acting as a perpetuating system.[30] In mice, the c-kit gene might play a critical role in this process, since inhibition of the c-kit function, by injection of an anti-c-kit monoclonal antibody, results in the growth of unpigmented hair.[3] Another possibility is that functional hair bulb melanocytes die in early catagen, possibly by apoptosis.[31] Amelanotic melanocytes of ORS or another unidentified precursor pool might migrate to the hair bulb at the beginning of anagen. A third, but less likely, hypothesis is that bulb melanocytes leave the follicular epithelium at catagen and reenter at anagen. This cell migration might be linked with secretion of inductive signals, such as fibroblast growth factor 2 (FGF-2) and neurotrophins, by keratinocytes.[32]

The mechanisms implied in the control of melanogenic activities during the hair cycle are unknown. A better understanding of epithelial mesenchymal interactions during hair follicle development will notably be a key to resolve the mystery of hair follicle pigmentation[33] and may provide new clues in the understanding of acquired hair pigmentation disorders.

In conclusion, the melanocyte population of the skin appears as a bicompartmental system, with a follicular and an epidermal component. The main difference is that follicular melanocyte activity and proliferation are linked with the hair follicle cycle, whereas epidermal melanocyte activity is regulated mainly by UV-exposure. Epidermal melanocytes usually do not proliferate. However, exchanges may occur between these two compartments. It is important to emphasize that follicular melanocytes that migrate into the epidermis lose their particular behavior and have their activity regulated by UV exposure. It is therefore likely that the distinctive features between the follicular and epidermal melanin units are largely due to environmental influences rather than to intrinsic differences of the melanocytes themselves. The chemical signals arising from the dermal papilla and from the follicular keratinocytes are probably quite different from those coming from the epidermal keratinocytes and from the upper dermis.

Murine mutations of coat colors

The wide range of genetically determined variations in coat color of the laboratory mouse provides an excellent model for the study of gene action within many biological processes.[34] Over many years more than 150 distinct mutations that affect pigmentation either directly or indirectly have been identified in murine models.[35] These mutations occur at more than 60 different loci. About 25% of the known genes involved in melanin formation have already been cloned and characterized. Many of these gene products have been shown to be involved in various clinical pigmentary diseases in man and many also play important roles in immune responses to malignant melanoma.

Mutations that affect melanocyte development and migration

Differentiation, proliferation and migration of melanocytes and their precursors, the melanoblasts, require a series of events. The genes involved in these processes along with their putative functions and associated pigmentary diseases are summarized in Table 1. The specific transcription factors Pax3, MITF and SOX10 play a regulatory role in the early embryonic development of the pigmentary system. A certain number of growth factors and their receptors appear also predominant. Steel factor (c-kit ligand), also known as mast cell/stem cell (SCF) growth factor, binds to its receptor (c-kit) to initiate a cascade of signal transduction events that upregulate melanoblast proliferation. C-kit ligand is essential as a survival factor for active migrat-

ing and proliferating melanoblasts. Pax3 regulates MITF[36] whereas MITF regulates genes for c-kit, tyrosinase, TRP-1 and TRP-2. Endothelin 3, the endothelin B receptor, seems also to be essential for development of epidermal and follicular melanocytes.[35]

Mutations that affect melanosome biogenesis

Several loci that encode structural melanosomal proteins have been characterized. These genes include those of the silver, beige, pale ear, pallid, mocha and pearl loci. Mice homozygotes for the silver mutations have variably pigmented hair. Melanin may be completely absent or be present only at the tip or at the base of the hair. The number of melanin granules in the hair is reduced, owing to premature death or loss of melanocytes from the hair follicles. The product of the silver locus contains a putative signal protein and a transmembrane domain and is thought to be inserted in the melanosomal membrane.

Mutations in some of these genes lead to abnormal pigmentation because of the dysfunctional melanosomes produced, but also lead to pleiotropic effects owing to malfunction of other related organelles such as lysosomes and/or platelets that also require those gene products for their function.[35] The beige gene product is a large cytosolic product termed LYST (lysosomal trafficking regulator). LYST has been proposed to have a role in regulating fusion with lysosomes. The pale-ear gene encodes an integral membrane protein, the function of which is currently unknown. The pallid gene encodes the erythrocyte protein 4.2 found on the surface of erythrocytes, platelets, kidney and brain. AP-3 is a new adaptor protein complex that has recently been identified in mammalian cells. The mammalian AP-3 complex is composed of four subunits termed β3 adaptin, δ-adaptin, μ3 and J3. The AP-3 complex has a functional role in cargo-selective transport via an alternative trafficking pathway from the Golgi to the vacuole-lysosome/melanosome. The mocha gene encodes mouse δ-adaptin and the pearl gene is likely to encode mouse β3A adaptin.[37]

Table 1   Genes controlling hair pigmentation and associated diseases.[35]

Mouse locus	Human disease	Encoded protein
Genes that affect melanocyte embryogenesis		
Steel	Piebaldism	Stem cell factor (SCF)
c-kit (SCF receptor)	Piebaldism	Tyrosine kinase receptor
Splotch	WS type 1 and 3	*Pax3* transcription factor
Microphthalmia	WS type 2	Microphthalmia transcription factor
Piebald-lethal	WS type 4	Endothelin B receptor
Dom	WS type 4	SOX10 transcription factor
Genes that affect melanosome structure and function		
Silver	Hair silvering?	Pmel 17 (melanosome matrix protein)
Beige	Chediak–Higashi syndrome	LYST (lysosomal membrane protein)
Pale ear	Hermanski–Pudlak syndrome	HPS (lysosomal membrane protein)
Pallid	Platelet storage pool disease	Protein 4.2 pallidin
Mocha	Unknown	δ subunit AP-3 complex
Pearl	Unknown	β subunit AP-3 complex
Pink-eyed dilution	OCA-2	P protein (membrane transporter)
OA-1	Ocular albinism type 1	OA-1 (melanosome membrane protein)
Genes that affect melanosome transport		
Ashen	Unknown	RAB-related GTPase
Dilute	Griscelli disease	MYH 12 myosin type Va
Genes that affect melanogenic enzymes		
Albino/platinum	OCA 1	Tyrosinase (melanogenic enzyme)
Brown	OCA 3	TRP-1 (melanogenic enzyme)
Slaty	OCA 4?	TRP-2 (melanogenic enzyme)
Mottled	Menkes' disease	ATP7A (copper transporter)
Genes that affect regulation of melanogenesis		
Extension	Red hair/phototype 1	MC1-R (MSH receptor)
Agouti	Hair pigmentation	ASP (Agouti signal protein)

OCA = Oculocutaneous albinism
WS = Waardenburg syndrome

Mutations that affect melanogenic enzymes

Proper pigmentation depends on the production of competent melanogenic enzymes. The tyrosinase-related protein family includes tyrosinase itself and two similar proteins, TRP-1 and TRP-2. The albino mutation affecting the tyrosinase gene induces the albino phenotype characterized by a lack of melanin pigment in epidermal and follicular melanocytes and in the pigmented retinal epithelium resulting in pink eyes. The TRP-2 gene maps to the slaty locus. Mice homozygote for the slaty mutation produce a dark-gray-brown rather than black eumelanin. The TRP-1 gene maps to the brown locus. Mice homozygous for a loss of function mutation of TRP-1 produce brown rather than black eumelanin.

Tyrosinase and tyrosinase-related proteins contain two atoms of copper. Mutations in the copper-transport mechanism encoded by the *X*-linked mottled locus produce a pigmentation phenotype. Male mice hemizygous for mottled mutations have pale pigmentation of the coat in association with severe defects.

Table 2 Correlations of hair color with biochemical aspects in human hair (simplified data, from ref. 11).

	Red hair	Blond hair	Brown hair	Black hair
Mutations	Unknown MC1-R gene?	Unknown	Unknown	Unknown
Tyrosinase level	Elevated	Slightly elevated	Normal	Normal
Total amount of melanins	No correlation between the total amount of melanin or the tyrosinase level with the visual aspect of hair			
Type of melanins	Pheomelanins predominant or mixed type	Various proportions of both types of melanins		Eumelanins predominant with small amounts of pheomelanins

Mutations that affect regulation of melanogenesis

Synthesis of the two types of melanin that color hair and skin is regulated by the action of the peptide hormone α-melanocyte-stimulating hormone (α-MSH). Two loci, extension (e) and agouti (a) control the switch between eumelanogenesis and pheomelanogenesis. The extension locus encodes the MSH receptor MC1-R. The agouti locus encodes the agouti signal protein (ASP). It is not yet completely understood how the switch to produce eu- or pheomelanin is effected. Conditions under which there is over-stimulation of MSH receptor function elicit eumelanin production and a black phenotype, whereas, conversely, conditions under which function of the MSH receptor is abrogated or is overwhelmed by ASP overexpression result in the production of pheomelanin. Activation of MC1-R following the binding of melanotropic peptides stimulates eumelanin formation. ASP acts as a competitive inhibitor of α-MSH binding to human MC1-R.[38]

Genes that affect melanosome transport

The ashen gene encodes a RAB-related GTPase that may be involved in the regulation of melanosome transport.[39] The ashen mutation induces reduction in hair color. The dilute muta-tion results in a general lightening of the coat. Dilute melanocytes apparently lack dendrites; in fact, the dendrites are normal but invisible due to failure of transport melanosome in them. The 'dilute' gene encodes a novel myosin protein, myosin V. Melanosome transport occurs by binding to myosin V which acts as a molecular motor upon interaction with actin filaments.

Normal human hair colors

The relationship between the ultrastructural and biochemical aspects of hair and hair color is set out in Table 2.

It is only in Caucasians that the color of hairs ranges from shades of yellow and red to black. Most people over the world have black hairs. However, in all skin types, melanins are a mixture of both eu- and pheomelanins.

Tyrosinase activity

Tyrosinase activity determines the level of the melanogenetic activity of follicular melanocytes. The possibility that hair color could be related to a variability of tyrosinase activity between individuals has been raised; however, in human beings, results show that red hairs have the highest tyrosinase activities, compared to black and brown hair follicles. Blond hairs seem to have similar or slightly increased hair bulb tyrosinase level and activity, compared to black and brown hair follicles.[40,41] It has also been shown that tyrosine hydroxylase and DOPA oxidase activities are coordinated over a broad range of hair colors.[42] These results from different groups show that follicular melanocytes from red hair bulbs have the highest melanogenic activity. Besides, they show that the light color of blond hair is not due to the low tyrosinase and melanogenic activities, but rather to the chemical structure of the melanins produced.

Ultrastructural aspects

Pheomelanosomes are spherical, and contain microvesicular (vesiculoglobular) and proteinaceous matrices on which melanin deposition is spotty and granular. They are rich in vesicles, but lack an organized internal matrix. Many components of their eumelanotic counterparts are absent: TRP-1, TRP-2, p gene product and silver protein. Tyrosinase levels are reduced by a third.[43] Eumelanosomes are ellipsoidal and contain matrices with regular striations. The chemical analysis of melanins – that is, the ratio of eumelanin to pheomelanin – corresponds well to the fine structural differentiation of eumelanosomes and pheomelanosomes. In addition, 'mixed' melanosomes may also be encountered. They have features of both eumelanosomes (ellipsoidal shape, regular striations) and pheomelanosomes (spotty and granular melanization). Whether they are eumelanic, pheomelanic or mixed remains to be clarified.

Biochemical aspects

Analysis of melanins was applied to the study of human hair color.[12,44] In 17 subjects with hair color ranging from white to blond, the hair follicles were engaged in mixed type melanogenesis. In six subjects with brown and black hair, eumelanins were predominantly synthesized. Pheomelanins were predominantly synthesized in only three of nine red-haired subjects. This demonstrates that human hair color does not always reflect the melanogenesis type in human hair follicles. Furthermore, whatever the color, all

the human hair contained both eumelanin and pheomelanin, in various proportions. In addition, most natural melanins contain a certain amount of sulfur, which is typically associated with pheomelanin. As high as 3–5.3% sulfur has been found in human black hair, 2.3% in Scandinavian blond hair, and 8.8% in Irish red hair.[11,45]

Melanogenesis in human hair

Human red hair

In some hair, that can be termed pheomelanic hair, melanocytes contain pheomelanosomes and synthesize mostly pheomelanins. The sequences of melanization are identical to those occurring in the yellow mice hair follicles.[46]

In other human red hair, melanocytes synthesize both eu- and pheomelanins. A majority of melanocytes produce pheomelanosomes and also mosaic melanosomes. In addition, a second type produces eumelanosomes.

Human blond hair

Melanocytes produce eumelanosomes and synthesize both eu- and pheomelanins. Melanosomes are not fully melanized and melanin granules are smaller and less numerous than in dark-haired subjects. Thus, the ultrastructural aspect suggests that the light color in blond hair might be due to a quantitative decrease in the production and melanization of melanosomes – that is, as shown earlier, it is not due to a decrease in tyrosinase activity.[46]

Human black and brown hairs

Whatever the racial background, follicular melanocytes produce typical eumelanosomes with ultrastructural characteristics identical to those of the epidermal melanosomes of Caucasoids and negroids. Lighter-brown hairs have smaller melanosomes.

Senile gray and white hairs

Aging leads to graying and whitening of hair with a high variability between individuals.

Although the precise mechanisms, at the molecular level, are not fully understood, morphological studies provide interesting insights. They show that these color changes are due to a decrease in the number of hair follicle melanocytes. In the melanocytic zone of the senile gray hair bulb, the number of melanocytes appears normal or a little reduced, but the pigment cells contain very few melanosomes and seem to have little activity. In senile white hair, melanocytes are scarce and DOPA-negative, or entirely absent, and immunoreactive tyrosinase antigen cannot be detected in hair bulbs.[47] However, as suggested by the detection of tyrosinase mRNA, amelanotic melanocytes may be present in the outer root sheath.[48]

This decrease in the number of hair follicle melanocytes, resulting in graying, might be linked to a defect in redox-regulated melanin synthesis. This defect might increase the autocytotoxicity of certain metabolic intermediates within the pigment cells. Interestingly, BCL-2-deficient mice turn gray with the second hair follicle. As the BCL-2 gene inhibits most types of apoptotic cell death by regulating an anti-oxidant pathway at sites of free radical generation, BCL-2 might be a good candidate to explain premature graying in human beings.[49,50]

Genetic control of human hair color

In human beings, the genetic and molecular events that are responsible for the different skin and hair colors are nearly unknown. An attempt to correlate human phenotypes with the expression of the agouti gene failed.[51] Low levels of expression were found in all skin types. In contrast, variants of the MC1-R gene have been associated with red hair and fair skin.[52] However, both studies appear preliminary and need further confirmation. The functional consequences – that is, the ability to tan and the hair and skin color – associated with the different variants of MC1-R gene need to be defined further. The type of inheritance (recessive, dominant, or complex inheritance depending on interactions with variant genes at other loci) is unknown.

Clinical aspects

Various terms have been used to refer to decreased melanin content in the skin and hair. *Leukoderma* is a generic term that denotes a mild to marked decrease in normal color. *Hypomelanosis* refers to a leukoderma characterized by reduced or absent melanin content. The terms 'pigmentary dilution' and 'hypopigmentation' are synonymous with hypomelanosis. Amelanosis refers to hypomelanosis in which melanin pigmentation is totally absent. *Depigmentation* implies a loss of preexisting melanin pigmentation. *Leukomelanoderma* refers to melanin disturbances characterized by both hyper- and hypomelanosis in the same general area of skin. *Poliosis* is a term applied to a localized hypomelanosis of hair, whereas *canities* implies a more generalized pigmentary dilution of hair. Graying of hair is a localized or generalized hypomelanosis in which there is an admixture of normally pigmented and depigmented hair. Generalized graying of hair is a form of canities. Whitening of hair is the endpoint of canities.

Normal hair color is altered in many diseases; in most of them, hair color is decreased (Table 3). Genetic abnormalities at the different steps of the melanization process have been described, leading to hypomelanoses that most often affect both the skin and hair. We will briefly discuss the diseases with recent advances in their understanding that correlate with melanocyte biology.

Disorders of fetal melanoblast migration

Piebaldism

Piebaldism, or white spot disease (Figures 2 and 3), a dominant disease, is due to several different mutations at the W-locus, the gene encoding c-kit receptor.[53] Mutations cause a failure of melanocytes to colonize the fetal skin. Patients present a congenital and stable leukoderma with a characteristic distribution that involves the anterior trunk, extremities, the central portion of the eyebrows, and the midfrontal portion of the scalp with a resultant white forelock.

Table 3   Classification of hypomelanosis in human hair.

Category	Condition
Genetic	Phenylketonuria
	Homocystinuria
	Histidinemia
	Oculocutaneous albinisms
	Cross–McKusick–Breen syndrome
	Tietze's syndrome
	Menkes' syndrome
	Vitiligo
	Piebaldism
	Woolf's syndrome
	Ziprokowski–Margolis syndrome
	Waadenburg's syndrome
	Nevus depigmentosus
	Neurofibromatosis
	Kappa chain deficiency
	'Bird headed' dwarfism
	Premature aging syndromes: progeria, Werner's
	Rothmund–Thomson's
	Böök's syndrome
	Fish's syndrome
	Myotonia dystrophica
	Down's syndrome
	Pierre Robin syndrome
	Hallermann–Streiff syndrome
	Treachers Collins syndrome
Metabolic	Copper deficiency
	Iron deficiency
Endocrine	Hyperthyroidism
Nutritional	Chronic protein deficiency of loss
	Chronic kwashiorkor
	Chronic nephrosis
	Chronic ulcerative colitis
	Chronic malabsorption syndrome
	Vitamin B12 deficiency
Chemical and pharmacological agents	Hydroquinone
	Guanotitrofurazone
	Hydrogen peroxide
	Mephenesin carbamate
	Triparanol
	Fluorobutyrophenone
	Chloroquine and hydroxychloroquine
Physical agents	Burns, thermal, UV
	Ionizing radiation
	Trauma
Infection	Herpes zoster
Neoplastic	Leukoderma acquisitum centrifugum
	Leukoderma halo nevus or benign pigmented tumor
	Various types of leukoderma associated with melanoma
Miscellaneous	Alezzandrini
	Vogt–Koyanagi–Harada
	Senile canities and sudden whitening of hair
	Alopecia areata
	Heterochromia irides

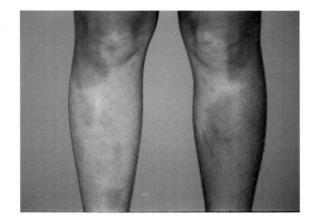

Figure 2

Piebaldism

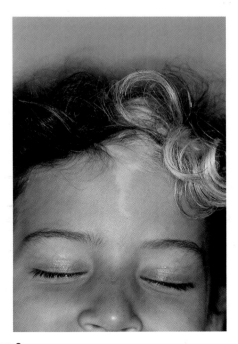

Figure 3

Piebaldism

Waardenburg syndromes

Waardenburg syndromes are rare autosomal dominant diseases, with four types (Figures 4 and 5). They are characterized by lateral displacement of the inner canthi and of the inferior lacrymal puncta (except for the type II), prominence of the root of the nose and of the medial portions of the eyebrows, congenital deafness, white forelock, and heterochromia irides. Furthermore, type III is associated with defects of arms and type IV with Hirsprung's disease. The syndromes are due to mutations of transcription factors (*Pax3* or MITF) or endothelin receptors.

Disorders of melanogenesis

Oculocutaneous albinism (OCA) is a recessive inherited disorder of the melanin pigmentary system characterized by a decrease or an absence of melanin in the skin, hair, and eyes (Figures 6 and 7). The outstanding characteristics are the 'milk-white' skin and hair color, photophobia, and nystagmus.

The negative tyrosine OCA, or OCA-1, is due to mutations of the tyrosinase gene.

The yellow mutant, or OCA-III, has the same clinical presentation as OCA-I at birth, but is characterized by yellow-red hair by 6 months. It is due to TRP-1 gene mutations.

Disorders of melanosomes

Mutations of the p-gene are associated with the *tyrosinase-positive OCA II*.

Chediak–Higashi syndrome

Chediak–Higashi syndrome (CHS) is a rare autosomal recessive disease characterized by OCA, severe recurrent infections, lymphoproliferative disorder, progressive peripheral neuropathy, and death before the age of 10 in the lack of allogenic bone marrow transplantation. The pigmentary dilution involves skin, hair and eyes. It is almost always present, but may be partial and overlooked in patients of fair-skinned ancestry. Melanocytes contain giant melanosomes and

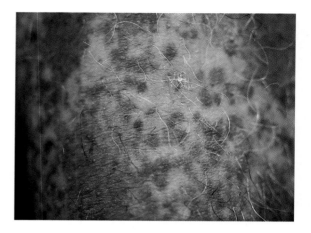

Figure 4

Waardenburg syndrome

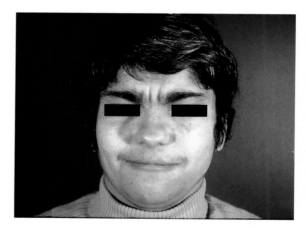

Figure 5

Waardenburg syndrome

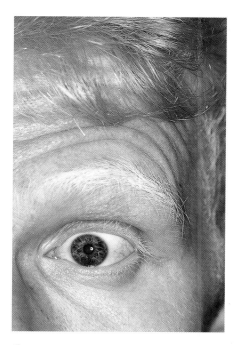

Figure 6

Ocutoculaneous albinism

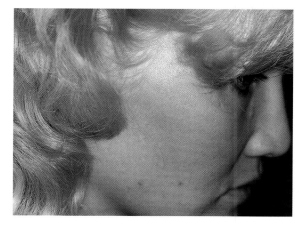

Figure 7

Ocutoculaneous albinism

leucocytes contain giant granules. Mutations at the LYST locus cause defects of the CHS protein, which is thought to be a component of a membrane-associated signal transduction complex regulating intracellular protein trafficking.[54]

Hermansky–Pudlak syndrome

Hermansky–Pudlak syndrome (HPS) or OCA with hemorrhagic diathesis is an autosomal disorder consisting of a triad of tyrosinase-positive OCA, hemorrhagic diathesis due to storage-pool-deficient platelets, and an accumulation of a ceroid-like material (Figure 8). The lysosomal defect results in the accumulation of ceroid-lipofucsin material in the lysosomes of macrophages of the lung and the gut, resulting in a restrictive lung disease and granulomatous colitis. Other manifestations include kidney failure and cardiac myopathy. The melanocytes contain macromelanosomes thought to be formed by the fusion of microvesicles. A gene associated with HPS has been cloned and encodes a novel protein, whose precise role remains undetermined. In HPS, the mutated protein might affect the membranes of melanosomes, lysosomes and platelet-dense bodies.[55,56]

Griscelli-Pruniéras syndrome

Griscelli–Pruniéras syndrome (GPS) is an autosomal recessive syndrome with silvery-gray colour dilution of skin and hair, associated with neurological and immunological defects (Figure 9). It is due to mutations of the actin-based motor protein myosin V which cause a disturbed transfer of melanosomes.[57,58] GPS illustrates the role of motor protein in melanosome transport and dendrite formation. During GPS, melanocytes are full of mature melanosomes with stubby dendrites; yet, there is still a limited transfer of melanosomes during GPS, a feature which suggests that other transporters of melanosomes exist.

Vitiligo

Vitiligo is an acquired disease characterized by achromic macules of various size, with a regular border and often symmetrical (Figures 10 and

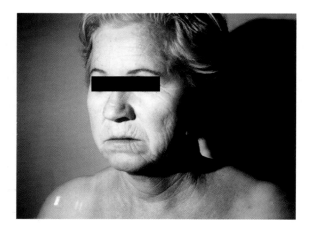

Figure 8

Hermansky–Pudlak syndrome

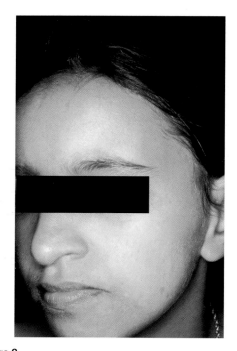

Figure 9

Griscelli-Pruniéras syndrome

11). The lesional skin is characterized by the lack of epidermal melanocytes. In contrast, hairs present within the vitiligo macules often remain pigmented a long time before they become white. The precise etiopathogenic mechanisms that induce vitiligo lesions are unknown, although genetic and immunologic factors are supposed to play a role. However, biochemical abnormalities – autotoxicity of melanins, for example – might be involved in some cases of vitiligo. Indeed, whether vitiligo is a single disease or an entity which may be the result of different causes remains elusive. In addition, the reason why follicular melanocytes are to some extent intact at the first onset of the disease is unknown. Perhaps, the suggestion that the melanocyte populations of the epidermis and follicle are antigenically different is the beginning of an explanation.[26]

Another particular aspect of vitiligo is that follicular melanocytes are thought to have a potential role in treatment since they are thought to play a reservoir function. During vitiligo repigmentation, whether spontaneous or after PUVA therapy, scanning electron microscopy and hair-follicle split DOPA techniques show that hypertrophic pigmented melanocytes appear in the ORS of the hair follicle, and migrate from the infundibulum into the nearby epidermis. The migration is probably mediated by integrins, activated by cytokines, released as the result of UV exposure. It is supposed that photochemotherapy evokes its therapeutic effect by modulating cytokine release and extracellular production. However, it is unknown whether, in vivo, UV may stimulate hair follicle melanocytes like epidermal melanocytes, either directly, through UV-induced photoproducts and upregulation, or in an autocrine and paracrine manner, through nitrogen monoxide produced by both keratinocytes and melanocytes after UVB-irradiation.[59]

Conclusion

Establishment of cultures of human melanocytes has led to an explosion of knowledge concerning the biology of melanocytes. Routine culture of follicular melanocytes is probably for the near future and should lead to a similar progress in the understanding of the biology of follicular

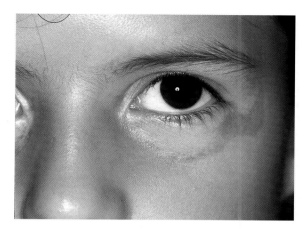

Figure 10

Vitiligo

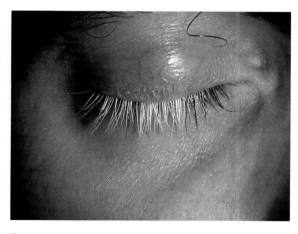

Figure 11

Vitiligo

melanocytes. In particular, the link between melanogenesis and hair cycle is perhaps a clue to understanding the relations between melanocytes and keratinocytes. The ability of hair follicles to migrate into the epidermis under certain circumstances may also give hope for the treatment of hypomelanoses.

References

1. Ortonne JP, Prota G: Hair melanins and hair color: ultrastructural and biochemical aspects. *J Invest Dermatol* 1993; **101**: 82S–89S.
2. Holbrook KA: The appearance, density and distribution of melanocytes in human embryonic and fetal skin revealed by the anti-melanoma monoclonal antibody HMB-45. *Anat Embryol* 1989; **180**: 443–455.
3. Nishikawa S, Kusakabe M, Yoshinaga K, et al.: In utero manipulation of coat color formation by a monoclonal anti-c-kit antibody: two distinct waves of *c-kit* dependency during melanocyte development. *EMBO J* 1991; **10**: 2111–2118.
4. Hemesath TJ, Roydon Price E, Takemoto C, Badalian T, Fisher DE: MAP kinase links the transcription factor Microphthalmia to c-kit signaling in melanocytes. *Nature* 1998; **391**: 298–301.
5. Hearing VJ, Tsukamoto K: Enzymatic control of pigmentation in mammals. *FASEB J* 1991; **5**: 2902–2909.
6. Bentley NJ, Eisen T, Goding CR: Melanocyte-specific expression of the human tyrosinase promoter: activation by the microphthalmia gene product and role of the initiator. *Mol Cell Biol* 1994; **14**: 7996–8006.
7. Ganss R, Schütz G, Beermann F: The mouse tyrosinase gene. Promotor modulation by positive and negative regulatory elements. *J Biol Chemistry* 1994; **269**: 29808–29816.
8. Bertazzo A, Costa C, Biasolo M, et al.: Determination of copper and zinc levels in human hair: influence of sex, age, and hair pigmentation. *Biological Trace Element Research* 1996; **52**: 37–53.
9. Kobayashi T, Urabe K, Winder A, et al.: DHICA oxidase activity of TRP1 and interactions with other melanogenic enzymes. *Pigment Cell Res* 1994; **7**: 227–234.
10. Aroca P, Garcia-Borron JC, Solano F, et al.: Regulation of distal mammalian melanogenesis. I. Partial purification and characterization of a DOPAchrome converting factor: DOPAchrome tautomerase. *Biochem Biophys* 1990; **1035**: 266–275.

11. Prota G: Progress in the chemistry of melanins and related metabolites. *Med Res Rev* 1988; **8**: 525–526.

12. Jimbow K, Alena F, Dixon W, Hara H: Regulatory factors of pheo- and eumelanogenic compartments. *Pigment Cell Res* 1992; **2**: 36–42.

13. D'Ischia M, Napolitano A, Prota G: Peroxidase as an alternative to tyrosinase in the oxidative polymerization of 5,6-dihydroxyindoles to melanin(s). *Biochem Biophys* 1991; **1073**: 423–430.

14. Jimbow K, Quevedo WC Jr, Fitzpatrick TB, et al.: Biology of melanocytes. In: Fitzpatrick TB, Eisen AZ, Wolff K, Freedberg IM, Austen KF (eds). *Dermatology in General Medicine*, 4th edn. New York, MacGraw-Hill, 1993: 261–271.

15. Chakraborty AK, Mishima Y, Inazu M, Hatta S, Ichihashi M: Melanogenic regulatory factors in coated vesicles from melanoma cells. *J Invest Dermatol* 1989; **93**: 616–620.

16. Rosemblat S, Sviderskaya EV, Easty DJ, et al.: Identification of a melanosomal membrane protein encoded by the pink-eyed dilution (type II oculocutaneous albinism) gene. *Proc Natl Acad Sci USA* 1994; **91**: 12071–12075.

17. Donatien PD, Orlow SJ: Interactions of melanosomal proteins with melanin. *Eur J Biochem* 1995; **232**: 159–164.

18. Gardner JM, Nakatsu Y, Gondo Y, et al.: The mouse pink-eyed dilution gene: association with human Prader–Willi and Angelman syndromes. *Science* 1992; **257**: 1121–1124.

19. Kippenberger S, Bernd A, Bereiter-Hahn J, Ramirez-Bosca A, Kaufmann R: The mechanism of melanocyte dendrite formation: the impact of differentiating keratinocytes. *Pigment Cell Res* 1998; **11**: 34–37.

20. Yamamoto O, Bhawan J: Three modes of melanosome transfers in caucasian facial skin: hypothesis based on an ultrastructural study. *Pigment Cell Res* 1994; **7**: 158–169.

21. Tang A, Eller MS, Hara M, et al.: E-cadhedrin is the major mediator of human melanocytes adhesion to keratinocytes *in vitro*. *J Cell Science* 1994; **107**: 983–992.

22. Hara M, Yaar M, Tang A, et al.: Role of integrins in melanocyte attachment and dendricity. *J Cell Science* 1994; **107**: 2739–2748.

23. Staricco RG: Amelanotic melanocytes in the outer sheath of the human hair follicle and their role in the repigmentation of regenerated epidermis. *Ann NY Acad Sci* 1963; **100**: 239–255.

24. Narisawa Y, Kohda H, Tanaka T: Three-dimensional demonstration of melanocyte distribution of human hair follicles: special reference to the bulge area. *Acta Derm Venereol (Stockh)* 1997; **77**: 97–101.

25. Tobin DJ, Colen SR, Bystryn JC: Isolation and long-term culture of human hair-follicle melanocytes. *J Invest Dermatol* 1995; **104**: 86–89.

26. Tobin JD, Bystryn JC: Different populations of melanocytes are present in hair follicles and epidermis. *Pigment Cell Res* 1996; **9**: 304–310.

27. Hirobe T: Structure and function of melanocytes: microscopic morphology and cell biology of mouse melanocytes in the epidermis and hair follicle. *Histol Histopathol* 1995; **10**: 223–237.

28. Lindner G, Botckkarev NV, Ling G, van der Veen C, Paus R: Analysis of apoptosis during hair follicle regression (catagen). *Am J Pathol* 1997; **151**: 1601–1617.

29. Sugyiama S, Kubita A: Melanocyte reservoir in the hair follicles during the hair growth cycle: an electron microscopic study. In: Kobori T, Montagna T (eds). *Biology and Diseases of the Hair*. Baltimore, University Park Press, 1976: 181–200.

30. Vegesna V, Withers HR, Taylor JM: The effect on depigmentation after multi-fractionated irradiation of mouse resting hair follicles. *Radiat Res* 1987; **111**: 464–473.

31. Tobin DJ, Hagen E, Botchkarev A, Paus R: Do hair bulb melanocytes undergo apoptosis during hair follicle regression (catagen)? *J Invest Dermatol* 1998; **11**: 941–947.

32. Yaar M, Eller MS, Di Benedetto P, et al.: The trk family of receptors mediates nerve growth factor and neurotrophin-3 effects in melanocytes. *J Clin Invest* 1994; **94**: 1550–1562.

33. Hardy MH: The secret life of the hair follicle. *Trends Genet* 1992; **8**: 55–61.

34. Jackson IJ: Molecular and developmental genetics of mouse coat color. *Ann Rev Genet* 1994; **28**: 189–217.

35. Alhaidari Z, Olivry T, Ortonne JP: Melanocytogenesis and melanogenesis: genetic regulation and comparative clinical diseases. *Veterinary Dermatol* 1999; **10**: 3–16.

36. Tachibana M: A cascade of genes related to Waardenburg syndrome. *J Invest Dermatol*, Symposium Proceedings 1999; **4**: 126–129.

37. Odorizzi G, Cowles CR, Emr SD: The AP-3 complex: a coat of many colours, *Trends Cell Biol*, 1998; **8**: 282–288.

38. Suzuki I, Im S, Tada A, et al.: Participation of the melanocortin-1 receptor in the UV-control of pigmentation. *J Invest Dermatol*, Symposium Proceedings 1999; **4**: 29–34.

39. Hearing VJ: Biochemical control of melanogenesis and melanosomal organisation. *J Invest Dermatol*, Symposium Proceedings 1999; **4**: 24–28.

40. King RA, Olds DP, Witkop CJ: Characterization of human hair bulb tyrosinase. Properties of normal and albinoenzyme. *J Invest Dermatol* 1978; **171**: 136–139.

41. Burchill SA, Ito S, Thody AJ: Tyrosinase expression and its relationship to eumelanin and phaeomelanin synthesis in human hair follicles. *J Derm Science* 1991; **2**: 281–286.

42. Wolfram LJ, Albrecht L: Chemical and photobleaching of brown and red hair. *J Soc Cosmet Chem* 1987; **82**: 179–191.

43. Kobayashi T, Vieria WD, Potterf B: Modulation of melanogenic protein expression during the switch from eu- to pheomelanogenesis. *J Cell Sci* 1995; **108**: 2301–2309.

44. Thody AJ, Higgins EM, Wakamatsu K: Pheomelanin as well as eumelanin is present in human epidermis. *J Invest Dermatol* 1991; **97**: 340–344.

45. Arnaud JC, Boré P: Isolation of melanin pigments from human hair. *J Soc Cosmet Chem* 1981; **32**: 137–152.

46. Cesarini JP: Hair melanin and hair color. In: *Hair and hair diseases*. Berlin, SW Klauss, 1990: 165–197.

47. Lloyd T, Garry FL, Manders EK, Marks JG: The effect of age and hair colour on human hair bulb tyrosinase activity. *Br J Dermatol* 1987; **116**: 485–489.

48. Tadaka K, Sugiyama K, Yamamoto I, Oba K, Takeuchi T: Presence of amelanotic melanocytes within the outer root sheath of senile white hair. *J Invest Dermatol* 1992; **99**: 629–633.

49. Hockenberg DM, Oltvai ZN, Yin XM, Milliman CL, Korsmeyer SI: Bcl-2 functions in an antioxidant pathway to prevent apoptosis. *Cell* 1993; **75**: 241–251.

50. Veis DJ, Sorenson CM, Shutter JR, Korsmeyer SJ: Bcl-2-deficient mice demonstrate fulminant lymphoid apoptosis, polycystic kidneys, and hypopigmented hair. *Cell* 1993; **75**: 229–240.

51. Wilson BD, Ollmann MM, Kang L: Structure and function of ASP, the human homolog of the mouse agouti gene. *Hum Mol Genet* 1995; **4**: 223–230.

52. Valverde P, Healy E, Jackson I, Rees JL. Thody A: Variants of the melanocyte-stimulating hormone receptor gene are associated with red hair and fair skin in human. *Nature Gen* 1995; **11**: 328–330.

53. Spritz RA: Molecular basis of human piebaldism. *J Invest Dermatol* 1994; **103**: 137–140.

54. Nagle DL, Karim MA, Woolf EA, et al.: Identification and mutation analysis of the complete gene for Chediak–Higashi syndrome. *Nature Genet* 1996; **14**: 307–311.

55. Oh J, Bailin T, Fukai K, et al.: Positional cloning of a gene for Hermansky–Pudlak syndrome, a disorder of cytoplasmic organelles. *Nature Genet* 1996; **14**: 300–306.

56. Gardner JM, Wildenberg SC, Keiper NM, et al.: The mouse pale ear (ep) mutation is the homologue of human Hermansky–Pudlak syndrome. *Proc Natl Acad Sci USA* 1997; **94**: 9238–9243.

57. Pastural E, Barrat FJ, Dufourq-Lagelousse R, et al.: Griscelli maps to chromosome 15q21 and is associated with mutations in the myosin Va gene. *Nature Genet* 1997; **16**: 289–292.

58. Rogers SI, Gelfand V: Myosin cooperates with microtubule motors during organelle transport in melanophores. *Curr Biol* 1998; **8**: 161–164.

59. Ortonne JP, MacDonald DM, Micoud A, Thivolet J: PUVA-induced repigmentation of vitiligo: histoenzymological (split dopa) and ultrastructural study. *Br J Dermatol* 1979; **101**: 1–13.

Section II

REGULATORY FACTORS IN THE FOLLICLE

5
Androgens: the main regulator of human hair growth

Valerie Anne Randall

Introduction

Androgens or 'maleness' were first reported to affect human hair growth by Aristotle. Since then the paradoxical variety of responses human hair follicles have to androgens and the difficulties caused by the common hair disorders of hirsutism (male pattern hair growth in women) and androgenetic alopecia have been recognized. This chapter will review the function of human hair, the current knowledge of the importance of androgens in human hair growth, the mechanism of androgen action in various types of human hair follicles and the current model of how androgens regulate follicles to change the type of hair produced. Further details of androgenetic alopecia and hirsutism and their treatment can be seen in Sections 3 and 7 respectively of this book.

The functions of human hair

Hair growth is a specific feature of mammals that has contributed significantly to their success. Hair has important functions in thermoregulation and camouflage; these often need to be altered in line with seasonal changes, for example the thick, white, winter coats of arctic foxes contrast with their short brown, summer coats.[1] Hair also forms an important protective physical barrier and plays a role in social and sexual communication, for example the distinctive mane of the male lion; hair follicles are also often specialized as neuroreceptors, for example, whiskers.

Human hair growth is so reduced compared with that of other mammals that we have been termed the 'naked ape'.[2] The insulation and cam-

ouflage roles have virtually disappeared though their evolution can be seen in the seasonal patterns of human hair growth,[3] and the erection of hairs, 'goosebumps', in response to cold. The main functions of human hair are protection and communication. Hairs that are obvious in children are mainly protective; the eyebrows and eyelashes stop foreign bodies entering the eyes and scalp hair may prevent sun damage and physical injury to the scalp and back of the neck,[4,5] or even protect from cold since the scalp has little adipose tissue.[4] Human hair plays a very significant, although often not now fully appreciated, role in human social and sexual communication whatever the genetic background or culture. This is reflected in the ritual head-shaving of Christian and Buddhist monks and many prisoners, the religiously uncut hair of Sikhs and the standard short hair cuts of soldiers.

The arrival of visible pubic and axillary hair signals puberty in both sexes[6–8] and their associated apocrine glands produce secretions yielding odours involved in sexual communication.[9] Mature masculinity is signalled by the greater terminal hair on the chest, upper pubic triangle and limbs and, particularly, in the beard; this explains the significant psychological stress suffered by hirsute women. The involvement of the beard in male threatening display behaviour[4] may explain the modern custom of removing it daily in the less openly aggressive Western world. Whether the common loss of scalp hair in androgenetic alopecia in men is a natural progression of a secondary sexual characteristic or a pathological process is unclear. Nevertheless, in the current youth-orientated Western culture the social communication role of hair, plus the association of androgenetic alopecia with ageing, lead to a negative effect on the quality of life. This is discussed further by Randall in Chapter 10.

Changing the type of hair produced

Like other mammals human hairs are produced all over the skin, except for the palms, soles and lips. Their size and colour may vary over an individual's skin; this is particularly obvious in children where long, pigmented *terminal* scalp hair contrasts with the tiny, almost colourless *vellus* hair on the face. Many mammals also change the type of hair produced in different areas of the body within an individual, either regularly in seasonal changes, or, on maturity, like the development of the lion's mane.[1] In human beings, dramatic, although quite slow, changes take place during puberty when terminal hairs replace vellus ones in the axillae and pubis in both sexes and on the face, chest and abdomen in men[6–8] (Figure 1). The hair follicle possesses a very important and unique mechanism, the hair cycle, to accomplish these changes.[10,11] For further details see Chapter 6 by Paus et al. This involves the destruction of the original lower follicle and its total regeneration to form another follicle, which can produce a hair with different characteristics. Currently it is unclear how different a hair can be from its immediate predecessor because most major changes in human hair growth take place over several years. The full production of a beard[12] is not established until around 30 years of age and ear canal hair[13] takes until fifty years of age to be established. Similarly, the miniaturization process of male-pattern baldness appears to take many years[14] (Figure 1).

The type of hair produced, particularly its length, greatly depends on the length of the *anagen* or growing phase of the cycle. For example, long scalp hairs are produced by follicles with growing periods of over 3 years,[11,15] whereas anagen on the finger may last only 1.5–3 months.[15] The cell biology and biochemistry of the local interactions involved in the control processes of the hair cycle are, however, not understood, although there is currently much interest[16] with the ultimate aim being the ability to regulate the anagen phase and hence the length of the cycle and final hair length.

Seasonal changes in human hair growth

Hair follicles are under hormonal regulation because of the importance of co-ordinating changes in mammalian coat insulation and colour to the environment, and the social and sexual communication roles to the appropriate stage in the life cycle. Seasonal changes are co-ordinated to day length, and to a lesser extent temperature, in the same way as seasonal breeding activity. Changes are translated to the follicle via the pineal and hypothalamo-pituitary route through the influence of gonadal, thyroid and corticosteroid hormones.[1]

Regular, seasonal changes during the year in human hair growth have only been recognized comparatively recently.[3,17,18] Androgen-dependent beard and thigh hair growth increased significantly in the summer in English Caucasian men with indoor occupations,[3] falling to its lowest in January and February (Figure 2). This may reflect changes in circulating androgen levels, since these have been reported to rise in European men in the summer.[19–21]

Scalp hair showed a single annual cycle with over 90% of hairs growing in the spring, falling to about 80% at the end of summer. This was paralleled by an increase in the number of hairs shed per day, which more than doubled (Figure 3). Considering that most people's scalp hair follicles will be in anagen for at least 2–3 years, such a seasonal effect is quite remarkable. To date it is unclear which hormones regulate this; nevertheless, any investigations of hormonal effects on human hair growth or therapies to treat human hair disorders need to be performed for at least a year to separate any effects from normal seasonal variation.

Effects of androgens on human hair growth

Androgens are the main normal regulator of human hair growth. Nevertheless other hormones including those of the thyroid, pregnancy, prolactin and melanocyte stimulating hormone (α-MSH), also influence hair growth in humans

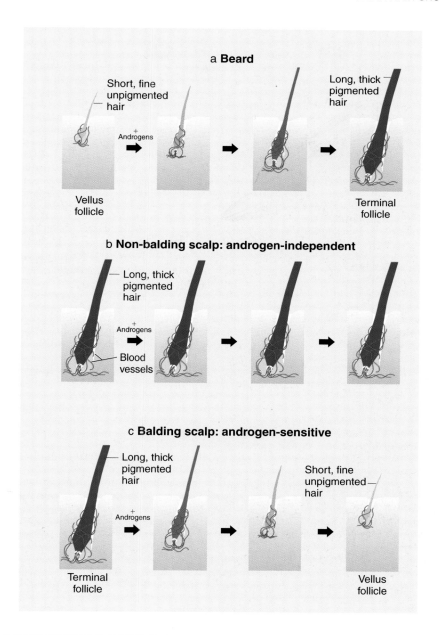

Figure 1

The paradoxically differing effects of androgens on human hair follicles. (a) After puberty androgens stimulate the gradual production of pigmented terminal hair in many regions, such as beard, axilla and pubis, which previously grew only small, fine vellus hairs. (b) Other follicles producing terminal hair in children remain unaffected, for example eyelashes and non-balding scalp. (c) In genetically predisposed individuals, androgens may cause, simultaneously, the opposite gradual transformation of terminal to vellus follicles, leading to balding. Modified from Randall et al, 1991.[41]

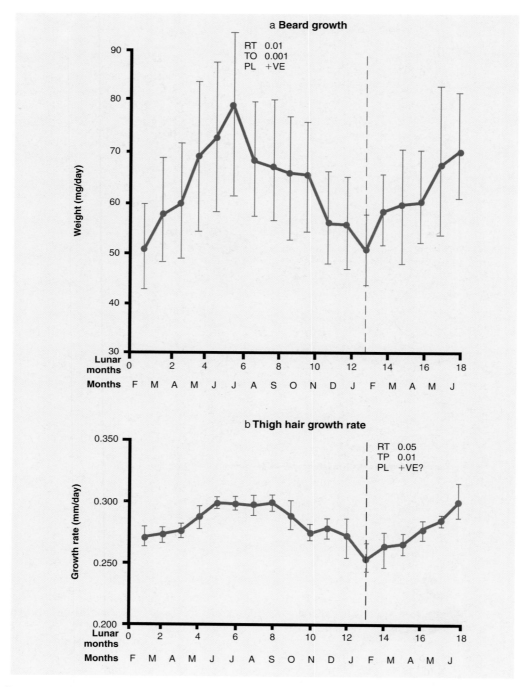

Figure 2

Androgen-dependent hair growth showing significant seasonal changes during the year. The rate of beard (a) and thigh (b) hair growth is faster in the summer in Caucasian men aged 18–39 years living in the north of England. This natural seasonal effect means that investigations of treatment to alter hair growth must be carried out for at least a 12-month period. RT, runs test; TP, turning points; PL, phase length. Data redrawn from Randall and Ebling (1991).[3]

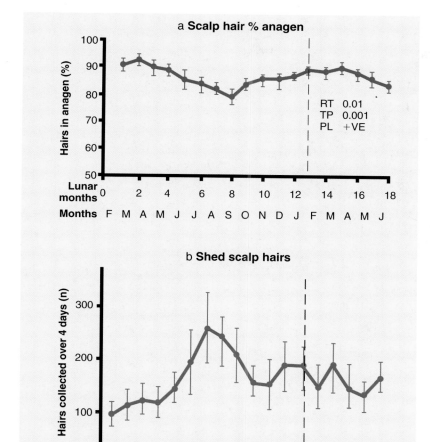

a Scalp hair % anagen

RT 0.01
TP 0.001
PL +VE

b Shed scalp hairs

Figure 3

Human scalp hair growth shows significant seasonal changes. The percentage of hair follicles in anagen (growing) on the scalp decreases (a) and the number of hairs shed per day increases in the autumn (b) in 14 Caucasian men aged 18–39 living in the north of England (mean ± SEM). This seasonal effect means that clinical investigations of human hair growth need to be carried out over at least a 12-month period. RT, runs test; TO, turning point; PL, phase length. Data redrawn from Randall and Ebling (1991).[3]

and other species.[22] Poor nutritional status also has dramatic inhibitory effects on hair growth due to the high energy load of the intensive cell division to produce new hairs.[3]

One of the first signs of puberty is the gradual replacement of tiny vellus hairs with larger, more pigmented *intermediate* hairs in the pubis and later the axillae;[7,8] eventually larger and darker terminal hairs are produced (see Figure 1). These changes parallel the pubertal rise in plasma androgens, which occurs earlier in girls than

boys.[23,24] Later, similar changes occur on the male face and this, plus an extended pubic diamond, chest hair and greater hair on the limbs, readily distinguishes the sexually mature adult man (Figure 4). The changes in all areas are gradual, often progressing over many years. Beard growth increases rapidly during puberty but continues to rise until the mid-thirties[12] (Figure 5), while terminal hair on the chest or auditory canal may not appear until many years after puberty.[13]

In marked contrast, androgens have no

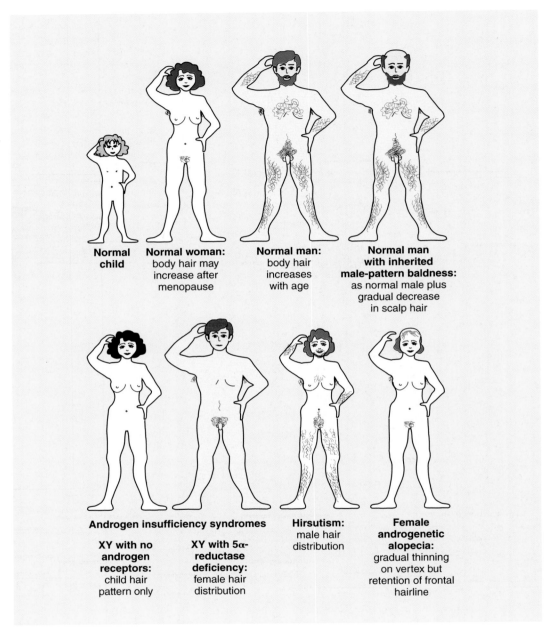

Normal child

Normal woman: body hair may increase after menopause

Normal man: body hair increases with age

Normal man with inherited male-pattern baldness: as normal male plus gradual decrease in scalp hair

Androgen insufficiency syndromes

XY with no androgen receptors: child hair pattern only

XY with 5α-reductase deficiency: female hair distribution

Hirsutism: male hair distribution

Female androgenetic alopecia: gradual thinning on vertex but retention of frontal hairline

Figure 4

The variation of human hair growth with different endocrine conditions. The protective terminal hairs of childhood on the scalp, eyelashes and eyebrows are augmented during puberty by axillary and pubic hair growth in both sexes, plus beard, chest and greater body hair in men. None of this occurs without functional androgen receptors and only axillary and pubic hair is formed in the absence of 5α-reductase type 2. In genetically predisposed individuals, androgens may also cause inhibition of scalp hair growth, particularly in men. Raised circulating androgens or idiopathic causes such as increased follicle sensitivity may lead to hirsutism, otherwise known as male-pattern hair distribution in women. Modified from Randall 1998.[42]

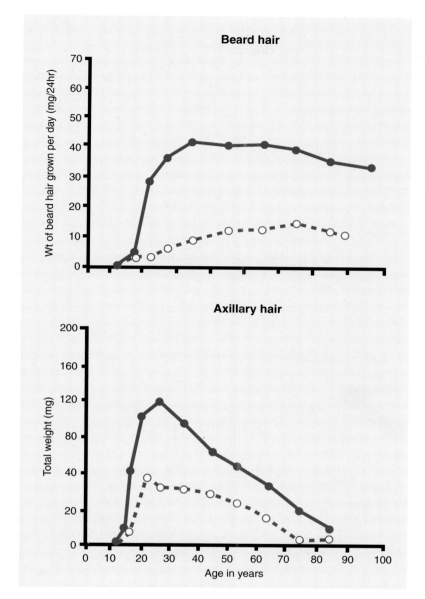

Beard hair

Wt of beard hair grown per day (mg/24hr)

Axillary hair

Total weight (mg)

Age in years

Figure 5

Intrinsic differences in androgen stimulation between beard and axillary hair follicle growth. Both axillary and beard growth are stimulated during puberty but beard growth is maintained until old age, while axillary hair growth in both sexes falls in early adulthood. Data redrawn from Hamilton, 1958[12] show beard and axillary hair growth in Caucasian (——●——) and Japanese (– – – O – – –) men

obvious effect on many follicles that produce terminal hairs in childhood such as the eyelashes or many scalp follicles (see Figure 1). Paradoxically, in individuals with a genetic predisposition, androgens progressively inhibit large terminal scalp follicles, which are gradually replaced by tiny vellus ones, causing balding of the scalp, in other words, androgenetic alopecia[14,25,26] or male-pattern baldness (see Figure 1). (This is discussed in more detail in Chapter 10 by Randall). Apart from the role of androgens, the precise mechanisms of these responses within the hair follicle are not well understood, although they are currently the focus of much investigation.

Intrinsic response to androgens by individual follicles

Responses to androgens are intrinsic to the individual follicle. Not only does the response range from stimulation to inhibition depending on the body site but sensitivity to the hormone also varies within individual areas. For example, clearly defined patterns of pigmented facial hair first develop above the mouth and centre of the chin in both young men and hirsute women before expanding across the face; regression in androgenetic alopecia also occurs in a patterned, progressive manner[14] (see Chapter 10). Similarly, female circulating androgen levels are high enough to promote axillary and the female pubic pattern of terminal hair but male patterns of body hair normally require the higher adult male levels.[7,8,23,24] In addition, although beard growth is maintained at high levels until old age, axillary hair growth increases until around 30 years of age and then falls again in both sexes[12] (see Figure 5).

Androgens appear to promote and amplify the individual follicle's genetic programming. This end-organ response is the basis for hair-transplant surgery[27] for androgenetic alopecia. In hair-transplantation, skin from 'non-balding' regions of the scalp, such as the nape of the neck, is transplanted to the balding vertex, where the follicles retain their innate lack of androgen response and continue to produce terminal hairs, while miniaturization progresses in the vertex follicles behind them. Presumably, this different genetic programming occurs during development. Interestingly, the dermis of the frontal-parietal scalp (the human balding regions) of the quail chick has been shown to develop from the neural crest, while the occipital-temporal scalp arises from the mesoderm.[28] If this development also occurs in humans it may explain the different scalp regional responses to androgens.

Neither beard growth[12] nor androgenetic alopecia[25] return to prepubertal levels if men are castrated after puberty, suggesting that the altered gene expression may not need androgen to persist, at least to some extent and once sufficiently triggered, although it is necessary for further development. On the other hand, male beard growth shows seasonal variation, presumably by short-term response to fluctuating hormone levels,[3] and antiandrogen treatment with cyproterone acetate causes regression of hirsutism.[29,30] This indicates a dependence on androgens to maintain the status quo as well as to stimulate progression. The difference between these observations may result from the length of time that the androgen effect had been established; for example, if chronic inflammation has caused fibrosis below the shortened balding follicle,[31] it seems much less likely that the follicle could reform a terminal hair follicle, regardless of stimulus.

Mechanism of androgen action in hair follicles

Hair growth in androgen insensitivity syndromes and 5α-reductase type 2 deficiency

All steroid hormones act by diffusing through the plasma membrane and binding to specific intracellular receptors; these hormone–receptor complexes undergo conformational changes, exposing DNA binding sites. The activated complexes then bind to specific hormone response elements in the DNA, promoting the expression of specific hormone-regulated genes (Figure 6). The mechanism of androgen action is more complex. In many tissues such as the classical androgen target organ, the prostate, testosterone, the major circulating androgen, is metabolized intracellularly by the enzyme, 5α-reductase, to 5α-dihydrotestosterone. This 5α-dihydrotestosterone binds and activates the androgen receptor. In other androgen-dependent tissues such as skeletal muscle, however, testosterone itself binds the same receptor, while androgens are aromatized to oestrogens acting via the oestrogen receptor in some organs such as the brain.[22]

The essential nature of both androgens and androgen receptors in much human hair growth is shown by the absence of any changes in body or scalp hair growth after puberty in individuals without functional androgen receptors, that is those with the androgen insensitivity syndrome;[32] this occurs despite normal or raised androgen levels. Individuals with the complete form exhibit no pubic, axillary, chest or beard terminal hair and do not develop androgenetic alopecia (see Figure 4).

Although all hair follicles require intracellular androgen receptors to respond to androgens, there appears to be divergence in the requirement for 5α-reductase activity to produce intracellular 5α-dihydrotestosterone for the androgen response.[33] Individuals with 5α-reductase type 2 deficiency do not develop male patterns of body hair growth despite their circulating androgens; they only produce female patterns of pubic axillary hair, although their body shape becomes masculinized at puberty[34] (see Figure 4). They have not yet been reported to exhibit male-pattern baldness either, but this is more difficult to interpret. For many years they were said not to suffer from acne but a more recent investigation showed normal sebum production in 5α-reductase deficiency and reported some acne.[35]

Male secondary sexual hair growth, therefore, does appear to require intracellular 5α-reductase type 2 as well as androgen receptors, suggesting the classical mechanism of androgen action via 5α-dihydrotestosterone.[32] In contrast, pubic and axillary hair follicles are not only more sensitive to androgens but also may be using testosterone intracellularly, unless 5α-dihydrotestosterone is being formed by 5α-reductase type 1.[33] Cultured dermal papilla cells from pubic and axillary hair follicles do not form much 5α-dihydrotestosterone, unlike beard cells.[36] This would suggest testosterone itself was active. Whichever occurs, the mechanism of androgen action appears to differ between the male secondary sexual follicles and those found in both sexes, even though androgens are initiating similar changes in both follicles.

Current model for androgen action in the hair follicle

The mesenchyme-derived dermal papilla plays an important regulatory role in the follicle, altering many parameters and determining the type of hair produced.[37,38] Hair follicles appear to partially recapitulate embryogenesis during the hair cycle (compare chapters by Wu-Kuo and Chuong (Chapter 2) and Paus et al (Chapter 6)). Since steroids act via the mesenchyme in many developing steroid-dependent tissues,[39,40] androgens have been proposed to act on the other components of the follicle via the dermal papilla.[22,41] This hypothesis, summarized in Figure 7, involves circulating androgens entering the dermal papilla via its blood capillaries where they bind to androgen receptors within the dermal papilla cells of androgen-dependent hair follicles. Whether or not they would first be metabolized intracellularly to 5α-dihydrotestosterone would depend on the site of the follicle; for example, beard follicle cells would first metabolize testosterone with 5α-reductase type 2, but axillary and pubic cells would not[22,23,41,42] (see Figure 6).

In this hypothesis, the androgen-receptor complex would alter the gene expression of the dermal papilla cells so that they changed their production of regulatory factors for the other cell types of the follicle, particularly the keratinocytes and melanocytes. These factors could be soluble growth factors and/or extracellular matrix proteins.[22,41] Targets could also include the cells of the follicular connective tissue sheath, the dermal vasculature and even dermal papilla cells themselves, since all these would be altered in the formation of a differently sized follicle; the production of autocrine stimulatory factors by beard and scalp dermal papilla cells has recently been reported.[42] This would mean that the direct androgen target cells would be the dermal papilla cells, while other follicular components would be controlled indirectly by androgens. This would seem a realistic model since androgens have such widely differing effects on follicles in different body sites, including whether or not 5α-reductase type 2 is necessary for stimulation of hair growth. It is hard to imagine these responses being so well controlled if each target cell in the follicle had to respond directly to androgens.

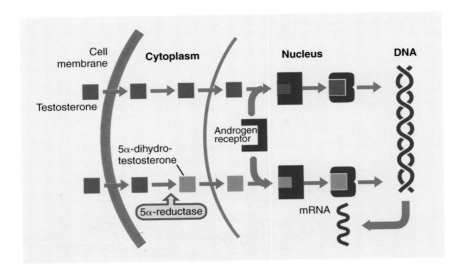

Figure 6

The mechanism of androgen action. Androgens from the blood diffuse through the plasma membrane. Inside the cell, testosterone may bind to the specific intracellular androgen receptor or be metabolized to the more potent androgen, 5α-dihydrotestosterone, by 5α-reductase enzyme. The androgen receptor binds 5α-dihydrotestosterone more strongly than testosterone. The hormone–androgen receptor complexes undergo a conformational change exposing their DNA binding sites. This enables them to bind to specific hormone response elements (HREs) in the DNA altering the expression of specific androgen-dependent genes and hence the production of specific proteins. In human hair growth, androgen receptors are needed for all body hair growth and androgenetic alopecia, but 5α-reductase type 2 is not required for pubic and axillary hair growth.

This hypothesis has now received much experimental support. High-affinity, low-capacity androgen receptors have been identified in cultured dermal papilla cells from androgen target follicles including beard[43] and balding scalp;[44] these cells contain higher levels than those from control, non-target follicles. They have also been located in the dermal papilla using immunohistochemistry but not elsewhere in the follicle using a monoclonal antibody technique,[45] although a recent study reported staining in both the papilla and the outer root sheath using a polyclonal antibody technique.[46] Important corroboration also comes from studies of the metabolism of androgens by cultured dermal papilla cells since this reflects hair growth in 5α-reductase deficiency (see Figure 4). In these studies, beard, but not pubic, cells produce 5α-dihydrotestosterone[34,47,48] corresponding to the absence of beard but the presence of pubic hair in these patients.

There is also substantial evidence from bioassays that cultured dermal papilla cells can secrete proteinaceous factors that promote growth in other dermal papilla cells,[41,49] outer root sheath cells,[50] transformed epidermal keratinocytes[51] and endothelial cells.[52] Interestingly, testosterone in vitro altered the mitogenic capacity of dermal papilla cells in line with its effect on hair growth in vivo. Testosterone stimulated beard, but not non-balding scalp, cells to produce greater mitogenic capability for beard dermal papilla cells[49] and outer root sheath cells;[50] in marked contrast, testosterone decreased the mitogenic capacity of androgenetic alopecia scalp dermal papilla cells from both men[51] and the stump-tailed macaque.[53] This reflection of the paradoxical in vivo responses of hair follicles to androgens in these in vitro experiments with cultured dermal papilla cells from two species also strongly supports the hypothe-

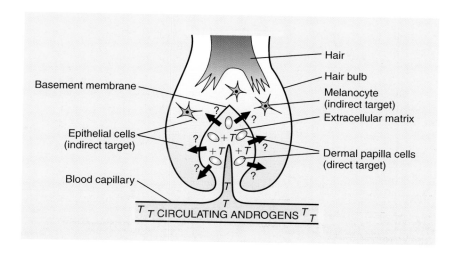

Figure 7

The current model of androgen action in the hair follicle. In this model, androgens from the blood enter the hair follicle via capillaries in the dermal papilla. They are bound by androgen receptors in the dermal papilla cells of androgen-sensitive follicles, stimulating an alteration in their production of regulatory paracrine factors. In some follicles binding to the receptors is preceded by metabolism to 5α-dihydrotestosterone. These paracrine factors then alter the activity of other follicular cells, including keratinocytes and melanocytes. *T*, testosterone, *?*, unknown paracrine factors. Reproduced from Randall, 1998.[42]

sis that androgens act via the follicular dermal papilla. Research is currently focused on identifying androgen-regulated factors but, to date, only insulin-like growth factor (IGF-1) has been reported as altered in vitro by androgens.[50] Several other factors have been suggested to play a role in hair growth[16] but so far only stem cell factor (SCF) is produced in higher amounts by androgen-dependent beard cells than in control non-balding scalp cells,[54] presumably in response to androgens in vitro. Since SCF is the ligand for the cell surface receptor, *c-kit* (discussed further by Castanet and Ortonne, Chapter 4), recently found on human hair follicle melanocytes,[55] this may play a role in androgen-potentiated changes in hair pigmentation.

Summary and conclusions

Androgens are clearly key regulators of human hair growth with intriguingly different effects on follicles from various parts of the body. The responses are intrinsic to the follicles themselves. The obvious strong contrasts between the stimulation of beard growth and inhibition of scalp hair are also further refined by progressive effects within these areas themselves as seen by the slow, gradual manifestation of balding in androgenetic alopecia. The length of the response to androgens also varies depending on the site, with beard growth being maintained into old age, while axillary growth is greatest around 30 years of age and then declines. These differences, and the marked racial variations in the amount of androgen-dependent hair growth, suggest that androgen responses depend on gene expression in individual follicles.

The effects of androgens are all dependent not only on the presence of circulating androgens but also of specific intracellular androgen receptors. However, only some follicles also require the presence of 5α-reductase type 2; an enzyme that can be inhibited by specific enzyme inhibitors, which are now being used clinically (see Chapter 13 by Price). The hypothesis that androgens act on the follicle by altering the production of paracrine regulators, such as growth factors and extracellular matrix, has received considerable support. Further investigation into the finer aspects of the mechanism of androgen action and the identification of specific paracrine factors secreted by the dermal papillae under hormonal regulation may enable us to understand the paradoxical variety of androgenic effects on human hair growth and facilitate the development of novel therapeutic regimens to control androgen-dependent hair disorders.

Acknowledgements

The assistance of Mr Chris Bowers and Mrs Jenny Braithwaite in the production of the figures and Mrs Christine Dove and Mrs Jayne Dunn in the preparation of the manuscript is gratefully acknowledged.

References

1. Ebling FG, Hale PA, Randall VA: Hormones and hair growth. In: Goldsmith LA (ed.). *Biochemistry and Physiology of the skin*, 2nd edn. Oxford, Clarendon Press, 1991: 660–696.
2. Morris D: *The Naked Ape.* London, Jonathon Cape Ltd, 1969.
3. Randall VA, Ebling EJG: Seasonal changes in human hair growth. *Br J Dermatol* 1991; **124**: 146–151.
4. Goodhart CB: The evolutionary significance of human hair patterns and skin colouring. *Advancement Sci* 1960; **17**: 53–58.
5. Ebling FJG: The mythological evolution of nudity. *J Hum Evolut* 1985; **14**: 33–41.
6. Reynolds EL: The appearance of adult patterns of body hair in man. *Ann NY Acad Sci* 1951; **53**: 576–584.
7. Marshall WA, Tanner JM: Variations in pattern of pubertal change in girls. *Arch Dis Child* 1969; **44**: 291–303.
8. Marshall WA, Tanner JM: Variations in the pattern of pubertal changes in boys. *Arch Dis Child* 1970; **45**: 13–23.
9. Giacometti L: Facts, legends and myths about the scalp throughout history. *Arch Dermatol* 1967; **95**: 629–635.
10. Dry FW: The coat of the mouse (*Mus Musculus*) *J Genet* 1926; **16**: 32–35.
11. Kligman AG: The human hair cycle. *J Invest Dermatol* 1959; **33**: 307–316.
12. Hamilton JB: Age, sex and genetic factors in the regulation of hair growth in man: a comparison of Caucasian and Japanese populations. In: Montagna W, Ellis RA (eds.). *The Biology of Hair Growth.* New York, Academic Press, 1958: 399–433.
13. Hamilton JB: A secondary sexual character that develops in men but not in women upon aging of an organ present in both sexes. *Anat Record* 1946; **94**: 466–467.
14. Hamilton JB: Patterned loss of hair in man; types and incidence. *Ann NY Acad Sci* 1951; **53**: 708–728.
15. Saitoh M, Sakamoto M: Human hair cycle. *J Invest Dermatol* 1970; **54**: 65–81.
16. Stenn KS, Combates NJ, Eilertson KJ, et al.: Hair follicle growth controls. In: Whiting DA (ed.). *Dermatol Clinics 14: Update on Hair Disorders.* Philadelphia, WB Saunders, 1996: 543–558.
17. Orentreich N: Scalp hair replacement in men. In: Montagna W, Dobson RL (eds.). *Advances in the Biology of Skin, Vol. 9, Hair Growth.* Oxford, Pergaman Press, 1969; 99–108.
18. Courtois M, Loussouarn G, Howseau S, et al.: Periodicity in the growth and shedding of hair. *Br J Dermatol* 1996; **134**: 47–54.
19. Reinberg A, Lagoguey M, Chauffourinier JM, Cesselin F: Circannual and circadian rhythms in plasma testosterone in five healthy young Parisian males. *Acta Endocrinol* 1975; **80**: 732–743.
20. Smals AGH, Kloppenberg PWC, Benrad THJ: Circannual cycle in plasma testosterone levels in man. *J Clin Endocrinol Metab* 1976; **42**: 979–982.
21. Bellastella A, Criscuoco T, Mango A, Perrone L, Sawisi AJ, Faggiano M: Circannual rhythms of LH, FSH, testosterone, prolactin and cortisol during puberty. *Clin Endocrinol* 1983; **19**: 453–459.
22. Randall VA: Androgens and human hair growth. *Clin Endocrinol* 1994; **40**: 439–457.
23. Winter JSD, Faiman C: Pituitary-gonadal relations in male children and adolescents. *Paed Res* 1972; **6**: 125–135.
24. Winter JSD, Faiman C: Pituitary-gonadal relations in female children and adolescents *Paed Res* 1973; **7**: 948–953.
25. Hamilton JB: Male hormone stimulation is a prerequisite and an incitant in common baldness. *Am J Anat* 1942; **71**: 451–480.
26. Hamilton JB: Effect of castration in adolescent and young adult males upon further changes in the proportions of bare and hairy scalp. *J Clin Endocrinol Metab* 1960; **20**: 1309–1318.
27. Orentreich N, Durr NP: Biology of scalp hair growth. *Clin Plast Surg* 1982; **9**: 197–205.

28. Ziller C: Pattern formation in neural crest derivatives. In: Van Neste D, Randall VA (eds.). *Hair Research for the Next Millennium*. Amsterdam, Elsevier, 1996; 1–5.

29. Sawers RA, Randall VA, Iqbal MJ: Studies on the clinical and endocrine aspects of antiandrogens. In: Jeffcoate SL (ed.). *Current Topics in Endocrinology 1: Androgens and Antiandrogen Therapy*. Chichester, John Wiley, 1982: 145–168.

30. Jeffcoate W: The treatment of women with hirsutism. *Clin Endocrinol* 1993; **39**: 143–150.

31. Kligman AM: The comparative histopathology of male-pattern baldness and senescent baldness. *Clin Dermatol* 1988; **6(4)**: 108–118.

32. Quigley CA: The androgen receptor: physiology and pathophysiology. In: Nieschlag E, Behre HM (eds.). *Testosterone: Action, Deficiency, Substitution*. Berlin, Springer-Verlag, 1998: 33–106.

33. Randall VA: The role of 5α-reductase in health and disease. In: Sheppard M, Stewart P (eds.). *Baillières Clinical Endocrinology and Metabolism 8: Hormones, enzymes and receptors*. 1994: 405–431.

34. Wilson JD, Griffin JE, Russell DW: Steroid 5α-reductase 2 deficiency. *Endocrinol Rev* 1993; **14**: 577–593.

35. Imperato-McGuinley J, Gautier T, Cai L, Yee B, Epstein J, Pochi P: The androgen control of sebum production. Studies of subjects with dihydrotestosterone deficiency and complete androgen insensitivity. *J Clin Endocrinol Metab* 1993; **76**: 524–528.

36. Hamada K, Thornton MJ, Liang I, Messenger AG, Randall VA: Pubic and axillary dermal papilla cells do not produce 5α-dihydrotestosterone in culture. *J Invest Dermatol* 1996; **106**: 1017–1022.

37. Oliver RF, Jahoda CAB: The dermal papilla and maintenance of hair growth. In: Rogers GE, Reis PR, Ward KA, Marshall RC (eds.). *The Biology of Wool and Hair*. London, Chapman & Hall, 1989: 51–67.

38. Jahoda CAB, Reynolds AJ: Dermal-epidermal interactions; adult follicle-derived cell populations and hair growth. In: Whiting DA (ed.). *Dermatology Clinics 14. Update on Hair Disorders*. Philadelphia, WB Saunders, 1996; 573–583.

39. Oka T, Yoshimura M: Paracrine regulation of mammary gland growth. In: Franchimont P (ed.). *Clinics in Endocrinology, vol 15*. London, WB Saunders, 1986: 79–99.

40. Cunha GR, Donjacour AA, Cook PS, et al.: The endocrinology and developmental biology of the prostate. *Endocrinol Rev* 1987; **8**: 338–362.

41. Randall VA, Thornton MJ, Hamada K, et al.: Androgens and the hair follicle: cultured human dermal papilla cells as a model system. *Ann NY Acad Sci* 1991; **642**: 355–375.

42. Randall VA: Androgens and hair. In: Nieschlag E, Behre HM (eds.). *Testosterone: Action, Deficiency, Substitution*, 2nd edn. 1998: 167–186.

43. Randall VA, Thornton MJ, Messenger AG: Cultured dermal papilla cells from androgen-dependent human follicles (e.g. beard) contain more androgen receptors than those from non-balding areas. *J Endocrinol* 1992; **133**: 141–147.

44. Hibberts NA, Randall VA: Dermal papilla cells from human balding scalp hair follicles contain higher levels of androgen receptors than those from non-balding scalp. *J Endocrinol* 1998; **156**: 59–65.

45. Choudhry R, Hodgins MB, Van der Kwast TH, Brinkman AO, Boersma WJA: Localisation of androgen receptors in human skin by immunohistochemistry: implications for the hormonal regulation of hair growth, sebaceous glands and sweat glands. *J Endocrinol* 1992; **133**: 467–475.

46. Sawaya ME, Price VH: Different levels of 5α-reductase type I and II, aromatase and androgen receptor in hair follicles of women and men with androgenetic alopecia. *J Invest Dermatol* 1997; **109**: 296–301.

47. Itami S, Kurata S, Takayasu S: 5α-reductase activity in cultured human dermal papilla cells from beard compared with reticular dermal fibroblasts. *J Invest Dermatol* 1990; **94**: 150–152.

48. Thornton MJ, Liang I, Hamada K, Messenger AG, Randall VA: Differences in testosterone metabolism by beard and scalp hair follicle dermal papilla cells. *Clin Endocrinol* 1993; **39**: 633–639.

49. Thornton MJ, Hamada K, Messenger AG, Randall VA: Beard, but not scalp, dermal papilla cells secrete autocrine growth factors in response to testosterone in vitro. *J Invest Dermatol* 1998; **111**: 727–732.

50. Itami S, Kurata S, Takayasu S: Androgen induction of follicular epithelial cell growth is mediated via insulin-like growth factor I from dermal papilla cells. *Biochem Biophys Res Commun* 1995; **212**: 988–994.

51. Hibberts NA, Randall VA: Testosterone inhibits the capacity of cultured cells from human balding scalp dermal papilla cells to produce keratinocyte mitogenic factors. In: Van Neste DV, Randall VA (eds.). *Hair Research for the Next Millennium*. Amsterdam, Elsevier, 1996: 303–306.

52. Hibberts NA, Sato K, Messenger AG, Randall VA: Dermal papilla cells from human hair follicles secrete factors (e.g. VEGF) mitogenic for endothelial cells. *J Invest Dermatol* 1996; **106**: 341.

53. Obana N, Uno H: Dermal papilla cells in macque alopecia trigger a testosterone-dependent inhibition of follicular cell proliferation. In: Van Neste DV, Randall VA (eds.). *Hair Research for the Next Millennium*. Amsterdam, Elsevier, 1996: 307–310.

54. Hibberts NA, Messenger AG, Randall VA: Dermal papilla cells derived from beard hair follicles secrete more stem cell factor (SCF) in culture than scalp cells or dermal fibroblasts. *Biochem Biophys Res Commun* 1996; **222**: 401–405.

55. Randall VA, Jenner TJ, DeOliveira I: The human hair follicle contains several populations of melanocyte-lineage cells with differential expression of three melanocyte-lineage markers, *c-kit* and Bcl-2. *J Invest Dermatol* (submitted).

6
Control of the hair follicle growth cycle

Ralf Paus, Sven Müller-Röver and Ian McKay

The hair cycle

The life of a mature hair follicle can be divided into three important phases of pattern formation: The first occurs during hair follicle morphogenesis (Figure 1: Stages 1–8), when two tiny clusters of apparently homogenous epithelial and mesenchymal cells develop into a highly organized mini-organ with the capacity to produce hair fibres.[1] The second is seen after completion of hair follicle morphogenesis, that is, when the hair cycle is initiated, which, surprisingly, starts not with growth but with the first phase of hair follicle regression (catagen), followed by a so-called 'resting' phase (telogen). The third phase of pattern formation is seen during the subsequent growth stage of the hair cycle (anagen) (see Figure 1: showing catagen, telogen and anagen), which recapitulates morphologically, at least in part, hair follicle morphogenesis.[2] Following this first cycle, these phases are repeated continuously through the animal's life. The main characteristics of each phase of the hair cycle are summarized in Table 1.

Catagen

Since it is a commonly held concept that hair cycling starts with hair growth (anagen), it deserves special emphasis that the life-long cyclic transformation of the hair follicle (catagen → telogen → anagen → catagen …) commences *not* with an extended growth phase including proliferation and hair fibre production, *but* with a period of patterned organ involution.[2] During catagen, the hair follicle undergoes a dramatic process of regression and partial organ suicide during which the central and proximal outer root sheath and the inner root sheath as well as the hair matrix are deleted. This rapid, stringently regulated form of organ involution by massive, yet highly controlled apoptosis of follicular keratinocytes in precisely predetermined regions of the hair follicle[3] may be viewed as a striking example of *inverse* pattern formation.

Catagen-associated follicular regression is characterized by the termination of pigment production, substantial extracellular matrix-remodelling and condensation of the dermal papilla, which may be controlled by intra- and perifollicular protease/antiprotease systems[2–5] and interconnected adhesion receptors such as cadherins and neuronal cell adhesion molecule (NCAM).[6–8] The shortening of the regressing epithelial strand and the upwards movement of the dermal papilla within the connective tissue sheath is probably dependent on massive apoptosis of the majority of hair matrix keratinocytes,[3] in combination with strong cell adhesion of the remaining keratinocytes,[9] for example as a result of epithelial cadherins.[7,8]

An instructive example of a de-regulated upwards movement of the dermal papilla caused by a combined apoptosis and adhesion defect is the *hairless* mouse mutation. In these mice, in addition to the occurrence of massive and abnormally located apoptosis, the epithelial strand seems to rip apart because of an adhesion defect. The dermal papillae, as well as remnants of the regressing epithelial strand, remain in the deep subcutis and start to develop into cysts.[10,11] As a consequence, the remnants of the distal part of the hair follicles fail to develop into a regular telogen follicles and degenerate into sack-like structures, which are connected to the epidermis forming dermal cysts. Thus, the protective zinc-

Table 1   Synopsis of key stages of the hair cycle.

Stage	Key characteristics	Human scalp	
		Duration*	Percentage*
Anagen	• **Growth phase** • Construction of the 'fibre production unit': hair matrix, inner root sheath • Hair shaft production via massive proliferation of keratinocytes of the hair matrix and fast differentiation in the pre-cortical matrix • Pigmentation of the hair shaft via follicular melanogenesis • Neuronal plasticity • Remodelling of the hair follicle immune system (e.g. development of the immune privilege of the hair matrix)	1–6 years	80–90%
Catagen	• **Regression phase** • Programmed, apoptosis-driven regression of the proximal hair follicle: deconstruction of the fibre production unit • Follicular melanogenesis is switched off including partial melanocyte apoptosis • Club hair development • Condensation and upward movement of the dermal papilla • Massive remodelling of the follicular basement membrane • Phagocytosis of excess basement membrane by macrophages (?)	Weeks (?)	<1%
Telogen	• **Resting phase** • Maturation of the club hair (?) • Several progenitor cells remain in the secondary hair germ and the bulge region	3–9 months	10–20%
Exogen	• (Hypothetical) phase of *active* hair shedding	?	?

*periods and percentages vary – on human body with site; in animals with species.

finger transcription factor that is coded by the normal *hairless* gene appears to be crucial for controlling the inverse pattern formation of catagen, namely for regulating the necrobiology and topobiology of the regressing hair follicle.[10,11]

Although only the proximal part of the hair follicle (i.e. below the insertion of the arrector pili muscle) is generally considered to be affected by the catagen-associated regression, it has been recently demonstrated in mice that the so-called 'permanent' part of the distal follicular epithelium above the insertion of the arrector pili muscle (which includes the bulge, the main seat of the epithelial stem cells of the hair follicle— see Chapter 3 by Cotsarelis) also undergoes substantial apoptosis during catagen.[3]

Telogen

Although hair follicle morphogenesis is partially similar to anagen development, it is by no means identical to it since anagen hair follicles develop from pre-existing telogen follicles, and not de novo. These telogen follicles already represent a complex combination of distinct, highly differentiated cells of mesenchymal, epithelial and neuroectodermal origin, such as keratinocytes of the outer root sheath and the secondary hair germ, including the epithelial stem cells of the hair follicle (see Chapter 3 by Cotsarelis), fibroblasts of the dermal papilla and the perifollicular connective tissue sheath, melanocytes, sebocytes, Langerhans' cells and T cells, and perifollicular endothelial and mast cells as well as macrophages. Merkel cells.[12] In contrast to the developing hair bud, a telogen hair follicle is already highly innervated and vascularized. The telogen follicle also shows substantial proliferative and metabolic activity. In addition, the duration of telogen is lightly variable and subject to modulation by numerous extra- and intrafollicular signals (Figure 2, Table 2). Finally, there is evidence to suggest the extension of the newly formed 'club hair' that is characteristic of telogen

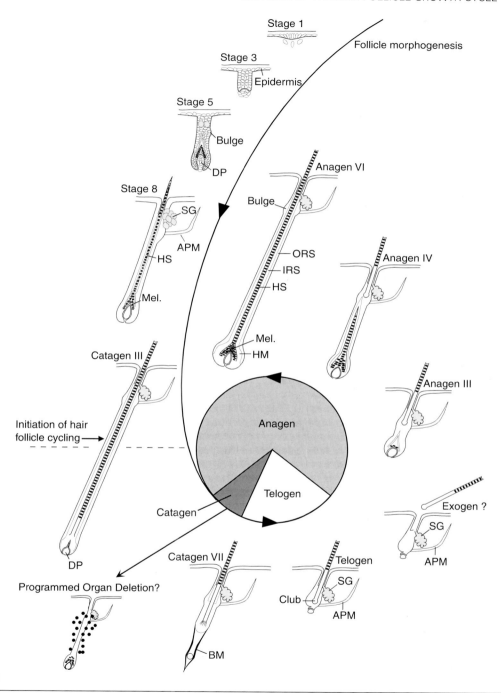

Figure 1

Schematic representation of key stages of hair follicle development and cycling, modified after Stenn et al.[4]
Stages 1–8 represent distant stages of hair follicle development.[1]
Anagen, growth phase; catagen, regression phase; telogen, resting phase; exogen, active shedding phase of the hair shaft;
APM, arrector pili muscle; BM, basement membrane; DP, dermal papilla; HS, hair shaft; HM, hair matrix; IRS, inner root
sheath; mel, melanin; ORS, outer root sheath; SG, sebaceous gland.

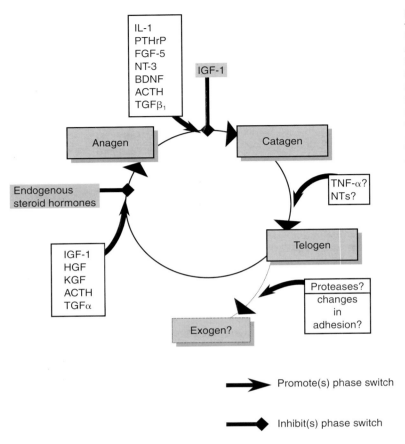

Figure 2

Modulators of hair growth.
ACTH, adrenocorticotrophin; BDNF, brain-derived neurotrophic factor; FGF-5, fibroblast growth factor-5; HGF, hepatocyte growth factor; IGF-1, insulin-like growth factor-1; IL-1, inter-leukin-1; KGF, keratinocyte growth factor; NT, neurotrophin, PTHrP, parathyroid hormone-related peptide; TGF, transforming growth factor; TNFα, tumour necrosis factor-α

follicles, is an actively regulated process (see below).[4,9] Thus, telogen cannot really be regarded as the 'resting phase' that it once was thought to be.

Anagen

For the production of a new hair shaft, an entirely new 'factory for fibre production' is established in the form of the anagen hair bulb.[5] Various stimuli such as injection of cyclosporin A or plucking of the hair, i.e., a mild wounding of the hair follicle epithelium, easily induce hair growth (anagen).[2,4,5] It is an important feature of anagen that not only the hair shaft is growing but that most epithelial hair follicle compart-ments undergo proliferation, with hair matrix

keratinocytes located around the dermal papilla showing the highest proliferative activity. In addition, the newly formed hair shaft is pig-mented by the follicle pigmentary unit,[5,9] while the production unit that generates the hair shaft and contains the pigment producing hair follicle melanocytes enjoys a special immune privi-lege.[12]

Telogen as the 'pre-regeneration state' of the hair follicle cycle

It remains mysterious why the hair follicle, immediately after being constructed during mor-phogenesis, is already de-constructed again. Perhaps, telogen is best viewed as the 'pre-

Table 2   Selected intrinsic hair cycle control signals in mice.*

	Inhibitors	Promotors
	Anagen inhibition and/or catagen induction and/or telogen prolongation	**Anagen induction, promotion, prolongation and/or catagen inhibition**
Hormones	• Glucocorticosteroids • PTHrp • Estrogen	• ACTH • PTH (7–34)
Growth factors	• BDNF • BMP-4 • EGF • FGF-2 • FGF-5 • NT-3, NT-4 • TGFα • TGF-β1	• FGF-7 • HGF/SF • IGF-1
Cytokines	• IL-1 • IL-6	
Neuropeptides		• Substance P

*ACTH, adrenocorticotropic hormone; BDNF, brain-derived neurotrophic factor; BMP, bone morphogenic protein; EGF, epidermal growth factor; FGF, fibroblast growth factor; HGF/SF, hepatocyte growth factor/scatter factor; IGF, insulin-like growth factor; NT, neurotrophin; PTHrp, parathyroid hormone-related peptide; TGF, transforming growth factor; IL, interleukin.

regeneration state' of the follicle, that is, whenever a hair follicle seeks to regenerate itself following severe damage, it enters into catagen in order to deconstruct itself and to become a telogen hair follicle, again. In fact, rapid catagen induction is the most effective way to return to the *telogen state* and to reconstruct a new fibre factory.[13] In addition, the return to telogen by partial organ suicide at the end of each extended period of hair growth may also be associated with the inherent risk of hair shaft production going awry. Since hair shafts are extremely durable biostructures compared with other epithelial products they must be prevented from entering the perifollicular skin, which would cause a vigorous, inflammatory foreign body reaction.[35] Thus, returning to the *telogen state* during the hair cycle will routinely limit fibre production.

Furthermore, returning to the *telogen state* might be important for the prevention of follicle-derived skin cancer.[35] A huge amount of trichocytes have to be generated to produce a hair shaft; therefore, the hair matrix displays one of the highest rates of proliferation in any mammalian tissue, even outranking that of many malignant tumours. Comparisons with other very

rapidly proliferating tissues, such as bone marrow and mucosal epithelium suggest there should be a high risk of malignant degeneration—particularly when taking into account the very high rate of intrafollicular melanogenesis during anagen stages III–VI, with its associated generation of oxygen radicals and toxic intermediates of melanogenesis. In contrast to this expected risk, malignant tumours of hair matrix keratinocytes or melanocytes are extremely rare, if they ever occur at all. Thus, re-entering the *telogen state* during cycling may be crucial for the prevention of malignant degeneration.[35]

The proposed telogen default state, therefore, is more than a mere 'resting' state, and is clinically important, since it may be pharmaceutically targeted, for example by hair drugs that prolong anagen for the treatment of alopecia or effluvium,[21] or that 'freeze' follicles in telogen for the management of hirsutism.

Exogen

In most mammalian species, a new hair shaft is generated *before* the old hair shaft is shed in order to assure that the animal is never naked.[9] Since the process of active hair shedding may well represent a separate and distinctive phase of the hair cycle, the intriguing term 'exogen' has been proposed to single out this hair cycle stage.[4,9] One key effector molecule in the control of active hair shedding (exogen) may be the adhesion receptor desmoglein 3.[13] Mice with a targeted disruption of desmoglein 3 display *normal* hair follicle morphogenesis and normal onset of telogen. However, in contrast to wild-type control mice, they display a wave-like pattern of hair loss from head to tail because the telogen hair shafts are not appropriately anchored in the outer root sheath by desmoglein 3. By entering into anagen, new hair shafts are grown and lost again during the consecutive telogen. Thus, desmoglein 3 expression on those keratinocytes that surround the club hair appears to be of critical importance for keeping the hair shaft anchored during telogen.[18]

Programmed Organ Deletion (POD)

Total hair follicle deletion occurs under pathological conditions in the form of scarring alopecias, for example as a result of ionizing radiation, *lichen planopilaris* or *lupus erythematodes*.[5,19] Nevertheless, it has been demonstrated in the murine system that hair follicles can also undergo a *physiological* process of total follicle destruction.[20] This process of programmed organ deletion (POD) eliminates a very small number of isolated hair follicles in the apparently normal skin of non-infected, non-traumatized mice, where the distal outer root sheath of individual follicles becomes surrounded by a dense inflammatory cell infiltrate, consisting mainly of activated macrophages. In a very few follicles, these immune cells infiltrate the bulge region, which represents the major seat of the epithelial stem cells[34] (discussed by Cotsarelis in Chapter 3). The induction of pathological apoptosis in this region of the outer root sheath may subsequently lead to total destruction of the hair follicle. The molecular controls of programmed organ deletion remain to be identified. Nevertheless, the concept of physiological programmed organ

deletion of the hair follicle has important clinical implications, since currently the only way to achieve permanent hair removal (e.g. for the therapy of hirsutism) is to destroy the entire follicle by electroepilation or laser application. Careful induction of follicular programmed organ deletion may be the most effective way to treat such unwanted hair growth.

Clinical relevance of the hair cycle

Most patients presenting with hair growth disorders in clinical practice suffer from unwanted hair loss (effluvium or alopecia) or unwanted hair growth (hirsutism or hypertrichosis). Very simplistically, one might classify most cases of common hair loss (e.g. androgenetic alopecia, alopecia areata, non-androgenetic causes of telogen effluvium) as processes of premature termination of anagen associated with premature entry into catagen, while hypertrichosis and hirsutism depend at least partially on overly extensive anagen prolongation and/or catagen inhibition.[21] Therefore, clinically it is critically important to dissect the molecular controls of the anagen–catagen transformation of the hair cycle.

Hair cycle hypotheses

During the last decades, only relatively few hypotheses have been proposed to explain the basic characteristics of hair follicle cycling. Several elements have to be covered by a comprehensive hair cycle theory.[2,35] Firstly, it must include an explanation of how pattern formation during hair follicle morphogenesis is established and how it is linked to repetitive pattern formation during cycling (transformation of a large anagen stage VI hair follicle into a small telogen follicle and back again into a large anagen VI follicle etc.). Secondly, a comprehensive hair cycle theory must explain the striking autonomy and periodicity of hair cycling (i.e. what is the 'oscillator' of the hair cycle clock that forces the follicle periodically to enter into anagen–catagen–telogen?). Thirdly, each theory must explain the induction/

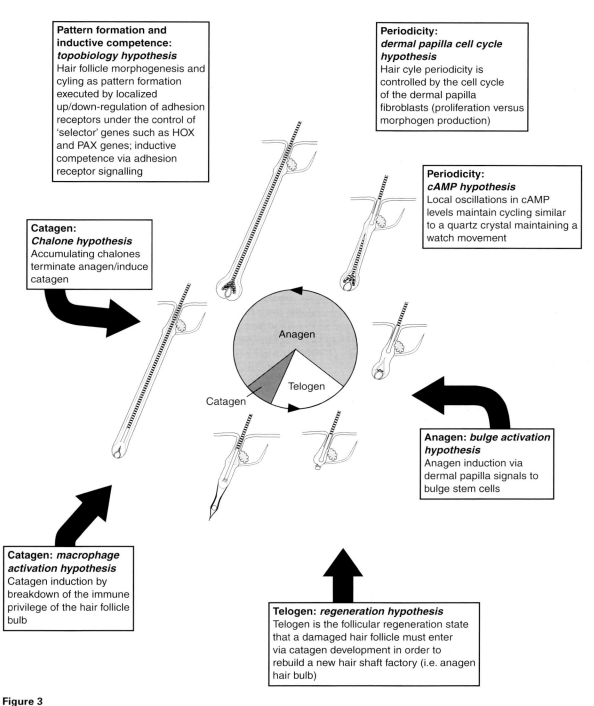

Pattern formation and inductive competence: *topobiology hypothesis*
Hair follicle morphogenesis and cyling as pattern formation executed by localized up/down-regulation of adhesion receptors under the control of 'selector' genes such as HOX and PAX genes; inductive competence via adhesion receptor signalling

Periodicity: *dermal papilla cell cycle hypothesis*
Hair cyle periodicity is controlled by the cell cycle of the dermal papilla fibroblasts (proliferation versus morphogen production)

Periodicity: *cAMP hypothesis*
Local oscillations in cAMP levels maintain cycling similar to a quartz crystal maintaining a watch movement

Catagen: *Chalone hypothesis*
Accumulating chalones terminate anagen/induce catagen

Catagen: *macrophage activation hypothesis*
Catagen induction by breakdown of the immune privilege of the hair follicle bulb

Anagen: *bulge activation hypothesis*
Anagen induction via dermal papilla signals to bulge stem cells

Telogen: *regeneration hypothesis*
Telogen is the follicular regeneration state that a damaged hair follicle must enter via catagen development in order to rebuild a new hair shaft factory (i.e. anagen hair bulb)

Anagen

Telogen

Catagen

Figure 3

Hair cycle hypotheses

termination phase of each stage (what induces and what terminates anagen, catagen and telogen?).[2,35] Figure 3 summarizes several hypotheses that address these three issues at least in part.

The topobiology hypothesis

According to this hypothesis,[7] the segmentation or regionalization of skin is probably established—similar to all other organ systems that have been investigated—by overlapping gradients of 'selector' genes such as Homeobox (HOX) or Paired Box (PAX) genes.[7,22–25] Indeed, there is increasing evidence that adhesion receptors are key effector molecules of selector genes.[7,22–25] The selector gene-controlled modulation of adhesion receptor expression (e.g. on the aggregating fibroblasts of the dermal papilla) may lead to selective cell sorting (e.g. by expressing NCAM[7]) or to selective binding of specific components of the extracellular matrix (e.g. by integrins). In addition, binding of adhesion receptors to their ligands may dramatically modulate the gene and protein expression patterns[26] of key cell populations in hair-cycle control, including alterations of the cellular phenotype and feedback loops for the control of selector gene expression. This may not only alter the three-dimensional form of follicular cell subpopulations but also their competence to elaborate or react to morphogens.[7] Cell sorting by means of distinct cell adhesion profiles, also seems to play a role during later hair follicle morphogenesis and again during anagen development, since the selective expression of epithelial adhesion receptors (e.g. E- and P-cadherin) on distinct compartments of the follicle separates hair matrix, inner and outer root sheaths and likely serves important signalling functions.[8,27–29]

Macrophage activation hypothesis

These hypotheses[30–32] have emphasized the role of 'activated' macrophages in catagen development, which appear to accumulate around the regressing hair follicle and might drive catagen development, for example by eliminating excess basement membrane or by secreting catagen-promoting factors. In contrast, they could be responding to some hair follicle-derived stimulus, for example resulting from the disruption of the connective tissue sheath during catagen. It is far from clear, however, whether macrophages are functionally important in catagen control,[12,33] even though their role in hair follicle cycling certainly deserves to be clarified.

The bulge activation hypothesis

In their landmark paper, Cotsarelis et al.[34] identified the bulge region of the outer root sheath as a site of epithelial stem cells in murine hair follicles. According to their hypothesis, the stem cells of the bulge are activated by a signal emanating from the dermal papilla, leading to the generation of a population of very rapidly proliferating keratinocytes ('transient amplifying cells'). Consecutively, the transient amplifying cells construct the new anagen hair bulb.[34] The *bulge activation hypothesis* is a persuasive scenario of how an anagen hair follicle is constructed, and runs its course from anagen stages I–VI (see Figure 1). Likewise, this hypothesis develops reasonably well how dermal papilla, bulge and hair matrix may interplay during the three-dimensional development of the hair follicle. Exhaustion of the proliferative potential of these cells is proposed as the *trigger* of catagen.[34] Nevertheless, it remains to be explained convincingly why the dermal papilla secretes the initial signal for anagen induction, and why this occurs in a periodic fashion; also, the bulge activation hypothesis fails to explain how the putative exhaustion of the proliferative potential of hair matrix cells can bring about all the other catagen-associated follicular transformations, such as epithelial cell and melanocyte apoptosis, extensive remodelling of the hair follicle, extracellular matrix, immune system and innervation and inhibition of melanogenesis.[2]

Hair cycle periodicity

Since most hair diseases are, at least in part, cycling disorders, from a clinical point of view, it is of critical importance to understand how the hair follicle is forced to enter in a highly rhythmic fashion into the repetitive process of anagen–catagen– telogen transformations.[21] Several hypotheses address the difficult problem of how this periodicity may be established, and what the nature of the oscillator, the genuine 'hair cycle clock', might be (Figure 3).[35] To describe this 'hair cycle clock', the workings of a quartz clock may be invoked as a metaphor for the basic principles of hair follicle cycling. An unknown molecular 'battery' may provide the initial impulse to start oscillations in one or more follicular cell populations. Oscillations are then counted by an intracellular mechanism. A threshold may be reached at which time one or more cell populations change their phenotype and their secretory activities leading to a phase change in the hair cycle.

The Chalone hypothesis

In the earliest hypothesis for the nature of such a counting mechanism, Herman Chase suggested that hair follicle cycling may be based on an inhibition/des-inhibition system.[36] During each anagen phase, an unknown endogenous mitotic inhibitor or *chalone* was postulated to accumulate gradually in the epithelial hair bulb. After reaching a threshold of activity, this mitotic inhibitor would terminate anagen and induce catagen by shutting off keratinocyte proliferation in the bulb; the activity of this mitotic inhibitor would then slowly decrease during telogen, down to a level that des-inhibits anagen development.[2] This visionary concept appears still to be relevant since inhibition/des-inhibition systems are now recognized to drive numerous comparable developmental systems, including feather and tooth development.[37]

The dermal papilla cell cycle hypothesis

According to this hypothesis,[2,35] dermal papilla fibroblasts secrete a 'cocktail' of dermal papilla morphogens, which induce and maintain anagen, only so long as these fibroblasts are in the G0/G1 phase of their cell cycle. Continued secretion of dermal papilla morphogens requires feedback signals from the hair matrix, which may also modulate the composition of the dermal papilla morphogen 'cocktail'. Although this linkage of the cell cycle machinery and the 'hair cycle clock' offers the most comprehensive hair cycle hypothesis proposed so far, this hypothesis needs to be tested further, since conflicting data have been reported concerning the precise hair cycle stage during which dermal papilla fibroblast proliferation occurs in human, sheep and rodent skin.[2,38,39]

The cAMP hypothesis

In this hypothesis[2] the nature of the oscillator is explained in analogy to the pulsatile secretion of melatonin from the pineal.[40] There, the 'battery' is represented by daylight, the impulse is cAMP, the 'oscillator' is a combination of the cAMP-response element binding proteins (CREB) transcription factor and its inhibitor, inducible cAMP early repressor (ICER), and the output is pulsatile melatonin secretion.[40] This mechanism of oscillation could apply to one or more cell populations in the hair follicle (and may even be driven by the cell cycle, as in the dermal papilla cell cycle hypothesis). Certainly, there are photoperiodic effects on hair growth,[5,9] and CREB has already been implicated in feather development,[41] although neither CREB nor ICER expression have been studied during hair follicle morphogenesis or cycling. Indeed, modulators of cAMP levels such as ACTH and capsaicin also modulate the hair cycle.[14,42–44] One possible candidate for the 'accumulating chalone' invoked by Chase[36] might be telomerase, which has been shown to be involved in a well-known intracellular counting mechanism: for example, oscillatory mechanisms involving cAMP may be coupled to changes in telomerase activity through the cell cycle. Telomerase has actually been demonstrated to accumulate almost exclusively in the actively dividing portions of the hair bulb in anagen hair follicles, and to diminish in catagen hair follicles.[45]

Conclusions and future directions

Based on the clinical importance of hair cycle modulation, alopecias may become preventable or treatable by anagen prolongation and/or inhibition of premature catagen induction.[21] Candidate signalling pathways that might be manipulated for this purpose are listed in Table 2 and Figure 2. Provided that exogen (active hair shedding) is, indeed, a separately controlled phase of the hair cycle,[9] the inhibition of exogen, for example by targeted suppression of *desmoglein 3* down-regulation, may help to reduce the cosmetically and psychologically disturbing effects of telogen effluvium, since exogen inhibition would prevent hair shaft shedding even though the follicles remain in telogen.

Conversely, unwanted hair growth (e.g. hypertrichosis, hirsutism) may be reduced by catagen induction, and/or by arresting the hair follicle in the *telogen state* after hair shaft depilation by commercially available waxes or depilation cremes. In addition, *permanent* hair removal may be achieved by eliminating the hair follicle via the therapeutic induction of programmed organ deletion.[20]

Although many basic principles of hair follicle growth control await clarification, several simple and clinically relevant postulates for the treatment of hair diseases can be defined.[46] Although the hair cycle can be modulated by numerous extrinsic and intrinsic factors,[4,5,9,21,46] the hair cycle clock is located in the skin itself. Thus, effective hair cycle control should in principle be achievable by *topical* drug application. The most promising topical formulations are applications targeted to the hair follicle itself, for example by the use of appropriate liposome preparations.[47]

The activities that such clinically useful, topically applicable hair drugs should exhibit may best be classified into the following three classes:[46]

(1) *Inhibitors/stimulators of keratinocyte apoptosis* (control of catagen-associated hair bulb involution);
(2) *Inhibitors/stimulators of morphogen secretion by the dermal papilla* (modulation of the stage-specific milieu of cytokines, growth factors etc.);
(3) *Inhibitors/stimulators of morphogen recognition by hair matrix and follicular epithelial stem cells* (targeted inhibition/activation of relevant receptors).

It is reasonable to expect that combinations of hair drugs from *different* hair drug classes will be considerably more effective in clinical hair growth management than the currently favoured forms of monotherapy (e.g. with minoxidil or finasteride).

Summary

The hair follicle growth cycle is characterized by at least three different stages: after completion of morphogenesis, the follicle initially undergoes dramatic apoptosis-driven involution (catagen) to enter telogen, which is followed by active hair follicle growth and production of a pigmented hair shaft (anagen). Whenever a follicle is reversibly damaged, it tends to return to the *telogen default state* by catagen induction. Active shedding of the hair shaft may be interpreted as a separate phase of hair follicle cycling, termed *exogen*. The only escape for the hair follicle from its life-long, repetitive entry into cycles of anagen–catagen–telogen–anagen ... and so on, may be to die by a process termed programmed organ deletion (POD), during which the entire hair follicle is irreversibly removed by macrophage-driven attack on the bulge, the site of epithelial stem cells in the hair follicle. Although the hair follicle growth cycle is now appreciated to be modulated by a multitude of growth-regulatory factors that switch the local signalling milieu, the basic 'hair cycle clock' that periodically drives these cyclic transformations of the intra- and perifollicular signalling milieu has still not been identified. Yet, several hypothetical scenarios briefly covered here may guide future experimental work to reveal the molecular nature of the elusive 'hair cycle clock'.

Acknowledgements

The compilation of this chapter was suggested in part by a grant from EU RP and IAM (Brite-Euram III: BE97–4301).

References

1. Philpott MP, Paus R: Principles of hair follicle morphogenesis. In: Chuong CM: *Molecular Basis of Epithelial Appendage Morphogenesis*, Austin, Texas, Landes, 1998.
2. Stenn K, Nixon AJ, Jahoda CAB, Mckay I, Paus R: What controls hair follicle cycling? *Exp Dermatol* 1999; **8**: 229–236.
3. Lindner G, Botchkarev VA, Botchkarev NV, Ling G,

van der Veen C, Paus R: Analysis of apoptosis during murine hair follicle regression (catagen). *Am J Pathol* 1997; **151(6)**: 1601–1617.

4. Stenn KS, Combates NJ, Eilersten KJ, et al.: Hair follicle growth controls. *Dermatol Clinics* 1996; **14**: 543–558.

5. Paus R, Cotsarelis G: The biology of hair follicles. *N Engl J Med* 1999; **341**: 491–497.

6. Müller-Röver S, Botchkarev VA, Peters EJM, Panteleyev A, Paus R: Distinct patterns of NCAM expression are associated with defined stages of murine hair follicle morphogenesis and regression. *J Histochem Cytochem* 1998; **46**: 1401–1410.

7. Müller-Röver S and Paus R: Topobiology of the hair follicle: adhesion molecules as morphoregulatory signals during hair follicle morphogenesis. In: Chuong CM: *Molecular Basis of Epithelial Appendage Morphogenesis*, Austin, Texas, Landes, 1998.

8. Müller-Röver S, Tokura Y, Welker P, et al.: E- and P-cadherin expression during murine hair follicle development and cycling. *Exp Dermatol* 1999; **8**: 237–246.

9. Stenn K, Parimoo S, Prouty S: Growth of the hair follicle: a cycling and regenerating biological system. In: Chuong CM: *Molecular Basis of Epithelial Appendage Morphogenesis*, Austin, Texas, Landes, 1998.

10. Panteleyev AA, van der Veen C, Rosenbach T, Müller-Röver S, Sokolov VE, Paus R: Towards defining the pathogenesis of the hairless phenotype. *J Invest Dermatol* 1998; **110**: 902–907.

11. Panteleyev AA, Botchkareva NV, Sundberg JP, Christiano AM, Paus R: The role of the hairless (hr) gene in the regulation of hair follicle catagen transformation. *Am J Pathol* 1999; **1555**: 159–171.

12. Paus R, van der Veen C, Eichmüller S, Kopp T, Hagen E, Müller-Röver S, et al.: Generation and cycling remodeling of the hair follicle immune system in mice. *J Invest Dermatol* 1998; **111**: 7–18.

13. Paus R, Handjiski B, Eichmüller S, Czarnetzki BM: Chemotherapy-induced alopecia in mice. Induction by cyclophosphamide, inhibition by cyclosporine A, and modulation by dexamethasone. *Am J Pathol* 1994; **144**: 719–734.

14. Paus R, Heinzelmann T, Schultz KD, Furkert J, Fechner K, Czarnetzki BM: Hair growth induction by substance P. *Lab Invest* 1994; **71**: 134–140.

15. Straile W, Chase H, Arsenault C: Growth and differentiation of hair follicles between periods of activity and quiescence. *J Exp Zool* 1961; **148**: 205–221.

16. Johnson E: Moulting cycles. *Mammalian Rev* 1972; **1**: 198–208.

17. Pinkus H: Factors in the formation of club hair. In: Browne AC, Crounse RG: *Hair, Trace Elements and Human Illness*. New York, Praeger, 1980.

18. Koch PJ, Mahoney MG, Cotsarelis G, Rothen-

berger K, Lavker RM, Stanley JR: Desmoglein 3 anchors telogen hair in the follicle. *J Cell Sci* 1998; **III**: 2529–2537.

19. Hermes B, Paus R: 'Vernarbende' Alopezien. Anmerkungen zur Qualifikation, Differentialdiagnose und Pathobiologie. *Hautarzt* 1998; **49**: 462–472.

20. Eichmüller S, van der Veen C, Moll I, Hermes B, Hofmann U, Müller-Röver S, et al.: Perifollicular, inflammatory cell infiltrates: physiological degeneration of selected hair follicles by 'programmed organ deletion'. *J Invest Dermatol* 1997; **108**: 654a.

21. Paus R: Control of the hair cycle and hair diseases as cycling disorders. *Curr Opin Dermatol* 1996; **3**: 248–258.

22. Edelman GM: *Topobiology: An Introduction to Molecular Embryology*. New York, Basic Books, 1988.

23. Edelman GM: Morphoregulation. *Dev Dyn* 1992; **193**: 2–10.

24. Edelman GM, Jones FS: Developmental control of N-CAM expression by Hox and Pax gene products. *Philos Trans R Soc Lond B Biol Sci* 1995; **349**: 305–312.

25. Dhouailly D, Prin F, Kanzler B, Viallet JP: Variations of cutaneous appendages: regional specification and cross-species signals. In: Chuong CM: *Molecular Basis of Epithelial Appendage Morphogenesis*, Austin, Texas, Landes, 1998.

26. Aplin AE, Howe A, Alahari SK, Juliano RL: Signal transduction and signal modulation by cell adhesion receptors: the role of integrins, cadherins, immunoglobulin-cell adhesion molecules, and selectins. *Pharmacol Rev* 1998; **50**: 197–263.

27. Hirai Y, Nose A, Kobayashi S, Takeichi M: Expression and role of E- and P-cadherin adhesion molecules in embryonic histogenesis. II. Skin morphogenesis. *Development* 1989; **105**: 271–277.

28. Fujita M, Furukawa F, Fujii K, Horiguchi Y, Takeichi M, Imamura S: Expression of cadherin cell adhesion molecules during human skin development: morphogenesis of epidermis, hair follicles and eccrine sweat ducts. *Arch Dermatol Res* 1992; **284**: 159–166.

29. Hardy MH, Vielkind U: Changing patterns of cell adhesion molecules during mouse pelage hair follicle development. 1. Follicle morphogenesis in wild-type mice. *Acta Anat* 1996; **157**: 169–182.

30. Parakkal PF: Role of macrophages in collagen resorption during hair growth cycle. *J Ultrastruct Res* 1969; **29**: 210–217.

31. Westgate GE, Craggs RI, Gibson WT: Immune privilege in hair growth. *J Invest Dermatol* 1991; **97**: 417–420.

32. Paus R, Czarnetzki BM: Neue Perspektiven der Haarforschung: Auf der Suche nach der Haarzyklusuhr. *Hautarzt* 1992; **43**: 264–271.

33. Paus R, Müller-Röver S, Christoph T: Hair follicle immunology: a journey into *terra incognita*. *J Invest Dermatol Symp Proc* 1999; [In press]

34. Cotsarelis G, Sun TT, Lavker RM: Label-retaining cells reside in the bulge area of pilosebaceous unit: implications for follicular stem cells, hair cycle, and skin carcinogenesis. *Cell* 1990; **61**: 1329–1337.

35. Paus R, Müller-Röver S, Botchkarev VA: Chronobiology of the hair follicle: hunting the 'hair-cycle clock'. *J Invest Dermatol Symp Proc* 1999; [In press]

36. Chase HB: Growth of the hair. *Physiol Rev* 1954; 113–126.

37. Chuong CM: Feather morphogenesis: a model of the formation of epithelial appendages. In: Chuong CM: *Molecular Basis of Epithelial Appendage Morphogenesis*, Austin, Texas, Landes, 1998.

38. Sholley MM, Cotran RS: Endothelial DNA synthesis in the microvasculature of rat skin during the hair growth cycle. *Am J Anat* 1976; **147**: 243–254.

39. Bassukas ID, Kiesewetter F, Schell H, Hornstein OP: In situ [³H]thymidine labelling of human hair papilla: an in vitro autoradiographic study. *J Dermatol Sci* 1992; **3**: 78–81.

40. Foulkes NS, Borjigin J, Snyder SH, Sassone-Corsi P: Rhythmic transcription: the molecular basis of circadian melatonin synthesis. *Trends Neurosci* 1997; **20**: 487–492.

41. Widelitz RB, Jiang TX, Noveen A, Ting-Berreth SA, Yin E, Jung HS, et al.: Molecular histology in skin appendage morphogenesis. *Microsc Res Tech*. 1997; **38(4)**: 452–465.

42. Paus R, Maurer M, Slominski A, Czarnetzki BM: Mast cell involvement in murine hair growth. *Dev Biol* 1994; **163**: 230–240.

43. Maurer M, Fisher E, Handjiski B, Barandi A, Meingasser J, Paus R: Activated skin mast cells are involved in hair follicle regression (catagen). *Lab Invest* 1997; **77**: 319–332.

44. Slominski A, Botchkareva NV, Botchkarev VA, Chakraborty A, Luger T, Uenalan M, et al.: Hair cycle-dependent production of ACTH in mouse skin. *Biochim Biophys* 1998; **1448**: 147–152.

45. Ramirez RD, Wright WE, Shay JW, Taylor RS: Telomerase activity concentrates in the mitotically active segments of human hair follicles. *J Invest Dermatol* 1997; **108**: 113–117.

46. Paus R: Principles of hair cycle control. *J Dermatol (Tokyo)* 1998; **25**: 793–802.

47. Li L, Hoffman RM: Model of selective gene therapy of hair growth: liposome targeting of the active Lac-Z gene to hair follicles of histocultured skin. *In Vitro Cell Dev Biol* 1995; **31**: 11–13.

7

Signalling molecules in human hair follicle cell populations

Ulrike Blume-Peytavi and Nathalie Mandt

Introduction

The last few years have witnessed an acceleration in understanding the epidermal–mesenchymal signalling within the hair follicle itself, as well as in the interplay between the hair follicle and the perifollicular vascular, nervous and immune system.[1-6] It is well established that hair follicle development, initiation of hair cycling and hair growth control mechanisms involve a wide variety of cellular regulation processes such as cell proliferation and differentiation, cellular adhesion and spreading, migration, apoptosis, and chemotaxis (see Chapters 2 and 6 by Chuong and Wu-kuo and Paus et al respectively). Moreover, increasing knowledge has been achieved in hair follicle biology, especially in the field of signal transduction and in the significance of signalling molecules, such as cytokines, growth factors and angiokines (see Chapter 8 by Philpott).

Members of the following growth factor families have been documented to be involved in hair cycle processes:

- Epidermal Growth Factor family (EGFf)[7,8]
- Heparin-Binding Growth Factor family including Fibroblast Growth Factor family (FGF-1, -2, -4, -5, KGF)[7,9] and Vascular Endothelial Growth Factor (VEGF)[10-13]
- Transforming Growth Factor family (TGFs, BMPs)[14-15]
- Plateled-Derived Growth Factor family (PDGFAA, PDGFBB)[16]
- Insulin-like Growth Factor family (IGF-1, IGF-2)[17-19]
- Colony Stimulating Factors (GM-CSF)[3,20]
- Many other unclassified growth factors, for example HGF.[21,22]

In addition, cytokines, such as interleukin (*IL*)-*1*, tumour necrosis factor (*TNF*)α and interferon (*IFN*)γ have been demonstrated as powerful modulators of hair follicle activity, causing mainly induction of catagen-like changes and growth arrest.[23] The role of selected growth factors and cytokines in the development, growth and cycling of the human hair follicle is summarized in Table 1. Several of these growth factors and cytokines are supposed to act as paracrine or autocrine regulators; however, within the pilosebaceous unit it seems that only the cascade of different individual factors leads to the effective regulation of the hair growth cycle.

Molecular signals involved in both the development of new hair follicles and the hair cycle are key concerns in hair research; a main aim is to identify *key molecules* involved in switch-on and switch-off mechanisms for the different phases of the human hair cycle. Reliable in vitro techniques are currently used to study these aspects in the human hair follicle as follows:

- Culture of individual epithelial and mesenchymal cell populations of the human hair follicle, such as follicular and interfollicular keratinocytes, dermal papilla cells, fibrous sheath fibroblasts, germinative cells, and sebocytes,
- Co-culture techniques of individually grown cell populations, and
- Whole-organ culture of microdissected individual human hair follicles.

Histochemical, biological and molecular investigations using these tools have, and are continuing to, contribute to elucidate the role of cell-cell and cell-matrix signalling, as well as the central role of cytokines, growth factors and adhesion molecules in hair growth regulatory mechanisms.

Table 1 The role of selected growth factors and cytokines in hair follicle development, hair growth and hair cycle activity.*

Signalling molecules	Function in hair development, hair growth and hair cycle activity
EGF	• Delays follicular development • Retards hair growth and cycling • Induces follicle regression and catagen-like changes in vitro • Stimulates elongation but thereafter causes thickening/vacuolization of the lower outer root sheath, upward migration of the matrix, cell-club hair-like structure formation
TGFα	• Controls normal positional development of the hair follicle • Retards hair growth in vitro in mice
aFGF and bFGF	• Angiogenic, together with VEGF, possibly responsible for formation and maintenance of perifollicular blood vessels • Important for skin appendage morphogenesis and the formation of skin appendage domains, induce the expansion of further bud domain, specifically expressed in feather germs
FGF4 (host oncoprotein)	• Necessary for follicular development and for epithelial regeneration • Induces placode formation, present in dermal condensation independent from epidermis, also present in epithelial placode thereafter, induces the expansion of further bud domain
FGF5	• Hair elongation inhibitor • Initiates transition from anagen phase into catagen
VEGF	• Probably responsible for the maintenance of the perifollicular capillaries in anagen
TGFβ-1,2,3	• Inhibits follicular development • Gene overexpression in the epidermis leads to marked reduction of epidermal and follicular proliferation and decreased number of hair follicles in mice
BMP-2, BMP-4	• In development expressed on the dermal condensation independent from the presence of epidermis, also present in epithelial placode thereafter • Necessary for epithelial regeneration
NGFβ	• Probably trophic functions for neurons • Probably responsible for maintenance of perifollicular nerves in anagen
TNFα	• Probably responsible for inducing apoptosis, unable to induce hair regeneration
PDGF-A, B	• PDGFs are pleiotropic • Important in follicular development and vasculogenesis • Mitogenic for mesenchymal cells • Stimulates hair canal development

* Data from refs 1, 5, 8, 10–13, 15, 16–18, 24–27.

The dermal papilla is believed to be crucial in orchestrating hair follicle activity, especially the regulation of cell proliferation and differentiation of hair follicle matrix, possibly by emiting specific signals inducing different stages of the hair cycle. Therefore, most studies have focused on the mesenchymal component of the human hair follicle. These have demonstrated that dermal papilla cells synthesize several cytokines, growth factors and some, yet unidentified, secreted bioactive soluble molecules,[28–30] which probably initiate and control the intrafollicular epithelial and mesenchymal interactions.

The most interesting stage of the hair cycle is the catagen stage, which is the initialization of programmed cell death, leading to telogen, with subsequent hair loss. Apparently it is a very active and a highly regulated stage of the hair cycle involving the inhibition of cellular divisions, cell death, cessation of hair growth and resorption of the lower two-thirds of the hair follicle. It has been suggested that it occurs as a consequence of decreased expression of anagen-maintaining cytokines (e.g. IGF-1, bFGF and VEGF) and the increased expression of cytokines promoting destructive processes (e.g. TGFβ, IL-1, TNFα).[24,31,33]

Insulin-like Growth Factor-1 (IGF-1) is currently

regarded as one of the most important growth factors for the maintenance of the hair follicle in anagen. IGF-1 is present in the dermal papilla and possibly acts on neighbouring structures such as bulbar and follicular keratinocytes. Recent studies have demonstrated that IGF-1 stimulates keratinocyte proliferation and differentiation and protects against apoptosis in vitro.[19] Indeed IGF-1 stimulates hair follicle growth and prevents the transition to catagen in vitro.[18] Nevertheless, it has been suggested that IGF-1 may be a morphogen not a mitogen owing to the distribution of IGF-1 and its receptors in the hair follicle.[19]

Basic Fibroblast Growth Factor (bFGF) and *Vascular Endothelial Growth Factor (VEGF)* are suggested to be responsible for the creation and proper functioning of perifollicular capillaries in anagen. *Vascular Endothelial Growth Factor (VEGF)* is regarded as the most important positive regulator of angiogenesis and vascular permeability; its significance has also been demonstrated in the human hair follicle.[11,12] Human cultured dermal papilla cells synthesize large amounts of this cytokine, which is possibly responsible for the regulation of hair vascularization. VEGF is upregulated by proinflammatory IL-1α, IL-1β and GM-CSF. In addition, growth factors known to behave, in general, as angiogenic, such as TGF-β1, PDGFAA, as well as the catagen-preventing IGF-I, significantly stimulated VEGF mRNA expression in human dermal papilla cells. It seems highly likely that the growth factors necessary for the induction and maintenance of the anagen phase may also sustain the function of perifollicular capillaries. Therefore, the strong relationship between proinflammatory cytokines and VEGF secretion provides new insights into the significance of altered vascular supply during the different phases of the growth cycle, and in the course of many inflammatory processes affecting the human hair follicle. Cultured human dermal papilla cells synthesize significant amounts of *granulocyte macrophage-colony stimulating factor (GM-CSF)*; these are up-regulated by proinflammatory cytokines IL-1α, IL-1β and TNF-α in a time-dependent manner.[35] It seems likely, therefore, that the dermal papilla via its production of GM-CSF may play a crucial role in the pathogenesis of inflammatory processes in the human hair follicle; it is possible that GM-CSF may be involved in the regulatory mechanisms of the intrinsic cycling capacity of each hair follicle.

Transforming Growth Factor β1 (TGF-β1) partially inhibits follicular proliferation and hair follicle growth in vitro.[21,35] Thus, early catagen changes could be caused by this factor, which is highly expressed on follicular structures.[4,14,35]

Recently, whole organ culture methods showed that *Interleukin-1α (IL-1α)*, *Interleukin-1β (IL-1β)*, *Tumor Necrosis Factor-α (TNF-α)* (potent) and *Tumor Growth Factor-β (TGF-β)* (mild) are inhibitors of hair follicle growth in vitro, whereas *Interleukin-4 (IL-4)* and *Interferon-γ (IFN-γ)* did not affect hair follicle growth.[4,20] The dermal papilla may serve as a source for IL-1β in the human hair follicle[37] since dermal papillae cells synthesize significant amounts in vitro. IL-1β is able to completely abrogate hair follicle growth.[23,37] In contrast, IL-4, a Type 2 cytokine, mainly augmenting antibody production, was not found to affect hair follicle growth in vitro.[20] It has been reported that IL-1α inhibits growth of cultured human hair follicles, although no changes in morphology have been described.[23] Interestingly, IL-1α was recently detected in sebaceous glands in vivo.[38] In addition, it was shown previously that non-stimulated cultured human sebocytes that were maintained under serum-free conditions express IL-1α mRNA and produce marked amounts of IL-1α protein.[39] However, further research is required to investigate the interaction between cells of the pilar apparatus and cells of the sebaceous gland to elucidate fully the complex cytokine network within the pilosebaceous unit leading to effective signalling and correct co-ordination of interactive growth processes of the human hair follicle. Furthermore, an additional target of hair follicle research in the future will be the investigation of intracellular signalling events linking the well-known action of cytokines and growth factors at the plasma membrane level to downstream events taking place at the nuclear level.

The follicular expression of cytokines and growth factors and their corresponding receptors identified by studies of cultured human hair follicle cell populations, is summarized schematically in Figure 1 and detailed in Table 2. These results provide evidence for the significant role of the autocrine and paracrine activity of dermal papilla cells and follicular keratinocytes.

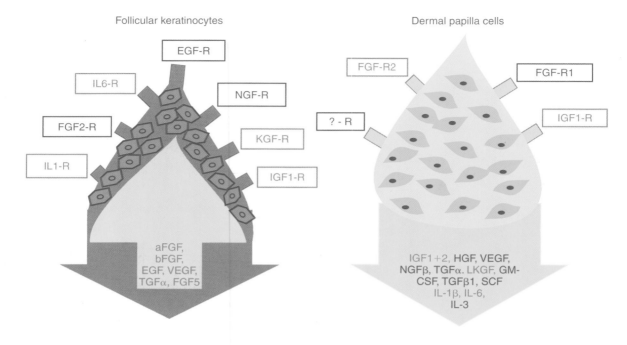

Figure 1

Epithelial-mesenchymal interaction in the human hair follicle: possible intrafollicular autocrine and paracrine signalling molecules and their corresponding receptors in dermal papilla cells and follicular keratinocytes.

Conclusions

The follicular localization of growth factors, cytokines and their receptors as found in the whole organ culture model, in cultured individual hair follicle cell populations in vitro, and in in vivo investigations, together with the data on the regulatory effects of these molecules on hair follicle growth in vitro, are beginning to be moulded into an integrated model of pilosebaceous regulation (Table 2). Pro-inflammatory cytokines, such as IL-1α, IL-1β, IL-4, IL-6, and GM-CSF, the angiokine VEGF and growth factors such as IGF-I, HGF, KGF, NGF, TGF-β1, and PDGF-AA have been identified as the most interesting candidates. Based on the research in the current literature, speculations can be made on

the roles of these different signalling molecules in the control of the hair cycle. Three groups can be distinguished:

(1) *Initiation of the anagen phase*: IGF-1, EGF, TGFα, bFGF and VEGF, as strongly mitogenic factors for keratinocytes and endothelial cells;
(2) *Maintenance of the mature anagen follicle*: IGF-1 and VEGF as stimulating proliferation, vascularization, and differentiation processes;
(3) *Induction of catagen* and *hair follicle degradation*: IL-1, IL-4, TNFα, TNFβ, FGFs and TGFβ with their action as growth-inhibiting and pro-apoptotic cytokines.

Improving our knowledge of the role of growth factors and cytokines in hair follicle biology

Table 2 Expression of the most important signalling molecules in the human hair follicle and in cultured human hair follicle cell populations and their regulatory effects*

Signalling molecule	Cell population or structure	Effect, function	Corresponding receptor
Hepatocyte Growth Factor (HGF)	DP, DPC	• Stimulates follicular proliferation in vitro • Enhanced mRNA expression by IL1-α, TNF-α, TPA but suppressed by TGF-β	HGF-receptor • Only in follicular epithelium of mice
Interleukin-1β H(IL-1B)	Human HF	• Negative on growth • Condensation of dermal papilla, vacuolisation of precortical matrix, abnormal keratinization of the hair fibre and inner root sheath	IL-1 receptor I • Human follicular epithelium • Probably ORS follicular matrix cells
Insulin growth factor (IGF-1)	DP, DPC	• Strongly stimulates keratinocyte proliferation and protects against apoptosis in vitro	IGF-R • Probably on follicular and matrix keratinocytes;
IGF-2	Not on ORS	• Stimulates follicular cells' metabolism, mitogenesis and differentiation	
Insulin growth factor binding protein (IGFBP)	or highly proliferative matrix KC	• Maintains anagen and prevents transition to catagen in vitro	
Stem cell factor (SCF)	DPC	• Localization-dependent secretion	c-kiv. Identified on melanocytes
Transforming Growth Factor-β (TGF-β) superfamily	Hair follicle	• Inhibits keratinocyte proliferation and hair growth in vitro	TGF-β receptor • Several receptors with wide follicular distribution
Vascular Endothelial Growth Factor (VEGF)	DP, DPC	• Stimulation of endothelial cells • Probably responsible for hair vascularisation	VEGF receptor • Human tissue
Epidermal growth factor (EGF)	ORS in vitro and in vivo	• Stimulates proliferation of ORS • Negative on growth of human hair follicles	EGF receptor • ORS, bulb matrix
Tumor necrosis factor (TNFα, TNFβ)	Human HF	• Inhibits hair growth in vitro, shorten anagen and induce catagen, causes catagen-like changes in vitro	TNF receptor • Becomes highly expressed in catagen follicles
TNFα		• Condensation of dermal papilla, vacuolisation of percortical matrix, abnormal keratinization of the hair fibre and inner root sheath	

*Data from refs 1, 4, 8, 10, 12, 18, 20, 22, 24, 37, 40, 41
†DP, dermal papilla; DPC, dermal papilla cells; HF, hair follicle; ORS, outer root sheath; KC, keratinocytes; IRS, inner root sheath.

seems, therefore, to be an essential direction in improving our understanding of pathogenic mechanisms and developing new therapeutic approaches in hair follicle disorders in the future, based on selective targeting.

References

1. Little J, Westgate G, Evans A, Granger S: Cytokine gene expression in intact anagen hair follicles. *J Invest Dermatol* 1994; **103**: 715–720.
2. Akiyama M, Smith L, Holbrook K: Growth factor and growth factor receptor localisation in the hair follicle bulge and associated tissue in human fetus. *J Invest Dermatol* 1996; **106**: 391–396.
3. Blume-Peytavi U: Control of the human hair cycle: Function of the dermal papilla and its significance. *Z Hautkr* 1996; **6**: 410–415.
4. Hoffmann R, Eicheler W, Huth A, et al.: Cytokines and growth factors influence hair growth in vitro. Possible implications for the pathogenesis and treatment of alopecia areata. Arch Dermatol Res 1996; **288**: 153–156.
5. Paus R, Peters EMJ, Eichmüller S, Botchkarev VA: Neural mechanisms of hair growth control. *J Invest Dermatol* 1997; **2**: 61–68.
6. Danilenko DM, Ring BD, Pierce GF: Growth factors and cytokines in hair follicle development and cycling: recent insights from animal models and the potentials for clinical therapy. *Mol Med Today* 1996; **2**: 460–467.
7. Du Cross DL: Fibroblast growth factor and epidermal growth factor in hair development. *J Invest Dermatol* 1993; **101**: 106S–113S.
8. Philpott MP, Kealey T: Effects of EGF on the morphology and patterns of DNA synthesis in isolated human hair follicles. *J Invest Dermatol* 1994; **102**: 186–191.
9. Herbert JM, Rosenquist T, Götz J, Martin GR: FGF5 as a regulator of the hair growth cycle: evidence from targeted and spontaneous mutations. *Cell* 1994; **78**: 1017–1025.
10. Lachgar S, Charveron M, Gall Y, Plouet J, Bonafe JL: Vascular endothelial cells: Targets for studying the activity of hair follicle cell-produced VEGF. *Cell Biol Toxicol* 1996a; **12**: 331–334.
11. Lachgar S, Moukadiri H, Jonca F, et al.: Vascular endothelial growth factor is an autocrine growth factor for hair dermal papilla cells. *J Invest Dermatol* 1996; **106**: 17–23.
12. Kozlowska U, Blume-Peytavi U, Kodelja V, et al.: Vascular Endothelial Growth Factor expression in various compartments of the human hair follicle. *Arch Dermatol Res* 1998; **290**: 661–668.

13. Kozlowska U, Blume-Peytavi U, Kodelja V, et al.: Vascular endothelial growth factor induced by proinflammatory cytokines (IL-1α,β) in cells of the human pilosebaceous unit. *Dermatology* 1998; **196**: 89–92.
14. Massague J: The transforming growth factor beta family. *Ann Rev Cell Biol* 1990; **6**: 597–641.
15. Chuong CM, Widelitz RB, Ting-Berrath S, Jiang TX: Early events during avian skin appendage regeneration: dependence on epithelial-mesenchymal interaction and order of molecular reappearance. *J Invest Dermatol* 1996; **107**: 639–646.
16. Takakura N, Yoshida H, Kunisada T, Nishikawa S, Nishikawa SI. Involvement of platelet-derived growth factor receptor-α in hair canal formation. *J Invest Dermatol* 1996; **107**: 770–777.
17. Philpott M, Sanders D, Kealey T: Cultured human hair follicles and growth factors. *J Invest Dermatol* 1995; **104**: 44S–45S.
18. Philpott M, Sanders D, Kealey T: Effects of insulin and insulin-like growth factors on cultured human hair follicles: IGF-I at physiologic concentrations is an important regulator of hair follicle growth in vitro. *J Invest Dermatol* 1994; **102**: 857–861.
19. Rudman S, Philpott M, Thomas GA, Kealey T: The role of insulin-like growth factor I in human skin and its appendages: Morphogen as well as mitogen? *J Invest Dermatol* 1997; **109**: 770–777.
20. Philpott M, Sanders T, Bowen J, Kealey T: Effects of interleukins, colony-stimulating factor and tumour necrosis factor on human hair follicle growth in vitro: A possible role for interleukin-1 and tumour necrosis factor-alpha in alopecia areata. *Br J Dermatol* 1996; **135**: 942–948.
21. Shimaoka S, Tsuboi R, Jindo T, et al.: Hepatocyte growth factor/scatter factor expressed in follicular papilla cells stimulates human hair growth in vitro. *J Cell Physiol* 1996; **165**: 333–338.
22. Jindo T, Tsuboi R, Imai R, Takamori K, Rubin JS, Ogawa H: Hepatocyte growth factor/scatter factor stimulates hair growth of mouse vibrissae in organ culture. *J Invest Dermatol* 1994; **103**: 306–309.
23. Harmon C, Nevins T: Il-1α inhibits human hair follicle growth and hair fibre production in whole-organ cultures. *Lymphokine and Cytokine Res* 1993; **12**: 197–203.
24. Little J, Redwood KL, Granger S, Jenkins GJ: In vivo cytokine and receptor gene expression during the rat hair growth cycle. Analysis by semi-quantitative RT-PCR. *Exper Dermatol* 1996; **5**: 202–212.
25. Lyons KM, Hogan BL: Involvement of bone morphogenetic protein-4 (BMP-4) and Vgr-1 in morphogenesis and neurogenesis in the mouse. *Development* 1991; **111**: 531–542.
26. Noji S, Koyama E, Myokai F, et al.: Differential expression of three chick FGF receptor genes,

FGFR1, FGFR2 and FGFR3, in the limb and feather development. *Prog Clin Biol Res* 1993; **383**: 645–654.

27. Widelitz RB, Jiang TX, Noveen A, Chen C-WJ, Choung C-M: FGF induces new feather buds from developing avian skin. *J Invest Dermatol* 1996; **107**: 797–803.

28. Francz P, Bayreuther K, Limat A, Noser F: Differentiating dermal papilla fibroblasts express specific cellular and secreted proteins in vitro. *Ann NY Acad Sci* 1991; **642**: 501–502.

29. Limat A, Hunziker T, Waelti E, Inaebnit S, Wiesmann U, Braathen LR: Soluble factors from human hair papilla cells and dermal fibroblasts dramatically increase the clonal growth of outer root sheath cells. *Arch Dermatol Res* 1993; **285**: 205–210.

30. Thornton MJ, Hamada K, Messenger AG, Randall VA: Androgen-dependent dermal papilla cells secrete autocrine growth factor(s) in response to testosterone unlike scalp cells. *J Invest Dermatol* 1998; **111**: 727–732

31. Seiberg M, Marthinuss J, Stenn K: Changes in expression of apoptosis associated genes in skin mark early catagen. *J Invest Dermatol* 1995; **104**: 78–82.

32. Mandt N, Geilen CC, Schudrowitz A, et al.: Evidence of Interleukin-1β and Interleukin-4 induced apoptosis in human follicular keratinocytes in vitro. Possible role in the initiation of catagen. Symposium Proceedings of the Second Intercontinental Meeting of Hair Research Societies. *J Invest Dermatol* 1999; [in press]

33. Hoffman R, Wenzel E, König A, Happle R: Expression and regulation of Il-1 and Il-1-RA in cultured dermal papilla cells. *J Invest Dermatol* 1995; **105**: 467.

34. Tavakkol A, Elder J, Griffiths C, et al.: Expression of growth hormone receptor, insulin-like growth factor (IGF-1) receptor mRNA and proteins in human hair follicle. *J Invest Dermatol* 1992; **99**: 343–349.

35. Blume-Peytavi U, Kozlowska U, Kodelja V, Sommer Ch, Orfanos CE: Dermal papilla cells differentially express and synthesize Granulocyte Macrophage Colony Stimulating Factor (GM-CSF). *Arch Dermatol Res* 1998; **403**: 105.

36. Philpott MP, Westgate GE, Green M, Kealey T: An in vitro model for the study of the human hair growth. *Ann New York Acad Sci USA* 1991; **642**: 148–166.

37. Xiong Y, Harmon CS: Interleukin-1beta is differentially expressed by human dermal papilla cells in response to PKC activation and is a potent inhibitor of human hair follicle growth in organ culture. *J Interferon Cytokine Res* 1997; **17**: 151–157.

38. Boehm KD, Yun JK, Strohl KP, Elmets CA: Messenger RNAs for the multifunctional cytokines interleukin-1 alpha, interleukin-1 beta and tumor necrosis factor-alpha are present in adnexal tissues and in dermis of normal human skin. *Exper Dermatol* 1995; **4**: 335–341.

39. Zouboulis CC, Xia L, Akamatsu H, et al.: The human sebocyte culture model provides new insights into development and management of seborrhoea and acne. *Dermatology* 1998; **196**: 21–31.

40. Hibberts N, Messenger A, Randall V: Dermal papilla cells derived from beard hair follicles secrete more stem cell factor (SCF) in culture than scalp cells or dermal fibroblasts. *Biochem Biophys Res Commun* 1996; **222**: 401–405.

41. Barch J, Mercuri F, Werther G: Identification and localization of insulin-like growth factor-binding protein (IGFBP) messenger RNAs in human hair follicle dermal papilla. *J Invest Dermatol* 1996; **106**: 471–475.

The roles of growth factors in hair follicles: investigations using cultured hair follicles

Michael P Philpott

Background to hair follicle culture in vitro

Several in vitro models have been developed to study hair follicle biology, ranging from mono-layer cell culture through to whole skin organ maintenance. All of these models have been used widely and have generated significant hair growth data, which are reviewed elsewhere.[1,2] The aim of this chapter is to focus on the culture of isolated hair follicles and how these hair folli-cle models have been used in studies to deter-mine the role of growth factors in hair follicle biology. In this chapter, the way combined studies using in vitro follicle models, along with RT-PCR and immunohistochemistry, have led to the proposal of some simple hair growth regula-tory models will be discussed.

There has always been considerable interest in developing methods of hair follicle isolation and culture and this is reflected in the number of dif-ferent approaches taken to achieve this goal. Several early reports described the in vitro growth of embryonic hair follicles in isolated skin plugs.[3–9] The ability of these skin plugs to sustain prolonged hair growth was, however, generally found to decrease both with time in culture and with increasing age of the embryo from which the skin is removed. So much so that by birth very little in vitro hair growth was usually observed. Likewise, the in vitro maintenance of hair follicles in post-embryonic skin resulted in limited, suboptimal rates of hair growth.[10] More-over, a significant disadvantage of using skin plugs that contain several hair follicles is that they do not permit detailed biochemical and

morphological analysis of individual hair foll-icles. Furthermore, there is usually considerable outgrowth of cells from the skin plug itself, making data difficult to interpret.

Studies on individual isolated hair follicles have always been difficult to perform owing to the problems of obtaining sufficient numbers of follicles with which to work. Individual microdis-sected mouse hair follicles have been used to study the increase in hair follicle bulb length with time in culture[11] and morphological studies have been carried out on microdissected rat hair foll-icles.[12] All these studies demonstrated that intact hair follicles could be isolated and, when placed in culture, would continue to grow for between 24–48 hours. However, these models were never used to any significant degree to investigate hair biology as such. A significant advance in the use of in vitro follicles as a model with which to investigate hair biology was made by Buhl and colleagues[13] who showed that the growth of cul-tured vibrissae follicles was stimulated by the agent minoxidil, thus demonstrating that cul-tured hair follicles may be used to investigate factors that regulate hair growth.

Following on from these studies both Kondo[14] and Philpott et al[15] reported new methods for the isolation of human hair follicles from facelift skin, and showed that these follicles could be success-fully maintained in vitro. In our studies[15–17] iso-lated human hair follicles could be maintained in vitro for up to 9 days during which time they underwent in vivo patterns of cell proliferation and differentiation, giving rise to a keratinized hair fibre at rates similar to that seen in vivo. Moreover, it was demonstrated in our early studies that cultured human hair follicles were highly responsive to exogenous growth factors[15,16] Subsequently, in vitro cultured follicles have been widely used to investigate the role of growth factors in hair biology (Table 1).

Epidermal growth factor and transforming growth factor-alpha

Both epidermal growth factor (EGF) and transforming growth factor-alpha (TGF-α) have been implicated strongly in the regulation of hair growth. In vivo studies have shown that when EGF is injected into newborn mice, hair growth is inhibited[18] and that when injected[19] or infused[20] into sheep, hair growth is inhibited and the fleece is shed. Light and electron microscopy[20,21] have shown that in sheep, these depilatory infu-

sions of EGF trigger the hair follicles to switch from anagen to catagen. On the basis of these studies, it has been suggested that EGF, or its related TGF-α, may be important regulators of the hair growth cycle in vivo, especially during the switch from anagen to catagen.

In vitro, both EGF and TGF-α have also been shown to have a 'depilatory-like' effect on cultured human hair follicles.[15,22] Moreover, the in vitro data also appears to mimic the in vivo changes seen in sheep, and also some aspects of the in vivo switch from anagen to catagen. Detailed analysis of the in vitro data, however, suggests that this switch from anagen to catagen may in fact be an artifact. It has been shown that in vitro EGF stimulates the marked proliferation of a population of basal cells that reside in the outer root sheath of the hair follicle.[22] Activation of these outer root sheath cells results in the marked thickening of the hair follicle outer root sheath that, in effect, squeezes the hair follicle

Table 1 Cultured hair follicles and growth regulatory factors.

Growth factor	Result	Reference
Cyclosporin A	Prolongs growth of cultured follicles	77
1,25 (OH)2 D3	Biphasic, stimulates growth at low concentration, inhibits growth at high concentration	78
EGF/TGF-α	Stimulates outer root sheath proliferation, mimics in vivo depilation reported in sheep	22
EGF/TGF-α	Stimulates collagenase release from follicle organoids	79
FGF-1 (aFGF)	Accelerates entry into catagen in absence of insulin	(unpublished data)
FGF-I (aFGF)	Stimulates ORS keratinocyte outgrowth	(unpublished data)
FGF-2 (bFGF)	Stimulates ORS keratinocyte outgrowth	(unpublished data)
IL-1α	Inhibits hair follicle growth	69, 70
IL-1β	Inhibits hair follicle growth	69, 70
KGF	Delays catagen in absence of insulin	(unpublished data)
KGF	Stimulates ORS keratinocyte outgrowth	(unpublished data)
IGF-I	Stimulates follicle growth in absence of insulin	41
IGF-I	Prevents entry into catagen	41
IGF-I	Stimulates growth of red deer follicles (mane)	48
IFN	Stimulates HLA-DR in ORS	80
HGF	Stimulates mouse and human follicle growth	50, 51
Minoxidil	Stimulates whisker growth	13
Oestrogen	Inhibits hair follicle growth	14
PDGF	Stimulates connective tissue sheath	(unpublished data)
13-cis-retinoid acid	Regulates hair fibre/hair sheath interactions	81
Testosterone	Inhibits hair follicle growth	14
Testosterone	Stimulates growth of red deer follicles (mane)	48
TGF-β	Inhibits hair follicle growth	15
TNF-α	Inhibits hair follicle growth	69

matrix cells upward within the hair follicle. As a result of this expansion of the outer root sheath, and the upward movement of the matrix cells, normal patterns of cellular interaction between the dermal papilla and the germinative epithelium are disrupted. Thickening of the outer root sheath has also been reported in vivo — in sheep injected with EGF.[20,21] In vivo such disruption to hair follicle architecture would probably trigger the hair to enter the resting telogen stage of its hair growth cycle. It is possible therefore, that the anagen to catagen switch reported in vivo may be secondary to the EGF-stimulated disruption of normal hair follicle epithelial-mesenchymal interactions.

If the EGF-induced hair cycle seen in sheep is a response to follicle disruption, what role, if any, does EGF or a related ligand play in the biology of the hair follicle? From our own studies it has been suggested that EGF plays an important role in the regeneration and down-growth of the new anagen follicle following telogen. This proposal is based on both in vitro and in vivo data. Firstly, in vitro EGF has been shown to activate a highly proliferative population of outer root sheath cells and this results in expansion of the outer root sheath. Secondly, during the hair growth cycle, as follicles re-enter anagen from their resting telogen stage, there is a marked increase in cell proliferation in the outer root sheath[23] and the epidermis also thickens simultaneously.[24] This suggests that a common ligand may activate both the basal outer root sheath and intrafollicular epidermal cells. EGF and TGF-α are excellent candidate molecules for this as both EGF and TGF-α are reported to stimulate keratinocyte proliferation in vitro[25] and epidermal thickening in vivo.[26] Third, immunohistochemistry and radioligand binding assays have shown that EGF receptors are localized to the bulge region of the outer root sheath in embryonic human hair follicles[27] and to the outer root sheath of adult human hair follicles.[28] Finally, Cotsarellis et al[29] have suggested that hair follicle stem cells reside in the bulge of rodent hair follicles and that, with the onset of anagen, the dermal papilla activates these stem cells to regenerate a new anagen follicle. Therefore, we speculate that EGF or a related ligand may be important in generating down-growth of the hair follicle during early anagen; whether these cells are stem cells remains open to debate and requires further detailed investigation.

Insulin-like growth factors (IGFs)

The insulin-like growth factors, IGF-I and IGF-II, are potent mitogens and regulators of cellular differentiation in many tissues and cell types.[30,31] Both IGF-I and IGF-II stimulate the proliferation of cultured keratinocytes and dermal fibroblasts.[32–34] IGF-I mRNA has been detected by both Northern blot and polymerase chain reaction (PCR) in keratomed human skin and cultured dermal fibroblasts, but not in cultured keratinocytes. IGF-I receptor mRNA has, however, been detected by PCR in both cultured fibroblasts and keratinocytes as well as in dermatomed skin.[35] These early observations led to the suggestion that IGF-I may be an important autocrine/ paracrine regulator of cellular proliferation and differentiation in the skin. This was later supported by the observation that, in transgenic knockout mice made null for the IGF-I receptor, abnormal patterns of growth and differentiation in the skin and hair follicles were reported.[36] Moreover, in patients suffering from acromegaly, elevated levels of growth hormone (GH) resulted in a marked thickening of the epidermis.[37] GH is known to up-regulate IGF-I expression in the liver and GH receptors have also been reported in the skin. Therefore, thickening of the epidermis in acromegaly may be mediated via GH upregulation of IGF-I in the skin.

Early immunohistochemical studies reported IGF-I expression in rat hair follicles;[38] however, detailed distribution patterns were not reported. Messenger[39] reported that cultured human beard dermal papilla fibroblasts, which, in vivo, are essential for hair growth,[40] secrete IGF-I into their tissue culture medium and suggested that IGF-I may be an important hair follicle growth factor. In our experiments,[15–17] in vitro growth of isolated human hair follicles required supraphysiological (10 μg/ml) levels of insulin. Since insulin at supraphysiological concentrations is known to act via the IGF-I receptor[30,31] we, therefore, investigated the effects of IGF-I on cultured human hair follicles maintained in the absence of insulin. IGF-I was found to be 1000-fold more potent at maintaining hair follicle growth in vitro than insulin. Moreover, we observed that, in the absence of insulin and IGF-I, hair follicles entered catagen,[41] however, this was prevented by IGF-I.

This data strongly points to IGF-I being an important regulator of hair follicle growth and also indicates a key role in hair cycle control. Since systemic IGF-I levels remained constant, we proposed that the hair growth cycle may be controlled by regulation of IGF-I receptor (IGF-IR) expression.[41]

Evidence that IGF-IR expression is regulated during the hair growth cycle has been obtained from both RT-PCR and immunohistochemical studies.[42,43] Immunohistochemistry[43] showed that IGF-I is present in both dermal papilla and the epithelial cells of the hair follicle (outer root sheath and matrix). However, IGF-I receptor is only expressed in dermal papilla and the terminally differentiating cells of the hair follicle (precortical matrix and outer root sheath) and is not expressed in either the germinative epithelium or the basal cells of the outer root sheath. Moreover in catagen hair follicles IGF-I receptor expression in the dermal papilla is absent. Further, Little et al[43] and Ralf Paus (personal communication) showed using semi quantitative RT-PCR that in both the rat and the mouse IGF-I receptor mRNA is regulated in a hair cycle dependent manner with marked downregulation of IGF-IR mRNA with the onset of catagen. In conclusion, combined in vitro follicle studies as well as immunohistochemistry and RT-PCR indicate that the IGF-I/IGF-IR signalling pathway plays an important role in the hair growth cycle.

Our observation that in the absence of IGF-I hair follicles enter catagen suggests that IGF-I signalling is important in maintaining hair follicles in anagen. The mechanisms by which this may occur, however, are unclear. The patterns of IGF-I and IGF-1R expression in the hair follicle suggest that IGF-I may not act directly as a mitogen on the germinative cells but instead acts on the dermal papilla, stimulating production of other growth factors that may be mitogenic for the germinative cells. Candidate molecules that may be induced by IGF-I include KGF (FGF-7) and VEGF, both of which are known to be produced by the dermal papilla.[1,44] Using cultured hair follicles we have attempted to identify candidate growth factors that are able to replace IGF-I as stimulators of hair follicle growth. To date, however, we have been unable to identify any growth factor that can replace IGF-I apart from IGF-II and insulin (at supraphysiological concentrations). Interestingly, we have identified factors that may control the rate of catagen regression (see fibroblast growth factors in later discussion). The patterns of IGF-I receptor expression in the suprabasal terminally differentiating cells of the hair follicle and the outer root sheath indicate that IGF-I may also play an important role in regulating terminal differentiation. Another important role for IGF-I in the hair follicle may also be to prevent apoptosis. It is well known that IGF-I is a potent anti-apoptotic growth factor[45] and this may also be its function in the hair follicle. Moreover, when isolated human hair follicles are cultured in the absence of IGF-I there is a marked increase in apoptotic cells (personal observation).

Additional data that also supports our hypothesis of IGF-I as a major hair follicle growth factor comes from the observations that IGF-I secretion by cultured beard dermal papilla cells is stimulated by testosterone,[46] suggesting that the androgen responsive growth of the beard may be mediated via IGF-I. Furthermore, in red deer, the growth of cultured follicles from the mane, an androgen-responsive target tissue, is stimulated by either testosterone or IGF-I.[47]

Finally, it has been reported recently that transgenic mice that overexpress IGF-I have accelerated rates of whisker growth.[48] On the basis of these observations we have proposed a simple model (Figure 1) for the actions of IGF-I in the hair follicle.

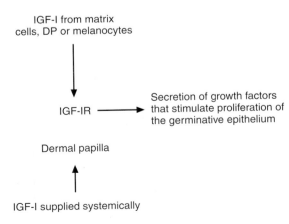

Figure 1

Proposed model for the role of IGF-I in regulating germinative epithelial cell proliferation.

Hepatocyte growth factor/scatter factor

Hepatocyte growth factor/scatter factor (HGF/SF) is a potent mitogen, morphogen and motogen of epithelial cells and plays an important role in mediating epithelial-mesenchymal signalling during embryonic development.[49] In hair follicles, HGF has been reported to stimulate the growth of both human and mouse follicles in vitro,[50,51] although in our culture system we have failed to observe any effect of HGF on hair follicle growth over a wide range of HGF concentrations. HGF mRNA has been shown by RT-PCR to be present in cultured dermal papilla fibroblasts, although protein secretion into dermal papilla-conditioned medium was not detected.[52] However, IL-1α, TNF-α and TPA are all reported to upregulate HGF mRNA expression in cultured dermal papilla cells and to stimulate dermal papilla secretion of HGF into conditioned medium. The exact role of HGF in the hair follicle is, however, unknown. IL-1α, TNF-α and TPA are all potent inhibitors of hair follicle growth in vitro (see later) and it is possible that HGF may modulate the activity of these growth factors in hair follicles.

Fibroblast growth factors

The fibroblast growth factor (FGF) family consists of at least nine members, which bind to high-affinity receptors that signal via tyrosine kinase.[53,54] Currently four FGF receptor (FGFR) genes have been identified; in addition, each gene can undergo splicing to generate several receptor isoforms.[55] Moreover, FGFs can also bind to low-affinity receptors that are heparin sulphate proteoglycans. FGFs are potent stimulators of cell proliferation and differentiation in several cells and tissues, they are therefore prime candidates to play an important role in regulating hair growth.

Both acidic FGF (FGF-1) and basic FGF (FGF-2) have been detected in the hair follicle. FGF-1 is localized to the IRS and FGF-2 to the basement membrane of the outer root sheath and hair follicle matrix.[56] The possible role of these growth factors in regulating hair follicle growth and differentiation is not known. Du Cros[57] has shown that FGF-1, when injected into mice, inhibits hair growth in the surrounding skin. This suggests that FGF-1 may be an inhibitor of hair growth, however, FGFs bind with great avidity to the extracellular matrix[58] and the localized inhibition reported by Du Cros may well be caused by localized binding of high concentrations of FGF.

The most significant advance with regard to the role of FGFs and hair growth has come from the generation of transgenic, knockout, mice made null for the FGF-5 gene. In these mice the onset of catagen is delayed, resulting in prolonged anagen and the growth of longer pelage hair fibres. The coats of these mice are similar to that seen in the Angora mouse and subsequent analysis revealed that the gene for FGF-5 in the Angora is mutated.[59] In situ hybridization studies in mice have shown that FGF-5 is expressed in the lower outer root sheath of the hair follicle and that its expression is activated at anagen stage VII and downregulated prior to the onset of catagen.[44] This suggests that FGF-5 is an important regulator of the onset of catagen. FGF-5 protein has not been reported in either the dermal papilla or hair follicle matrix. Nevertheless, FGF-5 binds to the FGFR$_1$ receptor, which has been localized in rodent hair follicles exclusively to the dermal papilla. This suggests that prior to catagen FGF-5 expression in the lower outer root sheath may activate or down-regulate gene expression by the dermal papilla.

Keratinocyte growth factor (FGF-7) is produced by dermal fibroblasts and acts in a paracrine fashion on keratinocytes.[60] In the hair follicle, immunohistochemistry and in situ hybridization have shown KGF to be localized to the dermal papilla.[44] FGF-7 can bind to both the FGFR-I and FGFR-II, which, in hair follicles, are expressed in the matrix cells of the follicle bulb.[44] This suggests that KGF produced by the dermal papilla may act in a paracrine fashion on the germinative cells of the hair follicle bulb. Moreover, in catagen hair follicles the dermal papilla is reported to be FGF-7 negative.

In transgenic KGF knockout mice[61] normal hair follicle growth and development is reported; however, by 2 months of age the mice develop greasy, matted coats that resemble the rough mutant mouse.[62] This observation suggests that, in the hair follicle, KGF may be redundant as a mitogenic factor but may play an important role in regulating hair fibre differentiation. It is reported that in KGF null mice, the greasy hairs appear in the male mice first. It has been suggested that KGF may be involved in androgen-dependent pathways;[63] however, in KGF-null mice male reproductive organs appeared normal. Transgenic mice that overexpress KGF, however, have marked abnormalities of their hair follicles and this results in abnormal patterns of hair growth.[64] Interpretation of these transgenic studies, especially with regard to hair follicle biology is difficult. Perhaps more important is the observation that, when KGF is injected either subcutaneously or intraperitoneally into the nude (*nu/nu*) mouse, hair growth is stimulated by prolonging the anagen phase of its hair cycle.[65]

In our own experiments we have investigated the effects of FGF-1, FGF-2, FGF-5 and KGF (FGF-7) on the growth of isolated human hair follicles both under normal anagen conditions but also in the absence of IGF-I (induced catagen). Under normal anagen growth conditions FGFs had no apparent affect on hair follicle growth; however, FGF-1, FGF-2 and FGF-7 were found to stimulate outgrowth of epithelial cells from the cut surface of the outer root sheath. This suggests that some members of the FGF family may be important mediators of re-epithelialization from the outer root sheath following wounding. In the absence of IGF-I hair follicles switch from anagen to catagen. In this model KGF (FGF-7) delayed progression into catagen, whereas aFGF (FGF-1) stimulated onset of catagen (Table 2). This in vitro data supports the in vivo KGF data, which suggests that KGF delays onset of catagen. Importantly, although FGFs were able to modulate anagen to catagen transition, none were able to replace IGF-I as a stimulator of hair follicle growth. This suggests that either IGF-I is a direct mitogen on germinative epithelial cells (which conflicts with our in vitro culture data), or some other growth factor, untested by us, is the major mitogen for germinative cells.

TGF-β

Members of the TGF-β family appear to play a crucial, but as yet unidentified, role in the embryonic development of the hair follicle.[66] In isolated human hair follicles we have shown that TGF-β1 is a potent inhibitor of hair follicle growth,[15]

Table 2 The effect of fibroblast growth factors on in vitro hair follicle transition from anagen to catagen.

Experimental conditions	% follicles in catagen after 7 days culture
Insulin (10 µg/ml)	8.6
– insulin	73
– insulin + aFGF (10 ng/ml)	88
– insulin + bFGF (10 ng/ml)	66
– insulin + KGF (10 ng/ml)	58

which suggests a possible role for this growth factor as a negative regulator of hair follicle growth. This is supported by RT-PCR analysis of TGF-β1 gene expression during the rat hair growth cycle,[42] which showed that, with the onset of early catagen gene expression for TGF-β1, is up-regulated. These same authors also reported that the receptor, betaglycan, was elevated during early anagen and decreased with the onset of catagen. This observation is important since the betaglycan receptor is believed to play an important role in sequestering TGF-β.[42] Moreover, with the onset of catagen breakdown of the connective tissue sheath surrounding the hair follicle may release TGF-β to bind to the TGF-β receptors type I and II, resulting in the inhibition of cell proliferation in the hair follicle bulb.

Interleukins, tumour necrosis factors, colony stimulating factors

There is strong evidence to suggest that the hair follicle may be an immune privileged tissue. Immunohistochemical studies carried out by Westgate et al[67] have shown that the transient epithelial portion of the hair follicle does not express MHC class I. Furthermore, the connective tissue sheath of the hair follicle is rich in proteoglycans, which is a common feature of other immune privilege sites in the mammalian body.[68] Moreover, with the onset of catagen some proteoglycans are lost from the sheath and this is associated with a marked influx of macrophages expressing activated MHC class II phenotype.

The authors suggest that this data indicates a role for the immune system in regulating hair growth. It is not clear from these studies, however, whether the influx of macrophages is secondary to the onset of catagen; in fact the authors suggest that cytokines were involved in signalling proteoglycan breakdown and mediating activation of macrophages.

Both ourselves and Harmon and Nevins have studied the effects of a range of interleukins and colony stimulating factors on the growth of cultured human hair follicles.[69,70] We have observed that both IL-1α and IL-1β as well as TNF-α are potent inhibitors of hair follicle growth in vitro and as such, may play a role in the regulation of the hair growth cycle. This is supported by the observation that in rat hair follicles mRNA for the TNF-α receptor increased during late anagen, which suggests a possible role in growth inhibition.[43] Moreover, TNF-α is also known to stimulate the expression of metalloproteinases[71] and may, therefore, be important in the degradation of the extracellular matrix during catagen.

Changes in hair follicle morphology induced by IL-1α, IL-1β and TNF-α are similar, and are characterized by rounding of the dermal papilla, vacuolation of the outer root sheath and matrix and the presence of melanin granules within the dermal papilla. These changes in morphology, with the exception of rounding of the dermal papilla, are not, however, characteristic of the onset of catagen, and suggest a more dystrophic change in the hair follicle. Interestingly, these dystrophic changes resemble some of the changes in hair follicle morphology reported in patients suffering from alopecia areata and suggest that IL-1α, IL-1β and TNF-α may play important roles in the pathophysiology of this disease.[72,73]

Hair growth regulation model

On the basis of both in vitro observations on the effects of growth factors on cultured human hair follicles and in vivo studies of mRNA expression and immunohistochemistry, we have attempted to produce a simple growth regulation model (Figure 2). In this model we proposed that the IGF-I/IGF-IR axis plays a central role in hair follicle cycling. Since IGF-I is known to be a potent

stimulator of mitogenesis and differentiation and also a potent inhibitor of apoptosis, we propose that, during anagen, IGF-I is an important hair follicle maintenance factor and that the onset of catagen is driven by down-regulation of the IGF-IR. Our data suggests that IGF-I may not, however, be a direct mitogen for the germinative epithelial cells but may act via the dermal papilla. Candidate hair follicle mitogens produced by the dermal papilla and which may be regulated by IGF-I include KGF and VEGF.

Our in vitro growth data also suggests that EGF/TGF-α signalling is important in activating hair follicle outer root sheath keratinocytes and that stimulation of these cells results in rapid down-growth of the anagen hair follicle. This action of EGF-TGF-α is also supported by in situ hybridization data, which shows that both EGFR and EGF mRNA are expressed in the outer root sheath and especially the bulge region of the hair follicle during early anagen. Whether these cells

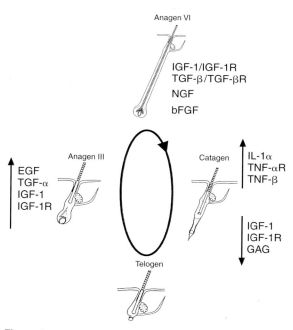

Figure 2

Hair growth regulatory model showing some of the key growth factors that may be important regulators of the hair growth cycle.

activated by EGF/TGF-α are hair follicle stem cells, remains to be determined.

With the onset of catagen hair follicle IGF-IR is down-regulated and IL-1α, TNF-α and TGF-β are up-regulated. All three of these growth factors are potent inhibitors of hair follicle growth in vitro and also induce apoptosis. It is likely, therefore, that these growth factors are important mediators of catagen. The fibroblast growth factors may be involved in the fine regulation of anagen to catagen transition. In vivo studies have shown that mice made null for FGF-5 delay entry into catagen and that therefore, FGF-5 may act in vivo by promoting catagen. Nevertheless, FGF-5 mice undergo a normal hair cycle, which suggests that FGF-5 is not the key, single, regulatory factor but acts in conjunction with other growth factors. In vitro we have shown that both KGF and bFGF (FGF-2) delay the onset of catagen in cultured hair follicles, maintained in the absence of insulin and IGF-I whereas aFGF (FGF-1) appears to promote catagen. These observations suggest that the role of the FGFs is to 'fine tune' the hair growth cycle.

Future goals: modelling the hair growth cycle in vitro

To date, virtually all research using in vitro cultured hair follicles has been based on the growth of anagen hair follicles. The reason for this is simple. Anagen follicles are very easy to isolate whereas, as a rule, only two or three catagen hair follicles are found for every 100 anagen follicles isolated. This, therefore makes gathering sufficient numbers of catagen hair follicles for meaningful experiments very difficult. As already discussed, follicles can be switched from anagen to catagen by insulin/IGF-I withdrawal. If these follicles are further maintained in vitro some appear to regress dramatically, giving rise to small 'telogen-like' follicles. Nevertheless, the numbers of follicles that survive to this state are very small (less than 5%) and this makes experimentation very difficult.

In order to overcome this problem we have begun to investigate the culture of neonatal rat vibrissae follicles, making use of the fact that in rodents the hair growth cycle is synchronized.[74,75]

Therefore, it is possible to predict the stage of cycle that hair follicles will be in from the age of the animal. Robinson et al[76] have shown that in vitro growth of mouse vibrissae follicles reflected closely both their in vivo origin but also the specific stage of the cycle at which the vibrissae were isolated. We have isolated vibrissa follicles from 12-day-old rats and confirmed, using histology, that these follicles are in the anagen stage of their first hair growth cycle. We have then maintained these follicles in vitro, on Gelfoam supports, for up to 23 days (35 days of age) and compared their histology with in vivo follicles from equivalent age littermates. It was found that 12-day-old follicles maintained in vitro for up to 23 days showed changes in morphology similar to those seen in freshly isolated pro-anagen follicles taken from 26-day-old littermates. These changes suggest that cultured rat vibrissa follicles retain cyclical activity in vitro and that eventually it will be possible to model the hair growth cycle in vitro.

Acknowledgements

I would like to thank Unilever Research for financial support. Most of my research presented in this chapter was carried out in Terence Kealey's laboratory in collaboration with Debbie Sanders.

References

1. Randall VA: The use of dermal papilla cells in studies of normal and abnormal hair follicle biology. In: Whiting DA (ed.). *Dermatologic Clinics: Update on Hair Disorders*, Volume 14. Philadelphia, WB Saunders Company, 1996: 585–594.

2. Philpott MP, Saunders DA, Kealey T: Whole hair follicle culture. In: Whiting DA (ed.). *Dermatologic Clinics: Update on Hair Disorders*, Volume 14. Philadelphia, WB Saunders Company, 1996: 595–607.

3. Strangeways DH: The growth of hair in vitro. *Arch Exp Zellforsch* 1931; **11**: 344.

4. Murray MR: Development of the hair follicle and hair in vitro. *Anat Rec* 1933; **57**: 74.

5. Hardy MH: The development of mouse hair in vitro with some observations on pigmentation. *J Anat* 1949; **83**: 364–384.

6. Hardy MH, Lyne AG: Studies on the development of wool follicles in tissue culture. *Aust J Biol Sci* 1956; **9**: 559–574.

7. Kollar EJ: An in vitro study of hair and vibrissae development in embryonic mouse. *J Invest Dermatol* 1966; **46**: 254–262.

8. Bartosova L, Rebora A, Moretti G, Cipriani C: Studies on rat hair culture. I. A re-evaluation of technique. *Arch Derm Forsch* 1971; **240**: 95–106.

9. Hardy MH, Van Exan RJ, Sonstegard KS, Sweeny PR: Basal lamina changes during tissue interactions in hair follicles—an in vitro study of normal dermal papilla and vitamin A-induced glandular morphogenesis. *J Invest Dermatol* 1983; **80**: 27–34.

10. Frater R, Whitmore PG: *In vitro* growth of post-embryonic hair. *J Invest Dermatol* 1973; **61**: 72–81.

11. Uzuka M, Takeshita C, Morikawa F: *In vitro* growth of mouse hair roots. *Acta Derm (Stockholm)* 1977; **57**: 217–219.

12. Frater R: The effect of rat serum on the morphology of rat hair follicles in tissue culture. *Arch Dermatol Res* 1980; **269**: 13–20.

13. Buhl AE, Waldon BS, Kawabe TT, Holland DVM: Minoxidil stimulates mouse vibrissae follicles in organ culture. *J Invest Dermatol* 1989; **92**: 315–320.

14. Kondo S, Hozumi Y, Aso K: Organ culture of human scalp hair follicles: effect of testosterone and oestrogen on hair growth. *Arch Dermatol Res* 1990; **282**: 442–445.

15. Philpott MP, Green MR, Kealey T: Human hair growth *in vitro*. *J Cell Sci* 1990; **97**: 463–471.

16. Philpott MP, Green MR, Kealey T: An in vitro model for the study of human hair growth. *Ann NY Acad Sci* 1991; **642**: 148–166.

17. Westgate GE, Gibson WT, Kealey T, Philpott MP: Prolonged maintenance of human hair follicles in vitro in serum-free defined medium. *Br J Dermatol* 1993; **129**: 372–379.

18. Moore GP, Panaretto BA, Robertson D: Effects of epidermal growth factor on hair growth in the mouse. *J Endocrinol* 1981; **88**: 293–299.

19. Chapman RE, Hardy MH: Effects of intradermally injected and topically applied mouse epidermal growth factor on wool growth, skin and wool follicles of merino sheep. *Aust J Biol Sci* 1988; **41**: 261–268.

20. Hollis DE, Chapman RE, Panaretto BA, Moore GPM: Morphological changes in the skin and wool fibres of merino sheep infused with epidermal growth factor. *Aust J Biol Sci* 1983; **36**: 419–434.

21. Hollis DE, Chapman RE: Mode of action of mouse epidermal growth factor on the wool follicles of merino sheep: an ultrastructural study. *Aust J Agric Res* 1989; **40**: 1047–1063.

22. Philpott MP, Kealey T: The effects of EGF on the morphology and patterns of DNA synthesis in isolated human hair follicles. *J Invest Dermatol* 1994; **102**: 186–191.

23. Bullough WS, Laurence EB: Mitotic activity of the follicle, In: Montagna W, Ellis RA (eds.). *The Biology of Hair Growth*, New York, Academic Press, 1958, 171–187.

24. Chase HB, Montagna W, Malone JD: Changes in the skin in relation to the hair growth cycle. *Anat Rec* 1953; **116**: 75–81.

25. Moore GPM, Panaretto BA, Carter NB: Epidermal hyperplasia and wool follicle regression in sheep infused with epidermal growth factor. *J Invest Dermatol* 1985; **84**: 172–175.

26. Sun T-T, Green H: Cultured epithelial cells of the cornea, conjunctiva and skin: absence of marked intrinsic divergence of their differentiated states. *Nature* 1977; **269**: 489–492.

27. Green MR, Couchman JR: Distribution and number of epidermal growth factor receptors in rat tissue during embryonic skin development, hair formation and the adult hair growth cycle. *J Invest Dermatol* 1984; **83**: 118.

28. Green MR, Basketter DA, Couchman JR, Rees DA: Distribution and number of epidermal growth factor receptors in skin is related to epithelial growth. *Dev Biol* 1983; **100**: 506–512.

29. Cotsarelis G, Sun T-T, Lavker RM: Label retaining cells reside in the bulge area of pilosebaceous unit: implications for follicular stem cells, hair cycle and skin carcinogenesis. *Cell* 1990; **61**: 1329–1337.

30. Daughaday WH, Rotwein P: Insulin like growth factors I and II peptide, messenger ribonucleic acid and gene structure, serum and tissue concentrations. *Endocrine Rev* 1989; **10**: 68–91.

31. Daughaday WH: The possible autocrine/paracrine and endocrine roles of insulin like growth factors of human tissues. *Endocrinol* 1990; **127**: 1–4.

32. Nickoloff BJ, Misra P, Morhenn VB, Hintz RL, Rosenfeld RG: Further characterisation of the keratinocyte somatomedin-C/insulin like growth factor I (SMC/IGF-1) receptor and the biological responsiveness of cultured keratinocytes to SM-C/IGF-I. *Dermatologica* 1988; **177**: 265–273.

33. Ristow H-J, Messmer TO: Basic fibroblast growth factor and insulin like growth factor-I are strong mitogens for cultured mouse keratinocytes. *J Cell Physiol* 1988; **137**: 277–284.

34. Neely EK, Morhenn VB, Hintz RL, Wilson DM, Rosenfeld RG: Insulin like growth factors are mitogenic for human keratinocytes and squamous cell carcinoma. *J Invest Dermatol* 1991; **96**: 104–110.

35. Tavakkal A, Elder JT, Griffiths CEM, et al.: Expression of growth hormone receptor, insulin-like

growth factor (IGF-I) and IGF-I receptor mRNA and proteins in human skin. *J Invest Dermatol* 1992; **99**: 343–349.

36. Liu J-P, Baker J, Perkins AS, Robertson EJ, Efstratiadis A: Mice carrying null mutations of the genes encoding insulin-like growth factor I (IGF-I) and type 1 IGF receptor (IGF1r). *Cell* 1993; **75**: 59–72.

37. Barkan AL, Beitins IZ, Kelch RP: Plasma insulin like growth factor-I/somatomedin-C in acromegaly: correlation with degree of growth hormone secretion. *J Clin Endocrinol Metab* 1988; **67**: 69–73.

38. Hansson HA, Nilsson A, Isgaard J, et al.: Immuno-histochemical localisation of insulin like growth factor-I in the adult rat. *Immunohistochemistry* 1988; **89**: 403–410.

39. Oliver RF: Whisker growth after removal of the dermal papilla and lengths of the follicle in the hooded rat. *J Embryol Exp Morphol* 1966; **15**: 331–347.

40. Messenger AG: Isolation, culture and in vitro behaviour of cells isolated from the papilla of human hair follicles. In: Van Neste D, Lachapelle JM, Antoine JL (eds.). *Trends in Human Hair Growth and Alopecia Research*. Amsterdam, Kluwer Academic Publishers, 1989; 57–67.

41. Philpott MP, Sanders DA, Kealey T: Effects of insulin and insulin-like growth factors on cultured human hair follicles; IGF-I at physiologic concentrations is an important regulator of hair follicle growth in vitro. *J Invest Dermatol* 1994; **102**: 857–861.

42. Rudman SR, Philpott MP, Kealey T: The role of IGF-I in human skin and its appendages: morphogen as well as mitogen. *J Invest Dermatol* 1997; **109**: 770–777.

43. Little JC, Redwood KL, Jenkins G, Granger SP. In vivo cytokine and receptor gene expression during the rat hair cycle-analysis by quantitative RT-PCR. *Arch Derm Res* 1996 (In press).

44. Rosenquist TA, Martin GR: FGF signalling in the hair growth cycle: expression of the FGF receptor and ligand genes in the murine hair follicle. *Devel Dynamics* 1996; **205**: 379–386.

45. Harrington EA, Bennett MR, Fanidi A, Evan GI: c-Myc induced apoptosis in fibroblasts is inhibited by specific cytokines. *EMBO J* 1994; **13**: 3286–3295.

46. Itami S, Kurata S, Takayasu S: Androgen induction of follicle epithelial cell growth is mediated via insulin-like growth factor-1 from dermal papilla cells. *Biochem Biophys Res Commun* 1995; **212**: 988–994.

47. Thornton MJ, Thomas DJ, Brinklow BR, Loudon ASI, Randall VA. Only androgen dependant hairs of red deer are stimulated by testosterone and IGF-I in vitro. *Br J Dermatol* 1994; **131**: 427A.

48. Su H-Y, Hickford JGH, The PHB, Hill AM, Frampton CM, Bickerstaffe R: Increased vibrissa growth in transgenic mice expressing insulin-like growth factor 1. *J Invest Dermatol* 1999; **112**: 245–248.

49. Sonnenberg E, Meyer D, Weidner KM et al: Scatter factor/hepactocyte growth factor and its receptor the c-met tyrosine kinase, can mediate a signal exchange between mesenchyme and epithelia during mouse development. *J Cell Biol* 1993; **123**: 223–235.

50. Jindo T, Tsuboi R, Imai R, Takamori K, Rubin JS, Ogawa, H: The effect of hepatocyte growth factor/scatter factor on human hair follicle growth. *J Dermatol Sci* 1995; **10**: 229–232.

51. Jindo T, Tsuboi R, Imai R, Takamori K, Rubin JS, Ogawa H: Hepatocyte growth factor/scatter factor stimulates hair growth of mouse vibrissae in organ culture. *J Invest Dermatol* 1994; **103**: 306–309.

52. Shimaoka S, Imai R, Ogawa H: Dermal papilla cells express hepatocyte growth factor. *J Dermatol Sci* 1994; **7**: S79–S83.

53. Rifkin DB, Moscatelli D: Recent developments in the cell biology of basic fibroblast growth factor. *J Cell Biol* 1989; **109**: 1–6.

54. Miyamoto M, Naruo K-I, Seko C, Matsumoto S, Kondo T, Kurokawa T: Molecular cloning of a novel cytokine cDNA encoding the ninth member of the fibroblast growth factor family, which has a unique secretion property. *Mol Cell Biol* 1993; **13**: 4251–4259.

55. Peters KG, Werner S, Chen G, Williams LT: Two FGF receptor genes are differentially expressed in epithelial and mesenchymal tissues during limb formation and organogenesis in the mouse. *Development* 1992; **114**: 233–243.

56. Du Cros DL, Isaacs K, Moore GPM: Distribution of acidic and basic fibroblast growth factors in ovine skin during hair follicle morphogenesis. *J Cell Sci* 1993; **105**: 667.

57. Du Cros DL: Fibroblast growth factor and epidermal growth factor in hair development. *J Invest Dermatol* 1993; **101**: 101S–106S.

58. Baird A, Walicke PA: Fibroblast growth factors. In Waterfield MD (ed.). Growth Factors. *Br Med Bull* 1989; **45**: 438–452.

59. Hebert JM, Rosenquist T, Gotz J, Martin GR: FGF5 as a regulator of the hair growth cycle: evidence from targeted and spontaneous mutations. *Cell* 1995; **78**: 1017–1025.

60. Finch PW, Cunha GR, Rubin JS, Wong J, Ron D: Pattern of keratinocyte growth factor and keratinocyte growth factor receptor expression during mouse fetal development suggests a role in mediating morphogenetic mesenchymal-epithelial interactions. *Develop Dynamics* 1995; **203**: 223–240.

61. Guo L, Degenstein L, Fuchs E: Keratinocyte growth

factor is required for hair development but not for wound healing. *Genes and Develop* 1996; **10**: 165–175.

62. Sundberg JP: *Handbook of Mouse Mutations with Skin and Hair Abnormalities: Animal Models and Biochemical Tools*. Boca Raton, Florida, CRC Press, 1994.

63. Yan G, Fukabori Y, Nikolaropoulis S, Wang F, McKeehan WL: Heparin binding keratinocyte growth factor is a candidate stromal to epithelial andromedin. *Mol Endocrinol* 1992; **6**: 2123–2128.

64. Guo L, Yu Q-C, Fuchs E: Targeting expression of keratinocyte growth factor to keratinocytes elicits striking changes in epithelial differentiation in transgenic mice. *EMBO J* 1993; **12**: 973–986.

65. Danilenko DM, Ring BD, Yanagihara D, et al.: Keratinocyte growth factor is an important endogenous mediator of hair follicle growth development and differentiation. *Am J Pathol* 1995; **147**: 145–154.

66. Paus R, Foitzik K, Welker P, et al.: Transforming growth factor-β type I and type II expression in murine hair follicle development and cycling. *J Invest Dermatol* 1997; **109**: 518–526.

67. Westgate GE, Craggs RI, Gibson WT: Immune privilege in hair growth. *J Invest Dermatol* 1991; **97**: 417–420.

68. Westgate GE, Messenger AG, Watson LP, Gibson WT: Distribution of proteoglycans during the hair growth cycle in human skin. *J Invest Dermatol* 1991; **96**: 191–195.

69. Philpott MP, Sander DA, Bowen J, Kealey T: Effects of interleukins, colony stimulating factor and tumour necrosis factor on human hair follicle growth in vitro: a possible role for interleukin-1 and tumour necrosis factor-a in alopecia areata. *Br J Dermatol* 1996; **135**: 942–948.

70. Harmon CS, Nevins TD: IL-1α inhibits human hair follicle growth and hair fibre production in whole-organ cultures. *Lymphokine Cytokine Research* 1993; **12**: 197–203.

71. Dayer J, Beutler B, Cami A: Cachectin/tumour necrosis factor stimulates collagenase and prostaglandin E2 production by human synovial cells and dermal fibroblasts. *J Exp Med* 1985; **162**: 2163–2168.

72. Macdonald-Hull S, Nutbrown M, Pepall L, Thornton J, Randall VA, Cunliffe WJ: Immunohistologic and ultrastructural comparison of the dermal papilla and hair follicle bulb from 'active' and 'normal' areas of alopecia areata. *J Invest Dermatol* 1991; **96**: 673–681.

73. Nutbrown M, Macdonald-Hull S, Cunliffe WJ, Randall VA: Abnormalities in the ultrastructure of melanocytes and the outer root sheath of clinically normal hair follicles from alopecia areata scalps. *J Invest Dermatol* 1995; **104**: 12S–13S.

74. Chase HB: Growth of the hair. *Physiol Rev* 1954; **34**: 113–126.

75. Ebling FJ, Johnson E: The control of hair growth. *Symp Zool Soc Lond* 1964; **12**: 97–130.

76. Robinson M, Reynolds AJ, Jahoda CAB: Hair cycle stage of the mouse vibrissa follicle determines subsequent fibre growth and follicle behaviour in vitro. *J Invest Dermatol* 1997; **108**: 495–500.

77. Taylor M, Ashcroft ATT, Messenger AG: Cyclosporin A prolongs human hair growth in vitro. *J Invest Dermatol* 1993; **100**: 237–239.

78. Harmon CS, Nevins TD: Biphasic effect of 1,25-dihydroxyvitamin D3 on human hair follicle growth and hair fiber production in whole-organ cultures. *J Invest Dermatol* 1994; **103**: 318–322.

79. Rogers GE, Martinet N, Steinert P, et al.: Cultivation of murine hair follicles as organoids in a collagen matrix. *J Invest Dermatol* 1987; **89**: 369–379.

80. McDonagh AJG, Snowden JA, Stierle C, et al.: HLA and ICAM-I expression in alopecia areata in vivo and in vitro: the role of cytokines. *Br J Dermatol* 1993; **129**: 250–256.

81. Williams D, Siock P, Stenn K: 13-*cis*-retinoic acid affects sheath-shaft interactions of equine hair follicles in vitro. *J Invest Dermatol* 1996; **106**: 356–361.

9

Human hair follicle grafts in nude mice: an important in vivo model for investigating the control of hair growth

Dominique Van Neste and Bernadette de Brouwer

Introduction

In recent years clinicians have become increasingly interested in the area of hair growth research. This upsurge of interest was triggered by the discovery of compounds showing some efficacy in maintaining hair in subjects with male pattern baldness (androgenetic alopecia).[1] During the processes of androgenetic alopecia, large terminal scalp follicles producing long, thick, pigmented hairs are gradually transformed to increasingly smaller follicles. Eventually, they become tiny vellus follicles forming short, thin, colourless hairs and spending much larger proportions of time resting (reviewed by Randall in Chapter 11). The mechanism for the induction of hair regrowth involves the initiation of anagen in dormant hair follicles as well as reverting a variable proportion of vellus follicles into terminal hair follicles. It is clear from the clinical-experimental approach that the hair dynamics on any given skin area is determined by five variables.[2,3]

(1) The absolute number of hair follicles liable to become functionally active;
(2) The duration of the anagen phase;
(3) The linear hair growth rate;
(4) The thickness of the hair fibres; and
(5) The delay before a new anagen hair appears at the skin surface after the shedding of the telogen hair.

This latter follicular stage has also been named *metanagen* because the follicle has reached a stage following anagen, and the club hair shedding named *exogen* because the detached hair fibre has irreversibly left the hair follicle. The remaining permanent portions may proceed with the early stages of anagen to develop a new lower follicle and form a new hair. This mimicry of the embryogenesis of the hair follicle occurs only after the cells of the dermal papilla have initiated a new hair matrix from close contact with the presumptive stem cell zone, which is found at the junction of the permanent and the impermanent portion of the follicle during telogen.

Hair follicles reflect the dynamic status of a living system. Any approach that would capture all the dimensions at once (global approach) but also allow a detailed analysis of each component (analytical approach) would be considered as an ideal candidate for experimental evaluation of human hair growth. It is clear that no in vitro model has yet been established that can reflect this level of complexity. Serendipity, however, introduced us to this field of experimental production of human hair, with studies of human skin grafts maintained on nude mice. Indeed, from observation of grafted benign naevi, we learned that functional hair follicles were maintained in the specimens.[4] These mice do not reject human material because they are athymic. This observation prompted us to start a research programme focused on human hair production by follicles from subjects with androgenetic alopecia using this experimental system.

Current understanding of the model system

This model has now been investigated sufficiently to establish that it is potentially very interesting for investigating human follicle biology.[4-11] After the grafting of human scalp specimens onto nude mice, the structure of the pilosebaceous apparatus is maintained (Figure 1) and the initiation of secondary germs can be seen histologically (Figures 2 and 3) suggesting that hair cycling could occur.[4] An important aspect of the model is that cell proliferation and differentiation in the hair matrix can be evaluated in a non-invasive way by measuring the hair diameter and linear growth rates since human hair can be collected from the surface of the grafted scalp.[5] Hair diameter is comparable with in situ distribution, reflecting the presence of vellus and terminal hair (Figure 4), and although linear growth rate is decreased by 25%, it maintains its correlation with the hair diameter as observed in situ; the thinner the hair the slower the growth rate.

Biochemical analysis has also shown that the protein content of hair fibres, as evaluated by the amino acid composition, is maintained in the experimental model.[6,7] Excitingly, when skin from patients with the genetic defect in amino

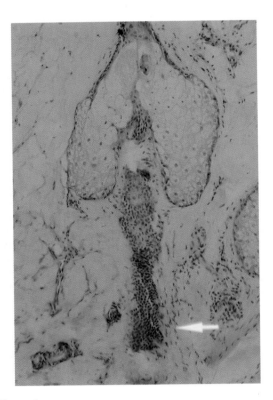

Figure 1

Human scalp graft onto nude mice: vellus-like hair follicle. A new anagen phase is initiated (arrow) from densely stained, small, nucleated epithelial cells deriving from the bottom of the permanent part of the hair follicle (stem cell zone) adjacent to the sebaceous gland. After a while a vellus-like hair follicle will eventually produce a thin, barely pigmented, hair shaft that will be visible at the surface (see Figure 4). (Reproduced with permission from Sundberg et al.,[14] in press.)

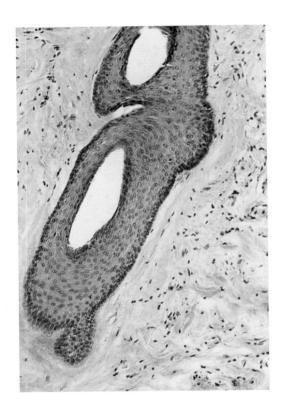

Figure 2

Human hair follicle budding: incipient stage. This phenomenon of budding occurs within the first 2–3 months after grafting of human scalp onto nude mice. The process is flanking the originally implanted hair follicle.

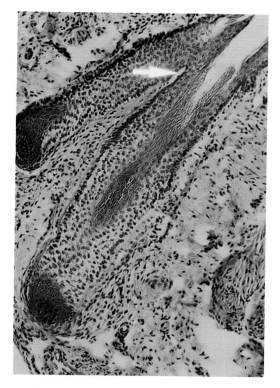

Figure 3

Human hair follicle: maturation stage. At a later stage of follicular budding than the one shown in Figure 2, two hair follicles can be observed merging into a single follicular canal (arrow).

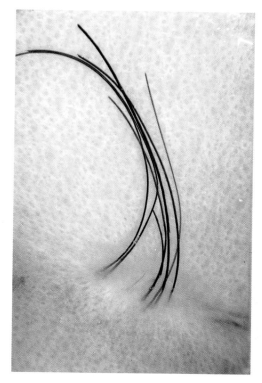

Figure 4

Human scalp graft onto nude mouse: surface view of vellus-like and terminal hair (1 month after clipping all visible hair). Terminal hair is characterized by its thickness and pigmentation. A thin and less pigmented hair follicle grows amidst the terminal hair shafts, From left to right there are two terminal hairs, a thin vellus-like hair and another five terminal hair shafts growing from a human scalp graft placed onto nude mouse skin. The latter shows a characteristic pattern of reflecting the acro-infundibula of empty hair follicles. (Reproduced with permission from Sundberg et al.,[14] in press.)

acid composition of hair, trichothiodystrophy (TTD) was used, the abnormality was continuously expressed after grafting on to the nude mouse system.[6,7]

When fetal scalp skin was transplanted to nude mice, cell commitment, induction of hair follicles and complete follicular morphogenesis occurred.[8] This is in marked contrast to in vitro studies where follicular morphogenesis occurs only after induction of the hair follicles has been initiated in situ. The density of hair follicles (hair number per unit area) in fetal scalp skin grafts is much higher because expansion of the scalp skin had not occurred as it has in a full adult individual.[7] Air-exposed fetal scalp grafts on to nude mice display accelerated maturation, and the samples exhibit a more advanced development stage compared with age-matched controls maintained in utero or in the absence of air exposure.[8]

Further investigations have shown that adult hair production is maintained for a long time, up to 6 months, compared with only up to about 10 days in vitro.[9] Follicular cycling has also been observed clearly using non-invasive monitoring methods. Continuous hair shaft production for more than 2 months was followed by cessation of hair growth, reflecting telogen; this was achieved by hair shedding (exogen) and then regrowth of hair from the same follicular opening, indicating new anagen and full cyclic activity.[10]

Since much human hair growth is altered by androgens (reviewed by Randall in Chapter 5), it is important to have an in vivo model where androgen effect can be investigated. Treatment with testosterone raising the female mouse serum level to the level of the human male body resulted in decreased hair production from the grafted male balding scalp samples. This indicates that the hormonal sensitivity of grafted follicles is maintained.[10] In addition, when a topical anti-androgen was applied on the balding scalp grafts maintained in the appropriate systemic hormonal environment, improved hair growth was reported.[11] These results all reflect what would be expected in the original human donor of the scalp skin.

Conclusions

In short, the human hair follicle keeps its structural integrity after grafting and can retain the ability to cycle. Some functional characteristics such as linear growth rate are modified at the phenotypic level, presumably reflecting differences in nutrition, growth factors, and so on in the new metabolic environment but, more importantly, the genetic mechanisms such as protein synthesis and hormonal response are maintained.

These findings, along with the results of several other studies[12–14] indicate that the model has a future for further investigation of hair follicle biology or for evaluation of new therapies on a clinically relevant human target.

It is hoped that this new area of experimental and clinical research will be of significant use for industrial and academic partners and will lead to a better experimental modelling of the human hair follicle biology.

References

1. Dawber R, Van Neste D: *Hair and Scalp Disorders. Common Presenting Signs, Differential Diagnosis and Treatment.* London, Martin Dunitz, 1995.
2. Van Neste D: Dynamic exploration of hair growth: critical review of methods available and their usefulness in the clinical trial protocol. In: Van Neste D, Lachapelle JM, Antoine JL (eds.). *Trends in Human Hair Growth and Alopecia Research.* Lancaster, Kluwer, 1989: 143–154.
3. Van Neste D: Hair growth evaluation in clinical dermatology. *Dermatology* 1993; **187**: 233–234.
4. Van Neste D, Warnier G, Thulliez M, Van Hoof F: Human hair follicle grafts onto nude mice: morphological study. In: Van Neste F, Lachapelle JM, Antoine JL (eds.). *Trends in Human Hair Growth and Alopecia Research.* Lancaster, Kluwer Academic Publishers, 1989: 117–131.
5. Van Neste D, De Brouwer B, Dumortier M: Reduced linear hair growth rates of vellus and of terminal hairs produced by human balding scalp grafted onto nude mice. *Ann NY Acad Sci* 1991; **642**: 480–482.
6. Van Neste D, Gillespie M, Marshall RC, Taieb A, De Brouwer B: Morphological and biochemical characteristics of trichothiosdystrophy-variant hair are maintained after grafting of scalp specimens on to nude mice. *Br J Dermatol* 1993; **128**: 384–387.
7. De Brouwer B, Föhles J, Van Neste D: Human hair production by scalp samples grafted onto nude mice. Biochemical data on normal human hair and the genetic defect trichothiodystrophy. *J Dermatol Sci* 1994; **7**: S39–S46.
8. Lane AT, Scott GA, Day KH: Development of human fetal skin transplanted to the nude mouse. *J Invest Dermatol* 1989; **93**: 787–791.
9. Pouteaux P, Van Neste D: What is new in scalp cosmetic surgery? In: Van Neste D, Randall VA (eds.). *Hair Research for the Next Millennium.* Amsterdam, Elsevier, 1996: 131–133.
10. Van Neste D, De Brouwer B, Tetelin C, Bonfils A: Testosterone conditioned nude mice: an improved model for experimental monitoring of human hair production by androgen dependent balding scalp grafts. In: Van Neste D, Randall VA (eds.). *Hair Research for the Next Millennium.* Amsterdam, Elsevier, 1996: 319–322.
11. De Brouwer B, Tételin C, Leroy T, Bonfils A, Van Neste D: A controlled study of the effects of RU 58841, a non-steroidal antiandrogen, on human hair production by balding scalp grafts maintained on to testosterone-conditioned nude mice. *Br J Dermatol* 1997; **137**: 699–702.
12. Van Neste D: The growth of human hair in nude mice. *Dermatol Clin* 1996; **14**: 609–617.

13. Van Neste D: The use of scalp grafts onto nude mice as a model for human hair growth: is there something new for hair growth drug screening programs? In: Maibach HI (ed.). *Dermatologic Research Techniques*, Boca Raton USA, CRC Press, 1996: 37–49.

14. Sundberg JP, Beamer WG, Uno H, et al.: Androgenetic alopecia in vivo models. *Pathobiology* (Submitted for publication, No. 99c31).

Section III

ANDROGENETIC ALOPECIA

10
The biology of androgenetic alopecia

Valerie Anne Randall

Introduction

Androgenetic alopecia is the most commonly occurring form of balding on the scalp. It involves the progressive loss of clearly visible terminal hair, which is replaced by nearly invisible fine, vellus hair in response to circulating androgens and particularly affects men. Despite also occurring in women, it is known as male-pattern baldness, common baldness, male pattern alopecia and androgen-dependent alopecia.

Although androgenetic alopecia is not life-threatening, it has been regarded as an important disorder for many years; the anxieties suffered by ancient Egyptian men were recorded on papyrus 4000 years ago[1] and Aristotle discussed the importance of 'maleness' and the testes in developing androgenetic alopecia. This reflects the very significant, although not always recognized, role of hair in human social and sexual communication, whatever the genetic background or culture. The ritual head shaving of Christian and Buddhist monks, and often prisoners, the standard short haircuts of soldiers and the religiously uncut hair of Sikhs are only a few examples of the social importance of hair. Moreover, adult body hair growth, namely pubic and axillary hair, signals sexual maturity in both sexes, and readily distinguishes the adult male from the female with beard, chest and upper pubic triangle (discussed further by Randall in Chapter 5). As a result, people with hair disorders such as androgenetic alopecia may suffer from marked psychological distress. A wide range of cures have been suggested over the years,[2] including goose droppings or arsenic derivatives! Only in the last few years, however, has there been sufficient understanding of the biology of the hair follicle, the complex variations in the effects of androgens on follicles depending on their body site, and the actual mechanisms of androgen action to enable the development of more successful modes of control.

This chapter will consider the patterns of hair loss in both sexes, its incidence and effects, the pathological processes of androgenetic alopecia, particularly in men, and possible forms of treatment.

Patterns of hair loss in androgenetic alopecia

In men

The gradual replacement of long, pigmented, terminal hairs on the scalp of many adult men by short, pale, vellus hairs occurs in a relatively precise pattern (Figure 1). The progression was first graded by Hamilton[3] from Type I for the prepubertal scalp with terminal hair growth on the forehead and all over the scalp, through gradual regression of the frontal hairline and thinning on the vertex, to Type VIII where the bald areas have fully coalesced to leave hair only around the back and sides of the head. Hamilton's classification was later modified by Norwood[4] to include variations on the middle grades IIIa, III vertex, IVa and Va (see Figure 1); this scale has now been used extensively during clinical trials of hair growth promoting agents.

Hamilton's original grading scale[3] was produced after he examined 312 Caucasian men and 214 women aged 20–89 years. He reported a very

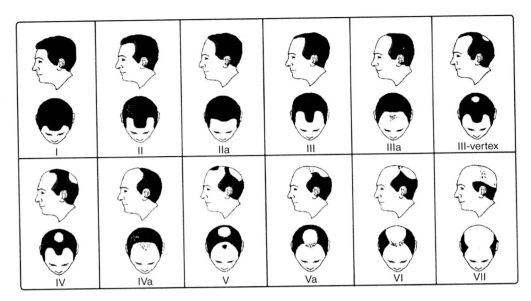

Figure 1

The pattern of hair loss in androgenetic alopecia in men. Androgens cause a gradual inhibition of hair growth on the scalp in genetically predisposed individuals; this is much more common in men than women. In men, the first signs are generally temporal regression, which spreads backwards and joins thinning regions on the vertex to give a bald crown. After Hamilton.[4]

common progression of the prepubertal scalp pattern to Type II in both sexes after puberty; this occurred in 96% of men and 79% of women. In addition, most men over 50 (58%) exhibited at least Type V, with further progression often occurring up to the age of 70 years.

In women

Interestingly, for a condition usually associated with men, Hamilton's study[3] revealed that, as well as a common postpubertal scalp pattern of Type II, about 25% of Caucasian women exhibited Type IV pattern by the age of 50 years, although there was no further development of this balding and no Types V–VIII were seen. Some women who had type II frontal recession appeared to return to the prepubertal pattern after 50 years of age.

Although the Hamilton male pattern can occur in women, the progressive diffuse loss of hair from the crown with retention of the frontal hairline described by Ludwig[5] is more common (Figure 2). Venning and Dawber[6] found that 80% of pre-menopausal women had thinning in the Ludwig pattern Stages I–III (see Figure 2) and 13% had Hamilton Type II–IV patterns when they examined 564 women aged over 20 years. After the menopause, the proportion exhibiting the male pattern increased to 37% and, although they did not progress beyond Hamilton Stage IV, some had marked M-shaped recession at both temples.

Incidence

Although there are no precise figures for incidence within a population, that in Caucasians is high. Estimates vary widely; it is often quoted as approaching 100%,[7] although other workers

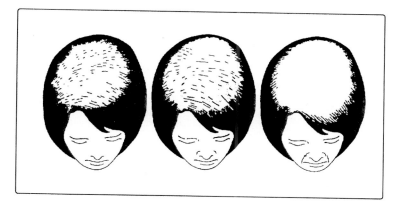

Figure 2

A common pattern of hair loss in women with androgenetic alopecia. The pattern of androgen-dependent hair loss in women differs from that in men (compare this with Figure 1). In women, the front hairline is normally retained and a general thinning on the vertex gradually becomes more pronounced until the vertex becomes bald. After Ludwig.[65]

suggest about 50% of men and women beyond 40 years of age exhibit androgenetic alopecia.[8] There is a marked racial variation in incidence; non-Caucasians often exhibit much less balding. Hamilton reported that most Chinese retained the prepubertal hairline after puberty and that baldness was less common, less extensive and started later in life than Caucasians.[3] Japanese men also began balding about 10 years later and exhibited a lower incidence (about 1.4 times).[9] Four times as many African-Americans also retained a full head of hair compared with Caucasians.[10] This racial variation is probably genetic as differences appear to be retained if the individuals move to other parts of the world.

Effects of androgenetic alopecia

Possible functions of androgenetic alopecia in men

Androgenetic alopecia is very common, with progression to Type II reported in 96% of Caucasian men.[3] It is also seen in other primates including the orang-utan and chimpanzee and has been well-studied in the stump-tailed macaque.[11] This suggests a natural progression of a secondary sexual characteristic rather than a disease. Thinking in comparative biological terms about human history when many men may have died early as a result of fighting, marked androgenetic alopecia would obviously clearly identify the surviving older male as a leader, like the silver-backed older male gorilla and the larger antlers on an older deer.

Other authors have speculated that the bald patch of an angry older dominant male would flush and look very aggressive to an opponent,[12] or give an advantage in close hand-to-hand fighting because there was less accessible hair to pull.[13] Whatever the potential benefit, the reduced incidence of androgenetic alopecia in Negro men suggests evolutionary pressure to retain scalp hair for protection from the sun in the Tropics.[10]

Negative effects of androgenetic alopecia on quality of life

In our youth-orientated culture, the association of hair loss with increasing age has negative connotations and, since hair plays such an important role in human social and sexual communication, male-pattern baldness often causes marked psychological distress and reduction in the quality of life, despite not being life-threatening or physically painful. This has been confirmed by several studies showing the negative effects of hair loss on men[14–19] and women.[20,21] These found that other people perceive men with visible hair loss as older, less physically and socially attractive, weaker and duller. People with hair loss also reported a poor self-image, a feeling of being older, and a loss of self-confidence. Although the majority of these studies focused on people already requesting medical treatment, a recent study by Girman and colleagues[19] has shown similar perceptions among those who appear more accepting of the condition, since they have never consulted anyone for potential treatment. Whatever its historical biological role, androgenetic alopecia reduces the quality of life in the affluent industrialized world of today.

Pathology of androgenetic alopecia

The progressive increase in patterned balding is the result of the gradual transformation of terminal follicles, producing the large, thick, pigmented scalp hairs of adolescence and childhood to smaller, vellus follicles forming short, fine, colourless vellus hairs (Figure 3). This is the reverse of the transformation of vellus follicles on many parts of the body, such as the face or axilla, to terminal follicles after puberty (discussed by Randall in Chapter 5). These are major changes in cell biological terms, with follicles passing through several cycles before the processes are completed (see Figure 3). Hair follicles are in anagen (the growing period) for most of the time in the normal scalp, with an average anagen length of 2–3 years and telogen of about 100 days.[22] This gives an anagen:telogen ratio of about 9:1, although there is some seasonal variation in people living in temperate regions[23,24] (discussed in Chapter 5). As androgenetic alopecia develops, the anagen phase shortens thus increasing the proportion of telogen hairs[25–27] (this can be detected before any balding) and causing shorter hairs to be produced,[27] miniaturization of the follicles is seen histologically[25,28] and the hairs produced are also thinner.[26,27] Most of the follicles are very short and small, with occasional resting terminal follicles, in balding scalp.

Studies of androgenetic alopecia may be complicated by the non-androgen-dependent hair thinning found in those over 50 years of age, known as *senescent balding*.[28] This also involves a progressive decrease in the number of anagen follicles[29] and hair diameter[30] but does not normally lead to baldness. Kligman suggested that both forms may occur together. He also proposed a pronounced inflammatory component in androgenetic alopecia but not in senescent balding.[28] The first indications of inflammatory involvement, Kligman reported, were focal perivascular degeneration in the lower one-third of the connective tissue sheath and perifollicular lymphohistiocytic infiltration at sebaceous gland level;[28] multinucleate giant cells may be seen later.[31] The sclerotic remains of the fibrous sheath may be seen below the shortened follicles as 'streamers'.[28] Although the damage to the connective tissue sheath caused by chronic inflammation may prevent the reformation of terminal hair follicles in long-term alopecia, this is currently the subject of much debate.

The arrector pili muscle reduces much more slowly than the follicle during the miniaturization processes[32] and the sebaceous gland, also an androgen-dependent tissue, becomes enlarged.[28] This means that the scalp often has an oily, more greasy appearance, since the long hairs that are normally coated by the sebum have been lost. There is also a reduced blood supply to the follicle[33,34] and nerve networks that have lost their follicular support may twist to form a type of encapsulated end-organ below the follicle.[35] Whether the reduced blood supply is induced after the reduction in follicle size or precedes it is currently unclear.

Pathogenesis

Role of androgens

Androgens are an essential factor in the development of androgenetic alopecia. Hamilton demonstrated that men who had never gone through puberty did not go bald, and that, although men castrated after puberty showed no further progression of their baldness, they did not regain the frontal hairline.[36–38] Hamilton analysed the importance of androgens by giving

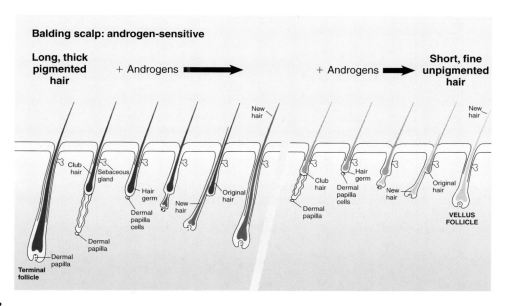

Figure 3

Diagrammatic representation of the miniaturization processes occurring in response to androgens on the scalp of an individual with a genetic predisposition to androgenetic alopecia. Androgens inhibit scalp hair follicles in balding regions by inducing them to produce progressively smaller, finer and less-pigmented hairs until the terminal hairs of childhood and early adulthood are replaced by the vellus hairs of androgenetic alopecia and the area appears bald. The follicles themselves become shorter and finer but must pass through a full hair cycle, probably a succession of cycles, to accomplish major changes.

testosterone proprionate replacement therapy to castrated men; this stimulated progressive balding, which halted during temporary withdrawal of the hormone in those with a family history of balding.[37] The importance of androgens is confirmed by the lack of androgenetic alopecia in individuals with androgen-insensitivity who lack functional androgen receptors.[39] These are genetic males (XY) who develop a mainly female phenotype despite normal or raised testosterone levels; moreover, as well as exhibiting no temporal regression or balding they do not even produce terminal hair in the female pubic pattern or in the axillae.

There is a widely held belief that baldness indicates increased male sexuality but there is little scientific evidence for this except for the clear link with normal androgen parameters. No relationship was found between androgenetic alopecia and other androgen-regulated parameters including muscle, bone and skin or sebum excretion rate and body hair growth in adult men.[40] Normal male testosterone levels have been reported in balding men[41,42] although with higher urinary dehydroepiandrosterone[41] or dehydroepiandrosterone sulphate;[42] other studies showed raised serum free testosterone.[43,44] Overall, normal male androgen levels appear to be sufficient to cause androgenetic alopecia, and this response appears to be related to the intrinsic sensitivity of the follicles themselves.

In women, circulating androgen levels appear to be related to the amount of hair loss,[45-51] presumably because the normal levels are much lower. Women presenting with androgenetic alopecia also often exhibit polycystic ovarian disease.[52]

Mechanism of androgen action in androgenetic alopecia

Androgens, like other steroid hormones, circulate in the blood and, since they are steroids, pass readily through the plasma membranes into cells where they bind specific, intracellular androgen receptors. The hormone–receptor complex undergoes a conformational change enabling it to bind to specific hormone-response elements in the DNA, activating specific gene expression and generally altering the production of specific proteins. The main circulating androgen in men, testosterone, is often metabolized intracellularly to other forms particularly 5α-dihydrotestosterone (5α-DHT) in many tissues, for example the classical target organ, the prostate.[53] The 5α-dihydrotestosterone binds to the androgen receptor with even greater affinity than testosterone and can activate both the receptor and appropriate gene expression (see Chapter 5). Testosterone itself seems to be active in some tissues such as skeletal muscle,[53] Recently, two isoforms of 5α-reductase, type 1 and type 2, have been identified, with type 2 being the classical form found in the prostate.[53]

The absence of balding in individuals with androgen-insensitivity syndrome who lack functional androgen receptors clearly demonstrates the need for androgen receptors within hair follicles for the miniaturization process of androgenetic alopecia to occur.[39] The role of the 5α-reductase enzymes necessary to metabolize testosterone to 5α-dihydrotestosterone has, however, been less clear.

Men with 5α-reductase deficiency type 2 only form terminal hair in the axillae and female pubic pattern, grow little or no beard or chest hair and are not reported to go bald.[54] Nevertheless, the various kindred with this deficiency around the world are generally from families that do not exhibit much balding; initial studies also reported that these individuals also did not have acne. Their sebum production has now been shown to be normal and acne has been reported.[55] Initial studies on androgen metabolism in androgenetic alopecia focused on whole skin or plucked hair follicles but, unfortunately, these are not very useful systems. Skin contains several androgen target tissues that may respond very differently to androgens, for example the tiny vellus hair follicles and enlarged sebaceous glands of the face of a woman with acne. Plucked hair follicles usually do not contain the dermal papilla, the key target in androgen action (discussed later) since this is retained in the skin. These facts make the results from whole-skin studies hard to interpret. Plucked hair follicles from all body sites metabolize testosterone to the less active androstenedione, regardless of the role of 5α-dihydrotestosterone in hair growth in that region; however, higher 5α-reductase activity by isolated balding follicles compared with non-balding ones was reported.[56]

Studies of the gene expression of the two 5α-reductases have not fully clarified matters. 5α-reductase type 1 activity has been associated with the sebaceous gland and scalp skin after puberty.[57] type 2, however, is expressed in scalp skin for a short period after birth.[58] The function of this time-limited expression is uncertain but it may be a type of imprinting mechanism on the scalp follicles. Nevertheless, the classical 5α-reductase type 2 enzyme appears to be involved in androgenetic alopecia, as well as beard and chest hair growth, since treatment with 5α-reductase type 2 inhibitor, finasteride, has either promoted hair regrowth or halted further progression of balding[59] (see also Chapter 13 by Price).

The current model for androgen action is based on the hypothesis put forward by Randall[60] (see also Chapter 5) that androgens act on the hair follicle by binding to androgen receptors in the mesenchyme-derived dermal papilla cells. The androgens then alter the expression of paracrine factors such as growth factors and/or extracellular matrix components. Presumably, with balding being the result of miniaturization of follicles, this would imply that androgens would either reduce the production of stimulatory factors or initiate the production of inhibitory factors. Cultured dermal papilla cells from human hair follicles with varying sensitivities to androgens have been studied throughout the 1990s. These studies have shown that androgen-stimulated cells, derived from beard, axilla, pubic and genital hair follicles contained androgen receptors[61] and metabolized testosterone in vitro, in line with hair growth in patients with 5α-reductase deficiency in vivo.[62–64] All these results support the concept that androgens act through the dermal papilla. Recently, dermal papilla cells have been cultured from human androgenetic alopecia hair follicles.[34] These cells also contained higher levels of specific androgen receptors than non-balding scalp, although the receptors had exactly the same pattern of binding affinity, indicating that they were not different receptors[65] (Figure 4).

Interestingly, testosterone stimulated mitogenic factor production by cultured beard dermal papilla cells[66,67] but when this experiment was repeated with human androgenetic alopecia cells testosterone caused a *reduction* in the amount secreted.[68] This also occurred in cells from the balding region of the stump-tailed macaque,[69] a type of monkey that exhibits androgen-dependent balding and which is often used as an animal model (see Chapter 14 by Uno). These results imply that further investigations to determine the nature of these molecules might lead to developing novel, more precise treatments for androgenetic alopecia.

Genetic involvement in androgenetic alopecia

Family history

The genetic involvement in androgenetic alopecia is pronounced. Male-pattern baldness runs in families[37] and Hamilton showed that the balding response to androgen replacement in castrated men depended on their family history, with those with no history of balding exhibiting no response.[37] This importance of genes concurs with the racial differences discussed earlier (see *Incidence*, p. 124). Although androgenetic alopecia is generally believed to be an autosomal dominant trait with variable penetrance,[70] no specific gene or set of genes have been identified so far, presumably because of the very high incidence. Genetic analysis focusing on those who exhibit advanced balding at an early age should

be the most rewarding since this is the most dramatic expression of the condition.

Intrinsic response of individual follicles

The paradoxically different effects of androgens on human hair follicles, varying from stimulation of beard follicles, apparent lack of effect on the eyelashes and inhibition of scalp follicles often in a single individual, clearly demonstrate the intrinsic response of the individual follicle. This is further emphasized by the range of sensitivity to androgens by scalp follicles, demonstrated by the slow, progressive nature of the miniaturization processes (see Figures 1, 2, 3). This individual, intrinsic response of human hair follicles to androgens is the basis for hair transplant surgery.[71] When androgen-insensitive hair follicles from 'non-balding' regions of the scalp, such as the nape of the neck, are transplanted to the balding crown, they retain their innate inability to respond and continue to produce terminal follicles, while miniaturization progresses in the androgen-sensitive vertex follicles behind them. This means that they will become progressively more isolated unless further transplants are carried out.

Although how this occurs is not yet understood, it seems likely that some genetic programming of androgen sensitivity occurs during development. Recently, the dermis of the frontal-parietal scalp (equivalent to the human balding regions) of the quail chick has been shown to develop from a different region to the (non-balding) occipital-temporal scalp dermis;[72] the frontal-parietal region arises from the neural crest, while the occipital-temporal region derives from the mesoderm. Since these areas have such different androgen responses in humans, a similar pattern in human scalp development may be involved with the different gene expression, causing the scalp regional responses to androgens in adults.

Androgenetic alopecia[37] does not return to prepubertal levels if men are castrated after puberty. This could suggest that the altered gene expression may not need androgen to persist once sufficiently triggered, although it is necessary for

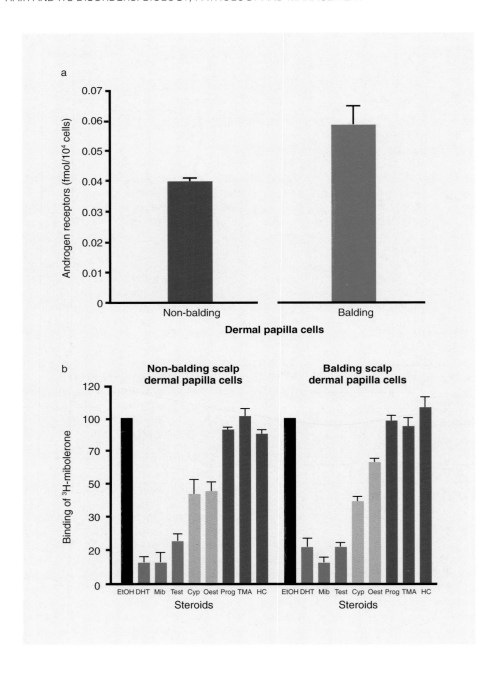

Figure 4

Cultured dermal papilla cells from human androgenetic alopecia hair follicles contain higher levels of androgen receptors than non-balding scalp cells (a), but their binding affinity for a range of steroids is the same indicating that the receptors are similar in type (b). EtOH, ethanol vehicle alone; DHT, 5α-dihydrotestosterone; Mib, mibolerone; Test, testosterone; Cyp, cyproterone acetate; Oest, 17β-oestradiol; Prog, progesterone; TMA, triamcinolone acetonide; HC, hydrocortisol. Taken from Hibberts, Howell and Randall, 1998.[65]

further development. Conversely, if chronic inflammation has caused fibrosis below the shortened balding follicle,[28] it seems unlikely that the follicle could reform a terminal hair follicle, regardless of stimulus. Recent studies using the 5α-reductase type 2 inhibitor, finasteride, have reversed miniaturization in some younger sufferers.[59] It may be that androgens manufactured in the adrenal glands are sufficient to maintain balding if not opposed.

Association with other diseases

Since androgenetic alopecia is so common, correlation with other diseases is not too helpful. Nevertheless, there has been some interest in relating it to other common male disorders involving androgens. A relationship between androgenetic alopecia and coronary heart disease has generally been inconsistent; however, two studies have related vertex balding in men below 55 years of age with the risk of myocardial infarction in a cross-sectional study[73] and rapidly progressing balding with coronary heart disease in a prospective study.[74] Whether this indicates a genetic link and/or dual end-organ increased sensitivity or whether the heart problems are caused by the psychological stress induced by early balding in the youth-orientated Western culture is unclear. Whatever the cause, early/rapidly progressing balding is an easy, non-invasive marker that could prove useful in screening for men with a tendency towards heart disease. A few studies have also explored whether androgenetic alopecia is associated with prostate cancer.[44] Since both have a high incidence in older men, the absence of any correlation so far could result from the case-control study design only involving older men; a prospective study involving men showing early or rapid balding would be necessary to see if there is any correlation.

Treatment of androgenetic alopecia

Numerous remedies have been suggested for androgenetic alopecia[2] over the years. Recently, spending some time upside down each day (presumably to increase blood flow to the head) and having a cow lick the balding area regularly (could this involve growth factors in saliva?) have been proposed. Although new suggestions need to be viewed with an open mind, established treatments are also wide-ranging; these include wigs and hair-pieces, surgery, modifiers of hormone action and non-hormonal therapy such as minoxidil (Table 1).

Surgery

All surgical methods are based on the different intrinsic responses of individual hair follicles as already discussed. The principle involves moving androgen-insensitive 'non-balding' (i.e. occipital

Table 1   Current forms of treatment for androgenetic alopecia.*

Approach	Treatment
Cosmetic	Wigs, hairpieces
Surgery	Hair transplants, scalp extension
Anti-hormonal therapy	Antiandrogens (e.g. cyproterone acetate) impractical for men because of side-effects
	5α-reductase Type 2 inhibitors – e.g. finasteride
Non-hormonal therapy	Biological response modifiers (e.g. minoxidil)

*Since androgen production is unaltered by these treatments, progression of the balding will extend unless the effects are blocked/countered continually.

and parietal) terminal follicles to the sites of the androgen-sensitive scalp follicles.[71] This has been carried out for many years by transplanting small biopsies with several follicles from areas such as the nape of the neck on to the frontal or vortex regions; more recently, variable size pieces ranging down to micrografts with one or two follicles have been used.[75] Once established, these expensive and painful treatments are long-lasting but the natural progression of the balding will continue and further transplants may be required to avoid the transplanted region being left surrounded by bald scalp.

Scalp extension is an alternative approach. The central bald skin is removed and the remaining hairy skin is stretched. Skin may be stretched before any surgery, but this is less popular due to the obvious head swelling involved during the stretching processes.

Hormonal treatments

Antiandrogens

The theoretically ideal approach of blocking the androgen receptor by antiandrogens is not really practical, since antiandrogens would block all androgen effects in the body. This would have unacceptable side-effects on masculinity and the potential to cause feminization of a male fetus in a pregnant woman. Nevertheless, cyproterone acetate, an antiandrogen with progestational effects, that has been used for hirsutism and acne in women in Europe and Canada for over 20 years, has also been used to treat female androgenetic alopecia. Generally 50–100 mg cyproterone acetate per day is used, combined with oestrogen to ensure contraception in premenopausal women. Although there are no large, controlled clinical studies, it appears to prevent further progression at least.[76] Cyproterone acetate is not available in the USA but spirolactone, an aldosterone antagonist with mild antiandrogenic effects, is often used as an alternative; spironolactone may have some clinical effect on progression but does not cause regrowth.[77]

5α-reductase inhibitors

The introduction of finasteride, a 5α-reductase type 2 inhibitor, that blocks the conversion of testosterone to 5α-dihydrotestosterone, is a recent, exciting, development in the treatment of androgenetic alopecia in men. Initially, finasteride was developed for the treatment of benign prostate hypertrophy where it is used at a dose of 5 mg per day.[78] Since it appears to be a safe treatment, double-blind clinical trials of the effects of 1 mg of finasteride orally per day on androgenetic alopecia in men have been conducted in the USA and elsewhere[59] (see Chapter 13 by Price for full details). Finasteride slowed the progression of hair loss and promoted hair growth in men under 40 with Stage II–V patterns in 6–12 months. Since both the endogenous hormonal trigger and the follicle's ability to respond to androgens continue to be present, any hormonal treatment must be continued for the effect to be maintained.

Whether or not finasteride would be useful in older men or those with more extensive balding is not yet known. Since plasma 5α-dihydrotestosterone levels are reduced during finasteride treatment,[59] it is unclear whether the inhibitor is working centrally blocking the action of 5α-reductase or within the balding follicles themselves. Nevertheless, topical application of 0.005% solution of finasteride twice daily caused some improvement in men and women under 40 years of age with early balding, suggesting a local effect.[79] Although the use of finasteride in women of child-bearing age is difficult, since there is, like with antiandrogens, the potential of abnormality in a male fetus, a trial in postmenopausal women is currently underway.

Non-hormonal therapy

The most frequently used non-hormonal treatment is minoxidil, initially devised as an antihypertensive drug and now available as an over the counter, topical treatment.[80] Minoxidil in a 2% solution applied topically to the scalp twice a day stimulated some hair regrowth in about 35% of men up to 50 years of age[81] and 63% of women up to 45 years of age;[81] again discontinuation of treatment leads to progression of baldness. Recently, a 5% solution produced somewhat greater effects.[82] These findings are reviewed by Dawber in Chapter 14. Although the precise mechanism of action is uncertain because minoxidil has many effects, including vasodilation, it can stimulate the growth of isolated hair follicles in culture in the absence of a blood supply,[83,84] suggesting that the capacity to open potassium channels may be the most important. Another potassium-channel opener, diazoxide, which is used for treating some pancreatic disorders may also promote hair growth in many areas, such as the back, as an unwanted side-effect, particularly in children.[85]

Summary and conclusions

Androgenetic alopecia is a common, progressive, androgen-dependent hair disorder that occurs in both men and women, often leading to marked negative effects on the quality of life. The progressive replacement of long, pigmented terminal hairs by tiny, colourless vellus ones is caused by the individual response of hair follicles to androgens. How androgens cause the paradoxical stimulation of hair growth in many areas, such as the beard, have no effect on others, such as the eyelashes and cause inhibition on the scalp is unclear. It is known that androgens act at the level of the hair follicle and require the presence of intracellular androgen receptors. In some androgen-responsive follicles such as the beard, the enzyme 5α-reductase type 2 is also necessary to metabolize testosterone 5α-dihydrotestosterone. This also seems to be involved in androgenetic alopecia. The current hypothesis for androgen action in the hair follicle is that androgens act via the dermal papilla. This suggests that androgens bind to receptors in dermal papilla cells, causing the alteration of their secretion of paracrine regulators such as growth factors that regulate other cells of the follicle. This is currently the subject of much research.

Pharmaceutical companies have been very interested in promoting hair growth since the realization from the side-effects of minoxidil, originally an antihypertensive drug, that hair regrowth could be stimulated. Most anti-hormonal treatment is unsuitable for men owing to antimasculinity side-effects. Nevertheless, the new development of the 5α-reductase type 2 inhibitor, finasteride, has opened up the use of hormonal treatments in men. Since finasteride and minoxidil act at different sites, it is possible that their combined effects would be greater; in the stump-tailed macaque, combined treatment in an androgenetic alopecia animal model produced an additive effect[86] (see Chapter 11 by Uno et al). Further drugs will probably be developed both as hormone and biological-response modifiers; combined 5α-reductase type 1 and type 2 inhibitors are also a possibility. Any therapy, however, will need to be taken for as long as the effect is required, since both the hormone and its target follicles are both still functional.

The recently developed culture of human androgenetic alopecia dermal papilla cells[34,65,68] appears to offer a useful system for identifying the regulatory paracrine factors whose gene expression is regulated by androgens. Identification of such factors could lead to other routes for therapeutic approaches. The most useful and practical route of application appears to be the topical approach since, theoretically at least, this should focus the treatment to the appropriate site and reduce any potential side-effects. The recent demonstration that the liposome method can deliver compounds into the cells of the hair bulb may offer a new route.[87] Overall, although there have been great improvements in our understanding of hair-follicle biology, the mechanism of androgen action in follicles and ways to treat androgenetic alopecia, everything is not yet clear; hopefully, the current interest and momentum in this area should result in even greater understanding and better treatments in the future.

Acknowledgements

The assistance of Mr Chris Bowers and Mrs Jenny Braithwaite in the production of the figures and Mrs Christine Dove and Mrs Jayne Dunn in the preparation of the manuscript is gratefully acknowledged.

References

1. Giacometti L: Facts, legends and myths about the scalp throughout history. *Arch Dermatol* 1967; **95**: 629–635.
2. Lambert G: *The Conquest of Baldness. The Wonderful Story of Hair.* London, Souvenir Press, 1961.

3. Hamilton JB: Patterned loss of hair in man; types and incidence. *Ann NY Acad Sci* 1951; **53**: 708–728.

4. Norwood OTT: Male-pattern baldness. Classification and incidence. *South Med J* 1975; **68**: 1359–1370.

5. Ludwig E: Classification of the types of androgenic alopecia (common baldness) arising in the female sex. *Br J Dermatol* 1977; **97**: 249–256.

6. Venning VA, Dawber R: Patterned androgenic alopecia. *J Am Acad Dermatol* 1988; **18**: 1073–1078.

7. Dawber RPP, de Berker D, Wojnarowska F: Disorders of hair. In: Champion RH, Burton JL, Durns DA (eds.). *Rook/Wilkinson/Ebling Textbook of Dermatology*, 6th edn. Oxford, Blackwell Science, 1988: 2869–2973.

8. Olsen EA: Androgenetic alopecia. In: Olsen EZ (ed.) *Disorders of Hair Growth, Diagnosis and Treatment*. New York, McGraw-Hill, 1994: 257–283.

9. Takashima I, Iju M, Sudo M: Alopecia androgenetica—its incidence in Japanese and associated conditions. In: Orfanos CE, Montagna W, Stuttgen G (eds.). *Hair Research Status and Future Aspects*. New York, Springer Verlag, 1981: 287–293.

10. Setty LR: Hair patterns of the scalp of white and negro males. *Am J Phys Anthropol* 1970; **33**: 49–55.

11. Montagna W, Uno H: The phyologeny of baldness. In: Baccaredla-Boy A, Morretti G, Fray JR (eds.). *Biopathology of Pattern Alopecia*. Basel, Karger, 1968: 9–24.

12. Goodhart DB: The evolutionary significance of human hair patterns and skin colouring. *Adv Sci* 1960; **17**: 53–59.

13. Ebling FJG: Age changes in cutaneous appendages. *J Appl Cosmetol* 1985; **3**: 243–250.

14. Terry RL, Davis JS: Components of facial attractiveness. *Percept Motor Skills* 1976; **42**: 918–923.

15. Cash TF: The psychological effects of androgenetic alopecia in men. *J Am Acad Dermatol* 1992; **26**: 926–931.

16. Franzoi SL, Anderson J, Frommelt S: Individual differences in men's perceptions of and reactions to thinning hair. *J Soc Psychol* 1990; **130**: 209–218.

17. Maffei C, Fossati A, Reialdi F, Ruia E: Personality disorders and psychopathologic symptoms in patients with androgenetic alopecia. *Arch Dermatol* 1994; **130**: 868–872.

18. Wells PA, Willmoth T, Russel RJH: Does fortune favour the bald? Psychological correlates of hair loss in males. *Br J Psychol* 1995; **86**: 337–344.

19. Girman CJ, Rhodes T, Lilly FRW, Guo SS, Siervogel RM, Patrick DL, et al.: Effects of self-perceived hair loss in a community sample of men. *Dermatology* 1998; **197**: 223–229.

20. Cash TF: Psychological effects of androgenetic alopecia on women: comparisons with balding men and with female control subjects. *J Am Acad Dermatol* 1993; **29**: 568–575.

21. Van der Dank J, Passchier J, Knegt-Junk C, Wegen-Keijser MH, Nieboer C, Stolz E, et al.: Psychological characteristics of women with androgenetic alopecia: a controlled study. *Br J Dermatol* 1991; **125**: 248–252.

22. Kligman AG: The human hair cycle. *J Invest Dermatol* 1959; **33**: 307–316.

23. Randall VA, Ebling EJG: Seasonal changes in human hair growth. *Br J Dermatol* 1991; **124**: 146–151.

24. Courtois M, Loussouarn G, Howseau S, et al.: Periodicity in the growth and shedding of hair. *Br J Dermatol* 1996; **134**: 47–54.

25. Brun-Falco O, Christophers E: Hair root patterns in male-pattern alopecia. In: Baccareda-Boy A, Moretti G, Fray JR (eds.). *Biopathology of Pattern Alopecia*. Basel, Kargel, 1968: 141–145.

26. Rushton DH, Ramsay ID, Norris MJ, Gilkes JJH: Natural Progression of male-pattern baldness in young men. *Clin Exper Dermatol* 1991; **16**: 188–192.

27. Whiting DA: Diagnostic and predictive value of horizontal sections of scalp biopsy specimens in male-pattern androgenetic alopecia. *J Am Acad Dermatol* 1993; **28**: 757–763.

28. Kligman AM: The comparative histopathology of male-pattern baldness and senescent baldness. *Clin Dermatol* 1988; **6(4)**: 108–118.

29. Pecoraro OV, Astore I, Barman JM: The pre-natal and postnatal hair cycles in men. In: Baccareda-Boy A, Moretti G, Fray JR (eds.). *Biopathology of Pattern Alopecia*. Basel, Kargel, 1968: 29–38.

30. Ebling FJG: Age changes in cutaneous appendages. *J Appl Cosmetol* 1985; **3**: 243–250.

31. Douritz JM, Silvers DN: Giant cells in male pattern alopecia: a histological marker and pathogenic clue. *J Cutan Pathol* 1979; **6**: 108–113.

32. Maguire HC, Kligman AM: Common baldness in women. *Geriatrics* 1963; **18**: 329–334.

33. Crovato F, Morreti G, Bertamino R: In Baccareda-Boy A, Moretti G, Fray JR (eds.). *Biopathology of Pattern Alopecia*. Basel, Kargel, 1968: 191–199.

34. Randall VA, Hibberts NA, Hamada K: A comparison of the culture and growth of dermal papilla cells derived from normal and balding (androgenetic alopecia) scalp. *Br J Dermatol* 1996; **134**: 437–444.

35. Giacometti L, Montagna W: The nerve fibres in male-pattern alopecia. In: Baccareda-Boy A, Moretti G, Fray JR (eds.). *Biopathology of Pattern Alopecia*. Basel, Kargel, 1968: 208–216.

36. Hamilton JB: Age, sex and genetic factors in the regulation of hair growth in man: a comparison of Caucasian and Japanese populations. In: Montagna

W, Ellis RA (eds.). *The Biology of Hair Growth.* New York, Academic Press, 1958: 399–433.

37. Hamilton JB: Male hormone stimulation is a prerequisite and an incitant in common baldness. *Am J Anat* 1942; **71**: 451–480.

38. Hamilton JB: Effect of castration in adolescent and young adult males upon further changes in the proportions of bare and hairy scalp. *J Clin Endocrinol Metab* 1960; **20**: 1309–1318.

39. Quigley CA: The androgen receptor: physiology and pathophysiology. In: Nieschlag E, Behre HM (eds.). *Testosterone: Action, Deficiency, Substitution.* Berlin, Springer-Verlag, 1998: 33–106.

40. Burton JL, Ben Halim MM, Meyrick G: Male-pattern alopecia and masculinity. *Br J Dermatol* 1979; **100**: 507–512.

41. Phillipou G, Kirke J: Significance of steroid measurements in male-pattern alopecia. *Clin Exper Dermatol* 1981; **6**: 53–58.

42. Pitts RL: Serum elevation of dehydroepiandrosterone sulphate associated with male-pattern baldness in young men. *J Am Acad Dermatol* 1987; **16**: 571–573.

43. Cipriani R, Ruzza G, Foresta C, Veller-Fornasa C, Peserico A: Sex hormone binding globulin and saliva testosterone levels in men with androgenetic alopecia. *Br J Dermatol* 1983; **109**: 249–252.

44. Denmark S, Wahnefried W, Lesko S, et al.: Serum androgens: associations with prostate cancer risk and hair patterning. *J Androl* 1997; **18**: 495–500.

45. Buiazzi M, Calandra P: Testosterone elimination in female patients with acne, chronic alopecia and hirsutism. *Ital Gen Rev Dermatol* 1968; **8**: 241.

46. Ludwig E: The role of sexual hormones in pattern alopecia. In: Baccareda-Boy A, Moretti G, Fray JR (eds.). *Biopathology of Pattern Alopecia.* Basel, Kargel, 1968: 50–60.

47. Kuhn BH: Male-pattern alopecias and/or androgenetic hirsutism in females. Part III Definition and aetiology. *J Am Med Wom Ass:* 1972; **27**: 357.

48. Miller JA, Darley CR, Karleavitsas K, Kirkby JD, Munro DD: How sex hormone binding globulin levels in young women with diffuse hair loss. *Br J Dermatol* 1982; **106**: 331–336.

49. De Villez RL, Dunn J: Female androgenic alopecia. The 3α-17β androstanedial glucuronide/sex hormone binding globulin ratio as a possible marker for female-pattern baldness. *Arch Dermatol* 1986; **122**: 1011–1014.

50. Georgala G, Papasotirion V, Stavropoulos P: Serum testosterone and sex hormone binding levels in women with androgenic alopecia. *Acta Dermatol Venerol (Stockh)* 1986; **66**: 532.

51. Moltz L: Hormonal diagnostik der sogenannten androgenetischen Alopezie der Fru. *Gebuts Frauenheil* 1988; **48**: 203–206.

52. Futterweit W, Dunif Y, Yeh H-C, Kingsley P: The prevalence of hyperandrogenism in 109 consecutive female patients with diffuse alopecia. *J Am Acad Dermatol* 1988; **19**: 831.

53. Randall VA: The role of 5α-reductase in health and disease. In: Sheppard M, Stewart P (eds.). Baillières Clinical Endocrinology and Metabolism, vol. 8 Hormones, Enzymes and Receptors. 1994: 405–431.

54. Wilson JD, Griffin JE, Russell DW: Steroid 5α-reductase 2 deficiency. *Endocrinol Rev* 1993; **14**: 577–593.

55. Imperato-McGuinley J, Gautier T, Cai L, Yee B, Epstein J, Pochi P: The androgen control of sebum production. Studies of subjects with dihydro-testosterone deficiency and complete androgen insensitivity. *J Clin Endocrinol Metab* 1993; **76**: 524–528.

56. Schweikert H, Wilson JD: Regulation of human hair growth by steroid hormones. I Testosterone metabolism in isolated hair. *J Clin Endocrinol Metab* 1974; **40**: 413–417.

57. Chan W, Zouboulis C, Orfanos C: The 5α-reductase system and its inhibitors. Recent development and its perspective in treating androgen-dependent skin disorders. *Dermatology* 1996; **193**: 177–182.

58. Thigpen AE, Silver RI, Guileyarlo JM, Casey ML, McConnell JD, Russell DW: Tissue distribution and ontogeny of steroid 5α-reductase isoenzyme expression. *J Clin Invest* 1993; **92**: 903–910.

59. Kaufman KD, Olsen EA, Whiting D, Savi R, De Villez R, Bergfeld W, et al. and the Finasteride Male Pattern Hair Loss Study Group: Finasteride in the treatment of men with androgenetic alopecia. *J Am Acad Dermatol* 1998; **39**: 578–589.

60. Randall VA: Androgens and human hair growth. *Clin Endocrinol* 1994; **40**: 439–457.

61. Randall VA, Thornton MJ, Messenger AG: Cultured dermal papilla cells from androgen-dependent human follicles (e.g. beard) contain more androgen receptors than those from non-balding areas. *J Endocrinol* 1992; **133**: 141–147.

62. Itami S, Kurata S, Takayasu S: 5α-reductase activity in cultured human dermal papilla cells from beard compared with reticular dermal fibroblasts. *J Invest Dermatol* 1990; **94**: 150–152.

63. Thornton MJ, Liang I, Hamada K, Messenger AG, Randall VA: Differences in testosterone metabolism by beard and scalp hair follicle dermal papilla cells. *Clin Endocrinol* 1993; **39**: 633–639.

64. Hamada K, Thornton MJ, Liang I, Messenger AG, Randall VA: Pubic and axillary dermal papilla cells do not produce 5α-dihydrotestosterone in culture. *J Invest Dermatol* 1996; **106**: 1017–1022.

65. Hibberts NA, Howell AE, Randall VA: Dermal papilla cells from human balding scalp hair follicles contain higher levels of androgen receptors than those from non-balding scalp. *J Endocrinol* 1998; **156**: 59–65.

66. Itami S, Kurata S, Takayasu S: Androgen induction of follicular epithelial cell growth is mediated via insulin-like growth factor I from dermal papilla cells. *Biochem Biophys Res Commun* 1995; **212**: 988–994.

67. Thornton MJ, Hamada K, Messenger AG, Randall VA: Beard, but not scalp, dermal papilla cells secrete autocrine growth factors in response to testosterone in vitro. *J Invest Dermatol* 1998; **111**: 727–732.

68. Hibberts NA, Randall VA: Testosterone inhibits the capacity of cultured cells from human balding scalp dermal papilla cells to produce keratinocyte mitogenic factors. In: Van Neste DV, Randall VA (eds.). *Hair Research for the Next Millennium.* Amsterdam, Elsevier, 1996: 303–306.

69. Obana N, Uno H: Dermal papilla cells in macaque alopecia trigger a testosterone-dependent inhibition of follicular cell proliferation. In: Van Neste DV, Randall VA (eds.). *Hair Research for the Next Millennium.* Amsterdam, Elsevier, 1996: 307–310.

70. Bergfeld WF: Androgenetic alopecia: an autosomal dominant disorder. *Am J Med* 1955; **98**: 955–985.

71. Orentreich N, Durr NP: Biology of scalp hair growth. *Clin Plast Surg* 1982; **9**: 197–205.

72. Ziller C: Pattern formation in neural crest derivatives. In: Van Neste D, Randall VA (eds.). *Hair Research for the Next Millennium.* Amsterdam, Elsevier, 1996: 1–5.

73. Lesko SM, Rosenberg L, Shapiro S: A case-control study of baldness in relation to myocardial infarction in men. *J Am Med Assoc* 1993; **269**: 988–1003.

74. Herrera CR, D'Agostino RB, Gerstman BB, Bosco LA, Belanger AJ: Baldness and coronary heart disease rates in men from the Framingham study. *Am J Epidemiol* 1995; **142**: 828–833.

75. Unger WP: What's new in hair replacement surgery. In: Whiting DA: *Dermatol Clinics, vol. 14 Update on Hair Disorders.* Philadelphia, WB Saunders, 1996: 783–802.

76. Mortimer CH, Rushton H, James KC: Effective medical treatment for common baldness in women. *Clin Exp Dermatol* 1984; **9**: 342–348.

77. Burke B, Cunliffe WJ: Oral spirolactone therapy for female patients with acne, hirsutism or androgenic alopecia. *Br J Dermatol* 1985; **112**: 124–128.

78. Gormbey GJ, Stener E, Briskewitz RC, Imperato-McGinley J, Walsh PC, McConnell J: The effect of finasteride in men with benign prostate hyperplasia. *N Engl J Med* 1992; **327**: 1185–91.

79. Mazzarella F, Loconsole F, Commisa A, Mastrolonardo M, Vena GA: Topical finasteride in the treatment of androgenic alopecia. Preliminary evaluations after a 16-month therapy course. *J Dermatol Treat* 1997; **8**: 189–192.

80. Shapiro J, Price VH: Hair regrowth: therapeutic agents. In: *Dermatol Clinics, vol. 16. Dermatologic Therapy.* Philadelphia, WB Saunders 1998: 341–356.

81. De Villez R, Jacobs J, Szpunar C, et al.: Androgenetic alopecia in the female: treatment with 2% minoxidil solution. *Arch Dermatol* 1994; **130**: 303–308.

82. Price VH, Menefee E: Changes in hair weight and hair count in men with androgenetic alopecia, after application of 5% and 2% topical minoxidil, placebo, or no treatment. In: Van Neste D, Randall VA (eds.). *Hair Research for the Next Millennium.* Amsterdam, Elsevier, 1996: 67–71.

83. Buhl AE, Waldon BS, Kawabe TT, Holland JM: Minoxidil stimulates mouse vibrissae follicles in organ culture. *J Invest Dermatol* 1989; **92**: 315–320.

84. Jenner TJ, Davies GC, Carr RD, Godfredsen C, Thornton MJ, Randall VA: The potassium-channel openers, minoxidil and diazoxide, stimulate hair growth in whole organ culture. *Eur Hair Res Soc* 1999; **14**.

85. Koblenzer PJ, Baker L: Hypertrichosis lanuginosa associated with diazoxide therapy in prepubertal children: a clinicopathologic study. *Ann NY Acad Sci* 1968, **150**: 373–382.

86. Diani A, Mulholland MJ, Skull KL, et al.: Hair growth effects of oral administration of finasteride, a steroid 5α-reductase inhibitor, alone and in combination with topical minoxidil in the balding stump tail macaque. *J Clin Endocrinol Metab* 1992; **74**: 345–350.

87. Hoffmann RM, Li LN: The feasibility of targeted selective gene therapy of the hair follicle. *Nat Med* 1995; **1**: 705–706.

11

Androgenetic alopecia in the stump-tailed macaque: an important model for investigating the pathology and antiandrogenic therapy of male-pattern baldness

Hideo Uno, Koji Imamura and Huei-ju Pan

Introduction

Androgenetic alopecia, a common progressive form of scalp hair loss (discussed by Randall in Chapter 5), occurs in human beings and other primates such as the stump-tailed macaque. Human androgenetic alopecia, as its name implies, is clearly androgen-dependent[1] (see also Randall, Chapter 10).

The frontal alopecia in stump-tailed macaques develops during their pubertal elevation of testosterone and its metabolite, 5α-dihydro-testosterone; its androgenetic nature is further confirmed by both preventive and growth effects of antiandrogens on the macaque alopecia. In our earlier studies, an inhibitor of the enzyme that converts testosterone to the more potent 5α-dihydrotestosterone, 5α-reductase, prevented the development of alopecia in peripubertal macaques; thus potent 5α-dihydrotestosterone rather than testosterone plays a major role in the follicular regression of this unique species-specific phenomenon.[2,3] A potent inhibitor of human type II 5α-reductase, finasteride, caused significant reduction of serum levels of 5α-dihydrotestosterone and simultaneously induced hair regrowth in balding macaques[4] as also seen in men with androgenetic alopecia.[5,6] However, an inhibitor of human type I 5α-reductase (MK386) failed to affect hair growth in the alopecic macaque.[7] A potent blocker of binding to the androgen receptor, RU58841[8] also induced a significant degree of hair regrowth in the balding macaques[9–11] confirming the importance of androgens in macaque alopecia. Thus, this naturally occurring macaque alopecia is a unique model of human androgenetic alopecia; it has been used not only for clinical screening of hair growth agents but also studied to help elucidate the fundamental aspects of follicular regression in androgenetic alopecia.

Androgens are believed to act on the hair follicles via the regulatory mesenchyme-derived dermal papillae situated within the follicle bulb. In studies using follicular cell culture systems, dermal papilla cells appear to exhibit characteristics consistent with a major role in androgen-stimulated follicular growth in human beard as well as follicular regression in both human and macaque alopecia.[10,12–17] This system has also been used to investigate the effects of antiandrogens on follicular growth or regression.[12]

The macaque alopecia model has contributed to developing therapeutic approaches for alopecia and to our fundamental knowledge about the nature of androgenetic alopecia, and will continue to do so. However, our recent comparative studies on the histopathology of human and macaque androgenetic alopecia revealed critical differences in pathological manifestations between these two counterparts.[19]

In this review, the role of androgens and therapeutic effects of 5α-reductase inhibitors and antiandrogens on the macaque model in both *in vivo* and *in vitro* studies will be the main focus. Fundamental pathobiological differences between the macaque and human androgenetic alopecias and future directions for the development of improved regimens for androgenetic alopecia will also be discussed.

Development of novel, endocrine-based treatments for androgenetic alopecia

The roles of testosterone or 5α-dihydrotestosterone in the development of specific organs or pathological conditions induced by either excess or deficit of androgens became evident several decades ago. Our current understanding is greatly indebted to a series of studies on male pseudohermaphroditism resulting from an inborn deficiency of a steroid 5α-reductase enzyme, and the availability of specific inhibitors of this enzyme plus a new androgen receptor blocker.[8,19–22] Testosterone and 5α-dihydrotestosterone share the same receptor, the androgen receptor, in various organs. However, 5α-dihydrotestosterone has a much higher binding affinity than testosterone for the receptor although increasing the concentration of testosterone enables it to reach a high binding rate equivalent to 5α-dihydrotestosterone.[23] The initial studies on the production sites of 5α-dihydrotestosterone and its physiological significance in the prostate gland and skin were first reported around 1968.[24–28] The skin is known as one of the major conversion sites of testosterone to 5α-dihydrotestosterone by the enzyme 5α-reductase.[29–32] After puberty, 5α-dihydrotestosterone acts specifically in the prostate, seminal vesicles, and skin tissues, particularly on some hair follicles exhibiting secondary sexual hair growth in the male sebaceous glands and genital fibroblasts. Since Hamilton's earlier work, androgenetic alopecia has been known as an epigenetic follicular regression caused by the elevation of androgens to adult levels; prepubertal castration prevented this inherited phenomenon.[33] Furthermore, male pseudohermaphrodites with low 5α-dihydrotestosterone levels exhibit no postpubertal growth of the prostate, male pattern sexual hair growth, or temporal recession of scalp hair, otherwise they develop a typical male body form with a reduced phallus.[19,22] However, after the cloning of two forms of the gene of 5α-reductase from rat as well as human prostate, 5α-dihydrotestosterone is known to be produced by these two isozymes.[33] Although there are some contradictory data, the tissue distributions of these two isozymes have been explored in organs of various species including human scalp skin and hair follicles in balding and non-bald subjects.[35–43]

From early 1980, a group of pharmaceutical scientists worked on the synthesis of a series of compounds called 4-azosteroids which specifically inhibit 5α-reductase in the prostate.[20,21,44,45] Shortly after, we found that topical application of one of these compounds, 4 MA, prevented postpubertal hair loss and suppressed activity of 5α-reductase in the balding scalp skin of the macaque.[2,3] Later, finasteride, a 4-azosteroid, was shown to specifically inhibit human type II 5α-reductase, but type I and type II isozymes in rat.[36,46] Recently, MK386 (Merck Laboratory), a specific inhibitor of human type I 5α-reductase, induced no effect on hair growth in alopecic macaques.[7] Although currently there is wide variation in effect owing to species variations in pharmacological response to the isozymes, different delivery routes and varied doses, these compounds should enable further advances in our knowledge and hence improved therapeutic approaches for androgenetic alopecia, hirsutism, acne, and prostatic lesions.

In early 1990, a new specific potent blocker of the androgen receptor, the antiandrogen RU58841, was synthesized.[8,47] This seemed particularly useful for various androgen-induced skin lesions owing to its topical usage. In our macaque studies, topical RU58841 induced significant hair regrowth a relatively short time after its application. The effect was dose-dependent, requiring relatively high concentrations; doses less than 5% solution showed only minimal effect.[9,10] However, owing to its potent activity more in vivo studies are needed to evaluate the systemic antiandrogenic effects of RU58841.[11]

Frontal alopecia of the stump-tailed macaque

Serum levels of testosterone and 5α-dihydro-testosterone in the macaques show a similar pattern in their postpubertal elevation in human counterparts in both sexes.[48-50] In our longitudinal and cross-sectional studies, androgen levels in prepubertal macaques, from 6 months to late 3 years, remained within the base level, averaging 0.4 ng/ml of serum in both male and female. Around 4 years, equivalent to human pubertal age, androgen levels of testosterone and 5α-dihydrotestosterone elevated to adult levels in both sexes; testosterone in males climbed to 3.5–9 ng/ml and in females to 0.5–1 ng/ml. 5α-dihydrotestosterone in males elevates to 0.8–1.2 ng/ml and in females to 0.6–1.2 ng/ml (Figure 1).

The scalp hair of the macaque progressively develops after birth and at adolescence (3.5–4 years of age), long and thick terminal hair densely covers the entire scalp. Around 4 years,

thinning and shortening of hair begins to appear in the frontal scalp of both male and female macaques. Within a few years after puberty, hair thinning progresses evenly in the entire frontal region and hair changes to short and less pigmented, almost invisible hair called vellus hair (Figure 2). A micromorphometric (folliculogram) analysis of the frontal hair follicles revealed that prepubertal follicles were mostly large anagen follicles characterized as terminal type. However, while the alopecia develops, the follicles gradually decrease in length and size; these miniature follicles called vellus type are largely in the telogen phase (Figure 3, at pretreatment stage). These transformed vellus follicles can produce only fine short hair. These changes are similar to those seen in human androgenetic alopecia (see Randall, Chapter 10). Using these physiological paradigms, global appearances of hair, the changes of follicular sizes, and population of telogen and anagen follicles (folliculogram analysis), we evaluated the effects of various 5α-reductase inhibitors and antiandrogens on hair and follicular regrowth.

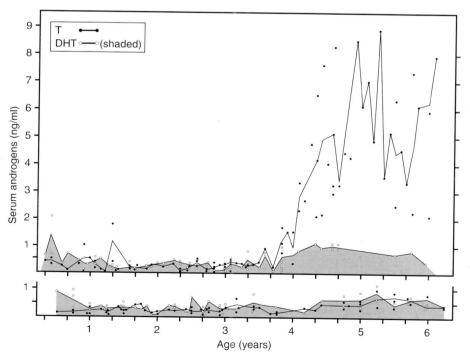

Figure 1

Serum levels of testosterone (T) and 5α-dihydrotestosterone (DHT) of male and female stump-tailed macaques, from the age of 4 months–6 years. Serum androgen levels increase at around 4 years of age in stump-tailed macaques. Male, upper panel; female, lower panel; T, solid line; DHT, shaded section. Concentration measured in ng/ml serum.

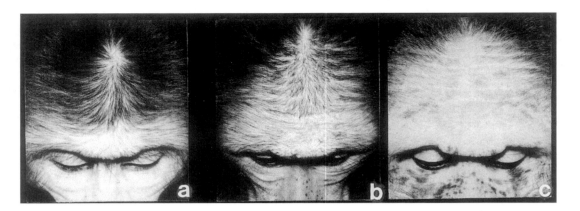

Figure 2

Progressive frontal alopecia in stump-tailed macaques. Scalp of female macaque aged 3 years 3 months showing long hairs densely covering entire scalp: (a) frontal scalp of 5-year-old male showing (b) thinning and shortening of hair; (c) frontal scalp of a male aged 7 years 7 months showing advanced stage of baldness furnished with short and thin vellus hair.

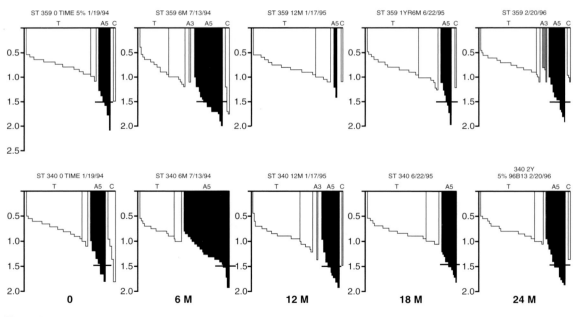

Figure 3

Effects of topical RU58841, an antiandrogen, on macaques' scalp hair follicles assessed by micromorphometry. Folliculo-grams at pre-treatment time (0 months) and 6, 12, 18, and 24 months after treatment with topical RU58841 (5% solution) in two adult stump-tailed macaques. Typical bald patterns at time 0 changed to marked signs of follicular growth; increased size of follicles in both telogen (T, white bar) and anagen (A5, black bar) and an increased population of anagen follicles were seen at 5 months. After 11–24 months, patterns of follicular growth regressed (upper panel) or slightly progressed at 11 months and thereafter, maintained at 18 and 24 months (lower panel). T, telogen; A3, anagen stage III; A5, anagen stage V; C, catagen.

5α-reductase inhibitors in macaque and human androgenetic alopecia

Topical application of 5α-reductase inhibitors

The effect of an inhibitor of 5α-reductase was examined by us in periadolescent stump-tailed macaques; 4 MA (N, N-diethyl-4-methyl-3-oxo-4-aza-5α-androste-17β-carboxamide, Merck Laboratory) was applied topically to the frontal scalp of macaques aged 2.5–4.3 years for 26 months. The daily dose was 7 mg of 4 MA dissolved in 0.5 ml DMSO solution; controls received the vehicle alone.[3] During the period of treatment, the serum levels of testosterone, 5α-dihydrotestosterone and androstanediol showed no significant differences between control and 4 MA-treated monkeys, but the activity of 5α-reductase in frontal scalp skin was markedly decreased in the 4 MA-treated group. Treated monkeys consistently produced a greater weight of hair in shaved samples taken from the frontal scalp at every 2-month period than did control monkeys. The folliculogram analysis revealed that, at the pretreatment age (2.5–4.3 years), all monkeys showed non-bald patterns. After 2 years of treatment, all control monkeys developed frontal alopecia and folliculograms showed typical patterns of alopecia. In contrast, 4 MA-treated monkeys maintained similar patterns of folliculogram to the pretreatment stage and showed no developmental signs of follicular regression.[2,3]

During the critical age for development of alopecia, consistent presence of the 5α-reductase inhibitor in the scalp skin successfully prevented the development of alopecia and follicular regression in postpubertal macaques. This was the first evidence that suppressed activity of 5α-reductase in scalp skin prevents alopecia development in androgenetic alopecia. However, 4 MA was discarded from therapeutic development owing to adverse systemic effects. Recently, topical application of finasteride, another 5α-reductase type II inhibitor, in human alopecia subjects failed to show any effect on hair regrowth.[51] The doses used for this human study, 0.01% and 0.05% solutions, were much lower than our topical dose of 4 MA (1.4% solution) in the macaque. In this human study, despite the low dose of topical finasteride, the serum levels of 5α-dihydrotestosterone reduced to 31% in 0.01% and 39% in 0.05%. However, the oral administration of finasteride or MK386 in the macaque studies suggested that over 70% reduction of serum 5α-dihydrotestosterone was necessary to induce the effect on hair regrowth.[4,7] Similar reductions in serum 5α-dihydrotestosterone were found in human alopecia studies with the use of oral administration of finasteride.[5,6]

Oral administration of 5α-reductase inhibitors

Adult stump-tailed macaques of both sexes were treated orally with finasteride at 1 mg/kg/day or placebo (lactose powder) for 6 months. During this period, the average weight of hair shaved from the frontal scalp every month was 10–25% heavier in finasteride-treated monkeys than the placebo group. Although there was a wide range of positive results in folliculogram analysis, seven out of ten monkeys treated with finasteride had increased numbers of terminal follicles (26–350%) and increased anagen follicles (35–366%) at 6 months compared with pretreatment; in controls, eight out of ten monkeys showed a rather decreased population of terminal and anagen follicles. The serum levels of 5α-dihydrotestosterone reduced to 86% in males and 48% in females compared with those of baseline and control values; testosterone levels increased moderately in males.[4,5]

In human androgenetic alopecia, oral finasteride (1 mg/day) showed a significantly increased hair count in balding scalp and also induced a 69% reduction of serum 5α-dihydrotestosterone. Increasing to 5 mg/day showed a slightly greater hair count but the reduction of 5α-dihydrotestosterone was similar to the 1 mg/day group. A lower dose, 0.2 mg/day, had generally weaker effects than the 1 mg/day group.[5,6] Details of human treatment with finasteride can be seen in Price, Chapter 13.

Systemic reduction of 5α-dihydrotestosterone levels, more than 68%, appeared to be necessary for hair and follicular regrowth in the bald scalp of stump-tailed macaques, as well as human androgenetic alopecia. Orally administered finasteride caused a suppression of testosterone to 5α-dihydrotestosterone conversion within organs, while, at the same time, scalp follicles received less circulating 5α-dihydrotestosterone. Together with the results of our studies of follicular cell culture (discussed later), we speculated that finasteride enters the dermal papilla cells in the follicles of bald scalp and that the reduced amount of 5α-dihydrotestosterone availability suppresses the production of follicular regressive factors in the dermal papilla cells.[10,53] The androgen inhibition of keratinocyte stimulation was also observed in a cell-culture system using dermal papilla cells from human androgenetic alopecia.[16]

MK386 (Merck Laboratory) is known to specifically inhibit human type I 5α-reductase.[54,55] MK386 reduced serum 5α-dihydrotestosterone in men, but to a lesser extent than finasteride. Interestingly, oral administration of MK386 (1 mg/kg/day) induced no signs of hair regrowth in macaques, although the serum level of 5α-dihydrotestosterone was reduced by about 33%.[7] The reduction of serum 5α-dihydrotestosterone by MK386 is much less than the 70% caused by finasteride. The follicles in human alopecia contain both type I and type II 5α-reductase, with both isozymes approximately 2-fold higher in frontal follicles than occipital ones in both men and women.[43] Our recent studies in the macaque follicular cell-culture system showed that finasteride inhibited testosterone-induced suppressive growth of keratinocytes but that MK386 had negligible effect.[18] Thus, we speculate that type II-dependent 5α-reductase plays a major role in androgenetic regression of scalp follicles, although we have to rely on further molecular genetic studies to determine the precise actions of the 5α-dihydrotestosterone receptor complex.

Topical application of the androgen-receptor blocker, RU58841, in macaque alopecia

The non-steroidal compound, RU58841, has approximately 2-fold higher binding affinity than testosterone in the hamster flank organ but the rate reverses in the hamster prostate.[23] Moreover, Battmann and co-workers showed that topical application of RU58841 significantly reduced the size of hamster flank organs in a dose-dependent manner.[8] Thus, RU58841 was suggested as a potential specific topical anti-androgen for the treatment of acne, androgenetic alopecia and hirsutism.

In our studies on macaque alopecia, RU58841 solutions, 5%, 3%, 1%, and 0.5%, and our vehicle solution (50% propylene glycol: 30% isopropanol: 2% isopropyl myristate: 18% water), were applied topically, once daily, to four or five monkeys in each group for 6 months. Thereafter, three monkeys from the groups of RU58841, 0.5% and 5%, and the vehicle solution, were treated continuously for 24 months in order to examine the longer-term effects on hair growth. Marked increases in density, thickening, and length of hair were observed in monkeys taking 5% RU58841 solution at 3 months. After 5 months, folliculogram analysis showed an average 2–3 fold increase in the population of follicles, which had enlarged to terminal size and were in anagen phase compared with the state before treatment.[9,10] At 3 months, the number of cells undergoing DNA synthesis in the follicles significantly increased compared with those before treatment. This dramatic effect of RU58841 on hair regrowth was dose-dependent. Concentrations below 5% showed no appreciable effect; a 3% solution induced a moderate effect in only one case and the remaining four showed very minimal effects in both hair and follicular growth. The lowest doses of 1% and 0.5% revealed minimal or no effects. In the longer-term studies, all cases in the 5% group showed progressive hair growth, which occurred continuously from 3–7 months, and thereafter these hairs were maintained so long as application continued. However, after the initial growth, the folliculogram patterns did not correspond with the external appearance of hair growth; at 11, 18, and 24 months after treatment, the follicular growth either reversed or just maintained the early remarkable growth patterns observed at 5 months (see Figure 3). No placebo effects were noticed in either short- or long-term application.

The concentrations of RU58841 and its endogenous metabolites in the serum of monkeys treated with a 5% solution were

12 ng/ml and 39 ng/ml in two monkeys at 3 months; the remaining two monkeys at 3 months and all four monkeys at 6 months contained only the detection level of 5 ng/ml or below. The serum levels of testosterone, 5α-dihydrotestosterone, and luteinizing hormone (LH) showed no significant changes during the entire treatment period. The lobular size of the prostate, measured by magnetic resonance imaging (MRI) analysis, in macaques treated with topical 5% RU58841 showed no difference compared with the placebo group; however, the seminal vesicles showed a slight size reduction. There were no detectable changes in body weight or the hematological and blood chemistry data.

Topical application of this androgen receptor blocker can suppress androgenetic follicular regression, but it appears to have no long-term continuous stimulatory effects on follicular cell proliferation. After the initial dramatic effect, the hair maintained its density and length so long as the treatment continued. Regressive changes that occurred within 3 months after treatment ceased in both global photographic appearance and folliculogram patterns. Nevertheless, the blocker had no direct stimulatory effects on follicular germ cell proliferation, unlike a hypertrichotic agent such as minoxidil.[52,56] In our preliminary study, combined treatment of RU-58841 with minoxidil induced remarkable effects of hair growth as early as 1 month after treatment and continuous progressive effects have been observed.[57] Although RU58841 is a good candidate for therapy of androgenetic alopecia because of its unique properties and the successful results in the macaque alopecia, further studies are required to detect any possible systemic side-effects before it can be used in human androgenetic alopecia.

Effect of testosterone and antiandrogens in follicular cell culture

Cultured dermal papilla cells derived from human beard follicles express the activity of 5α-reductase type II isozyme.[38,58] In co-cultured cell systems, testosterone stimulated DNA synthesis of the outer root sheath cells when the cells were co-cultured with beard dermal papilla cells and cyproterone acetate, while other antiandrogens abolished the effect of testosterone.[13] Recently, Thornton and co-workers[17] suggested that beard dermal papilla cells secrete autocrine growth factors in response to testosterone. Thus, dermal papilla cells are known to play a major role in androgen-dependent follicular growth in beard hair (discussed in Chapter 5 by Randall).

In contrast, in androgenetic alopecia, androgens trigger follicular regression in both human and macaque scalp. Dermal papilla cells in alopecic follicles presumably may produce regressive factors to the follicular cells under androgen stimulation. To test this hypothesis, we first established the cell culture of primary follicular dermal papilla cells and outer root sheath cells derived from the follicles of macaque scalp.[59] Testosterone caused no inhibitory nor stimulatory effects on cell proliferation of dermal papilla cells from bald frontal or hairy occipital scalp, outer root sheath cells from scalp follicles, or keratinocytes from human neonatal foreskin. However, testosterone-induced inhibition of outer root sheath cell growth occurred when the cells were co-cultured with dermal papilla cells derived from bald frontal scalp follicles. Interestingly, this inhibitory effect was not found using dermal papilla cells derived from juvenile prebald frontal scalp or hairy occipital adult scalp.[10,53]

For practical reasons, in further studies, we used readily available keratinocytes from human neonatal foreskin; these keratinocytes responded similarly to outer root sheath cells when co-cultured with dermal papilla cells (Figure 4). Conditioned medium was obtained by the cell-culture insert system (transwell) in which dermal papilla cells and keratinocytes were separated by collagen mesh in the same culture medium containing testosterone. This conditioned medium inhibited keratinocyte growth when serially diluted in parallel to the dilution rate; addition of testosterone to the conditioned medium further enhanced the suppressive effect (Figure 5). These data strongly suggest that, in response to testosterone, balding follicle dermal papilla cells secrete factors that suppress keratinocyte proliferation into the medium. After heating the conditioned medium the effect was lost. This heat-unstable factor(s), yet unidentified, is apparently secreted by the dermal papilla cells and

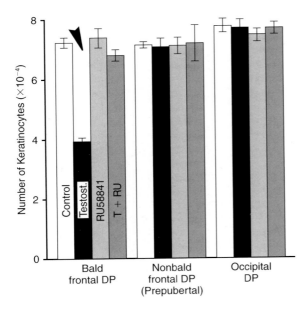

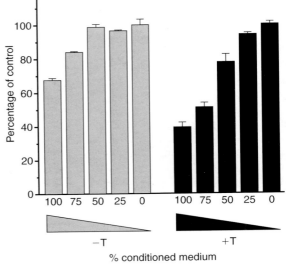

Figure 4

Balding, but not non-balding, macaque dermal papilla cells responded to testosterone by reducing their stimulatory effects on keratinocyte growth. Macaque dermal papilla cells and human foreskin keratinocytes were co-cultured in transwells with KGM medium for 7 days with or without (control) testosterone (10^{-10}M) and/or RU58841 (10^{-10}M). Dermal papillae were obtained either from bald frontal follicles (left column), from non-bald frontal follicles of juvenile (center), or hairy occipital scalp of adult macaques (right). Suppression of keratinocyte proliferation by testosterone occurred only in wells co-cultured with dermal papilla cells derived from bald scalp (second bar of left column, arrow head); RU58841 blocked the effect of testosterone.

Figure 5

Dose-responsive inhibitory effect of androgen-stimulated macaque balding dermal papilla cell-conditioned media on human keratinocytes. Conditioned media were obtained from dermal papilla cells from bald frontal follicles co-cultured in transwells with keratinocytes in the presence of testosterone. Charcoal-treated conditioned medium was serially diluted with KGM and keratinocytes were incubated with testosterone (black bar) or without testosterone (white bar) for 3 days. Suppressive effects on keratinocyte proliferation showed a linear correlation with dilution rates of conditioned medium, particularly in wells with added testosterone.

exists as a soluble form in the co-cultured medium. Using the same system, both the androgen receptor blocker, RU58841, and the type II 5α-reductase inhibitor, finasteride, reduced testosterone-induced suppressive growth of keratinocytes (Figure 6). RU58841 was more effective, reducing the response by 56.5 + 8.8% compared with 21.7 + 3.2% by finasteride; MK386, type I 5α-reductase, had a negligible effect.[11] Our preliminary data showed that

5α-dihydrotestosterone was slightly more potent than testosterone and that RU58841 abolished the effects of both equally.

Dermal papilla cells in the frontal follicles of the stump-tailed macaque apparently have a genetic predisposition to produce follicular regressive factors under androgen stimulation. Nevertheless, the expression of this genetic system needs to be primed by the elevation of androgens during puberty.

Comparison of the histopathology of the macaque and human androgenetic alopecia

The histopathological changes of the human androgenetic alopecia have been described by many investigators. Besides a miniaturization of follicles, fibrogranulomatous or collagenous streamers are seen beneath the follicles, together with focal perivascular and perifollicular inflammatory cell infiltrations, and varying degrees of dermal fibrosis have been reported (Table 1). Our recent study of 27 cases of bald and 6 non-bald human scalps detected similar histopathological changes.[9] More frequent and severe manifestations of these pathological changes are found in advanced cases rather than early stages of the alopecia. The most unique change in human androgenetic alopecia is the presence of fibrogranulomatous or collagenous streamers beneath the vellus follicles (Figure 7). In normal scalp skin, a fibrous streamer is a remnant of the lower portion of the perifollicular connective tissue sheath while a follicle undergoes involution during catagen. When a new follicle grows from the secondary germ, the streamer becomes a structural guide for a growing anagen follicle. However, in androgenetic alopecia, streamers are not simple remnant of fibrous tissue, but

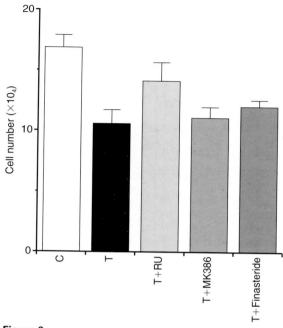

Figure 6

Both an antiandrogen and to a lesser extent a 5α-reductase type II inhibitor reduced the androgen inhibitory effect on proliferation. Dermal papilla cells from bald follicles and keratinocytes were co-cultured in transwells with testosterone (black bar) or without testosterone (white) (10^{-9}M). In some co-culture wells, either RU58841, finasteride, or MK386 was added with the same concentration of testosterone (10^{-9}M), respectively. Compared with the suppressive rate of keratinocyte proliferation by testosterone alone, RU58841 blocked the effect of testosterone at 56.5 + 8.9%, finasteride, 21.7 + 3.2%, and MK386, 7.6 + 5.7% (no effect).

Table 1 Histopathology of human androgenetic alopecia.

Shrinkage of anagen bulb	Van Scott and Ekel, 1958[60]
Dermal inflammatory foci	Maguire and Kligman, 1962[61]
Transformed vellus follicles	Montagna, 1963[62]
Reduced number of follicles	Giacometti, 1965[63]
Elastosis, transformation to vellus follicle	Allegra, 1968[64]
Increased telegen follicles	Braun-Falco and Christopheras, 1968[65]
Fibrous streamer beneath vellus follicle	Lattanand and Johnson, 1975[66]
Inflammatory perivascular infiltrate	
Sclerotic streamer beneath vellus follicle	Rook and Dawber, 1982[67]
Shortening of anagen phase	
Dermal inflammation	Headington and Novak, 1984[68]
Fibrovascular streamer	Kligman, 1988[69]
Perivascular inflammatory infiltrate	
Perifollicular CD-4, CD-8, T-cell infiltrate	Jaworsky et al, 1992[70]
Fibrous streamer and mast-cell degranulation	
Dermal inflammation	Whiting, 1993,[71] 1998[72]
Increased vellus follicles	

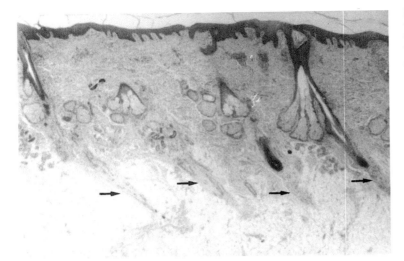

Figure 7

Streamers beneath the vellus follicles in the bald scalp of human androgenetic alopecia (arrowed), seen on low-power magnification.

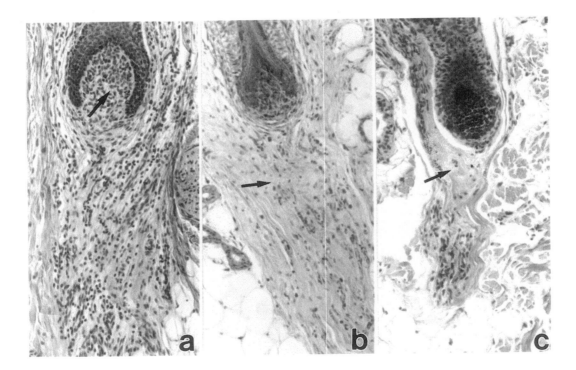

Figure 8

High-power view of streamers underneath vellus anagen follicles. (a) Angiofibrous streamer with infiltration of many lymphocytes and a few plasma cells. Dermal papilla cells in dilated papilla region showing densely packed small round cells (arrowed); with (b) streamer consisting of dense collagenous tissue with capillaries and few infiltrated cells (c) streamer showing hyalinized scarring tissue underneath anagen follicle.

involve various pathological changes such as angiogranulomatous, angiofibrous changes with dense collagen fibres and hyalinized scarring changes (Figure 8 a–c). Although the follicles in androgenetic alopecia undergo progressive shrinkage in size, the follicular structure remains normal and the follicle is capable of continuing its cyclic growth; these vellus follicles have a short anagen phase. In alopecia skin, the abnormal streamers underneath the follicles appear to be a structural barrier for the down-growth of anagen follicles. Moreover, severe inflammatory involvement in the streamers causes suppressive growth of the follicular bulb and dermal papilla cells (see Figure 8a). Dense collagenous or hyalinized scarring streamers block the growth of follicles (Figure 8b and c). These follicular structures naturally resist any therapeutic effect for follicular growth. Moreover, associations of focal perivascular and perifollicular inflammatory cell infiltrations are often seen in alopecic skin. Regional dermal fibrotic changes with or without elastosis are also seen in the late stage of the alopecia.[69] It is not easy to conceive that androgen causes such diverse pathological changes in alopecic skin, particularly since the progressive process of human androgenetic alopecia is very slow and expansive. Scalp hair loss does not occur evenly and has three major patterns, frontal, temporal and vertex types.[1] Once it begins, it gradually expands to the surrounding scalp resulting in a loss from most of the scalp in a period of about 10 years.

In the macaque, alopecia develops evenly in the entire frontal scalp during a relatively short period after the elevation of androgens during puberty. In the macaque alopecia, the histopathological changes comprise simply of a miniaturization of the follicles, with those vellus follicles remaining in telogen for a long period. There is no inflammatory involvement in the dermis and no abnormal streamers underneath the follicles, unlike the human counterpart.

Summary and future directions

Macaque alopecia has been used to study androgenetic follicular regression and for the screening of pharmacological agents stimulating hair growth. The results of 5α-reductase inhibitors and androgen receptor blockers on macaque androgenetic alopecia are summarized in Table 2. Both 5α-reductase type II inhibitors and the antiandrogen stimulated hair regrowth in the macaque alopecia but not the 5α-reductase type I inhibitor (MK386). However, presumably because of the different pathological backgrounds between macaque and human alopecia, macaque alopecia responded more strongly and homogeneously than human alopecia (Table 3). There is no doubt that 5α-dihydrotestosterone triggers follicular regression in both species. Subsequent or simultaneous involvement of dermal inflammatory and fibrotic processes in human alopecic skin may be caused by other insidious complications such as autoimmune cascade, ultraviolet (UV) insult, or porphyria associated with photosensitivity. Furthermore, in human androgenetic alopecia, therapeutic approaches cannot simply rely on either hypertrichotic or antiandrogenic agents or even a combination of both. For further therapeutic improvement, it may be necessary to use combined treatment with antiandrogenic and anti-inflammatory, as well as anti-fibrotic agents; hypertrichotic agents, such as minoxidil, or other potassium channel openers in addition, may enhance efficacy.

For the therapeutic use of agents opposing androgen action, demasculinizing side-effects have to be monitored carefully, particularly for long-term usage. Sensitivity to such effects is naturally much higher in the fetus compared with the adult. Clinically, finasteride (Proscar, Merck) is not currently used for androgenetic alopecia in women because of potential risk to a male fetus, although cyproterone acetate, and other antiandrogens, have been used to treat female hirsutism for many years, in combination with estrogen to ensure contraception. Topical rather than oral antiandrogens for the treatment of alopecia may reduce the rate of systemic antiandrogenic side-effects, although relatively high doses of both RU58841 and finasteride are needed to induce satisfactory effects on hair growth in macaque alopecia or in fuzzy rats used as an acne model.[73] More studies on the lowering of the applied dose of these agents are needed, and the development of new vehicles with enhanced skin penetration or with specific carrier molecules, for example.

Studies using follicular cell culture support the

Table 2 Effects of hair growth in stumptailed macaques.

	Evaluation (photo, hair weight)	Folliculogram	Serum T, DHT
5α-reductase inhibitor			
4 MA (topical)	Prevented baldness (2-year)	No pattern of regression	No change
Finasteride (oral)	Increased hair weight (6 M)	Increased, enlarged anagen	DHT 70% ↓
MK386 (oral)	Unchanged hair weight (6M)	ND	DHT 30% ↓
Androgen receptor blocker			
RU58841 (topical)	Marked hair regrowth (2-year)	Increased, enlarged anagen	No change

M, months; ND, no difference; DHT, dihydrotestosterone.

Table 3 Comparison of human and macaque androgenetic alopecia.

Human alopecia	**Macaque alopecia**
Postpubertal, genetic trait, gender difference	Postpubertal, high prevalence, no gender difference
Regional pattern: vertex, frontal, temporal types pattern	Androgen-dependent frontal scalp, uniform
Follicular regression, slowly expansive for man	Follicular regression, evenly occurring for a short time
Pathology	**Pathology**
Vellus follicle, long telogen phase	Vellus follicle, long telogen phase
Streamer granulomatous, angiofibrous, hyalinized scarring	Rare appearance of fibrous streamer
Perivascular, perifollicular inflammatory focidermal fibrosis	No inflammatory and fibrotic foci in dermis
Response to treatment	**Response to treatment**
Frequent individual variation	Little individual variation

concept that dermal papilla cells play a major role in androgen-induced follicular regression in both human and macaque alopecia. The co-culture cell system with dermal papilla cells and follicular cells or keratinocytes has been a useful tool for the elucidation of androgenetic follicular regression. It is also an incomparable system to identify presumptive suppressive factors secreted from the dermal papilla cells and to explore transcriptive genes for androgenetic follicular regression. These cell-culture systems may also be useful for screening potential therapeutic agents, particularly those interfering with androgen action.

Conclusion

The effects of antiandrogens strongly support the androgenetic property of macaque alopecia.

After human and macaque studies, 5α-reductase type II inhibitors became new therapeutic drugs for human androgenetic alopecia; an effective topical antiandrogen, RU58841, in the macaque, has not yet been explored in human alopecia. In the macaque, RU58841, a potent blocker of the androgen receptor, showed much greater effect on hair growth than an inhibitor of human type II 5α-reductase, finasteride, although direct comparison is inappropriate because of the different routes, topical versus oral, and doses applied. Furthermore, folliculogram analysis revealed that RU58841 induced significant follicular growth only initially up to 5 months, although hair was maintained during treatment. This suggests that 5α-dihydrotestosterone-induced follicular regression occurs more prominently in early and mid-anagen follicles than late anagen. Blocking the androgen receptor or suppressing 5α-dihydrotestosterone production seems to reduce the regressive factor in these growing follicles but, unlike hypertrichotic agents, antiandrogenic agents have no continuous stimulatory effects on follicular cell proliferation. Actually, combined treatment with both RU58841 and minoxidil induced more significant growth in our studies than the single use of each agent.

Nonetheless, the complexity of the pathological changes manifested in human androgenic alopecia appears to hamper the effects of these hair growth-stimulating agents. Thus, results obtained from the macaque, which has no such complications, usually show much greater and homogeneous effects than those obtained in human alopecia. The pathological changes associated with regressed follicles in human androgenetic alopecia have been described by many investigators. However, more studies on the histogenesis of inflammatory streamers, dermal lymphocytic infiltrations, and the process of focal fibrotic changes are necessary to fully define this disorder. For further improvement of therapy, combined pharmacological interventions may be needed to reduce or prevent inflammatory and fibrotic processes in human alopecic skin.

References

1. Hamilton JB: Patterned loss of hair in man: Types and incidence. *Ann NY Acad Sci* 1951; **53**: 708–728.
2. Uno H: Biology of hair growth. In: Speroff L (ed.). *Seminars in Reproductive Endocrinology: Andrology in Women,* vol. 4. New York, Thieme-Stratton, 1986: 131–141.
3. Rittmaster RS, Uno H, Povar ML, Mellin TN, Loriaux DL: The effect of 4MA, a 5α-reductase inhibitor and anti-androgen, on the development of baldness in the stumptail macaque. *J Endocrinol Metab* 1987; **65**: 188–193.
4. Rhodes L, Harper J, Uno H, et al.: The effect of finasteride (Proscar) on hair growth, hair-cycle stage, and serum testosterone and dihydrotestosterone in adult male and female stumptail macaques (*Macaca arctoides*). *J Clin Endocrinol Metab* 1994; **78**: 991–996.
5. Kaufman KD: Clinical studies on the effects of oral finasteride, a type II 5α-reductase inhibitor, on scalp hair in men with male pattern baldness. In: Van Neste DJ, Randall VA (eds.). *Hair Research for the Next Millennium.* Amsterdam, Elsevier, 1996; 363–365.
6. Kaufman, KD, Olsen EA, Whiting D, et al.: Finasteride in the treatment of men with androgenetic alopecia. Finasteride male pattern hair loss study group. *J Am Acad Dermatol* 1998; **39**: 578–589.
7. Rhodes L, Primka R, Berman C, et al.: Effect of 1-year treatment with oral MK386, an inhibitor of type 1 5α-reductase, in the stumptailed macaque (*Macaca arctoides*). *J Invest Dermatol* 1995; **104**: 658.
8. Battmann T, Bonfils A, Branche C, et al.: RU58841, a new specific topical antiandrogen: a candidate of choice for the treatment of acne, androgenetic alopecia and hirsutism. *J Steroid Biochem Mol Biol* 1994; **8**: 55–60,
9. Uno H, Obana N, Cappas A, Bonfils A, Battmann T, Philibert D: Stimulation of follicular regrowth by androgen receptor blocker (RU58841) in macaque androgenetic alopecia. In: Van Neste DJ, Randall VA (eds.). *Hair Research for the Next Millennium.* Amsterdam, Elsevier, 1996. 349–353.
10. Obana N, Chang C, Uno H: Inhibition of hair growth by testosterone in the presence of dermal papilla cells from the frontal bald scalp of the postpubertal stumptailed macaque. *Endocrinology* 1997; **138**: 356–361.
11. Pan H, Wilding G, Uno H, Inui S, et al.: Evaluation of RU58841 as an anti-androgen in prostate PC3 cells and a topical anti-alopecia agent in the bald scalp of stumptailed macaques. *Endocrinology* 1998; **9**: 39–43.
12. Randall VA, Thornton MJ, Hamada K, et al.: Androgens and the hair follicle: cultured human dermal papilla cells as a model system. In: Stenn KS, Messenger AG, Baden HP (eds.). *The Molecular and Structural Biology of Hair. Ann NY Acad Sci* 1991; **642**: 355–375.
13. Itami S, Kurata S, Sonoda T, Takayasu, S: Mechanism of action of androgen in dermal papilla. In: Stenn KS, Messenger AG, Baden HP (eds.). *The Molecular and Structural Biology of Hair. Ann NY Acad Sci*, vol. 642. 1991: 385–395.
14. Itami S, Kurata S, Sonoda T, Takayasu S: Interaction between dermal papilla cells and follicular epithelial cells in vitro: effect of androgen. *Br J Dermatol* 1995; **132**: 527–532.
15. Randall VA: The use of dermal papilla cells in studies of normal and abnormal hair follicle biology. *Dermatol Clin* 1996; **14**: 585–594.
16. Hibberts NA, Randall VA: Testosterone inhibits the capacity of cultured balding scalp dermal papilla cells to produce keratinocyte mitogenic factors. In: Van Neste DJ, Randall VA (eds.). *Hair Research for the Next Millennium.* Amsterdam, Elsevier, 1996: 303–306.
17. Thornton MJ, Hamada K, Messenger AG, Randall VA: Androgen-dependent beard dermal papilla cells secrete autocrine growth factor(s) in

response to testosterone unlike scalp cells. *J Invest Dermatol* 1998; **111**: 727–732.

18. Imperato-McGinley J, Guerrero L, Gautier T, Peterson PE: Steroid 5α-reductase deficiency in man: an inherited form of male pseudohermaphroditism. *Science* 1974; **186**: 1213–1215.

19. Uno H, Ye F, Hachisuka H, Kurata S, Esaki T: Follicular and dermal pathology in androgenetic alopecia and its therapeutic sequela with minoxidil. *J Invest Dermatol* 1996; **106**: 948.

20. Rasmusson GH, Reynolds GF, Steriberg NG, et al.: Azasteroids: structure-activity relationships for inhibition of 5α-reductase and of androgen-receptor binding. *J Med Chem* 1986; **29**: 2298–2315.

21. Mellin TN, Busch RD, Rasmusson GH: Azasteroids as inhibitors of testosterone 5α-reductase in mammalian skin. *J Steroid Biochem Molec Biol* 1993; **44**: 121–131.

22. Imperato-McGinley J: 5α-reductase-2 deficiency. *Curr Ther Endocrinol Metab* 1997; **6**: 384–387.

23. Grino PB, Griffin JE, Wilson JD: Testosterone at high concentrations interacts with the human androgen receptor similarly to dihydrotestosterone. *Endocrinology* 1990; **126**: 1165–1172.

24. Bruchovsky N, Wilson JD: The conversion of testosterone to 5α-androstan-17βol-3-one by rate prostate in vivo and in vitro. *J Biol Chem* 1968; **243**: 2012–2021.

25. Bruchovsky N, Wilson JD: The intranuclear binding of testosterone and 5-androstan-17β-ol-3-one by rate prostate. *J Biol Chem* 1968; **243**: 5953–5960.

26. Gomez ED, Hsia SL: In vitro metabolism of testosterone-4 ^{14}C and androstene-3, 17-dione-4C in human skin. *Biochemistry* 1968; **7**: 24–32.

27. Fang S, Anderson KMJ, Liao S: Receptor proteins for androgens: on the role of specific proteins in selective retention of 17β-hydroxy-5α-androstan-3-one by rat ventral prostate in vivo and in vitro. *J Biol Chem* 1969; **244**: 6584–6598.

28. Gloyna RE, Wilson JD: A comparative study of the conversion of testosterone to 17β-hydroxy-5α-androstan-3-one (dihydrotestosterone) by prostate and epididymis. *J Endocrinol Metab* 1969; **29**: 970–977.

29. Sansone G, Reisner RM: Differential rates of conversion of testosterone to dihydrotestosterone in acne and in normal human skin: a possible pathogenic factor in acne. *J Invest Dermatol* 1971; **56**: 366–372.

30. Wilson JD, Walker JD: The conversion of testosterone to 5α-androstane-17βol-3-one (dihydrotestosterone) by skin slices of man. *J Clin Invest* 1969; **4**: 372–379.

31. Schweikert HU, Wilson JD: Regulation of human hair growth by steroid hormones: 1. Testosterone metabolism in isolated hairs. *J Clin Endocrinol Metab* 1974; **38**: 811–819.

32. Price VH: Testosterone metabolism in the skin. *Arch Dermatol* 1975; **111**: 1496–1502.

33. Anderson S, Russell DW: Structural and biochemical properties of cloned and expressed human and rat steroid 5α-reductases. *Proc Natl Acad Sci USA* 1990; **87**: 3640–3644.

34. Hamilton JB: Male hormone stimulation is a prerequisite and an incitant in common baldness. *Am J Anat* 1942; **71**: 451–480.

35. Anderson JS, Berman DM, Jenkin EP, Russell DW: Deletion of steroid 5α-reductase 2 gene in male pseudohermaphroditism. *Nature* 1991; **4**: 159–161.

36. Normington K, Russell DW: Tissue distribution and kinetic characteristics of rat steroid 5α-reductase isozymes. *J Biol Chem* 1992; **267**: 19 548–19 554.

37. Thigpen AE, Silverr RI, Guileyardo JM, et al.: Tissue distribution and ontogeny of steroid 5α-reductase isozyme expression. *J Clin Invest* 1993; **92**: 903–910.

38. Itami S, Kurata S, Takasayu S: 5α-reductase activity in cultured human dermal papilla cells from beard compared with reticular dermal fibroblasts. 1990; **94**: 150–152.

39. Levy MA, Brandt M, Sheedy KM, et al.: Cloning, expression and functional characterization of type I and type 2 steroid 5α-reductase from cynomologous monkey: comparisons with human and rat isoenzymes. *J Steroid Biochem Molec Biol* 1995; **52**: 307–319.

40. Mahendroo MS, Cala KM, Russell DW: 5α-reduced androgens play a key role in murine parturition. *Mol Endocrinol* 1996; **10**: 380–392.

41. Russell DW, Wiley EL, Whiting DA: Expression of 5α-reductase I and II in scalp skin in normal controls and in androgenetic alopecia. In: Van Neste DJ, Randall VA, (eds.) *Hair Research for the Next Millennium* London, Elsevier Science, 1996: 330–340.

42. Azzolina B, Ellsworth K, Andersson S, et al.: Inhibition of rat alpha-reductases by finasteride: evidence for isozyme differences in the mechanism of inhibition. *J Steroid Boichem Mol Biol* 1997; **61**: 55–64.

43. Sawaya ME, Price, VH: Different levels of 5α-reductase type I and II, aromatase, and androgen receptor in hair follicles of women and men with androgenetic alopecia. *J Invest Dermatol* 1997; **109**: 296–300.

44. Liang T, Heiss CE, Ostrove S, Rasmussen GH, Cheung A: NADPH-dependent binding of a 4-methyl-4aza-steroid to 5α-reductase of rat liver and prostate microsomes. *Endocrinology* 1983; **112**: 1460–1468.

45. Rasmusson GH, Reynolds GF, Utne T, et al.: Azasteroids as inhibitors of rat prostate 5α-reductase. *J Med Chem* 1984; **27**: 1690–1701.

46. Brooks JR, Baptista EM, Berman C, et al.:

Response of rat ventral prostate to a new and novel 5 alpha-reductase inhibitor. *Endocrinology* 1981; **109(3):** 830–836.

47. Teutsch G, Goubet F, Battmann T, et al.: Non-steroidal antiandrogens: synthesis and biological profile of high-affinity ligands for the androgen receptor. *J Steroid Biochem Molec Biol* 1994; **48:** 1–19.

48. Tanner JM: Growth and endocrinology of the adolescent. In: Gardener, LI (ed.). *Endocrine and Genetic Diseases of Childhood and Adolescence*, 2nd edn. Philadelphia, WB Saunders, 1975: 14–63.

49. Uno H: Stumptailed macaques as a model of male-pattern baldness. In: Maibach HI, Lowe NJ (eds.), *Models in Dermatology*, vol. 3, Basel, Karger, 1987, 159–169.

50. Uno H, Aslum PB, Bauers K, de Waal FBM: Serum androgens in stumptailed macaques (*Macaca arctoides*). In: Ehara A, (ed.). *Primatology Today*. Amsterdam, Elsevier, 1991: 419–420.

51. Rushton DH, Norris MJ, Ramsay ID: Topical 0.05% finasteride significantly reduced serum DHT concentrations but had no effect in preventing the expression of genetic hair loss in men. In: Van Neste DJ, Randall VA (eds.). *Hair research for the Next Millennium*. Amsterdam, Elsevier, 1996: 359–362.

52. Uno H: Stumptailed macaques as a model of male pattern baldness. In: Maibach HI, Lowe NJ (eds.). *Models in Dermatology* vol 3. Basel, 1987: 159–169.

53. Obana N and Uno H: Dermal papilla cells in macaque alopecia trigger a testosterone-dependent inhibition of follicular cell proliferation. In: Van Neste DJ, Randall VA (eds.). *Hair Research for the Next Millennium*, Amsterdam, Elsevier, 1996: 307–310.

54. Bakshi RK, Patel GF, Rasmusson GH, et al.: 4,7β-dimethyl-4-azacholestan-3-one (MK386) and related 4-azosteroid as selective inhibitors of human type 1 5α-reductase. *J Med Chem* 1994; **37:** 3871–3874.

55. Schwartz JI, Van Hecken A, De Schepper PJ, et al.: Effect of MK386, a novel inhibitor of type 1 5α-reductase, alone and in combination with finasteride, on serum dihydroxytestosterone concentrations in men. *J Clin Endocrinol Metab* 1996; **81:** 2942–2947.

56. Uno H, Cappas A, Brigham P: Action of topical minoxidil in the bald stumptailed macaque. *J Am Acad Dermatol* 1987; **16:** 657–668.

57. Imamura K, Bonfils A, Diani A, Uno H: The effect of topical RU58841 (androgen receptor blocker) combined with minoxidil on hair growth in macaque androgenetic alopecia. *J Invest Dermatol* 1998; **110:** 679.

58. Itami S, Kurata S, Sonoda T, Takayasu S: Characterization of 5 alpha-reductase in cultured human dermal papilla cells from beard and occipatal scalp hair. *J Invest Dermatol* 1991; **96:** 57–60.

59. Kurata S, Uno H, Allen-Hofman BL: Effects of hypertrichotic agents on follicular and non-follicular cells in vitro. *Skin Pharmacol* 1996; **9:** 3–8.

60. Van Scott EJ, Ekel TM: Geometric relationships between the matrix of the hair bulb and its dermal papilla in normal and alopecic scalp. *J Invest Dermatol* 1958; **31:** 281–287.

61. Maguire HC, Kligman AM: The histopathology of common male baldness. In: Pillsbury DM, Livingood C (eds.). *Proceedings of the XII International Congress of Dermatology*. Amsterdam, Excerpta Medica Foundation, 1962: 1438–1444.

62. Montagna W: The phylogenetic significance of the skin of man. *Arch Dermatol* 1963; **88:** 1–19.

63. Giacometti L: The anatomy of the human scalp. In: Montagna W (ed.). *Advances in Biology of Skin*, vol. 6. New York, Appleton-Century-Crofts, 1965: 97–111.

64. Allegra F: Histology and histochemical aspects of the hair follicles in pattern alopecia. In: Baccaredda-Boy A, Moretti G, Frey JR (eds.). *Biopathology of Pattern Alopecia*. Basel, Karger, 1968: 107–128.

65. Braun-Falco O, Christopheras E: Hair root pattern in male-pattern alopecia. In: Baccaredda-Boy A, Moretti G, Frey JR (eds.). *Biopathology of Pattern Alopecia*. Basel, Karger, 1968: 141–146.

66. Lattanand A, Johnson WC: Male-pattern alopecia: a histopathological and histochemical study. *J Cutan Pathol* 1975; **2:** 58–64.

67. Rook A, Dawber R: Diseases of the hair and scalp. In: (?eds.). *Hair Patterns: Baldness and Hirsutism*. Oxford, Blackwell Scientific, 1982.

68. Headington JT, Novak E: Clinical and histologic studies of male pattern baldness treated with topical minoxidil. *Curr Ther Res* 1984; **36:** 1098–1106.

69. Kligman AM: The comparative histopathology of male-pattern baldness and senescent baldness. *Clin Dermatol* 1988; **6:** 108–118.

70. Jaworsky C, Kligman AM, Murphy GF: Characterization of inflammatory infiltrates in male pattern androgenetic alopecia: implications for pathogenesis. *Br J Dermatology* 1992; **127:** 239–246.

71. Whiting DA: Diagnostic and predictive value of horizontal sections of scalp biopsy specimens in male-pattern androgenetic alopecia. *J Am Acad Dermatol* 1993; **28:** 755–763.

72. Whiting DA: Male-pattern hair loss: current understanding. *Internat J Dermatol* 1998; **37:** 561–566.

73. Ye F, Imamura K, Imanishi N, Rhodes L, Uno H: Effects of topical antiandrogen and 5α-reductase inhibitors on sebaceous glands in male fuzzy rats. *Skin Pharmacol* 1997; **10:** 288–297.

Differences in the mechanisms of androgen action in hair follicles from women and men with androgenetic alopecia

Marty E Sawaya

Introduction

Androgen-stimulated progressive balding of the scalp, or androgenetic alopecia, occurs in both men and women. The extent of hair loss in women with androgenetic alopecia is thought to be less severe than the clinical presentation of men who have androgenetic alopecia; however, it is assumed that the hormonal basis is the same for both men and women, although no studies have been performed to confirm this hypothesis. The current understanding of the pathogenesis of androgenetic alopecia and the action of androgens in the hair follicle have been reviewed by Randall in Chapters 11 and 6, respectively. Androgens reach skin tissues through the bloodstream, then pass through the cell membrane into the cell, where they bind with specific intracellular androgen receptors. Hormone binding to the receptor causes a change in shape, exposing a DNA binding site and thus enabling the activation of specific gene transcription. Although testosterone is the main circulating androgen in men, it is often metabolized to the more potent 5α-dihydrotestosterone within many tissues such as the prostate (see Chapter 6). It is well known that 5α-dihydrotestosterone is the active androgen in some target tissues in the skin, and this has interesting implications in skin diseases such as hirsutism, androgenic alopecia, and acne.

5α-dihydrotestosterone is thought to be the main androgen involved in androgenetic alopecia, in which the hair follicle undergoes a miniaturization process through successive hair cycles, with hairs becoming shorter, finer and less pigmented. These are genetically marked hair follicles on the scalp; however, the opposite effect is seen in body hair, where the influence of androgens is thought to cause the hair follicles to produce thicker, longer and more pigmented, terminal hairs (see Chapter 6).

Current findings on the importance of androgens in human hair follicles

As the pharmaceutical companies thrust into new drug development for treating hair loss, the current major interest in androgenetic alopecia is strongly focused on the pharmacological modulation of androgen metabolism in the scalp, either through inhibition of 5α-reductase or the androgen receptor. It is now generally accepted that 5α-dihydrotestosterone is a key player in androgenetic alopecia, with evidence from the condition of male pseudohermaphroditism, where individuals lack or have markedly decreased 5α-reductase type II enzyme levels, leading to suppressed 5α-dihydrotestosterone, and do not develop androgenetic alopecia.[1]

The latest development in therapeutics in treating androgenetic alopecia, finasteride, a specific inhibitor of 5α-reductase type II, is already in the marketplace; its effects are discussed by Price in

Chapter 13. There are a host of other similar agents in clinical development that inhibit 5α-reductase and alter the metabolic pathway of this androgen; this emphasizes the importance of 5α-dihydrotestosterone in these androgen-related skin disorders.

Interest in 5α-reductase has provoked efforts to develop new compounds that effect 5α-dihydrotestosterone synthesis, and the finding of two isoenzymes of 5α-reductase allows different possibilities for selective reduction of 5α-dihydrotestosterone.

Since androgen metabolism and androgen receptor content may vary between men and women with androgenetic alopecia and might account for the different clinical presentation of androgenetic alopecia between the genders,[1] these parameters have been investigated.

Androgen receptor content, 5α-reductase and aromatase activity in scalp hair follicles in men and women with androgenetic alopecia

Previous reports on the metabolism of androgens and estrogens by human target tissues and organs have shown that the metabolizing enzymes are critical for determining the cellular effects of steroids. Studies of androgen metabolism in isolated frontal anagen hair follicles of young men with androgenetic alopecia have shown that they have a greater capacity to form 5α-dihydrotestosterone compared with those from non-balding men with androgenetic alopecia.[2]

The levels of 5α-reductase type I and II, the cytochrome P_{450} aromatase enzyme, and the androgen receptor in hair follicles of women and men with androgenetic alopecia have recently been investigated. Patients with androgenetic alopecia (12 men and 12 women; Ludwig I or II; men with Hamilton II-III grade hair loss) aged 18–33 years old were selected for frontoparietal and occipital biopsies. The biopsies were microdissected to obtain the hair follicles for biochemical and molecular analysis as previously described.[1]

Results shown in Tables 1–3, indicated that both women and men with androgenetic alopecia have higher levels of androgen receptor and 5α-reductase type I and II in frontal hair follicles than in their own occipital hair follicles, whereas higher levels of aromatase are found in their occipital follicles. Overall, marked quantitative differences in levels of androgen receptor and the three enzymes have been found (and verified with immunohistochemical localization of many of these factors) in the outer root sheath of hair follicles in both men and women.[1] In the past it was always emphasized that the dermal papilla was the main area of the hair follicle that is actively engaged in androgen metabolism; however, new findings suggest that other areas of the hair follicle, such as the outer root sheath, are actively engaged and interactive with other areas of the hair follicle to control and regulate hair growth.[3–7]

The androgen receptor content was evaluated in female frontal hair follicles in an early stage of hair loss and found to be approximately 40% lower than in male frontal hair follicles. The androgen receptor is the key factor that mediates androgen action by its molecular effects on transcription and translation of cellular proteins. Table 1 shows that the androgen receptor levels were 1.5 times greater in frontal than in occipital hairs of men.

Another important enzyme, aromatase, listed in Table 3, has important implications since androgens, such as 4-androstenedione, and testosterone can be metabolized locally in the hair follicle into estrogens, estrone and estradiol, respectively. The relevance of estrogens to hair growth continues to be established; however, it is postulated that since aromatase levels were six times greater in female frontal hair follicles than in male ones (see Table 3), it may be that aromatase can lower the level of androgens locally by shunting to the estrogen pathway. Further work continues in this area to establish the role of estrogens in regulating hair growth, especially now that it is recognized that there are two separate estrogen receptors, alpha and beta,[8] each of which could play specific roles in hair follicle regulation of growth.[9]

The results listed in Table 2 in women undergoing frontal hair biopsies indicate that, in women, approximately three times less 5α-reductase type I and II is found compared with that in the frontal hair follicles of men. The

Table 1 Androgen receptor levels in female and male hair follicles. Incubations were performed in triplicate as previously described,[1] with mean values given for 12 patients in each group in maximum binding capacity for androgen receptor levels. SD range is between 20 and 24.

Hair follicles	Nuclear androgen receptor levels (fmol/mg DNA)
Women	
Frontal	177
Occipital	132
Men	
Frontal	302
Occipital	226

Table 2 Type I and II 5α-reductase activity in hair follicles from women and men. Values given are the mean for the 12 patients in each group. Standard deviations (SD) ranged between 1.0–2.8. Incubations were performed in triplicate as previously described.[1]

Hair follicles	5α-reductase activity (pmol/min/0.5 mg protein)	
	Type I	Type II
Women		
Frontal	22.0	4.6
Occipital	13.0	2.8
Men		
Frontal	63.3	17.2
Occipital	29.4	6.9

Table 3 Aromatase levels in hair follicles from women and men. Enzyme activity is described in each group as the mean of 12 patients, with specific activity (pmol/min/0.5 mg protein), as previously described,[1] with SD range being 2.4–4.0.

Hair follicles	Aromatase activity (pmol/min/0.5 mg protein)
Women	
Frontal	18
Occipital	32
Men	
Frontal	3
Occipital	9

Still, the most popular enzyme to study in the pathway is 5α-reductase: a multitude of studies have emphasized the location of 5α-reductase in various body tissues.[10–15] Type I has been found primarily in skin,[10–13] while type II 5α-reductase has been found primarily in reproductive gonadal organs.[11–13] Studies by Sawaya and Price[16] emphasize that both 5α-reductase isoenzyme forms are found in hair follicles of both men and women and that both isoenzymes are important regulators of 5α-dihydrotestosterone synthesis. These studies[16] and others[14] have also revealed that there is less expression of type I 5α-reductase in the outer root sheath of hair follicles, with intense expression in distal lobular portions of the sebaceous glands. In contrast type II 5α-reductase is more common in the outer root sheath of hair follicles[15,16] as well as the ductal portion of the sebaceous gland.[16] This latter site is an interesting anatomical site that merges with the hair follicle, which may be important in acne since the duct of sebaceous glands is involved in the lipid-hormonal-microbial aspects of mediating the acne disease process.

In any case, the finding of both the 5α-reductase isoenzymes in hair follicles is important as new pharmacological agents approach the marketplace, some of these being specific for either type I, or type II, and some compounds acting as 'dual' 5α-reductase inhibitors. It is known that type I 5α-reductase is responsible for approximately one-third of the circulating 5α-dihydrotestosterone, whereas type II 5α-reductase is responsible for two-thirds of 5α-dihydrotestosterone in the circulation. This would indicate that type II 5α-reductase is the more important enzyme of the two. Based on the kinetic properties[10,12] of the two isoenzymes (Table 4), it suggests that finasteride, a type II 5α-reductase inhibitor that inhibits over 60% of circulating 5α-dihydrotestosterone, is an important therapeutic agent in treating androgenetic alopecia,[17] as discussed by Price in Chapter 13.

Conclusions

The study analysing scalp biopsies from men and women with androgenetic alopecia leads to several conclusions. Androgen receptor levels were found to be nearly 1.5 times greater in

same cellular enzymes and receptors are found in women and men, but the quantities of these factors vary between the genders; this fact may perhaps explain the different clinical presentations in patterns of hair loss.

Table 4   Biochemical differences between 5α-reductase type I and type II.

Characteristics	5α-reductase Type I	Type II
pH optimum	8.0	6.0
Km	24 µM	0.33 µM
Subcellular fraction	Microsomal	Microsomal and nuclear

frontal follicles of women and men than their occipital hair follicles; frontal follicles of women have approximately 40% fewer androgen receptor than frontal follicles of men. Two forms of 5α-reductase, type I and type II, are present in hair follicles of women and men with androgenetic alopecia. Moreover, even though type I is thought to be the primary form in skin, it is type II that may be important in contributing to the greater levels of 5α-dihydrotestosterone in hair follicles on the scalp. Women with androgenetic alopecia have approximately 40% more total 5α-reductase in frontal follicles compared with occipital follicles, but have less than 50% of the levels found in men with androgenetic alopecia. Frontal follicles of women have approximately 80% higher aromatase levels than frontal hair follicles of men with androgenetic alopecia. Men have nearly three times the levels of total and type II 5α-reductase in frontal follicles compared with occipital follicles, with minimal aromatase levels in frontal follicles. In scalp hair follicles, androgen receptors and enzymes localize primarily to the outer root sheath and fewer are found in dermal papilla.

The androgen receptor and the three important enzymes, 5α-reductase type I and II, and aromatase, are present in both men and women with androgenetic alopecia and are located, as seen by immunostaining, to the outer root sheath of the hair follicle, with less expression in the dermal papilla. The levels of these factors differ in women and men in different scalp regions. The author has studied many biopsies obtained from men from other scalp areas such as frontal, parietal, and vertex areas and compared these sites with the hairy occipital area, finding that, in men, the entire 'top' of the scalp is similar with regard to the quantities of these cellular factors affecting the hair follicle. The top of the scalp is now recognized to be a hormonally sensitive and responsive area. This differs dramatically from the occipital hairy scalp area, which is known to be 'resistant' to the effects of 5α-dihydrotestosterone and with regard to the expression of androgenetic alopecia. These latest studies give biochemical evidence to support these facts.[16]

The clinical studies help explain the various clinical patterns of androgenetic alopecia in women and men, while providing insight into the usually more severe expression of this trait in men. They also offer a biochemical basis for therapeutic strategies, as more compounds are being developed by a host of pharmaceutical companies to treat androgenetic alopecia in the near future.

References

1. Imperato-McGinley A, Guerrero J, Gautier T, et al.: Steroid 5α-reductase deficiency in man: an inherited form of male pseudohermaphroditism. *Science* 1974; **186**: 1213–1215.
2. Schweikert HU, Wilson JD: Regulation of human hair growth by steroid hormones II. Androstenedione metabolism in isolated hairs. *J Clin Endocrinol* 1974; **39**: 1012–1019.
3. Jahoda CAB, Horne KA, Oliver RF: Induction of hair growth by implantation of cultured dermal papilla cells. *Nature* 1984; **811**: 560–562.
4. Randall VA, Thornton MJ, Messenger AG, et al.: Hormones and hair growth: variations in androgen receptor content of dermal papilla cells cultured from human and red deer (*Cervus Elaphus*) hair follicles. *J Invest Dermatol* 1993; **101 (Suppl)**: 114S–120S.
5. Messenger AG: Isolation, culture and in vitro behaviour of cells isolated from papillae of human hair follicles. In Van Neste D, Lachapelle JM, Antonie JL (eds.): *Trends in human hair regrowth and alopecia research* Dordracht: Kluver Academic Publishers, 1989; 57–66.

6. Hamada K, Thornton MJ, Liang I, Messenger AG, Randall VA: The metabolism of testosterone by dermal papilla cells cultured from human pubic and axillary hair follicles concurs with hair growth in 5-α-reductase deficiency. *J Invest Dermatol* 1996; **106:** 1017–1022.

7. Randall VA, Hibberts NA, Hamada K: A comparison of the culture and growth of dermal papilla cells from hair follicles from non-balding and balding (androgenetic alopecia) scalp. *Br J Dermatol* 1996; **134:** 437–444.

8. Oh H-S, Smart RC: An estrogen receptor mediated pathway regulates the telogen-anagen hair follicle transition and influences epidermal cell proliferation. *Proc Natl Acad Sci USA* 1996; **93:** 12525–12530.

9. Couse JF, Lindzey J, Grandien K, Gustafsson JA, Korach KS: Tissue distribution and quantitative analysis of estrogen receptor-α (ERα) and estrogen receptor-β (ERβ) messenger ribonucleic acid in the wild-type and ERα-knockout mouse. *Endocrinology* 1997; **138:** 4613–4621.

10. Itami S, Kurata S, Sonoda T, et al.: Characterization of 5α-reductase in culture human dermal papilla cells from beard and occipital hair. *J Invest Dermatol* 1991; **96:** 57–59.

11. Anderson S, Bishop RW, Russell DW: Expression cloning and regulation of steroid 5α-reductase, an enzyme essential for male sexual differentiation. *J Biol Chem* 1989; **264:** 16249–16255.

12. Anderson S, Russell DW: Structural and biochemical properties of cloned and expressed human and rat steroid 5α-reductase. *Proc Natl Acad Sci USA* 1990; **87:** 3540–3644.

13. Thigpen AE, Silver RI, Guileyardo JM, et al.: Tissue distribution and ontogeny of steroid 5α-reductase isoenzyme expression. *J Clin Invest* 1993; *92:* 903–910.

14. Eicheler W, Dreher M, Hoffman R, et al.: Immunohistochemical evidence for differential distribution of 5α-reductase isoenzymes in human skin. *Br J Dermatol* 1995; *133:* 371–376.

15. Bayne EK, Flanagan J, Azzolina B, et al.: Immunolocalization of type 2 5α-reductase in human hair follicles. *J Invest Dermatol* 1997; **108:** 651.

16. Sawaya ME, Price VH: Different levels of 5α-reductase type I and II, aromatase, and androgen receptor in hair follicles of women and men with androgenetic alopecia. *J Invest Dermatol* 1997; **109:** 296–300.

17. Kaufman KD, Olsen EA, Whiting D, et al.: Finasteride in the treatment of men with androgenetic alopecia. *J Am Acad Dermatol* 1998; **39:** 578–589.

13
Clinical trials of oral finasteride

Vera H Price

Introduction

Androgenetic alopecia is a poorly-controlled, progressive form of balding on the scalp which occurs frequently in men and to a lesser extent in women. The biology, pathogenesis and established forms of treatment of androgenetic alopecia were reviewed by Randall in Chapter 10. Finasteride, a type II 5α-reductase inhibitor, is the first approved treatment for androgenetic alopecia that is specifically directed at the underlying pathophysiology. By inhibiting type II 5α-reductase,[1–3] finasteride blocks the conversion of testosterone to dihydrotestosterone (DHT) and decreases DHT levels in the systemic circulation and in target issues.[4–6] Finasteride has no affinity for the androgen receptor and has no antiandrogenic, androgenic, estrogenic, antiestrogenic, progestational, or other steroidal properties.[1–3] Finasteride, which was originally developed to treat prostatic disorders, at a dose of 5 mg per day, was introduced in 1992 for the treatment of benign prostatic hyperplasia (BPH). It was later introduced in 1998 at a dose of 1 mg per day for the treatment of androgenetic alopecia in men.

Overview of clinical trials

Phase III clinical studies for finasteride included three double-blind, placebo-controlled, randomized, multicenter trials that enrolled 1879 men aged 18–41 years with a spectrum of mild to moderate androgenetic alopecia. Two studies, one conducted at 33 sites in the USA and the second at 27 sites in 15 countries worldwide, enrolled men with predominantly vertex hair loss ($n = 1553$).[7] The third study involved men with anterior and mid-scalp hair loss ($n = 326$).[8]

(A single-center controlled hair weight study is in its third year, and 2 year data will be available shortly but not in time for this review.)

Study designs

All three trials began with a 1-year double-blind phase during which patients were randomized to treatment with either finasteride 1 mg/day or placebo. In the two vertex studies, 1215 men who completed the first 12 months elected to continue for a 12-month extension during which patients either continued to receive their original treatment or were switched to the alternative (Figure 1). The frontal study was followed by a 1-year open-label extension during which all patients received finasteride.

Evaluation methods

Efficacy was evaluated by four endpoints: hair count; patient self-assessment; investigator

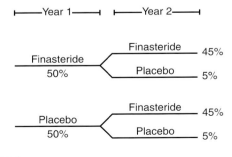

Figure 1

Design of controlled phase III vertex studies.

clinical assessment; and global photographic assessment.

Hair counts were obtained from color macrophotographs of a representative area of active scalp hair thinning. In men with vertex thinning, hair count was determined in a circular area 1-inch (5.1 cm^2) in diameter at the anterior leading edge of the vertex thinning area. In the frontal study, hair count was determined in a circular area (1 cm^2) in the thinning frontal parietal scalp. The site selected for hair counts was centered with a dot tattoo to ensure reproducibility,[7,9] and hair at this site was clipped to 1 mm prior to macrophotography. The macrophotographs were taken with dedicated preset camera systems with fixed focus, distance, and exposure, and were processed at a central quality-control center. After processing, the macrophotographs were enlarged into 8 × 10 inch (20.3 × 25.4 cm) color transparencies, for a final magnification of 5.84:1. At the end of the initial 1-year treatment, transparencies obtained at baseline, Month 6 and Month 12 were converted into dot maps of each visible hair by trained technicians blinded to patient, treatment, and time. At the end of the extension studies, dot maps were generated from Month 24 transparencies. Hair counts were then obtained from these dot maps by means of personal computer-based scanners and imaging software.

Patients also assessed hair growth by means of a validated self-administered questionnaire.[7,10] The six questions related to hair appearance and growth, slowing of hair loss, and satisfaction with the appearance of the frontal hairline, hair on top of the head, and the hair overall. In the vertex studies, an additional question related to the size of the bald spot.

Investigators subjectively rated change in the patient's hair from baseline on the following standardized seven-point scale: −3, greatly decreased; −2, moderately decreased; 1, slightly decreased; 0, no change; +1, slightly increased; +2, moderately increased; and +3, greatly increased.

Standardized color global photographs of the vertex or anterior/mid-scalp were taken, after the hair had been combed consistently for each patient, with the patient's head in a stereotactic device that ensured consistency of positioning and photographic distance.[9] At the end of the study, an expert panel of three dermatologists, blinded to patient and treatment, evaluated hair growth or loss by comparing baseline with follow-up photographs and rating the change with the seven-point scale used by the investigators. The photographic assessment, unlike the patient and investigator assessments, does not depend on memory recall and therefore decreases the placebo effect, while providing an objective measure of response to finasteride.

Results

Vertex studies

Of the 1553 patients enrolled in the two vertex studies, 779 were assigned to finasteride and 774 to placebo.[7] Data from the studies were combined for statistical analysis. Figure 2 shows changes in hair count during the initial year and the 1-year extension during which patients either continued to receive their original treatment or were switched to the alternative.

The increase in hair count achieved with finasteride during the first year was maintained during the second year in men who continued active treatment (see Figure 2). In contrast, further decrease in hair count occurred in men who continued on placebo in the second year. Hair count increased between Month 12 and Month 24 in the men switched from placebo to finasteride. At the same time, the beneficial effect of finasteride on hair count was reversed in men switched from finasteride to placebo at Month 12.

Analysis of responses on the patient self-assessment questionnaire indicated statistically significant improvement with finasteride beginning at Month 3 ($p < 0.05$) and persisting at all subsequent evaluations ($p < 0.001$). Mean investigator scores also showed significantly greater improvement with finasteride than with placebo ($p < 0.001$).

Assessment of standardized global photographs by the expert panel showed significantly greater improvement with finasteride than with placebo. At 24 months, 66% of patients were improved (increased scalp coverage) with finasteride compared with 7% for placebo. Global photographs of selected finasteride-treated patients are shown in Figure 3.

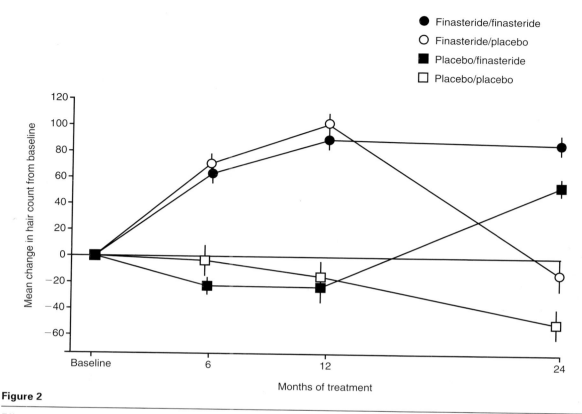

Finasteride/finasteride
Finasteride/placebo
Placebo/finasteride
Placebo/placebo

Figure 2

Effects of finasteride (1 mg/day) and placebo treatment on mean hair count in a circular area (1 cm^2) of scalp over 24 months in the vertex studies of men with androgenetic alopecia. Results are mean ± SEM/SD.

Frontal (anterior mid-scalp) studies

Figure 4 shows the effect of finasteride and placebo on hair count during the initial 12-month double-blind period and the subsequent 12-month open extension when everyone received finasteride.

Although the increase in hair count in patients with frontal (anterior mid-scalp) hair thinning treated with finasteride was not so great as the increase seen in the vertex studies, patients' self-assessments of efficacy were nearly identical in the frontal and vertex studies. Thus, the clinical significance of the hair-count increase achieved with finasteride was apparently similar in both the frontal and vertex areas of the scalp.

The mean investigator assessment for the finasteride-treated group was superior to that for the placebo-treated group at all time points. Similarly, the expert panel's evaluation of global photographs indicated greater improvement with finasteride compared with placebo. Global photographs of selected men treated with finasteride are illustrated in Figure 5. The improvement with finasteride after 12 months was maintained throughout the second year of treatment.

Finasteride in postmenopausal woman

Recently, the first trial of finasteride in women was carried out. Finasteride was not effective in a

a

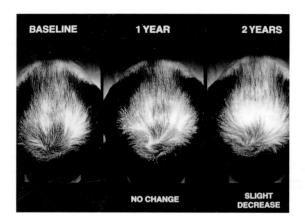

b

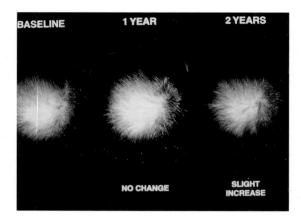

c

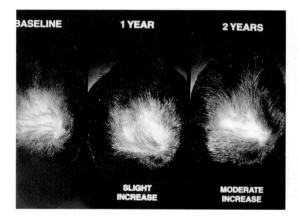

d

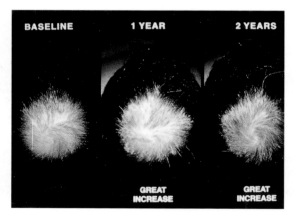

Figure 3

Global photographic assessments of individual men from the vertex studies showing the types of responses occurring after 12 and 24 months' treatment with oral finasteride at a dose of 1 mg per day.

1-year, placebo-controlled study in 137 post-menopausal women aged 49–59 years with androgenetic alopecia. The change in mean hair count did not differ significantly after 1 year of treatment with finasteride or placebo; in both groups, hair count decreased significantly from baseline to Month 12. Global photographic assessments further documented the lack of improvement in hair growth with finasteride.

No studies have been performed in women of childbearing age since finasteride is contra-indicated in women who are, or may be, pregnant

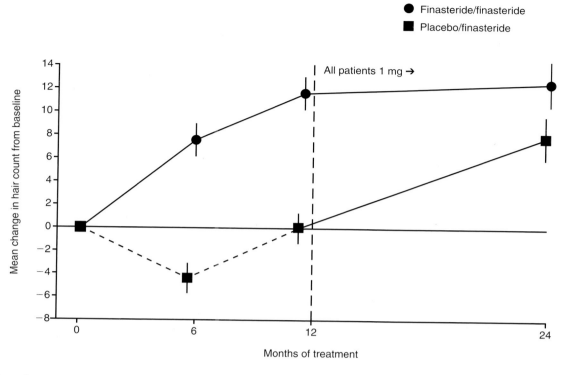

● Finasteride/finasteride
■ Placebo/finasteride

Figure 4

Effects of finasteride (1 mg/day) and placebo treatment on mean hair count in a circular area (1 cm^2) of scalp in frontal studies. Results are mean ± SEM/SD.

because of the potential risk of a genital birth defect in a male fetus.

Safety in clinical trials

Data from the phase III trials in men with androgenetic alopecia support the safety of finasteride demonstrated in large clinical trials and postmarketing surveillance in men with benign prostatic hypertrophy (BPH).[11,12]

During the initial 1-year period, the main drug-related adverse experiences were the following three sexual adverse events: decreased libido; erectile dysfuntion; and ejaculation disorder (primarily a decrease in ejaculate volume). Each occurred in less than 2% of men treated with

finasteride; moreover these adverse events also occurred in the placebo group (Table 1). These drug-related adverse experiences resolved in all men who stopped taking finasteride and also in men who continued treatment. Of the 17 men who experienced decreased libido, in 4 this disappeared after discontinuation of the drug and, in the remaining 13 men, resolved despite continuation of finasteride. Erectile dysfunction occurred in 12 men; this symptom ceased when treatment was halted in 3 men and resolved during drug continuation in 9 men. A slight decrease in ejaculatory volume occured in 11 men; this resolved in 2 when the drug was withdrawn and in 8 who continued on the drug, but is still present in 1 man who is continuing in the study.

A validated sexual function questionnaire

a

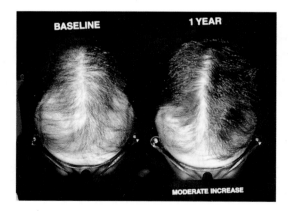

b

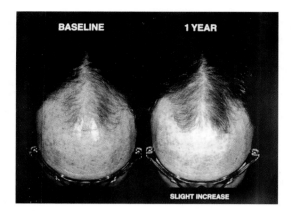

c

d

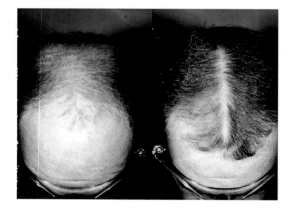

Figure 5

Global photographs of men in the frontal (anterior mid-scalp) study showing the types of responses occurring after 1 year of finasteride treatment.

demonstrated no effect of finasteride on the patients' overall satisfaction with their sex life. The incidence of these sexual adverse experiences did not increase during the extension studies.

Finasteride did not affect the fasting plasma lipid profile or the hypothalamic-pituitary-testicular axis and had no negative impact on bone density.

Table 1 Drug-related sexual adverse experiences each occurring in less than 2% of men in 24-month controlled Phase III trials of finasteride.

Adverse experience	Incidence	
	Finasteride	Placebo
Decreased libido	1.8 (17/945)	1.3 (12/934)
Erectile dysfunction	1.3 (12/945)	0.7 (7/934)
Ejaculation disorder	1.2 (11/945)	0.7 (7/934)

Summary

These clinical trials have shown that finasteride (taken orally at 1 mg/day) helps to slow the hair loss process and increases scalp coverage in men by increasing the length and girth of existing miniaturized hairs. It was not effective in postmenopausal women. In men who continued treatment for 2 years and longer, scalp coverage increased further as the responding hairs grew longer and darker. Men who have been followed in controlled extension studies for over 4 years show continued improvement. The best candidates for treatment are men with definite hair thinning and many miniaturized hairs. Those who are completely bald (have a totally smooth pate) may not respond (Norwood/Hamilton 6 and 7), and those with minimal thinning may not perceive the increased growth achieved with finasteride. All areas of scalp—frontal (anterior/mid-scalp) and vertex—are capable of responding to finasteride provided that miniaturized hairs are present at the start of treatment. Bitemporal recession is unlikely to disappear, however. If treatment with finasteride is discontinued, the beneficial effect is gradually lost within 12 months, as expected, since the underlying genetic predisposition to androgenetic alopecia remains. Finasteride is safe and well-tolerated.

Conclusion

Finasteride taken orally at a dose of 1 mg/day is a highly specific and effective new treatment for men with androgenetic alopecia. It will need to be continued long-term to maintain/extend benefits because the hormonal triggers and hair follicles' ability to respond are unaltered by treatment.

References

1. Liang T, Rasmusson GH, Brooks JR: Biochemical and biological studies with 4-aza-steroidal 5α-reductase inhibitors. *J Steroid Biochem* 1983; **19**: 385–390.
2. Liang T, Heiss CE, Cheung AH, et al.: 4-Aza-steroidal 5α-reductase inhibitors without affinity for the androgen receptor. *J Biol Chem* 1984; **259**: 734–739.
3. Rasmusson GH, Liang T, Brooks JR: A new class of 5α-reductase inhibitors. In: Roy AK, Clark JH (eds.). *Gene Regulation by Steroid Hormones II.* New York, Springer-Verlag, 1983: 311–334.
4. Dallob AL, Sadick NS, Unger W, et al.: The effect of finasteride, a 5α-reductase inhibitor, on scalp skin testosterone and dihydrotestosterone concentrations in patients with male pattern baldness. *J Clin Endocrinol Metab* 1994; **79**: 703–706.
5. Gormley GJ, Stoner E, Rittmaster RS, et al.: Effects of finasteride (MK-0906), a 5α-reductase inhibitor, on circulating androgens in male volunteers. *J Clin Endocrinol Metab* 1990; **70**: 1136–1141.
6. McConnell JD, Wilson JD, George FW, et al.: Finasteride, an inhibitor of 5α-reductase, suppresses prostatic dihydrotestosterone in men with benign prostatic hyperplasia. *J Clin Endocrinol Metab* 1992; **74**: 505–508.
7. Kaufman KD, Olsen EA, Whiting D, et al.: Finasteride in the treatment of men with androgenetic alopecia. *J Am Acad Dermatol* 1998; **39**: 578–589.
8. Leyden J, Dunlap F, Miller B, et al.: Finasteride in the treatment of men with frontal male pattern hair loss. (In press.)

9. Canfield D: Photographic documentation of hair growth in androgenetic alopecia. *Dermatol Clin* 1996; **14**: 713–721.

10. Barber BL, Kaufman KD, Kozloff RC, et al.: A hair growth questionnaire for use in the evaluation of therapeutic effects in men. *J Dermatol Treatment* 1988; **9(3)**: 181–186.

11. Gormley GJ, Stoner E, Bruskewitz RC, et al.: The effect of finasteride in men with benign prostatic hyperplasia. *N Engl J Med* 1992; **327**: 1185–1191.

12. Moore E, Bracken B, Bremner W, et al.: Proscar®: five-year experience. *Eur Urol* 1995; **28**: 304–309.

14
Update on minoxidil treatment of hair loss

Rodney Dawber

Introduction

During the last 25 years there has been a massive expansion of research into the pathogenesis and treatment of the whole spectrum of diseases causing hair loss. Much of this work has been stimulated by the finding that minoxidil, when given orally to control severe hypertension, caused very severe generalized, reversible hypertrichosis in the majority of patients treated, including on the bald scalp[1] (Figure 1). The increased hair growth occurs within 2–3 weeks and is lost within 2–3 months of stopping the drug. It is still available for the treatment of hypertension, being listed in most pharmacopoeias (Loniten, Pharmacia-Upjohn Ltd), although it has largely been replaced as a main-line antihypertensive by medicaments working on different principles and which do not induce significant hypertrichosis.

Minoxidil: mechanism of action

Minoxidil is a piperidinopyrimidine derivative that functions as a peripheral vasodilator.[2] When taken orally, approximately 15% of the parent substance is excreted in the urine; 85% is metabolized by the liver and excreted by the kidney, primarily as the glucuronide conjugate.[3] Its half-life is about 4 hours, although the antihypertensive effect is longer owing to retention by vascular smooth muscle.[3] Side-effects of oral therapy include renal sodium retention, reflex activation of the adrenergic system, with tachycardia, increased cardiac output, secondary myocardial oxygen demand, and pericardial effusions.[3] Electrocardiographic changes are relatively common, including flattening or inversion of T waves. In over 70% of patients, oral minoxidil treatment is associated with hypertrichosis, which is most prominent on the face and extremities. A topical preparation was developed to utilize this hair growth promotion. It has proven effective in patients with androgenetic alopecia, and possibly in those with alopecia areata.

The mechanism of action of topical minoxidil in hair growth, however, remains speculative, since it does not have any specific antiandrogen effect. In animal studies, minoxidil has not been found to stimulate testosterone secretion or adrenal androgen secretion; nor does it displace testosterone from the rat prostate cytosol androgen receptor.[4] In man, serum testosterone levels remain unchanged during therapy. Related to its vasodilating properties on oral administration, qualitative tests using laser Doppler velocimetry and photopulse plethysmography have shown increased cutaneous blood flow for about 1 hour after topical application of minoxidil.[5] Another well-designed study[6] did not show any increase in blood flow. To date, no cause-and-effect relationship between increased perfusion and hair growth has been proven.

Minoxidil has a direct mitogenic and morphological effect on epidermal cells;[7] it prolongs the survival time of cultured epithelial cells, and the time cultured keratinocytes can be passed after confluence. Minoxidil treatment of mouse vibrissae follicles in culture resulted in normalization of follicular morphology, decreased necrosis, and proliferation of matrix and inner root sheath cells.[8] In vitro studies of the follicles of the stump-tailed macaque showed a significant increase in DNA synthesis in follicular and

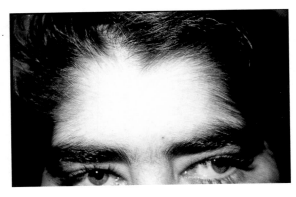

a

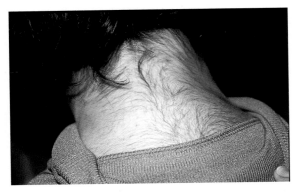

b

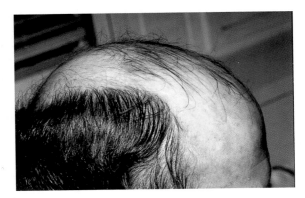

c

Figure 1

Severe (reversible) hypertrichosis due to oral minoxidil: **(a)** upper facial appearance (note long eyelashes); **(b)** increased neck hair in a previously relatively hairless individual; **(c)** increased growth on the bald scalp of a man with Hamilton VIII androgenetic alopecia.

perifollicular cells, but not in epidermal keratinocytes, following minoxidil treatment.[77] Hair bulbs with intact outer root sheath from plucked anagen hairs of men with androgenetic alopecia treated with topical minoxidil were studied by DNA flow cytometry and found to have a significant increase in proliferation index. These studies suggest a direct effect of topical minoxidil on the hair follicle cells.

Minoxidil sulphate appears to be the active metabolite responsible for stimulating hair growth.[9] Although it appears to work in vascular smooth muscle by opening potassium channels, this is still a speculative mechanism of action in hair follicles. Minoxidil acts on at least two sites in the hair follicle, leading to proliferation at the base of the bulb and differentiation above the dermal papilla. In vivo studies in the stump-tailed macaque show that topical minoxidil can reverse and prevent the balding process to some degree.[10] Adult animals with mild-to-advanced baldness and four pre-adolescent animals, which were either unaffected or showed only early baldness, were treated with 5% topical minoxidil 5 days per week for 10 months. Those adult animals treated with topical minoxidil had increased regrowth; pre-adolescent animals given minoxidil showed no signs of impending baldness, while all the control animals had advancing baldness. Histologically, the response to minoxidil showed an increase in the length and size of follicles, with an increase in the number of follicles in mid-to-late anagen phase. It is important to note that there is no evidence that minoxidil produces new follicles.

Clinical uses

Topical minoxidil is licensed for use in androgenetic alopecia in both sexes in most countries around the world. Its safety profile is such that it has become an over-the-counter product at 2% strength (men and women) and 5% (men only at the time of writing). It is also widely used by many clinicians for other than its licensed indications either alone or in combination with other treatments; the conditions treated include alopecia areata, anagen effluvium and certain scarring alopecias.

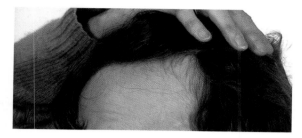

a

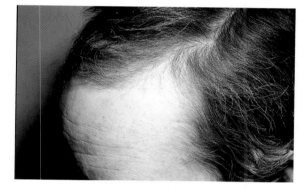

b

Figure 2

Androgenetic alopecia in a woman showing: **(a)** early Hamilton pattern frontal recession; and **(b)** 6 months later demonstrating increased hair growth ('infilling') owing to 2% minoxidil treatment twice daily for 6 months.

Androgenetic alopecia

Topical application of minoxidil increases the duration of the anagen phase of the hair cycle, leading to hairs that are progressively thicker and longer (Figure 2). The visible increase in hair density is mainly the result of partially miniaturized hairs responding to the treatment. It is appropriate to reflect back on the main studies that preceded minoxidil becoming a licensed product:

Multicentre studies involved 2294 men with male-pattern baldness, Hamilton patterns III–VI, between the ages of 18 and 50 years.[10] They received treatment with 1 ml of either 2% or 3% topical minoxidil or placebo twice daily; target area hair counts and clinical assessments were used to judge efficacy. Hair regrowth was not visually apparent until after 4–6 months of continuous use and tended to plateau for most men at about 1 year. After 1 year of therapy, Olsen et al showed that the mean target area terminal hair counts of patients treated with 2% topical minoxidil had increased 218 ± 158/inch diameter circle over the baseline mean of 126 ± 104/inch target circle.[2] While this 2.5-fold increase in terminal hairs was quite dramatic, the mean hair count was still far below the normal density of terminal hairs seen in the occipital area unaffected by male-pattern baldness (1246/inch). It is therefore not surprising that fewer than 5% of patients were noted to have dense regrowth; however, approximately 25–30% had moderate regrowth of hair with the use of topical minoxidil.[11]

Continued use of 2% minoxidil twice daily is necessary to maintain regrowth.[12] The mean terminal hair growth in patients continuously treated over a 5 year evaluation period declined slightly from the 1 year level but did not fall below baseline.[13] Those patients who cease topical minoxidil generally experience loss of the regrown hair within 3–4 months. Restarting the drug will usually regain the previously increased hair density.

There was no statistically significant difference between 2% and 3% topical minoxidil solution in the early clinical trials;[1] however, there was less efficacy with concentrations below 2%. Higher concentrations of topical minoxidil resulted in higher blood levels and, thus, for both safety and efficacy reasons, the 2% topical minoxidil preparation was chosen for initial licence approval around the world. However, the possible improved efficacy of 5% over the 1% or 2% topical minoxidil in alopecia areata raised the question of a potential overlooked dose effect in androgenetic alopecia. Subsequent studies[14] evaluating higher concentrations of topical minoxidil in the treatment of androgenetic alopecia have shown sufficient efficacy and lack of toxicity for it to be now available as a 5% solution. At this strength of topical application sufficient systemic absorption occurs for reversible hypertrichosis to be seen in a small minority: it is most commonly noted on the face, arms and buttocks.[15] After drug withdrawal, the excess hair disappears within a few months.

The results in women with androgenetic alopecia have been similar to those in men. Two hundred and fifty-six women, aged 18–45 years, with Ludwig I or II patterns were treated with 2% topical minoxidil or placebo twice daily for 32 weeks. Non-vellus hair counts in a 1 cm² target area on the top of the scalp showed a mean increase of 14% over baseline after 9 months of therapy (140.4 ± 3.9 to 163.1 ± 3.6). The investigators felt that 50% of the patients had minimal regrowth and 13% had moderate hair growth on 2% topical minoxidil compared with 33% and 6%, respectively, of patients on placebo (Figure 2). Jacobs et al[16] reported an improvement in 55% of women in a double-blind study comparing 2% minoxidil with placebo.

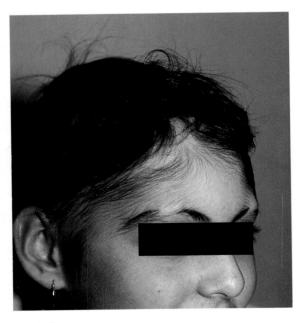

Figure 3

Alopecia areata. In this child frontal forehead hypertrichosis has developed as a result of overzealous topical minoxidil application beyond the scalp margin. (Courtesy of Dr D Van Neste, Brussels.)

The fact that 2% and 5% topical minoxidil are available over the counter in many countries testifies to the good safety profile. The side-effects are few and include allergic contact dermatitis in under 1% of patients and irritant dermatitis or folliculitis in 3–5%.[11] Hair growth on the forehead or cheeks is occasionally seen and represents either inadvertent transfer or spreading of the drug from the scalp (Figure 3) or local intravascular spread by the generous scalp blood supply. The total amount of the drug absorbed is less than 2%. No relevant haemodynamic effects have been observed in normotensive or hypertensive patients using topical minoxidil. Although many men on the topical minoxidil trials developed electrocardiographic changes, these changes occurred both in men on active drug and men on placebo; some of these abnormalities reversed while they were still on the drug. No cardiac problems were linked definitively to topical minoxidil; the background cardiac 'events' may have been associated with the underlying coronary artery disease possibly linked to vertex baldness.[17]

Combination therapies may prove to be beneficial in the future; Bazzano et al[18] found in a 1 year study that topical tretinoin and 0.5% minoxidil was equally as effective as 2% minoxidil alone. Vermoken[19] failed to show synergism between the anti-androgen cyproterone acetate and minoxidil; however, Diani et al[20] showed an increased effect of combined minoxidil and the topical anti-androgen finasteride compared with either alone. Pestana et al[21] found no additional effect when ultraviolet light and topical minoxidil were used to treat advanced male pattern baldness.

Alopecia areata

Early reports of a high success rate with topical minoxidil in alopecia areata[22] have been followed by double-blind and dose-response studies that were less encouraging. Topical 1% minoxidil in an open study of a mixed alopecia areata/alopecia totalis population[23] produced cosmetically acceptable regrowth in 20%. Tosti et al,[24] however, found no difference between 3% solution of minoxidil and placebo in moderate patchy alopecia areata. Price[25] showed cosmetically acceptable regrowth in three out of 11 patients on minoxidil and one out of 14 on placebo, in a double-blind study of 3% topical solution. In a continuation study a better response was seen at 64 weeks and Price[25] commented that the outcome was dependent on the initial severity. The highest response rate has been obtained by 5% topical minoxidil solution,[26] with demonstrable regrowth in 85% of 47 patients with severe alopecia areata, but this was cosmetically acceptable in only 6%. In an attempt to increase tissue minoxidil levels Fiedler-Weiss[26] used oral minoxidil 5 mg 12-hourly in an open trial; the result was a quicker response rate than with the 5% topical solution; but in only 18% was the regrowth cosmetically acceptable. Neither serum nor tissue minoxidil levels correlated with regrowth; this suggests that occlusion of the treated scalp or improvement in vehicle or topical minoxidil application would be unlikely to improve the response rate.

Topical minoxidil is yet another therapy for alopecia areata whose initial promising reports have not been substantiated. Once again, a few patients appear to recover some hair; however, this is rarely cosmetically useful and the evidence that there is a worthwhile treatment response is unconvincing. The controversy with regard to the use of minoxidil in alopecia areata can be summarized from three publications.

Oral minoxidil was evaluated in 65 patients with severe, treatment-resistant alopecia areata.[27] This study was performed to evaluate the maximal efficacy of minoxidil by circumventing the limitations of the topical preparation such as limited solubility and poor percutaneous absorption of minoxidil. Minoxidil was used as a single dose of 10 mg/day. Mean time to response was approximately 9 weeks and to 'cosmetic' response, approximately 35 weeks. Hair regrowth progressed more rapidly and became more extensive with oral minoxidil than with topical 5% minoxidil. Cosmetic response was achieved in 12 out of 65 (18%) treatment-resistant patients with extensive disease. Cosmetic regrowth was maintained during treatment, although minor episodes of hair loss occurred in some patients. Side-effects of oral minoxidil may be severe in hypertensive patients and include reflex tachycardia, oedema, transient T-wave changes seen on the electrocardiogram and, rarely, pericardial effusion. In normotensive patients, low-dose (10 mg/day) oral minoxidil was associated with periorbital oedema and swelling of the fingers, unless patients adhered strictly to a 2 g sodium diet. Women occasionally complained of headaches, depression, or lethargy. Patients occasionally complained of palpitations or tachycardia after ingestion of caffeine, alcohol, or decongestants. Facial hypertrichosis occurred in 11 out of 65 patients (17%). No electrocardiographic or echocardiographic abnormalities were found.

An extensive review of alopecia areata and its treatment by Fielder[28] concluded that topical minoxidil may be effective especially when used in the 5% concentration. However, Epstein,[29] in a letter to the editor in response to Fiedler's review, suggested that this review was not carefully balanced in its conclusions drawn from the literature quoted; he related four adequately controlled double-blind studies that failed to show any significant benefit of topical minoxidil in alopecia areata, which had not been considered. It is important to note in relation to this debate that, to the author's knowledge, Pharmacia-UpJohn Ltd do not have a product licence for the use of topical minoxidil in alopecia areata in any country.

There is much evidence that, whatever the conclusion in relation to the analysis of the minoxidil–alopecia areata literature, pragmatic clinicians frequently use it, often in combination with other agents. Topical 5% minoxidil combined with a topical steroid (0.05% betametasone dipropionate cream applied 30–60 min later) has been evaluated in a double-blind trial and was found to be superior to either drug used alone when treating severe, recalcitrant disease.[30] After 16 weeks of treatment to the entire scalp, fair to good regrowth was found in 56% of patients on combination therapy, 13% on placebo, 22% on steroids alone, and 27% on minoxidil alone. Cosmetic response following combination therapy was seen in 16% of patients with 100% scalp hair loss, 16% with 75–99% loss, 48% with 25–74% loss, and 63% with 0–24% loss. No systemic and only mild local irritant side-effects were seen. This apparent synergistic effect can be explained not only by the probably different mechanisms of action associated with each of the drugs, but possibly also by enhanced dermal residence time of minoxidil.

Topical minoxidil and anthralin has been

shown to be successfully combined to treat alopecia areata.[31] This combination was assessed in 49 patients who had been previous treatment failures to anthralin, minoxidil, or both, used as single-agent treatments. Minoxidil 5% solution was applied twice daily; anthralin 0.5% cream (Drithocreme®) was applied at night, 1 hour or more after the second minoxidil application. Both medications were applied to the entire scalp. Hair regrowth was seen in 38 out of 49 patients (78%) at week 12; cosmetic response was achieved in 5 out of 45 patients (11%) by week 24, at which point the study was terminated. Long-term cosmetic efficacy was not established; however, the five cosmetic responders continued treatment beyond 6 months, and four out of the five (80%) maintained cosmetic efficacy with continuing therapy for 84 weeks follow-up. Side-effects were limited to irritant reactions that were mild in all but one patient, who had to be discontinued from the study because of the dermatitis. No systemic minoxidil effects were noted despite some examples of enhanced systemic minoxidil absorption.[31]

Conclusions

One can conclude from the foregoing discussion that, despite the initial widespread use of topical minoxidil in almost every known cause of hair loss, it has only been found to have proven efficacy in androgenetic alopecia. It is still used in other conditions, particularly in relation to the mechanism by which it retains hairs in anagen for longer than normal. **Anagen effluvium** caused by tumour chemotherapy can be helped to some degree. Duvic et al[32] in a randomized trial of minoxidil in chemotherapy-induced alopecia, showed that the treatment with 2% minoxidil significantly decreased the interval from maximal hair loss to first regrowth, that is, the period of baldness was shortened by a mean of 50.2 days. The treatment of the common types of **scarring alopecia of the scalp**, such as lupus erythematosus, lichen planus, pseudopelade and folliculitis decalvans, is very difficult—most treatments used are only able to arrest such inflammatory pathology to a minor degree. Although there are no controlled trials, many clinicians feel

that topical minoxidil, by retaining unaffected hairs in anagen for a longer period of time, enables the overall density to be better than that of untreated individuals.

References

1. Burton JL, Marshall A: Hypertrichosis due to minoxidil. *Br J Dermatol* 1979; **101**: 593–594.
2. Olsen EA, Weiner MS, Delong ER, Pinnell S: Topical minoxidil in early male pattern baldness. *J Am Acad Dermatol* 1985; **13**: 185–192.
3. Linas SL, Nies AS: Minoxidil 1981. *Annals Intern Med* 1981; **94**: 61–65.
4. Parker LN, Lifrak ET, Odell WD: Lack of a gonadal or adrenal androgenic mechanism for the hypertrichosis produced by diazoxide, phenytoin and minoxidil. *Biochem Pharmacol* 1982; **31**: 1948–1950.
5. Wester RC, Maibach HI, Gur RH, Novak E: Minoxidil stimulates cutaneous blood flow in human balding scalps. Pharmacodynamics measured by laser doppler velocimetry and photopulse plethysmography. *J Invest Dermatol* 1984; **82**: 515–517.
6. Bunker CB, Dowd PM: Alterations in scalp blood flow after epicutaneous application of 3% minoxidil. *Br J Dermatol* 1988; **117**: 668.
7. Cohen RL: Direct effects of minoxidil on epidermal cells in culture. *J Invest Dermatol* 1984; **82**: 90–93.
8. Buhl AE, Waldon DJ, Kawabe TT, Holland JM: Minoxidil stimulates mouse vibrissoe follicles in organ culture. *J Invest Dermatol* 1989; **92**: 315–320.
9. Buhl AE: Minoxidil's action on hair follicles. *J Invest Dermatol* 1991; **96**: 735–745.
10. Uno H, Cappas A, Schlagel C: Cyclic dynamics of hair follicles and the effect of minoxidil on the bald scalps on stump-tailed macaques. *Am J Dermatopathol* 1985; **7**: 283–297.
11. Olsen EA: Treatment of androgenetic alopecia with topical minoxidil. *Res Staff Phys* 1989; **35**: 53–69.
12. Olsen EA, Delong ER, Weiner MS: Long term follow-up of men with male pattern baldness treated with topical minoxidil. *J Am Acad Dermatol* 1987; **16**: 688–695.
13. Olsen EA, Weiner MS, Amara IA, Delong ER: Five year follow-up of men with androgenetic alopecia treated with topical minoxidil. *J Am Acad Dermatol* 1990; **22**: 643–646.
14. Price VH, Menefac E: Quantitative estimation of hair growth: comparative changes in weight and hair count with 5% and 2% minoxidil, placebo and no treatment. In: Van Neste D, Randall VA (eds.):

Hair Research for the Next Millennium. Amsterdam, Elselvier 1996: 67–71.

15. Tosti A, Piraccini J: Androgenetic alopecia. *Int J Dermatol* 1999; **38**(Suppl 1): 1–7.

16. Jacobs JP, Szpunar CA, Warner ML: Use of topical minoxidil therapy for androgenetic alopecia in women. *Int J Dermatol* 1993; **32**: 758–760.

17. Lesko SM, Rosenberg L, Shapiro S: A case-controlled study of baldness in relation to myocardial infarction in men. *J Am Med Assoc* 1993; **269**: 998–1003.

18. Bazzano GS, Terezakis N, Gaylon W: Topical tretinoin for hair growth promotion. *J Am Acad Dermatol* 1986; **15**: 880–881.

19. Vermoken AJM: Reversal of androgenetic alopecia by minoxidil: lack of effect of simultaneously administered doses of cyproterone acetate. *Acta Derm Venereol* 1983; **63**: 268–270.

20. Diani AR, Mulholland MJ, Shull KL: Hair growth effects of oral administration of finasteride, a steroid 5α-reductase inhibitor, alone and in combination with topical minoxidil in the stump-tail macaque. *J Clin Endocrinol Metab* 1992; **74**: 345–347.

21. Pestana A, Olsen EA, Delong ER, Murray JC: Effect of ultraviolet light on topical minoxidil-induced hair growth of advanced male pattern baldness. *J Am Acad Dermatol* 1987; **16**: 971–973.

22. Fenton DA, Wilkinson JD: Alopecia areata treated with topical minoxidil. *J Roy Soc Med* 1982; **75**: 963–964.

23. Weiss VC, West DP, Fu TS, et al.: Alopecia areata treated with topical minoxidil. *Arch Dermatol* 1984; **120**: 457–459.

24. Tosti A, De Padova MP, Minghetti G, Veronesi S: Therapies versus placebo in the treatment of patchy alopecia areata. *J Am Acad Dermatol* 1986; **15**: 209–210.

25. Price VH: Topical minoxidil in extensive alopecia areata, including long-term efficacy. *J Am Acad Dermatol* 1987; **16**: 737–739.

26. Fielder-Weiss VC, Rumsfield JA, Buys CM, West DP, Wendrow A: Evaluation of topical minoxidil in the treatment of alopecia areata. *Arch Dermatol* 1987; **123**: 1488–1490.

27. Fielder VC, Alaiti S: Treatment of alopecia areata. In: *Update on Hair Disorders: Dermatol Clin* 1996; **14(4)**: 733–738.

28. Fielder VC: Alopecia areata. *Arch Dermatol* 1992; **128**: 1519–1529.

29. Epstein E: Alopecia areata, topical minoxidil and balanced reviews. *Arch Dermatol* 1993; **129**: 908–909.

30. Fielder VC: Alopecia areata: current therapy. *J Invest Dermatol* 1991; **96**: 69S–70S.

31. Fielder VC, Wendrow A, Szpunar GJ: Treatment-resistant alopecia areata response to combination therapy with minoxidil plus anthralin. *Arch Dermatol* 1990; **126**: 756–759.

32. Duvic M, Lemak NA, Valero V, Hymes SR: A randomised trial of minoxidil in chemotherapy-induced alopecia. *J Am Acad Dermatol* 1996; **35**: 74–78.

Section IV

ALOPECIA AREATA

15

Alopecia areata: aetiology and pathogenesis

Andrew G Messenger and Andrew JG McDonagh

Introduction

Alopecia areata is a common chronic inflammatory disorder of the hair and nails. Genetic factors are important in determining susceptibility and disease severity but it is unlikely that alopecia areata is caused by a single gene defect. In common with other inflammatory diseases, environmental factors may be involved in initiating disease expression. Research into the pathogenesis of alopecia areata has been concentrated in two main areas – the role of the immune system and the nature of the hair follicle pathology – but our understanding of the relationship between these is limited. In this article, the aetiology and pathogenesis of alopecia areata is reviewed. Some promising lines of research are now in progress and the future challenge is to formulate hypotheses on the pathogenesis that encompass the diversity of information now available from the various clinical and experimental studies.

Genetic factors

Family history

The importance of genetic factors in the aetiology of alopecia areata is underlined by the high frequency of a positive family history in affected individuals. In most reports, this has ranged from 10–20% of cases (Table 1), and the true figure may be greater because mild cases are often overlooked or concealed. In the patients studied by Colombe and colleagues[14] a family history of alopecia areata was more common in those with disease onset before the age of 30 years (37% compared with 7.1% in patients with onset after 30 years). There are also several reports of alopecia areata in twins, sometimes with concurrent onset.[15–19] A recent study found concordance of alopecia areata in 6 out of 11 sets of monozygotic twins but in none of 3 sets of dizygotic twins.[20] Except in occasional families, alopecia areata does not seem to be inherited in a

Table 1 Incidence of familial alopecia areata.

Investigator(s)	Region	No. of patients	Family history (%)
Sabouraud[1]	Paris	500	20
Brown[2]	London	135	20
Anderson[3]	Sheffield	114	19
Muller & Winkelmann[4]	Rochester, USA	736	10
Cunliffe et al.[5]	Newcastle	76	25
Gip et al.[6]	Stockholm	269	17
Sauder et al.[7]	Cleveland, USA	98	27
Friedmann[8]	Newcastle	151	28
Lutz & Bauer[9]	Bonn	167	6.6
De Waard-van der Spek et al.[10]	Rotterdam	209	17
Gollnick & Orfanos[11]	Berlin	149	11.4
van der Steen et al.[12]	Nijmegen/Munster	348	16
Shellow et al.[13]	Various regions, USA	820	42

Mendelian fashion and it is likely that the genetic basis is multifactorial in nature.

Genetic associations

Several genetic associations with alopecia areata have been described. Linkage between alopecia areata and HLA haplotypes has been studied most thoroughly but associations with further immune response genes and other genes have also been reported.

Histocompatibility antigens

Early studies on HLA class I failed to show consistent linkage to any particular antigen. In two families with a high prevalence of alopecia areata, the affected individuals within each family shared the same class I haplotype.[21,22] The haplotype was not the same in the two families (HLA–A2, B40 and HLA–Aw32, B18) but the observations suggest involvement of a locus within the MHC gene complex in predisposing to alopecia areata, at least in the families in question. In two further families from Israel, there was no association with class I haplotypes.[23] More consistent associations have been found between alopecia areata and class II haplotypes (Table 2), the majority of studies showing an increase in the frequency of DR4, DR5 (DR11) and

DQ3. Earlier studies using serological typing techniques suggested that DR4 and DR5 were associated with severe forms of alopecia areata. This severity association has been confirmed in more recent studies which used molecular typing methods. Colombe et al.[14] found an increase in the broad antigen DQ3 in all patients in their study, suggesting this may act as a susceptibility factor. The DQB1*0301 allele (a subtype of DQ3 which is in linkage disequilibrium with DR5) was associated with severe alopecia but not with newly diagnosed patchy disease. There was also a strong association between alopecia totalis/universalis and the DR11 allele DRB1*1104 (with a relative risk of 30:2) which was not present in less severe disease. The association with DQB1*0301 had previously been reported by Morling et al.[29] and Welsh et al.[30] The latter group also showed an increase in the frequency of DQ3, which was greater in alopecia totalis/universalis than in patchy alopecia. The role of the HLA system in alopecia areata has been reviewed in detail by Price and Colombe.[31]

Cytokine genes

Tarlow et al.[32] reported an association between the severity of alopecia areata and inheritance of allele 2 of a 5 allele polymorphism in intron 2 of the interleukin-1 receptor antagonist gene. This allele is also associated with severity in other chronic inflammatory disorders, including sys-

Table 2 HLA class II antigens in alopecia areata.

Investigator(s)	Region	No. of subjects	Association	Relative risk
Frentz et al.[24]	USA	22	DR4	2.3
			DR5	4.7
Friedmann[8]	UK	65	DR4	Not reported
Orecchia et al.[25]	Italy	127	DR4	3.1
Odum et al.[26]	Denmark	41	DR4	2.0
			DPW4	5.1
Duvic et al.[27]	USA	98	DR4	2.1
Zhang et al.[28]	UK	54	DR4	2.8
Morling et al.[29]	Denmark	20	DQB1*0301 (DQ7)	6.1
Welsh et al.[30]	USA	85		
		All	DQ3	4.2
		(AT/AU)	DQ3	12.1
Colombe et al.[14]	USA	131		
		All	DQ3	
		(AT/AU)	DRB1*1104 (DR11)	30.2
			DQB1*0301 (DQ7)	

AT, alopecia totalis; AU, alopecia universalis.

temic lupus erythematosus[33] and lichen sclerosus.[34] Interleukin-1 is a primary cytokine involved in mediating inflammatory responses. The IL-1 gene cluster on chromosome 2 includes genes for the pro-inflammatory IL-1 proteins, their cell membrane receptors and the anti-inflammatory IL-1 receptor antagonist. Polymorphisms within the IL-1 gene cluster may modulate IL-1 responses, although the function of the IL-1RA polymorphism is unknown. In addition to its role in inflammation, IL-1 may have a direct effect on hair growth. In hair follicle organ cultures IL-1 inhibits growth of the hair fibre[35] and induces morphological changes that resemble those seen in alopecia areata.[36]

Chromosome 21

There is an increased frequency of alopecia areata in Down's syndrome with up to 8.8% of patients affected[37,38] suggesting the involvement of genes on chromosome 21. There is an even stronger association with the autosomal recessive disorder autoimmune polyglandular syndrome Type 1 (APS-1, autoimmune polyendocrinopathy-candidiasis-ectodermal dystrophy) in which about 30% of sufferers also have alopecia areata.[39] The defective gene in APS-1 has been mapped to chromosome 21 but its function is not yet known.

Atopy

Several studies have suggested an association between alopecia areata and atopic disease[4,10,40–42] but none has used a control group to which the same criteria for defining atopy have been applied. It has also been claimed that alopecia areata is more severe in atopic subjects[40] but this was not found in a recent study from India.[43]

Miscellaneous associations

Associations have been reported with immunoglobulin heavy chain (Gm)[44] and light chain (Km)[45] allotypes in alopecia areata, raising the possibility of involvement of genes on chromosomes 2 or 14. Alterations of dermatoglyphic patterns in alopecia areata were described by Verbov[46] and Selmanowitz et al.[47] but the significance of these findings is unknown.

Autoimmunity

Alopecia areata is associated with several autoimmune diseases, such as myxoedema and pernicious anaemia. The idea that alopecia areata is itself an autoimmune disease was first suggested by Rothman following a paper presented by Van Scott.[48] Circumstantial evidence to support this idea comes from the immunopathology (see section on Immunopathology, below), the response to immunomodulatory therapy and HLA linkage studies. Also, in most series, patients with alopecia areata have had an increased frequency of circulating organ-specific and non-organ-specific autoantibodies compared with normal subjects and a variety of non-specific abnormalities in peripheral T cell numbers and function have also been reported (reviewed in [49]). Circulating autoantibodies to hair follicle tissue have been found in patients with alopecia areata.[50] These antibodies are also present in normal subjects albeit less frequently and at lower titre. They recognise various epithelial compartments within the hair follicle and appear to be targeted against intracellular antigens.[51] Antibody binding has not been demonstrated in vivo and it is not yet clear whether these autoantibodies play a primary role in the pathogenesis. Alopecia areata has been reported in patients with common variable immunodeficiency, a disorder with failure of functional antibody production. This fact argues against a primary role for antibodies in the pathogenesis.[52]

The best direct evidence implicating circulating immune factors in the pathogenesis of alopecia areata comes from the transplantation experiments carried out by Gilhar and colleagues.[53–55] Initially they showed that hair growth recovered in alopecic skin transplanted onto athymic nude mice.[53] They were unable to induce hair loss in the grafts by passive immunisation of recipient mice with alopecia areata serum.[54] However, in their most recent experiments (in which SCID rather than athymic nude mice were used as graft recipients) they showed that alopecia could be induced in grafted skin by the injection of autologous T lymphocytes that had been incubated with hair follicle extracts and antigen presenting cells.[55] T cells that had not been incubated with hair follicle extracts failed to cause hair loss. Taken together with the T cell depletion studies on the Dundee Experimental Bald Rat (DEBR) animal model (see section on DEBR, below) the results of these experiments strongly suggest that alopecia areata is a T cell mediated disease.

Environmental factors

The idea that alopecia areata is caused by infection, either directly or as a consequence of a remote 'focus of infection', has a long history and still cannot be ruled out. It was the predominant aetiological theory until well into the present century; indeed, sporadic reports associating alopecia areata with infective agents continue to appear. Most recently, Skinner and colleagues[56] reported finding mRNA for cytomegalovirus in alopecic lesions but this was not confirmed in a subsequent study from Italy.[57] There are occasional reports of epidemic alopecia areata,[58] although most date from the early part of this century and the clinical descriptions make it difficult to assess whether the subjects truly had alopecia areata or some other type of patchy hair loss. There are a few reports of alopecia areata in both husband and wife,[59,60] although this may be coincidence. There are also several reports of an apparent association between alopecia areata and various drugs but no single drug or class of drugs predominates and, once again, these associations may be coincidental. The 'external' factor that has most frequently been implicated in alopecia areata is psychological stress. The significance of such an association is difficult to establish because of the problems in performing a controlled investigation and the published evidence is conflicting to the extent that no firm conclusion can be reached.

Despite the anecdotal nature of much of the evidence it is possible that environmental factors are responsible for triggering alopecia areata in some patients. If this is the case it seems likely that a diversity of factors can operate in this way.

Pathology

Pathodynamics

Alopecia areata alters the dynamics of hair growth. This is important, firstly because it causes difficulty in interpreting the histopathology since disease-related features must be distinguished from changes that occur normally during the hair growth cycle and, secondly, because an understanding of the pathodynamic changes can provide clues to the nature of the hair follicle pathology.

The most detailed study of the early changes in alopecia areata was that carried out by Eckert and colleagues.[61] They determined anagen:telogen ratios in hairs plucked from demarcated concentric zones around the periphery of expanding bald patches. Loss of hair was preceded by a large increase in the proportion of telogen hairs. There was also an increase in the proportion of hairs showing dystrophic features. They concluded that the initial event in alopecia areata is precipitation of anagen follicles into telogen. Less severely affected follicles may remain in anagen for a time but these produce a dystrophic hair and eventually also undergo telogen conversion. In keeping with these observations, biopsies from the margins of expanding lesions of alopecia areata show most follicles in catagen or early telogen.[62] It is not clear whether follicles attain telogen status via a normal catagen stage. Exclamation mark hairs may have a well-formed club root identical to that of a normal telogen hair. However, the root is frequently narrowed and club hairs fall out more readily than normal, suggesting that anchoring of the hair within the follicle is defective. Anagen follicles in this site usually show peribulbar inflammation, although it may be necessary to take the biopsy peripheral to the patch of hair loss to encounter such follicles.

Van Scott[48] studied biopsies from patches of alopecia areata and found an average of 58% of follicles in anagen, suggesting that re-entry into anagen takes place. In early lesions, there was a reduction in the size of the lower follicle, with preservation of the upper part of the follicle and the sebaceous gland. In long-standing disease, the entire follicle became smaller. The matrix of these miniaturised anagen follicles was mitotically active and produced a normal inner root sheath. However, the cortex was incompletely keratinised. Van Scott interpreted these changes as indicating arrest of follicle development in anagen stage IV.[63] Our own findings have been in broad agreement with those of Van Scott.[62] Using horizontal sectioning of biopsies from alopecia totalis/universalis and from the centre of bald patches, we found that anagen follicles failed to develop beyond anagen stage III/IV. At this stage, the inner root sheath is a conical keratinised structure and the hair cortex has just started to differentiate beneath it. We suggested that follicles return prematurely to telogen from anagen stage III/IV and undergo repeated truncated cycles. As the disease activity subsides, follicles are able to progress further into anagen.

Except in very long-standing alopecia, hair follicles are retained, even in clinically hairless scalp. When alopecia areata has persisted for many years, particularly in the universal form, there may be a decline in follicle density, possibly associated with fibrosis of the perifollicular connective tissues.

Immunopathology

A perifollicular and intrafollicular inflammatory cell infiltrate is characteristic of alopecia areata. This is most striking early in the disease, when anagen hair bulbs appear to be affected preferentially. In established bald patches, the inflammatory infiltrate is often sparse but immunohistology will usually reveal lymphocytes within the dermal papilla and matrix epithelium of anagen follicles. In contrast to the inflammatory scarring alopecias, little or none of the inflammatory infiltrate is seen around the isthmus of the hair follicle, the proposed site for hair follicle stem cells.[64] This may explain why follicles are not destroyed in alopecia areata. The inflammatory infiltrate is composed mainly of activated T lymphocytes, with a preponderance of CD4 cells, with an admixture of macrophages and Langerhans cells.[65,66] In lesional anagen follicles, lymphocytic infiltration of the dermal papilla and bulbar epithelium may be accompanied by increased expression of HLA class I[67] and class II antigens[68] and of ICAM-1.[69,70] This is a common feature in inflammatory diseases characterised by lymphocytic infiltration and is thought to be secondary to the local release of T cell cytokines.

Hair follicle pathology

The inflammatory infiltrate in alopecia areata is concentrated in and around the bulbar region of anagen hair follicles. Cells of several different types and differentiation pathways are found in the hair bulb but it is unknown which of these forms the seat of the pathology. Based on the following observations, we suggested that matrix epithelium undergoing early cortical differentiation is the primary target of an immune attack on the hair follicle:

(1) These cells show vacuolar degeneration in lesional anagen follicles.[71,72] This explains the formation of the exclamation mark hair as it leads to a focal zone of weakness in the hair shaft, which then breaks on reaching the skin surface;

(2) The pathodynamic changes can be explained on this basis. The follicle is able to protect itself by reverting to telogen where cortical differentiation does not occur. The follicle reenters anagen normally but is restrained from developing beyond the stage when cortical differentiation commences, i.e. anagen stage III/IV;

(3) The pre-cortical region is the preferential site of aberrant MHC class I and II expression.

However, it is possible that the pathological changes in the pre-cortical matrix are secondary to dysfunction of the dermal papilla. This was first suggested by the work of Van Scott and Ekel[73] who showed alterations in the morphometric relationships between the dermal papilla and the hair bulb matrix in alopecia areata. More recently, ultrastructural abnormalities in cellular morphology within the dermal papilla have been described in hair follicles from both lesional and clinically non-lesional sites.[74]

The sparing of white hair sometimes seen in alopecia areata has led to suggestions that alopecia areata is primarily a disease of hair bulb melanocytes.[75] Alopecia areata also shows other pigmentary features including reduced pigmentation in regrowing hairs and an association with vitiligo. However, the melanocyte hypothesis does not explain why sparing of white hair is often a relative phenomenon and is sometimes absent.

Animal models

Dundee Experimental Bald Rat (DEBR)

This variant of the brown hooded rat arose as a spontaneous mutation in the University of Dundee, Scotland.[76] These animals grow a normal first coat of hair but then become progressively hairless. Histology of the skin confirms the persistence of hair follicles, mostly in a dystrophic anagen state. A perifollicular and intrafollicular lymphocytic infiltrate is a prominent feature, and vacuolar degeneration occurs in the cortex of some lesional anagen follicles. Increased expression of HLA class I and II molecules in the dermal papilla and precortical matrix is also seen in a pattern similar to that observed in human alopecia areata.[77] Hair regrowth in DEBR alopecia can be stimulated by photochemotherapy (PUVA), topical minoxidil, and systemic cyclosporin A. It may also be observed when bald scalp from these animals is transplanted on to athymic nude mice. Hair regrowth can be induced by depleting the animal of circulating T cells using monoclonal antibodies, implicating cellular immune mechanisms in the pathogenesis.[78]

C3H/HeJ mouse

A diffuse non-scarring alopecia with clinical and pathological features similar to alopecia areata was reported by Sundberg et al.[79] in a large production colony of C3H/HeJ mice. On the dorsal skin, the alopecia developed in circular areas with disease involvement restricted to anagen follicles. Pedigree analysis suggested the disease was inherited. Alopecia was commoner in ageing animals and the frequency was highest in mice selectively bred for inflammatory bowel disease.

Conclusions

As a result of its diverse associations and clinical presentations, it has been proposed that alopecia areata is a heterogeneous group of diseases and not a single entity. Given our current state of knowledge, it is impossible to determine whether or not this idea is correct. However, the available evidence suggests that alopecia areata is a multifactorial reaction pattern resulting from combinations of genetic and, possibly, environmental factors. Many genes may be involved and their relative contributions will inevitably differ from person to person. They may include genes controlling immune responses, inflammatory responses, interactions between the hair follicle and the immune system, and genes involved in regulating the hair cycle. Each of these factors plays a role but none, on its own, is sufficient to cause the disease. Thus, arguments over whether alopecia areata is primarily a disorder of the immune system or the hair follicle may be impossible to resolve because alterations in both immune function and hair follicle physiology may be necessary to cause clinical expression of the disease. The concept that the hair follicle is an immunologically privileged tissue,[80] not normally subject to immune surveillance, may provide the basis for a unifying hypothesis. A failure of follicular immune privilege, which might occur for a variety or combination of reasons, both intra- and extrafollicular, would then lead to an autoreactive attack on the hair follicle. In such a scenario, autoantibodies would not be a primary factor in establishing the disease but may still have a functional role. Understanding the part played by cell-mediated immunity against the follicular target is still at an early stage and this is an area ripe for study with the latest techniques in cellular and molecular immunology. We can look forward with reasonable confidence to increasing knowledge of the role of genetic factors in alopecia areata but the previously mentioned complexity in the pathogenesis suggests that achieving therapeutic advances may remain a laborious process.

References

1. Sabouraud R: Sur l'ètiologie de la pelade. *Arch Dermato-Syphiligraph Clin d'Hopital St Louis* 1929; **1**: 31–49.
2. Brown WH: The aetiology of alopecia areata and its relationship to vitiligo and possibly scleroder-mia. *Br J Dermatol* 1929; **41**: 229–323.
3. Anderson I: Alopecia areata: a clinical study. *Br Med J* 1950; **ii**: 1250–1252.
4. Muller SA, Winkelmann RK: Alopecia areata. *Arch Dermatol* 1963; **88**: 290–297.
5. Cunliffe WJ, Hall R, Stevenson CJ, Weightman D: Alopecia areata, thyroid disease and autoimmu-nity. *Br J Dermatol* 1969; **81**: 877–881.
6. Gip L, Lodin A, Molin L: Alopecia areata: a follow-up investigation of outpatient material. *Acta Derm Venereol* 1969; **49**: 180–188.
7. Sauder DN, Bergfeld WF, Krakauer RS: Alopecia areata; an inherited autoimmune disease. In: Brown AC, Crounse AG (eds.). *Hair, Trace Ele-ments and Human Disease.* New York, Praeger, 1980: 343–347.
8. Friedmann PS: Clinical and immunologic associ-ations of alopecia areata. *Semin Dermatol* 1985; **4**: 9–15.
9. Lutz G, Bauer R: Autoimmunity in alopecia areata. An assessment in 100 patients. *Hautarzt* 1988; **39**: 5–11.
10. De Waard-van der Spek FB, Oranje AP, De Raey-maecker DM, Peereboom-Wynia JD: Juvenile versus maturity-onset alopecia areata – a compar-ative retrospective clinical study. *Clin Exp Derma-tol* 1989; **14**: 429–433.
11. Gollnick H, Orfanos CE: Alopecia areata: pathogen-esis and clinical picture. In: Orfanos CE, Happle R (eds.). *Hair and Hair Diseases.* Berlin, Springer-Verlag, 1990: 529–569.
12. van der Steen P, Traupe H, Happle R, et al.: The genetic risk for alopecia areata in first-degree rela-tives of severely affected patients. An estimate. *Acta Derm Venereol (Stockh)* 1992; **72**: 373–375.
13. Shellow WV, Edwards JE, Koo JY: Profile of alope-cia areata: a questionnaire analysis of patients and family. *Int J Dermatol* 1992; **31**: 186–189.
14. Colombe BW, Price VH, Khoury EL, et al.: HLA class II antigen associations help to define two types of alopecia areata. *J Am Acad Dermatol* 1995; **33**: 757–764.
15. Omens DV, Omens HD: Alopecia areata in twins. *Arch Dermatol* 1946; **53**: 193.
16. Hendren OS: Identical alopecia areata in identical twins. *Arch Dermatol* 1949; **60**: 793–795.
17. Weidmann AI, Ziion LS. Mamelok AE: Alopecia areata occurring simultaneously in identical twins. *Arch Dermatol* 1956; **74**: 424–426.
18. Cole GW, Herzlinger D: Alopecia universalis in identical twins. *Int J Dermatol* 1984; **23**: 283.
19. Scerri L, Pace JL: Identical twins with identical alopecia areata. *J Am Acad Dermatol* 1992; **27**: 766–767.
20. Jackow C, Puffer N, Hordinsky M, et al.: Alopecia areata and cytomegalovirus infection in twins: genes versus environment? *J Am Acad Dermatol* 1998; **38**: 418–425.
21. Hordinsky MK, Hallgren H, Nelson D, Filipovich AH: Familial alopecia areata: HLA antigens and autoantibody formation in an American family. *Arch Dermatol* 1984; **120**: 464–468.
22. Valsecchi R, Vicari O, Frigeni A, et al.: Familial alopecia areata – genetic susceptibility or coinci-dence? *Acta Derm Venereol (Stockh)* 1985; **65**: 175–177.
23. Zlotogorski A, Weinrauch L, Brautbar C: Familial alopecia areata: no linkage with HLA. *Tissue Anti-gens* 1990; **36**: 40–41.
24. Frentz G, Thomsen K, Jakobsen BK, Svejgaard A: HLA-DR4 in alopecia areata. *J Am Acad Dermatol* 1986; **14**: 129–130.
25. Orecchia G, Belvedere MC, Martinetti M, et al.: Human leukocyte antigen region involvement in the genetic predisposition to alopecia areata. *Der-matologica* 1987; **175**: 10–14.
26. Odum N, Morling N, Georgsen J, et al.: HLA-DP antigens in patients with alopecia areata. *Tissue Antigens* 1990; **35**: 114–117.
27. Duvic M, Hordinsky MK, Fiedler VC, et al.: HLA-D associations in alopecia areata. DRw52a may confer disease resistance. *Arch Dermatol* 1991; **127**: 64–68.
28. Zhang L, Weetman AP, Friedmann PS, Oliveira DB: HLA associations with alopecia areata. *Tissue Antigens* 1991; **38**: 89–91.
29. Morling N, Frentz G, Fugger L, et al.: DNA poly-morphism of HLA class II genes in alopecia areata. *Disease Markers* 1991; **9**: 35–42.
30. Welsh EA, Clark HH, Epstein SZ, et al.: Human leukocyte antigen-DQB1*03 alleles are associated with alopecia areata. *J Invest Dermatol* 1994; **103**: 758–763.
31. Price VH, Colombe BW: Heritable factors distin-guish two types of alopecia areata. *Dermatol Clin* 1996; **14**: 679–689.
32. Tarlow JK, Clay FE, Cork MJ, et al.: Severity of alopecia areata is associated with a polymorphism in the interleukin-1 receptor antagonist gene. *J Invest Dermatol* 1994; **103**: 367–390.
33. Blakemore AIF, Tarlow JK, Cork MJ, et al.: Interleukin-1 receptor antagonist gene polymor-phism as a disease severity factor in systemic lupus erythematosus. *Arthritis Rheum* 1994; **37**: 1380–1385.
34. Clay F, Cork MJ, Tarlow JK, et al.: Interleukin 1 recep-

tor antagonist gene polymorphism association with lichen sclerosus. *Hum Genet* 1994; **94**: 407–410.

35. Harmon CS, Nevins TD: IL-1 alpha inhibits human hair follicle growth and hair fiber production in whole-organ cultures. *Lymphokine Cytokine Res* 1993; **12**: 197–203.

36. Philpott MP, Sanders DA, Bowen J, Kealey T: Effects of interleukins, colony-stimulating factor and tumour necrosis factor on human hair follicle growth in vitro: a possible role for interleukin-1 and tumour necrosis factor-alpha in alopecia areata. *Br J Dermatol* 1996; **135**: 942–948.

37. du Vivier A, Munro DD: Alopecia areata, autoimmunity and Down's syndrome. *Br Med J* 1975; **i**: 191–192.

38. Carter DM, Jegasothy BV: Alopecia areata and Down's syndrome. *Arch Dermatol* 1976; **112**: 1397–1399.

39. Betterle C, Greggio NA, Volpato M: Autoimmune polyglandular syndrome type 1. *J Clin Endocrinol Metab* 1998; **83**: 1049–1055.

40. Ikeda T: A new classification of alopecia areata. *Dermatologica* 1965; **131**: 421–445.

41. Penders AJM: Alopecia areata and atopy. *Dermatologica* 1968; **136**: 395–399.

42. Young E, Bruns HM, Berrens L: Alopecia areata and atopy. *Dermatologica* 1978; **156**: 306–308.

43. Sharma VK, Muralidhar S, Kumar B: Reappraisal of Ikeda's classification of alopecia areata: analysis of 356 cases from Chandigarh, India. *J Dermatol* 1998; **25**: 108–111.

44. Galbraith GM, Thiers BH, Pandey JP: Gm allotype-associated resistance and susceptibility to alopecia areata. *Clin Exp Immunol* 1984; **56**: 149–152.

45. Galbraith GM, Pandey JP: Km1 allotype association with one subgroup of alopecia areata. *Am J Hum Genet* 1989; **44**: 426–428.

46. Verbov J: Clinical significance and genetics of edipdermal ridges – a review of dermatoglyphics. *J Invest Dermatol* 1970; **54**: 261–271.

47. Selmanowitz VJ, Victor S, Warburton D, Orentreich N: Fingerprint arches in alopecia areata. *Arch Dermatol* 1974; **110**: 570–571.

48. Van Scott EJ: Morphologic changes in pilosebaceous units and anagen hairs in alopecia areata. *J Invest Dermatol* 1958; **31**: 35–43.

49. McDonagh AJG, Messenger AG: The pathogenesis of alopecia areata. *Dermatol Clin* 1996; **14**: 661–670.

50. Tobin DJ, Orentreich N, Fenton DA, Bystryn JC: Antibodies to hair follicles in alopecia areata. *J Invest Dermatol* 1994; **102**: 721–724.

51. Tobin DJ, Hann SK, Song MS, Bystryn JC: Hair follicle structures targeted by antibodies in patients with alopecia areata. *Arch Dermatol* 1997; **133**: 57–61.

52. Spickett G, Prentice AG, Wallington T, et al.: Alopecia totalis and vitiligo in common variable immunodeficiency. *Postgrad Med J* 1991; **67**: 291–294.

53. Gilhar A, Krueger GG: Hair growth in scalp grafts from patients with alopecia areata and alopecia universalis grafted onto nude mice. *Arch Dermatol* 1987; **123**: 44–50.

54. Gilhar A, Pillar T, Assay B, David M: Failure of passive transfer of serum from patients with alopecia areata and alopecia universalis to inhibit hair growth in transplants of human scalp skin grafted on to nude mice. *Br J Dermatol* 1992; **126**: 166–171.

55. Gilhar A, Ullmann Y, Berkutzki T, et al.: Autoimmune hair loss (alopecia areata) transferred by T lymphocytes to human scalp explants on SCID mice. *J Clin Invest* 1998; **101**: 62–67.

56. Skinner RBJ, Light WH, Bale GF, et al.: Alopecia areata and presence of cytomegalovirus DNA [letter]. *J Am Med Assoc* 1995; **273**: 1419–1420.

57. Tosti A, La Placa M, Placucci F, et al.: No correlation between cytomegalovirus and alopecia areata [letter]. *J Invest Dermatol* 1996; **107**: 443.

58. Williams N, Riegert AL: Epidemic alopecia areata. An outbreak in an industrial setting. *J Occupat Med* 1971; **13**: 535–542.

59. Swift S: Folie a deux? Simultaneous alopecia areata in a husband and wife. *Arch Dermatol* 1961; **84**: 94–96.

60. Zalka AD, Byarlay JA, Goldsmith LA: Alopecia à deux: simultaneous occurrence of alopecia in a husband and wife [letter]. *Arch Dermatol* 1994; **130**: 390–392.

61. Eckert J, Church RE, Ebling FJ: The pathogenesis of alopecia areata. *Br J Dermatol* 1968; **80**: 203–210.

62. Messenger AG, Slater DN, Bleehen SS: Alopecia areata: alterations in the hair growth cycle and correlation with the follicular pathology. *Br J Dermatol* 1986; **114**: 337–347.

63. Chase HB, Rauch H, Smith VW: Critical stages of hair development and pigmentation in the mouse. *Physiol Zoological* 1951; **24**: 1–8.

64. Cotsarelis G, Sun TT, Lavker RM: Label-retaining cells reside in the bulge area of pilosebaceous unit: implications for follicular stem cells, hair cycle, and skin carcinogenesis. *Cell* 1990; **61**: 1329–1337.

65. Perret C, Wiesner-Menzel L, Happle R: Immunohistochemical analysis of T-cell subsets in the peribulbar and intrabulbar infiltrates of alopecia areata. *Acta Derm Venereol (Stockh)* 1984; **64**: 26–30.

66. Wiesner-Menzel L, Happle R: Intrabulbar and peribulbar accumulation of dendritic OKT 6-positive cells in alopecia areata. *Arch Dermatol Res* 1984; **276**: 333–334.

67. Brocker EB, Echternacht-Happle K, Hamm H, Happle R: Abnormal expression of class I and

class II major histocompatibility antigens in alopecia areata: modulation by topical immunotherapy. *J Invest Dermatol* 1987; **88**: 564–568.

68. Messenger AG, Bleehen SS: Expression of HLA-DR by anagen hair follicles in alopecia areata. *J Invest Dermatol* 1985; **85**: 569–572.

69. Gupta AK, Ellis CN, Cooper KD, et al.: Oral cyclosporine for the treatment of alopecia areata. A clinical and immunohistochemical analysis. *J Am Acad Dermatol* 1990; **22**: 242–250.

70. McDonagh AJG, Snowden JA, Stierle C, et al.: HLA and ICAM-1 expression in alopecia areata in vivo and in vitro: the role of cytokines. *Br J Dermatol* 1993; **129**: 250–256.

71. Thies W: Vergleichende histologische Untersuchungen bei Alopecia areata und narbigatrophisierenden. *Archiv Für Klinische Und Experimentelle Dermatologie* 1966; **227**: 541–549.

72. Messenger AG, Bleehen SS: Alopecia areata: light and electron microscopic pathology of the regrowing white hair. *Br J Dermatol* 1984; **110**: 155–162.

73. Van Scott EJ, Ekel TM: Geometric relationships between the matrix of the hair bulb and its dermal papilla in normal and alopecic scalp. *J Invest Dermatol* 1958; **31**: 281–287.

74. Nutbrown M, MacDonald Hull SP, Baker TG, Cunliffe WJ, Randall VA: Ultrastructural abnormalities in the dermal papillae of both lesional and clinically normal follicles from alopecia areata scalps. *Br J Dermatol* 1996; **135**: 204–210.

75. Paus R, Slominski A, Czarnetzki BM: Is alopecia areata an autoimmune response against melanogenesis-related proteins, exposed by abnormal MHC class I expression in the anagen hair bulb? *Yale J Biol Med* 1993; **66**: 541–554.

76. Michie HJ, Jahoda CA, Oliver RF, Johnson BE: The DEBR rat: an animal model of human alopecia areata. *Br J Dermatol* 1991; **125**: 94–100.

77. Zhang JG, Oliver RF: Immunohistological study of the development of the cellular infiltrate in the pelage follicles of the DEBR model for alopecia areata. *Br J Dermatol* 1994; **130**: 405–414.

78. McElwee KJ, Spiers EM, Oliver RF: In vivo depletion of CD8[+] T cells restores hair growth in the DEBR model for alopecia areata. *Br J Dermatol* 1996; **135**: 211–217.

79. Sundberg JP, Cordy WR, King LEJ: Alopecia areata in aging C3H/HeJ mice. *J Invest Dermatol* 1994; **102**: 847–856.

80. Westgate GE, Craggs RI, Gibson WT: Immune privilege in hair growth. *J Invest Dermatol* 1991; **97**: 417–420.

16
Immunobiology of alopecia areata

Desmond J Tobin and Jean-Claude Bystryn

Introduction

Alopecia areata is a common cause of hair loss afflicting approximately 1–2% of the general population.[1] It is also expressed in non-human mammals.[2] The incidence in humans may be even higher as minor forms of the disorder are likely to go unreported. It is commonly manifested by patchy areas of complete hair loss on the scalp and other body parts but can progress to complete loss of all body hair (see García-Hernández and Camacho, chapter 21). Alopecia areata results from selective, largely reversible, damage to anagen hair follicles (HFs).[3] While not life-threatening, the disease is nonetheless serious because it is disfiguring and, in humans, can cause severe psychological and social problems, including loss of employment. Although the etiology of alopecia areata is unknown, an immune-mediated pathogenesis is suspected (reviewed by Messenger in chapter 15).[4,5] This hypothesis is based on several indirect and direct observations that are reviewed below. Nevertheless, much of the available data must be interpreted with caution since conclusions are often based on small numbers of patients, on poorly or uncontrolled studies, on differences whose significance has not been analysed statistically, and on results that are often contradictory. Part of this apparent confusion may be because the causes of alopecia areata might be multifactorial. Furthermore, there are no universally accepted criteria to describe the clinical manifestations in alopecia areata to be used in clinical research, although this situation should be greatly improved upon implementation of guidelines being developed by the National Alopecia Areata Foundation in San Rafael, California, USA. It is important to understand the cause(s) of alopecia areata when trying to discover effective treatments, and this knowledge is of wider biological interest since alopecia areata may be part of a still poorly understood form of autoaggression seen in other putative 'autoimmune' skin diseases.

A brief review of the immunology of alopecia areata is presented in this chapter. To critically review the evidence for and against an immune basis for alopecia areata, we first need to explore:

(1) The basic requirements for designating a disease as 'autoimmune'; and
(2) The immerging field of trichoimmunology.[6]

Criteria for an autoimmune designation in alopecia areata

The classic histology of alopecia areata—that is, a dense peribulbar lymphocytic infiltrate primarily affecting early anagen follicles—is one of the most consistent and reproducible immunological abnormalities in alopecia areata. The cellular infiltrate first becomes evident around bulbar vessels, particularly in the dermal papilla (DP) capillary network and consists mostly of T lymphocytes and, to a lesser extent, of macrophages (Figure 1) and Langerhans' cells. As the disease progresses, an increasingly dense infiltrate surrounds the bulb of early anagen hairs, and this is followed by invasion of the hair matrix and follicular epithelia. While it has been known for over 100 years that dystrophic HF in alopecia areata were associated with a leukocytic infiltrate, a paper by Van Scott in 1958[7] formally raised the possibility that alopecia areata was perhaps an autoimmune disorder. Before a disease can be accepted as autoimmune, certain basic conditions need to be met.[8]

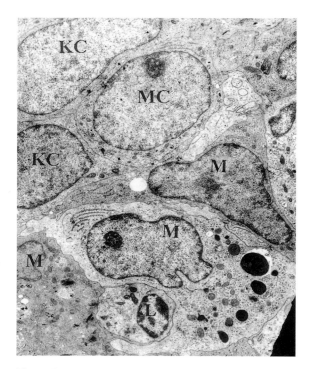

Figure 1

Immune cell infiltrate in alopecia areata. Infiltration of immune competent cells into the anagen hair bulb in a female with acute alopecia areata. Note presence of macrophages (M) in close association with a lymphocyte (L) and hair bulb melanocytes (MC). The macrophages contain melanin granules within phagolysosomes. KC, matrix keratinocyte. Magnification × 8000.

Requirements for classification as an autoimmune disease include the demonstration of:

(1) Unique antigen(s) in the affected organ;
(2) An autoimmune response (either antibody or T-cell response) to that antigen(s);
(3) An autoimmune response specifically associated with the disease;
(4) The autoimmune response producing rather than following the disease process; and
(5) The disease being able to be passively transferred by the autoantibody or T cells.

Indirect clues for autoimmunity include the association of the disease with a particular HLA haplotype, other autoimmune diseases, and a responsitivity to immunosuppression therapies. These are only clues, however, and should not, alone, be taken as evidence of an autoimmune etiology, since, for example, many inflammatory non-autoimmune diseases benefit from immuno-suppression.

Immunobiology of hair follicles

While much is known about the skin immune system (SIS), it is only very recently that a so-called hair immune system (HIS) has been proposed and that the immune status of the HF has been examined more systematically.[6] The skin emerged as a 'first-level lymphoid organ'[9] in the 1970s and, since then, much work has identified both cellular and humoral constituents of the SIS. During all this effort, the HF was oddly neglected. Oddly, because several observations suggest that the immune system could be involved with hair growth and cycling. First, HFs provide numerous ports of entry into the body for micro-organisms. The outward movement of the new hair shaft and displacement of the old club hair could open an access route for micro-organisms to the more proximal HF. Hair growth is affected by substances with immunomodulatory characteristics,[6] for example, cytokines, hormones, neuropeptides, and some drugs. HF regression during catagen is associated with dramatic alterations in the peri-follicular populations of both macrophages[10] and mast cells.[11] Lastly, some autoimmune diseases damage the HF.[12] Conversely, there is a lack of MHC class I expression[13,14] and Langerhans' cells[15] and T cells[16] in the proximal anagen hair bulb, suggesting this may be an immune privileged site.

Langerhans' cells are present in large numbers in the infundibulum, but there are very few below the level of the sebaceous gland and almost none in the hair bulb. Interestingly, they appear in the hair bulb during catagen,[15,16] early graying[18,19] and in alopecia areata.[20] The localization of Langerhans' cells, as the main antigen-presenting cell in the skin, in the upper HF, suggests that they operate there as key components of the 'sentinel receptor pathway'. T cells are another very important component of the SIS and human skin contains two populations; one mobile α/β TCR$^+$ intra-epidermal lymphocytes and a very minor subpopulation of γ/δ TCR[+]. This latter subpopulation is the predominant one in murine skin.[21] In the C57BL/6 mouse model for hair research,[6] the distribution of intra-epidermal T cells and Langerhans' cells is similar.[21] The reduction in the numbers of dendritic T cells below the insertion site of the arrector pili muscle may reflect reduced environmental exposure and/or the relative paucity of T-cell receptor stimulatory ligands in the more proximal HF. The relative number of CD4[+] and CD8[+] cells in the HF is also different depending on site. While these cells occur in very low numbers in the distal outer root sheath (ORS) above the sebaceous gland in the murine HF, they are extremely rare in the normal proximal murine HF.[16] By contrast, in the human anagen HF, a high density of CD4[+] cells (primarily helper/inducer T cells and a subpopulation of macrophages) is present in the infundibular ORS and these cells then decline dramatically toward the proximal HF.[22] CD4[+] cells are also present in the dermis, particularly around the distal ORS, and, interestingly, some may also be present in the anagen DP where they may exhibit a dendritic phenotype. A similar distribution of CD8[+] cells (cytotoxic/suppressor T cells) was observed, although no CD8[+] cells were observed in the DP.

Although not a classical immunocyte, skin mast cells have important immunomodulatory roles in the SIS. HF-associated mast cells are very common in the connective tissue sheath (CTS) or strategically located very close to the HF, where they secrete multiple cytokines with immunomodulatory activities, and can alter T-cell adhesion. They are not seen within the normal human follicular epithelium, although they can occasionally be detected in the DP.[22] Similarly, macrophages have antigen-presenting and immunomodulatory functions within the SIS, and are also detectable in the dermis, including the perifollicular CTS. They are usually not found in the HF epithelium. Like mast cells, they have a role in antimicrobial/parasitic defense, but may also secrete multiple immunomodulatory cytokines during HF regression.[10]

The HF immune system differs dramatically from the SIS in that the epithelium of proximal anagen HF lacks classical MHC class Ia (i.e. HLA-A, B, C) antigen.[6,13,14] All other nucleated cells express MHC class I, with the exception of the testes, eye, parts of the brain and fetotrophoblast. It has been proposed that, like these sites, the HF may enjoy immune privilege.[6,13] Anagen is associated with strong positive staining of class I antigens in the epidermis and the upper 'permanent' portion of the HF. In humans, the isthmus region displays a much reduced staining, where only basal keratinocytes are positive. In the lower HF, however, the ORS and inner root sheath (IRS) and all hair bulb keratinocytes express no detectable MHC class I,[13,14] and so, for so long as they exist, the IRS and the hair bulb matrix remain MHC class I-negative. In contrast, perifollicular CTS fibroblasts and immunocytes are MHC class I-positive. In humans, the DP is, for the most part, negative (i.e. except for endothelial and migratory cells) while DP cells in murine HF express MHC class I in anagen VI but not in catagen or telogen.[23] It has been suggested that the basement membrane-like material of the DP, and that encapsulating the HF, may provide a protective immune barrier to the lower HF. Similar basement membrane matrix barriers surround other tissues with immune privilege. Some believe that this may be a phsyical barrier inhibiting the trafficking of immunocytes between epithelium and mesenchyme.[13] Immune privilege appears to exist to prevent the inappropriate recognition of antigens that may result in the attack of cells presenting these antigens in the context of MHC. This is important in preventing the induction of autoimmunity if immunogenic autoantigens were to be exposed. Furthermore, such immunogenic antigens may be more likely to emerge from the hair bulb during the anagen phase of the hair cycle, since this is associated with major tissue remodeling. Early studies provide supporting evidence that the hair bulb provides an immunoprotective environment.[24] Experiments involved the grafting of black ear skin homografts between two inbred strains of spotted guinea pigs. When black skin was grafted onto incompatible white skin beds, the epidermal black color was soon lost from the donor graft, indicating that the donor epidermal melanocytes were rejected. Some time later, however, black hairs grew through the now white epidermis indicating that some foreign (e.g. black) HF melanocytes survived in the donated graft and repopulated the recipient, previously white-hair forming, HFs. Thus, the hair follicle appears to provide an immunologically privileged site.

Similar protection of HF melanocytes from autoimmune attack may also be seen in vitiligo. Here HF melanocytes are commonly spared, while many of the melanocytes in the epidermis are destroyed.[25] Importantly, repigmenting vitiligo commonly involves the replenishment of the epidermis in part with HF-derived melanocytes, as seen by the perifollicular nature of the repigmentation in many body sites.[25] It has been suggested that a major reason for immune privilege in the hair bulb is to block the recognition of melanocyte antigens since these are expressed only during certain stages of the hair growth cycle.[26] Thus, MHC class Ia antigen expression is lost from the HF at a time when melanogenesis is activated. This has particular relevance for alopecia areata, where melanocyte abnormalities have been detected.[3,27]

There is considerable interest in whether HF-associated immune responsivity changes as a function of the hair growth cycle. Recent studies indicate that, in mice at least, there is, indeed, such a hair growth cycle-associated alteration in the HIS.[6] Dendritic epithelial T cells are seen to increase significantly above telogen numbers in the epidermis and thereafter in the distal ORS, when the HF is in the anagen stage of the hair cycle. The stimulus for this change may be cytokines secreted from keratinocytes in the ORS of the anagen HF (e.g. IL-2). Using the C57BL/6 mouse model for hair research, Paus and co-workers reported little change in the numbers of Langerhans' cells during the hair growth cycle.[16] There is some evidence, however, that rare Langerhans' cells may be detected in the human hair bulb during normal catagen, where they appear to have a role in the removal of pigment incontinence from the regressing HF.[17] Langerhans' cells are also seen outside their usual anatomically-restricted sites in early canities,[18,19] where they may also interact with effete melanocytes, and in hair pathologies including alopecia areata.[3,20] Furthermore, murine anagen is associated with increased innervation of the skin, with the presence of sensory nerves rich in neuropeptides including calcitonin gene-related protein. This neuropeptide is known to modulate effectively skin and immune cell functions, including antigen presentation by Langerhans' cells.[28]

Hair cycle-dependent changes are also seen in macrophage numbers. In mice, a significant increase in MHC class II$^+$ macrophages is detected from telogen to early anagen VI, which returns to telogen values again by the anagen–catagen transition.[16] Macrophage activity has also been closely associated with human catagen, when these cells can be detected both perifollicularly and in the DP.[10] While the functional significance of these macrophage hair growth cycle-associated changes is unclear, they may be associated with a major change in the antigen-presentation capacity. Strikingly, despite the anagen-associated increase in antigen-presenting cells in mice, the contact hypersensitivity reaction is stronger in telogen than in anagen skin. For example, sensitization of C57BL/6 mice skin with picrylchloride, when all HFs are in telogen, results in a stronger contact dermatitis upon challenge with the allergen than if the HFs were in anagen[29] and may be related to the decreased ratio of Langerhans' cells to dendritic T cells during anagen. The HF appears to have a very effective anti-infection capacity. This is seen by the very rare occurrence of folliculitis on the human scalp, despite its approximately 100 000 individual HFs. Folliculitis in immunocompromised individuals is common, however, leading to a greatly increased risk of infection to the mammalian body through this entry port.

A deeper understanding of the HIS is particulalry important in the dissection of the immunopathology of alopecia areata. Moreover, the HF is a very attractive model system for studies on tolerance and immunosuppression in general, and provides an exceptionally accessible tissue to investigate the totally unknown signal transduction events associated with immunomodulatory drugs with hair growth effects, for example, glucocorticosteroids and immunosuppressive immunophilin ligands.

Evidence of an autoimmune etiology for alopecia areata

While it has been known for over 100 years that dystrophic HF in alopecia areata were associated with a leukocytic infiltrate, a paper by Van Scott in 1958 formally raised the possibility that alopecia areata was an autoimmune disorder.[7] It is only relatively recently, however, that there has been a widespread acceptance of an immune-mediated basis of alopecia areata.

Alopecia areata is associated with several immune abnormalities, some of which are non-selective, while others are specific and point to an immune abnormality directed selectively to a component of the anagen HF. These non-specific abnormalities include:

(1) The presence of a peri- and intrafollicular mononuclear infiltrate (see Figure 1);
(2) An increased expression of class I and II MHC antigens and of Langerhans' cells in hair bulbs;
(3) Deposits of immune reactants around HF;
(4) Effective therapies for alopecia areata have, as a common denominator, an immunosuppressive effect on immune cells in skin.

The specific abnormalities include abnormal antibody responses specifically directed to HF antigens. Nevertheless, no unequivocal statement about the etiology of alopecia areata can yet be made. Like many autoimmune diseases with predisposing HLA haplotypes, attempts have been also made to find associations with a particular HLA haplotype in alopecia areata. These have yielded conflicting results in the case of class I antigens, but increasingly convincing data is now being reported for associations with certain class II haplotypes.[30–32] The expression of some of these class II haplotypes appears to separate alopecia areata of different types.[32] Allied to HLA linkage studies, are observations that the severity of alopecia areata may be associated with the expression of some alleles of the IL-1 receptor antagonist gene,[33] which also occur in other inflammatory autoimmune disorders including systemic lupus erythematosus.[34]

Despite the HLA data, however, the only alopecia areata-associated conditions for which there is sufficient firm data are atopy[35] and Down's syndrome.[36] Alopecia areata, when associated with atopy, is reported to occur earlier in life, have a more severe course and prognosis, and respond less well to treatment. The incidence of alopecia areata appears to be increased in patients with Down's syndrome,[36] a condition associated with functional deficiencies in T-cell mediated immune response and decreases in

serum IgG levels. On average, 5% of patients with Down's syndrome have alopecia areata compared with approximately 0.1% of concurrent control mentally retarded patients.[36] Clinical severity and extent of alopecia areata lesions appears to correlate with the severity of mental retardation. The incidence of clinically evident thyroid abnormalities, such as Hashimoto's chronic lymphocyte thyroiditis, thyrotoxicosis, exophthalmic goiter, and myxedema, does not differ significantly in alopecia areata patients from that in historical controls.[37] In view of the contradictory reports, it is difficult to conclude that there is an association between thyroid disease and alopecia areata. There is also increasing evidence of an increase in the prevalence of diabetes mellitus, especially type I insulin-dependent diabetes, in relatives of patients with alopecia areata but not in the patients themselves.[38] These findings suggest a genetic association between the two diseases, whereby the expression of alopecia areata protects against the development of diabetes mellitus.

Many studies have concluded that the incidence of vitiligo is increased in alopecia areata.[39] Recent studies found no significant association between alopecia areata and vitiligo or with family history of vitiligo,[40] although there may be rare co-localization of vitiligo and alopecia areata. Increasing evidence now suggests that vitiligo may result from an intrinsic biochemical defect of the entire epidermal melanin unit in skin.[41]

Alopecia areata is a systemic disease because there is frequent involvement of organs other than the HF including the nails and eyes.[42,43] Thus, the defect may be extrinsic to HF. The prognosis of alopecia areata appears to be worse when nail changes are present. Eye abnormalities were reported to be detectable in up to 80% of patients with alopecia areata who otherwise had no ocular symptoms compared with 30% in normal concurrent controls.[42]

It should be emphasized, however, that the majority of patients with alopecia areata are in good health. It has been estimated that only 3–5% of patients with alopecia areata have another autoimmune or endocrine disease. Consequently, the association between alopecia areata and other autoimmune diseases is more the exception than the rule.

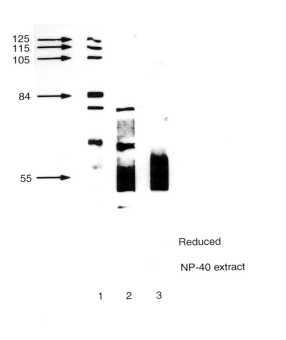

Reduced

NP-40 extract

1   2   3

1. Scalp Anagen Hair Follicle
2. Scalp Epidermis
3. Scalp Dermis

Figure 2

Hair follicles express antigens not found elsewhere in skin. Immunoblot analysis of proteins extracted from **(1)** HF, **(2)** epidermis and **(3)** dermis and reacted with normal human sera. Arrows indicate antigens uniquely expressed in HF.

Humoral immunity to hair follicles in alopecia areata

Various organ-specific autoantibodies are said to occur with increased frequency in alopecia areata.[44] These associations remain, for the most part, controversial. With the exception of thyroid autoantibodies, there are as many studies failing to show an association as there are showing an association. Recently, antibodies specifically directed to HF in alopecia areata have been demonstrated.[45–51] These observations indicate that, despite possible immune privilege during part of the hair growth cycle, HFs express unique antigens that can stimulate autoimmune responses. Antigens selectively expressed in HF are detectable by low titer 'natural' autoantibodies present in many normal individuals (Figure 2).[52] The nature of the HF antigens recognized by these IgM autoantibodies, and their clinical significance, remain to be established. Nevertheless, their frequency is unusually high, suggesting that HF are particularly immunogenic.

The most convincing evidence that alopecia areata is an autoimmune disease is that antibodies to HF-specific antigens are much more common and present in higher levels in patients with alopecia areata than in control individuals.[3,45–51] These antibodies can be detected by indirect immunofluorescence (Figure 3a) and immunoblotting (Figure 3b) in up to 90% of patients with alopecia areata but in less than one-third of control sera. Many 'alopecia areata' antibodies are directed specifically to HF and do not react with adjacent epidermis or dermis. By contrast, most control sera that reacted weakly with HF antigens also reacted with the epidermis. The 'alopecia areata' antibodies are directed to multiple structures within anagen HF and also to multiple antigens within each structure. The most common HF structures targeted include the ORS, followed by the matrix, IRS and hair shaft. Some targets are located in or near proliferating and differentiating areas of the anagen HF, and thus may have the potential to disrupt hair differentiation and growth.[45–51] During immunoblotting (see Figure 3b), alopecia areata antibodies react with multiple antigens of 44–60 kDa and 200–220 kDa solubilized from anagen HFs using 6 M urea.[45,46,50] These 'alopecia areata' anti-HF antibodies are predominantly IgG, unlike the IgM 'natural' autoantibodies that are more commonly detected in normal individuals. This observation suggests the occurrence of a switch in immunoglobulin isotype from IgM to IgG, which is indicative of the maturation of the antibody response to HF antigens. As in other autoimmune diseases, these IgG antibodies may have pathogenic potential.[52] Some of these antigens are also expressed by HF melanocytes and keratinocytes in vitro, supporting the involvement of melanocytes and keratinocytes as possible targets in alopecia areata.[51]

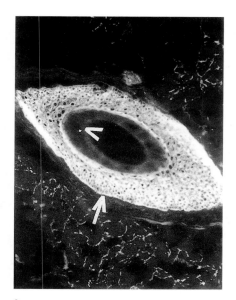

a

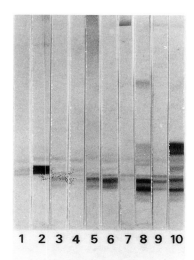

b

c

Figure 3

Patients with acute alopecia areata have antibodies to antigens expressed in anagen HF. **(a)** Indirect immunofluorescence analysis of HF structures targeted by 'alopecia areata' antibodies. Serum antibodies in a female patient with acute alopecia areata reacted with ORS (↑) but not the IRS (<) of anagen HF. **(b)** Immunoblot analysis of proteins extracted from anagen scalp HF reacted with sera from control individuals **(c)** including normal persons and patients with other inflammatory skin disease, and patients with acute alopecia areata **(a)**. Note that only patients with alopecia areata react to antigens in the 35–65 kDa range.

Further studies have shown that 'alopecia areata' antibodies target HF-specific keratins (Figure 4).[50] For example, a 44 kDa HF antigen, defined by alopecia areata affinity-purified antibody, co-localized in the anagen hair bulb with the 44/46 kDa hair-specific keratin (detected using AE13 monoclonal antibody[53]). Staining with both antisera was restricted to the precortex.[50] Confirmation of an anti-HF keratin antibody reactivity in acute alopecia areata was provided by finding that all alopecia areata sera tested, but no control sera, immunoprecipitated the 46 kDa hair-specific keratin (see Figure 4).

The biologic relevance of the HF antibodies in alopecia areata remains to be determined; however, their detection in two rodent models for alopecia areata[46,54] and, more recently, in dogs and horses with alopecia areata,[48,49]

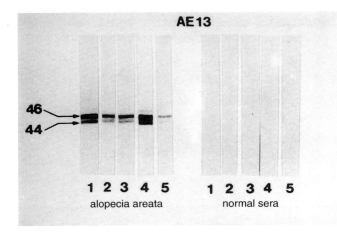

Figure 4

Identification of target antigens in alopecia areata. Immunoblot analysis of HF antigens immunoprecipitated by alopecia areata and normal sera. Note that only alopecia areata serum antibodies immunoprecipitated antigens identified as 44/46 kDa HF-specific keratins by monospecific antibody AE13.

suggests that alopecia areata-like hair loss is widespread in mammals and that similar immune mechanisms are involved in all cases. The basic question as to whether anti-HF antibodies are a cause or result of alopecia areata remains. Several observations suggest that anti-HF antibodies are not the result of the disease process. Firstly, high titer antibodies are not observed in normal individuals despite the release of HF antigens during the normal HF cycle or in scarring alopecias.[45,47] Secondly, in the C3H/HeJ mouse model of alopecia areata, the abnormal autoantibody response to HF is present both in affected mice and to a lesser degree in their, as yet, clinically unaffected littermates.[46] This suggests that the presence of antibodies to HF appears before the onset of hair loss and so may not be produced as a secondary response to HF damage in alopecia areata. Finally, it has been shown in a preliminary study that purified IgG from an alopecia areata-affected horse could adversely affect hair regrowth when passively transferred to normal mice. Interestingly, the passively transferred equine 'alopecia areata' IgG antibodies did not induce hair loss; rather HFs in treated skin were retained in the resting or telogen stage of the hair cycle around the site of antibody administration, while distant HFs apparently cycled normally.[46] This study, which needs to be confirmed, should be interpreted in light of an earlier study that reported the failure of passive transfer of whole serum

from human patients with alopecia areata to inhibit hair growth in human scalp skin grafted onto nude mice.[55]

Further involvement of a humoral immune response in alopecia areata is shown by the abnormal deposits of Ig and complement that are often present along the basement membrane zone of the lower half of HFs.[56] The deposits occasionally extending intercellularly to the adjacent ORS, were most common at the edge or active border of lesions, but were also present in uninvolved scalp. The most frequent immunoreactant deposited was C3, which was found in 75–100% of alopecia areata patients.[56,58] Deposits were rarely present along the basement membrane zone of epidermis overlying involved HFs, suggesting that the immune response is directed to an antigen localized to the lower half of HFs. The fact that deposits were present in uninvolved scalp, suggested that they precede (and may thus cause) rather than result from injury to HFs. Conversely, similar deposits have been reported in the scalp of normal individuals[57] and in some individuals with male-pattern alopecia.[56] Their presence in normal scalp has been ascribed to hair cycle-related changes in HF morphology since deposits are most common in catagen hairs with thickened and corrugated hyaline membrane. This observation raises the intriguing possibility that immune factors may be involved in the regulation of the hair cycle. It has been reported that some patients with alopecia areata have antibodies to endothelial cells[59] or to melanocytes.[51,60] They are discussed subsequently in this chapter in terms of the clues they provide to the identity of the cells that are the target of immune injury in alopecia areata.

Cellular immunity abnormalities associated with alopecia areata

Many consider T lymphocytes to be the effector agents involved in the induction, if not the maintenance, of alopecia areata. Alterations in the number and function of circulating peripheral T cells have been associated with alopecia areata, but again the findings are non-specific and often contradictory. The total number of circulating T cells is described as unchanged[61,62] in most studies. T suppressor cells are described as decreased[63] and T helper cells as unchanged[64] in most studies, resulting in an increase in the T helper (T_h)/T suppressor (T_s) ratio.[65] The T_h/T_s ratio appears to normalize in the regrowing phase of alopecia areata. Changes in the function of circulating T cells have also been described, although the nature of the change is inconsistent. Most studies report a decrease in mitogen-stimulated lymphoproliferative reponse for total T cells and T suppressor cells[65,66] but some studies show no change while others show opposite results. The reason for these conflicting results in the number and function of peripheral lymphoid cells in alopecia areata is unknown. Possible causes include: differences in the methods used to phenotype cells; in disease activity and/or severity in the patients studied; the small number of patients studied; and the small differences in the actual change present between alopecia areata and control patients.

The dense peribulbar lymphocytic infiltrate affecting early anagen follicles is one of the most consistent and reproducible immunological abnormalities in alopecia areata. The cellular infiltrate first becomes evident around bulbar blood vessels, particularly in the DP/capillary network[67] and consists mostly of T lymphocytes[68] and to a lesser extent of macrophages (see Figure 1) and Langerhans' cells.[69] An increasingly dense infiltrate surrounds the bulb of early anagen hairs and is followed by invasion of the hair matrix and follicular epithelia as the disease progresses. The infiltrate precedes or accompanies active lesions, and is most prominent in active disease. The infiltrate subsides in inactive disease and disappears in the regrowing phase. More than 75% of T cells are activated, as seen by the expression of DR antigens and IL-2 receptors.[70] Macrophages are present in lesser number with a T lymphocyte/macrophage ratio ranging from 2:1 to 7:1 regardless of disease stage.[69] It is believed that most of the cells infiltrating the hair bulb are cytotoxic T cells.[71] The T_h/T_s ratio in the infiltrate is approximately 2:1–4:1. This is elevated compared with normal skin where the ratio is approximately 1:1.[72] The T_h/T_s ratio in alopecia areata is similar to that in other inflammatory skin diseases, is similar in affected and unaffected HFs and tends to normalize in lesions treated with topical sensitizers.[73]

The implication of these observations is that there may be an immune response to antigens in the lower half of HFs or in peribulbar blood vessels in alopecia areata. The cell accumulation is selective, rather than passive, because the ratio of cells in the infiltrate differs from that present in the circulation of patients. This, together with the observation that the cells are activated, suggests that they are actively involved in an immune response. The presence of cellular infiltrates around unaffected HFs suggests the process precedes (and thus causes) rather than results from injury to HFs.

It has been reported more recently that alopecia areata may be transferred to human scalp explants, grafted onto SCID mice, by the injection of T cells (isolated from lesional alopecia areata skin), into the grafts.[74] Interpretation is, however, complicated by the observation that prior activation of these T cells by exposure, in vitro, to HF antigens was necessary, and it was not clear whether negative controls included non-HF skin tissue. In any case, these data support a role for T cells in the etiology of alopecia areata.

It has also been shown that alopecia areata-like hair loss can be induced experimentally in the C3H/HeJ alopecia areata murine model using full-thickness skin grafts.[75] Here, alopecia areata was serially transferred from alopecia areata-affected C3H/HeJ mice to normal littermates and C3H/OuJ mice, indicating that an immune response against HFs can be induced with suitable stimuli. The alopecia areata affected skin was thought to contain factors capable of activating hair loss by promoting host-derived mononuclear cells and by triggering an immune response against HFs in the grafted skin and host HFs. The suggestion here is that the immune system itself is the regulator of alopecia areata rather than any intrinsic defect of the HF itself and strongly suggests that anagen HF immune privilege, if it exists at all, is unable to resist the pathomechanism of alopecia areata.

Alopecia areata is associated with the abnormal expression of class I and II MHC antigens and Langerhans' cells in hair bulbs. Both are expressed abnormally within the bulb and matrix areas of HFs in active lesions of alopecia areata.[76] Class I MHC antigens are present in the absence of an intrabulbar cellular infiltrate and thus seem to precede, and consequently may play a role in, the accumulation of invading T cells. Class II MHC antigens, conversely, only appear to be expressed in the presence of an intrabulbar infiltrate and consequently are thought to be a secondary event.[70] Class II MHC antigens are known to be induced by IFN-γ, which is produced by activated T cells.[77] Langerhans' cells also accumulate intrabulbarly in progressive lesions of alopecia areata, particularly in the area between the DP and hair matrix.[67,69] Langerhans' cells have been reported to account for 5% of epithelial cells in HFs in progressive disease, as opposed to 1% in stationary lesions of alopecia areata or in normal individuals.[78]

The abnormal presence of Langerhans' cells and of MHC antigens, both of which are involved in antigen presentation in alopecia areata hair bulbs, may facilitate (and could be responsible for) the induction and elicitation of autoimmune responses to self antigens in hair bulbs. The presence of class I MHC antigens, which are necessary for interaction with cytotoxic T cells, may facilitate damage to hair bulb cells by cytotoxic T cells. The expression of class II MHC antigens, which are induced by immune injury, suggests that epithelial cells in affected hair bulbs are injured.

Another clue that alopecia areata is an autoimmune disease is that most effective therapies have as a common denominator the suppression or the functional modification of lymphocytes in the skin. Most, including corticosteroids,[79] UV light,[80] anthralin,[81] PUVA,[82] cyclosporin,[83] decrease the number of lymphocytes in skin. Topical sensitizers increase the number of lymphocytes in skin but change the composition of the infiltrate and, hence, presumably its functional behavior. This is illustrated by the effect of primary irritants, which increase the number of inflammatory cells in skin but have no beneficial effect on alopecia areata. Immunosuppressive therapy and contact sensitization also reduce the expression of class I and II MHC antigens and Langerhans' cells in hair bulbs,[83] and may have a beneficial effect on hair regrowth by 'normalizing' these parameters. The implication of these observations is that suppression or normalization of the cellular infiltrate around HFs is beneficial, and that, consequently, the cellular infiltrate is a cause rather than a result of the disease.

If alopecia areata is an autoimmune disease, then the hair bulb of anagen hairs appears to be the most likely target. Three different cell types in or near this structure have been implicated: cortical keratocytes;[3,84,85] melanocytes;[3,6,27,51,85,86] and endothelial cells.[59] Presently, there is insufficient information to determine which, if any, of these cells are the actual targets. There is clinical, histologic, immunohistochemical, and electron microscopic (EM) evidence that precortical keratinocytes are damaged in alopecia areata.[3,84–86] It is unknown, however, whether the injury is primary or secondary to damage to an adjacent cell. Using EM, the changes seen are cytoplasmic swelling and vacuolization, frank cellular necrosis and increased apoptosis. Deposits of granular necrotic debris are present, particularly above the basement membrane zone over the upper pole of the DP.[83] Another indication of keratinocyte damage is the aberrant expression of DR antigens. Aberrant DR expression is localized to the precortical matrix and presumptive cortex,[70,76] which are the sites of keratinocyte damage seen by EM. DR antigen expression is only seen in the presence of intrabulbar lymphocytic infiltrates, suggesting these cells are responsible for keratinocyte destruction.

Several observations suggest that melanocytes are targets of autoimmune responses in alopecia areata. Firstly, there is relative sparing of white, depigmented hairs in alopecia areata. Clinically this is seen by the phenomenon of rapid 'whitening' or 'graying' of hair of affected individuals.[87] The phenomenon indicates that those HFs that contain melanocytes and are able to produce a pigmented hair are preferentially attacked in alopecia areata. Secondly, hair bulb melanocytes are damaged in alopecia areata, as seen by the presence of melanophages around involved hair bulbs and within the cortical matrix (see Figure 1), and these may be the first cells in hair bulb to be attacked by infiltrating macrophages.[3,27,67,84] Others, however, report that melanocyte degeneration occurs only in the vicinity of necrotic keratinocytes, which they feel are primarily involved.[85] These differences may reflect the phase of the illness studied and the fact that melanocytes are more sensitive to injury than keratinocytes. Further evidence for selective damage to melanocytes is that regrowing hairs are often depigmented, and that using EM there is a decreased number and functional activity of melanocytes[86] at a stage where HFs have regained their capacity to make hair. There is a correlation between melanocyte activity in hair bulbs, which peaks during an early phase of anagen (III/IV), and the point where injury to HFs is believed to occur in alopecia areata.[26]

Melanocytes in locations other than hair are damaged in alopecia areata. This is particularly evident in the eye.[43] Galbraith and associates reported that antibodies to melanoma cells could be detected in alopecia areata patients by indirect immunofluorescence and western blotting.[60] Others, using a different technique and epidermal melanocytes did not find surface-reactive pigment cell antibodies in alopecia areata. However, antibodies to cytoplasmic antigens have been detected in cultured HF melanocytes.[50] Clearly these observations, which suggest that some alopecia areata patients have antibodies to distinctive pigment cell surface antigens, need to be explored further.

Endothelial cell involvement in alopecia areata is suggested by two observations, both in need of confirmation. Histologically, there is evidence that a perivascular infiltrate and endothelial cell damage are early events in alopecia areata, whereas infiltration of the hair bulb is reportedly sparse and seen in later phases of alopecia areata.[67] Antibodies to endothelial cells in alopecia areata have been reported in one study.[59]

Proposed mechanisms of immune injury in alopecia areata

The available data suggests, but does not prove, that alopecia areata is an autoimmune disease. Attempts to demonstrate specific T-cell responses to HF antigens have so far been unsuccessful or unconfirmed. The following hypothesis is proposed to link the various immunological abnormalities that have been observed to date. alopecia areata could result from an autoimmune response, involving both antibody and T cells, that is directed to self-antigens in keratinocytes and/or melanocytes in hair bulbs. The induction of such autoimmune responses would be facilitated by a decrease in suppressor T cells and in the T_h/T_s ratio in the circulation, and by an aberrant expression of Langerhans' cells and MHC class I antigens in the matrix and cortex of hair bulbs. The resulting immune responses would result in the deposition of Ig and complement around hair bulbs and in the infiltration of hair bulbs with immune cells. The increased expression of class I MHC on hair bulb cells would allow these cells to be attacked more easily by cytolytic T cells. The resulting immune injury would lead, when severe, to histologic evidence of cell death. When mild, it would result in expression of MHC class II antigens on damaged cells and switch off further maturation of HF cells, thus throwing the HF into catagen, leading to clinical hair loss. Inherent in this hypothesis is that antigenic properties of keratinocytes or melanocytes in hair differ qualitatively and/or quantitatively from similar cells in other locations in the epidermis and so may account for their selective destruction. This is supported by the expression of unique antigens in HF that are not detectable in similarly prepared extracts of epidermis or dermis (Figure 2).[88] Since alopecia areata affects preferentially matrix cells during the surge of mitotic activity associated with anagen III and IV, which is a phase associated with both the beginning of differentiation of cortical keratinocytes and the functional activation of melanocytes, it is possible that the relevant antigens are differentiation antigens[50] of keratinocytes or melanocytes. The observation that the abnormal deposits of immunoglobulin present around HFs are related to the hair cycle and that similar deposits are present in male pattern alopecia suggests the intriguing hypothesis that immune factors are involved in regulating the normal hair cycle by triggering entry into catagen.

Conclusion

The observations discussed in this chapter clearly demonstrate that an abnormal HF-specific immune response is associated with alopecia areata in humans and animals. The presence of tissue-specific autoantigens in HF, and of an abnormal antibody response to some of these antigens in alopecia areata, provides the underlying framework necessary to explain the selective damage to HF that occurs in alopecia areata. However, whether or not anti-HF antibodies or anti-HF T-cell clones have pathogenic potential still needs to be proven. Even if antibodies to HF are not a primary agent in the disease, their subsequent production could further damage or maintain HF pathology. The increasing sophistication of T-cell studies in alopecia areata research promises to define more clearly the involvement of these immunocytes in the pathogenesis of alopecia areata.

References

1. Safavi KH, Muller SA, Suman VJ, et al.: Incidence of alopecia areata in Olmsted County, Minnesota, 1975–1989. *Mayo Clin Proc* 1995; **70**: 628–633.
2. McElwee KJ, Boggess D, Olivry T, et al.: Comparison of alopecia areata in human and non-human mammalian species. *Pathobiol* 1998; **66**: 90–107.
3. Tobin JD: Morphological analysis of hair follicles in alopecia areata. *Microsc Res Tech* 1997; **38**: 443–451.
4. McElwee KJ, Tobin DJ, Bystryn J-C, et al.: Alopecia areata: an autoimmune disease? *Exp Dermatol* (In press).
5. Tobin DJ, Bystryn J-C: Immunity to hair follicles in alopecia areata. *J Invest Dermatol* 1995; **104**: 13s–14s.
6. Paus R: Immunology of the hair follicle. In: Bos JD

(ed.). *Skin Immune System*, 2nd edn. Boca Raton, CRC Press, 1997: 377–398.
7. Van Scott, EJ: Morphologic changes in philosebaceous units and anagen hairs in alopecia areata. *J Invest Dermatol* 1958; **31**: 35–45.
8. Rose NR: Characteristics of autoimmune disease. *J Invest Dermatol* 1991; **96**: 87S.
9. Fichtellius KE, Groth O, Lidén S: The skin, a first level lymphoid organ? *Int Arch Allergy Appl Immunol* 1970; **37**: 607–620.
10. Parakkal PF: Role of macrophages in collagen resorption during hair growth cycle. *J Ultrastruct Res* 1969: 29210–29217.
11. Paul R, Maurer M, Slominski A, Czarnetzki B: Mast cell involvement in murine hair growth. *Dev Biol* 1994; **163**: 230–240.
12. Wilson CL, Dean D, Wojnarowaska F: Pemphigus and the terminal hair follicle. *J Cutan Pathol* 1991; **18**: 428–431.
13. Westgate GE, Craggs RI, Gibson WT: Immune privilege and hair growth. *J Invest Dermatol* 1991; **97**: 417–420.
14. Harrist TJ, Ruiter DJ, Mihm MC, Bahn AK: Distribution of major histocompatibility antigens in normal skin. *Br J Dermatol* 1983; **109**: 623–633.
15. Jimbow K, Sato S, Kukita A: Langerhans' cells of the normal human pilosebaceous system. An electron microscopic investigation. *J Invest Dermatol* 1969; **52**: 177–180.
16. Paus R, van der Veen C, Echmuller S, et al.: Generation and cyclic remodeling of the hair follicle immune system in mice. *J Invest Dermatol* 1998; **111**: 7–18.
17. Tobin DJ: A possible role for Langerhans' cells in the removal of melanin from early catagen hair follicle. *Br J Dermatol* 1998; **138**: 795–798.
18. Kukita A, Sato S, Jimbow K: The electron microscopic study on dendritic cells in the hair matrix of human white and gray hair. *Jap J Derm Ser B* 1977; **81**: 777–787.
19. Tobin DJ, Cargnello J: Partial reversal of canities in a twenty-two year old Chinese male. *Arch Dermatol* 1992; **129**: 789–791.
20. Wiesner-Menzel L, Happle R: Intrabulbar and peribulbar accumulation of dendritic OKT 6-positive cells in alopecia areata. *Arch Dermatol Res* 1984; **276**: 333–334.
21. Paus R, Hofmann U, Eichmuller S, Czarnetzi BM: Distribution and changing density of γδ T cells in murine skin during the induced hair cycle. *Br J Dermatol* 1994; **130**: 281–289.
22. Christoph T, Audring H, Tobin DJ, et al.: Characteristics of the human hair follicle immune system. (Submitted for publication).
23. Paus R, Eichmüller S, Hofmann U, Czarnetzki BM, Robinson P: Expression of classical and non-

classical MHC class I antigens in murine hair follicles. *Br J Dermatol* 1994; **131**: 177–183.

24. Billingham RE, Silvers WK: A biologist's reflections on dermatology. *J Invest Dermatol* 1971; **57**: 227–240.

25. Cui J, Shen LY, Wang GC: Role of hair follicles in the repigmentation of vitiligo. *J Invest Dermatol* 1991; **97**: 410–416.

26. Paus R, Slominski A, Czarnetzki BM: Alopecia areata: an autoimmune-response against melanogenesis-related proteins, exposed by abnormal MHC class I-expression in the proximal anagen hair bulb? *Yale J Biol Med* 1994; **66**: 541–554.

27. Tobin DJ, Fenton DA, Kendall MD: Ultrastructural observations on the hair bulb melanocytes and melanosomes in acute alopecia areata. *J Invest Dermatol* 1990; **94**: 803–807.

28. Asahina A, Hosoi J, Murphy GF, Granstein RD: Calcitonin gene-related peptide modulates Langerhans' cell antigen-presenting function. *Proc Assoc Am Physicians* 1995; **107**: 242–244.

29. Hofmann U, Tokura Y, Takigawa T, Paus R: Hair cycle-dependent changes in skin immune function: anagen associated depression of sensitization for contact sensitivity in mice. *J Invest Dermatol* 1996; **106**: 598–604.

30. Frentz G, Thomsen K, Jakobsen BK, Svejgaard A: HLA-DR4 in alopecia areata. *J Am Acad Dermatol* 1986; **14**: 129–130.

31. Duvic M, Hordinsky MK, Fiedler VC, et al.: HLA-D locus associations in alopecia areata. DRw52a may confer disease resistance. *Arch Dermatol* 1991; **127**: 64–68.

32. Colombe BW, Price VH, Khoury EL, et al.: HLA class II antigen associations help to define two types of alopecia areata. *J Am Acad Dermatol* 1995; **33**: 757–764.

33. Cork MJ, Tarlow JK, Clay FE, et al.: An allele of the interleukin-1 receptor antagonist as a genetic severity factor in alopecia areata. *J Invest Dermatol* 1995; **104**: 15s–16s.

34. Chang DM: Interleukin-1 and interleukin-1 receptor antagonist in systemic lupus erythematosus. *Immunol Invest* 1997; **26**: 649–659.

35. De Weert J, Temmermann L, Kint A: Alopecia areata: a clinical study. *Dermatologica* 1984; **168**: 224–229.

36. Du Vivier A, Munro DD: Alopecia areata, autoimmunity and Down's syndrome. *Br Med J* 1975; **1**: 191–192.

37. Korkij W, Soltani K, Simjee S, et al.: Tissue specific autoantibodies and autoimmune disorders in vitiligo and alopecia areata: a retrospective study. *J Cutan Pathol* 1984; **11**: 522–530.

38. Wang SJ, Shohat T, Vadheim C, et al.: Increased risk for type I (insulin-dependent) diabetes in relatives of patients with alopecia areata (alopecia areata). *Am J Med Genet* 1994; **1**: 234–239.

39. Thompson DM: Alopecia areata, vitiligo, scleroderma and ulcerative colitis. *Proc R Soc Med* 1974; **67**: 48–50.

40. Schallreuter KU, Lemke R, Brandt O, et al.: Vitiligo and other diseases: coexistence or true association? Hamburg study on 321 patients. *Dermatology* 1994; **188**: 269–275.

41. Schallreuter KU, Blau N: GTP-cyclohydrolase and vitiligo. *Lancet* 1997; **25(350)**: 1254.

42. Horn RJ, Odom RB: Twenty nail dystrophy of alopecia areata. *Arch Dermatol* 1980; **116**: 573–574.

43. Tosti A, Colombati S, Caponeri GM, et al.: Ocular abnormalities occurring with alopecia areata. *Dermatologica* 1985; **170**: 69–73.

44. Friedmann PS: Alopecia areata and autoimmunity. *Br J Dermatol* 1981; **105**: 153–157.

45. Tobin DJ, Orentreich N, Fenton DA, Bystryn J-C: Antibodies to hair follicles in alopecia areata. *J Invest Dermatol* 1994; **102**: 721–724.

46. Tobin DJ, Sundberg JP, King LE, Boggess D, Bystryn JC: Autoantibodies to hair follicles in C3H/HeJ mouse model of alopecia areata. *J Invest Dermatol* 1997; **109(3)**: 329–333.

47. Tobin DJ, Hann SK, Song MS, Bystryn J-C: Hair follicle structures targeted by antibodies in alopecia areata. *Arch Dermatol* 1997; **133**: 57–61.

48. Tobin DJ, Olivry T, Bystryn J-C: Autoantibodies to trichohyalin in canine alopecia areata. *Adv Vet Dermatol* 1998; **3**: 355–362.

49. Tobin DJ, Alhaidari Z, Olivry T: Equine alopecia areata autoantibodies target multiple hair follicle antigens and may alter hair growth in passive transfer studies. *Exper Dermatol* 1998; **7**: 289–297.

50. Tobin DJ, Bystryn J-C: Alopecia areata is associated with antibodies to hair follicle-specific antigens located predominantly in the proliferative region of hair follicles. In: Neste DJJ, Randall VA (eds.). *Hair Research for the Next Millennium.* Amsterdam, Elsevier Science, 1996: 237–241.

51. Bystryn J-C, Tobin DJ: Alopecia areata is associated with antibodies to hair follicle melanocytes. *J Invest Dermatol* 1994; **102(4)**: 532.

52. Cohen IR, Cooke A: Natural autoantibodies might prevent autoimmune disease. *Immunol Today* 1986; **4**: 337–342.

53. Lynch MH, O'Guin WM, Hardy C, Mak L, Sun TT: Acidic and basic hair/nail ('hard') keratins: their co-localization in upper cortical and cuticle cells of the human hair follicles and their relationship to 'soft' keratins. *J Cell Biol* 1986; **103**: 2593–2606.

54. McElwee KJ, Pickett P, Oliver RF: The DEBR rat, alopecia areata and autoantibodies to the hair follicle. *Br J Dermatol* 1996; **134**: 55–63.

55. Gilhar A, Pillar T, Assay B, David M: Failure of

passive transfer of serum from patients with alopecia areata and alopecia universalis to inhibit hair growth in transplants of human scalp skin grafted on to nude mice. *Br J Dermatol* 1992; **126**: 166–171.

56. Bystryn J-C, Orentreich N, Stengel F: Direct immunofluorescence studies in alopecia areata and male pattern alopecia. *J Invest Dermatol* 1970; **73**: 317–320.

57. Igarashi R, Takeuchi S, Sato Y: Immunofluorescent studies of complement C3 in the hair follicles of normal scalp and scalp affected by alopecia areata. *Acta Dermatol Venereol* 1980; **60**: 33–37.

58. Igarashi R, Morohashi M, Takeuchi S, Sato Y: Immunofluorescence studies on complement components in the hair follicles of normal scalp and of scalp affected by alopecia areata. *Acta Dermatol Venereol (Stockholm)* 1981; **61**: 131–135.

59. Nunzi E, Hamerlinck F, Cormane RH: Immunopathological studies on Alopecia areata. *Arch Dermatol Res* 1980; **269**: 1–11.

60. Galbraith GMP, Miller D, Emerson DL: Western blot analysis of serum antibody reactivity with human melanoma cell antigens in alopecia areata and vitiligo. *Clin Immunol Immunopathol* 1988; **48**: 317–324.

61. Galbraith GMP, Thiers BH, Vasily DB, Fudenberg HH: Immunological profiles in alopecia areata. *Br J Dermatol* 1984; **110**: 163–170.

62. Baadsgaard O, Lindskov R: Circulating lymphocyte subsets in patients with alopecia areata. *Acta Dermatol Venereol (Stockholm)* 1986; **66**: 266–268.

63. Ledesma GN, York KK: Suppressor cell decrease in alopecia areata. *Arch Dermatol Res* 1982; **274**: 1–8.

64. Gu SQ, Petrini B, Ros AM, Thyresson N, Wasserman J: T lymphocyte subpopulations in alopecia areata and psoriasis: identification with monoclonal antibodies and Fc receptors. *Acta Derm Venereol* 1983; **63**: 244.

65. Majewski BBJ, Kohls MS, Taylor DR, et al.: Increased ratio of helper to suppressor T cells in alopecia areata. *Br J Dermatol* 1984; **110**: 171–175.

66. Orecchia G, Capelli E, Martinetti M, Cuccia Belvedere M, Rabbiosi G: Decreased in vitro lymphocyte stimulation and reduced sensitivity to IL-2 patients with alopecia areata. *Arch Dermatol Res* 1988; **280**: 47s–50s.

67. Peereboom-Wynia JD, van Joost T, Stolz E, Prins M: Markers of immunologic injury in progressive alopecia areata. *J Cut Pathol* 1986; **13**: 363–369.

68. Ranki A, Kianto U, Kanerva L, Tolvanen E, Johansson E: Immunohistochemical and electron microscopic characterization of the cellular infiltrate in alopecia areata, totalis and universalis. *J Invest Dermatol* 1984; **83**: 7–11.

69. Wiesner-Menzel L, Happle R: Intrabulbar and peribulbar accumulation of dendritic OKT6-positive cells in alopecia areata. *Arch Dermatol Res* 1984; **276**: 333–334.

70. Khoury EL, Price VH, Greenspan JS: HLA-DR expression by hair follicle keratinocytes in alopecia areata: evidence that it is secondary to the lymphoid infiltration. *J Invest Dermatol* 1988; **90**: 193–200.

71. Baadsgaard O, Lindskov R, Clemmensen OJ: In situ lymphocyte subsets in alopecia areata before and during treatment with a contact allergen. *Clin Exp Dermatol* 1987; **12**: 260–264.

72. Bos J, Zonneveld I, Das P, et al.: The skin immune system (SIS): distribution and immunophenotype of lymphocyte subpopulations in normal human skin. *J Invest Dermatol* 1987; **88**: 569–573.

73. Perret CM, Steijlen PM, Happle R: Alopecia areata. Pathogenesis and topical immunotherapy. *Int J Dermatol* 1990; **29**: 83–88.

74. Gilhar A, Ulmann Y, Berkutzki T, Assy B, Kalish RS: Autoimmune hair loss (alopecia areata) transferred by T lymphocytes to human scalp explants on SCID mice. *J Clin Invest* 1998; **101**: 62–67.

75. McElwee KJ, Boggess D, King LE Jr, Sundberg JP: Experimental induction of alopecia areata-like hair loss in C3/H/HeJ mice using full-thickness skin grafts. *J Invest Dermatol* 1998; **111**: 797–803.

76. Messenger A, Bleehen S: Expression of HLA-DR by anagen hair follicles in alopecia areata. *J Invest Dermatol* 1985; **85**: 569–572.

77. Volc-Platzer B, Leibl H, Luger T, et al.: Human epidermal cells synthesize HLA-DR alloantigens in vitro upon stimulation with gamma-interferon. *J Invest Dermatol* 1985; **85**: 16–19.

78. Kohchiyama A, Hatamochi A, Ueki H: Increased number of OKT-6-positive dendritic cells in the hair follicles of patients with alopecia areata. *Dermatologica* 1985; **171**: 327–331.

79. Abere W, Stingl G, Pogantich: Effects of glucocorticosteroids on epidermal cell induced immune responses. *J Immunol* 1984; **133**: 792–797.

80. Aprile J, Deeg HJ: Ultraviolet irradiation of canine dendritic cells prevents mitogen-induced cluster formation and lymphocyte proliferation. *Transplantation* 1986; **42**: 653–660.

81. Anderson R, Lukey PT, Dippenaar U, Eftychis HA: Dithranol mediates pro-oxidative inhibition of polymorphonuclear leukocyte migration and lymphocyte proliferation. *Br J Dermatol* 1987; **117**: 405–418.

82. Okamoto H, Takigawa M, Horio T: Alteration of lymphocyte function by 8-methoxypsoralen and long-wave ultraviolet radiation. I. Suppressive effects of PUVA on T-lymphocyte migration in vitro. *J Invest Dermatol* 1985; **84**: 203–205.

83. Havele C, Paetkau V: Cyclosporin blocks the action of antigen-dependent cytotoxic T lymphocytes

directly by an IL-2 independent mechanism. *J Immunol* 1988; **140**: 3303–3308.

84. Tobin DJ, Fenton DA, Kendall MD: Cell degeneration in alopecia areata: An ultrastructural study. *Am J Dermatopathol* 1991; **13(3)**: 248–256.

85. Messenger A, Slater D, Bleehen S: Alopecia areata: alterations in the hair growth cycle and correlation with the follicular pathology. *Br J Dermatol* 1986; **114**: 337–347.

86. Messenger AG, Bleehen SS: Alopecia areata: light and electron microscopic pathology of the regrowing white hair. *Br J Dermatol* 1984; **110**: 155–162.

87. Guin JD, Kumar V, Petersen BH: Immunofluorescence findings in rapid whitening of scalp hair. *Arch Dermatol* 1981; **117**: 576–578.

88. Tobin DJ, Orentreich N, Bystryn J-C: Antibodies to hair follicles in normal individuals. *Arch Dermatol* 1994; **130**: 395–396.

17
Cytokines in alopecia areata

Rolf Hoffmann

Introduction

Alopecia areata is a common type of hair loss with a lifetime risk of 1.7% in the general population[1] (US study). In clinical practice, most patients will present with reversible patchy hair loss, whereas others may develop complete baldness (alopecia areata totalis). Histopathological features of alopecia areata in humans include perifollicular lymphocytic infiltrates involving only anagen hair follicles, with subsequent miniaturization of the affected hair follicles.[2] Several animal species have been reported to develop hair loss resembling human alopecia areata, including dogs, cats, horses, rodents, and non-human primates.[3–5] In the larger species, however, alopecia areata is poorly characterized, the animals are outbred, and they are not readily available for study, which makes them of little practical use as research models. A reversible type of hair loss closely resembling human alopecia areata has been described in C3H/HeJ mice.[6] Hair loss in these mice is treatable either by steroids or, surprisingly, by allergic contact dermatitis (see later text). Microscopically, affected mice develop non-scarring alopecia with dystrophic anagen hair follicles surrounded by a mononuclear cell infiltrate with a predominance of $CD8^+$ lymphocytes and rather small numbers of $CD4^+$ T cells. Telogen hair follicles are not affected. Recently, circulating autoantibodies to hair follicle antigens, similar to those present in human patients with alopecia areata, have been found in C3H/HeJ mice with alopecia areata.[7,8]

Although the cause of alopecia areata is unknown at present, we are now able to define two common elements of all alopecia areata occurring in all mammalian species. These are: (1) the lymphocytic attack to the lower part of the anagen hair follicle; and (2) the ectopic expression of MHC class I[9,10] and class II[11] molecules on the epithelium of affected hair follicles, suggesting the local release of cytokines. Hence, two key pathogenetic factors leading to hair loss in alopecia areata can be discriminated in the form of cytokines and T cells. This review summarizes recent results obtained in different fields of research, and analyzes the data in view of the role of the pathogenesis of cytokines in alopecia areata.

Several clinical and experimental data point towards cytokines such as interleukin-1 (IL-1) as being crucial inducers of hair loss in alopecia areata. Cytokines play an important role in both physiology and pathophysiology of human skin, and it is possible that they co-ordinate the cyclical hair growth. In line with this concept, cytokine gene expression has been reported in anagen rat hair follicles and a crucial role for hair cycling has been proposed.[12] Here, the author summarizes recent results obtained in different fields of research that suggest that cytokines might be common mediators leading to reversible hair loss in alopecia areata and possibly in a variety of other inflammatory conditions affecting the scalp.

Cytokines are overexpressed in alopecia areata skin

The earliest clinical sign of alopecia areata is patchy hair loss, which is, in most cases, self-limited and reversible. The disease might progress, eventually leading to total loss of scalp and body hair but, even in such an event, a complete hair regrowth is still possible. Histologically the hair bulb is infiltrated and surrounded by mainly T helper cells. These lymphocytes do not destroy the hair follicle but rather initiate a 'switch off' mechanism of the hair cycle. This inhibitory effect persists as long as the lymphcytic infiltrate is present. Symptomatic treatment with immunosuppressive drugs such as cyclosporin A[13] or corticosteroids tends to diminish the lymphocytic infiltrate, and hair regrowth occurs. Several groups have detected, both at the protein,[14] and mRNA level, cytokines in skin biopsies from patients with alopecia areata. A consistent feature was the presence of cytokine of the Th1-type (IFN-γ, IL-2) and IL-1β.[15,16]

Cytokines inhibit hair growth in vitro

Since cytokines, such as IL-1β, have been found in the early stages of alopecia areata, it is conceivable to assume that they negatively influence hair growth. Single hair follicle cultures have been used to investigate the effect of various substances, including cytokines, on hair growth in vitro (see chapter 8 by Philpott).[17–20] The most potent inhibitors of hair shaft elongation so far investigated are IL-1α and IL-1β. Both cytokines are equally effective, and the inhibitory effect is completely abrogated by a 1000-fold molar excess of the IL-1 receptor antagonist, which is a natural antagonist of the interleukin-1 action, or by inhibitors of the cAMP pathway.[19]

Ultrastructural studies

In alopecia areata, electronmicroscopical examination has revealed initial changes within cells of the dermal papilla and the outer root sheath keratinocytes of affected hair follicles. These morphological changes were defined as a lack of structural organization within the dermal papilla and a marked polymorphism of the dermal papilla cells. The shape of the dermal papilla became more diamond-like.[21] Remarkably, all of these morphological changes observed in vivo can be induced by IL-1β stimulation of single human hair follicles in vitro.[22]

In a depilation-induced hair cycle, IL-1 is overexpressed in catagen

Changes in the local, cytokine-mediated signalling milieu of hair follicles (HF) have been implicated as major elements of hair cycle control, and several lines of clinical and experimental evidence point towards IL-1 as an important inducer of hair loss. To examine whether the steady state mRNA levels of gene expression of the IL-1 family parallel distinct phases of the murine hair cycle, the high degree of synchrony during depilation-induced HF cycling in mice was exploited to analyze the mRNA levels of IL-1α, IL-1β, IL-1-receptor antagonist, IL-1 receptor (R)-1 and IL-1-R-II by semiquantitative RT-PCR.[23] The results indicated that the induced murine hair cycle is associated with profound fluctuations in the steady-state mRNA levels of members of the IL-1 signalling system. Most interestingly, IL-1α and IL-1β transcript levels increased dramatically with the onset of spontaneous catagen (around Day 18) and peaked during telogen (Day 25). These fluctuations in the IL-1α and IL-1β transcript levels were paralleled by substantial expression changes of the corresponding signal transducing type I IL-1 receptor. Therefore, these findings are consistent with the concept that IL-1α, IL-1β, IL-1-RI and IL-1-RII might be involved in the control of catagen development.

Genetic background of alopecia areata

A hereditary component has been identified in patients with alopecia areata. It is most likely a polygenic disease. An increased frequency of autoimmune diseases has been found in patients with alopecia areata, most common associations being thyroid disease and vitiligo. The severity of the inflammatory response in alopecia areata may be determined by an interplay of pro- and anti-inflammatory cytokines. Recently, an increased frequency of the allele 2 of the interleukin-1 (IL-1) receptor antagonist gene was detected in patients with alopecia areata, especially in those with extensive hair loss.[24] Since the IL-1 receptor antagonist is the natural antagonist of IL-1, it has been assumed that patients who cannot secrete sufficient amounts of the IL-1 receptor antagonist, because of the gene polymorphism, may have a more progressive disease. In line with this concept is the recent observation of an additional gene polymorphism for a subtype of the IL-1α gene.[25] Patients with severe alopecia areata tend to have an IL-1 gene polymorphism that causes an exaggerated release of IL-1, which, in turn, may lead to a more progressive disease. A similar scenario has been supposed for TNF-α, because a gene polymorphism for the TNF-α gene has likewise been found in patients with severe alopecia areata as well.[26]

Animal models

The IL-1 family represents one of the most complex systems in cytokine biology. Two genes encode for the agonist molecules (IL-1α and IL-1β), a third gene encodes the IL-1 receptor antagonist, while two additional genes encode for the two types of the IL-1 receptor. As many cells express these five genes in vitro, the outcome of an IL-1 inducible event is therefore rather complex. To study this problem, animal models are needed. Transgenic mice overexpressing IL-1α in the epidermis are smaller in size and show an obvious cutaneous phenotype. Remarkably, these mice have patchy hair loss reminiscent of alopecia areata.[27]

Other diseases associated with hair loss

Patients suffering from T-cell lymphoma, such as the syringolymphoid hyperplasia with alopecia,[28] or other lymphomas, often develop severe but reversible circumscribed hair loss. During the leukemic stage of a cutaneous T-cell lymphoma the patients may become bald; however, hair regrowth starts upon treatment. The pathogenesis of this type of hair loss is unclear but several reports have shown an aberrant cytokine gene expression within both lymph nodes and serum from affected patients.[29,30] A remarkable feature is the overexpression of IL-1 in skin areas where the lymphoma cells enter the epidermis.[31]

Another example of an inflammatory scalp disease with hair loss is seborrhoeic eczema of the scalp.[32] This scalp disease typically induces diffuse hair loss, which is completely reversible upon treatment with topical steroids or ketoconazol. Furthermore, patchy hair loss resulting from syphilis is usually reversible and shows both clinical and histopathological features reminiscent of alopecia areata.[33,34]

Inflammatory scalp diseases may allow hair growth in alopecia areata

In cases where alopecia areata coincides with other inflammatory diseases of the scalp, in some instances there will be hair growth. To describe this striking response that is the opposite to the Köbner reaction, the anagrammatic term Renbök phenomenon has been proposed.[35] Examples of this phenomenon are psoriasis of the scalp and allergic contact dermatitis (ACD). The induction and periodic elicitation of an ACD is currently the most effective mode of treatment.[36] The underlying mechanism is still unexplained, but contrasting cytokine profiles have been found in treated versus untreated bald scalp. An increased expression of interferon-γ, IL-2 and IL-1β was found **before** treatment with the contact sensitizer, whereas IL-10, TNF-α[15] and TGF-β1[37] were the most abundant cytokines present within the scalp **after** treatment. Remarkably, IL-1β was reduced after successful treatment.

Similar to humans treated with the contact sensitizer squaric acid dibutylester (SADBE),[38] the C3H/HeJ mice can be sensitized with 2% SADBE and challenged with individually varying concentrations of the substance and they show clinical features of contact dermatitis for several days.[39] After SADBE treatment, there is a striking reduction of aberrant MHC class I expression on hair follicle keratinocytes in murine alopecia areata and a less conspicuous, but still distinct, reduction of ectopic MHC class II expression. These findings are consistent with the down-modulation of abnormal HLA-ABC and HLA-DR expression as observed in human alopecia areata after treatment with the contact allergen diphenylcyclopropenone (DCP).[9] The pronounced down-regulation of aberrant MHC class I expression can be related to the predominance of CD8+ cells in untreated murine alopecia areata, especially in the center of the inflammatory infiltrate being in direct contact with the hair follicle, as well as the reduced number of CD8+ cells after therapy. This again points towards an important role of a specific interaction between cytotoxic CD8+ T lymphocytes and MHC class I positive hair follicle keratinocytes in the pathogenesis of alopecia areata.

Discussion

Hair growth is a well-orchestrated process in which each hair follicle cycles between periods of active hair production and periods of rest. These cycles involve both epithelial and mesenchymal structures and recent advances have identified a variety of factors that might be encompassed during this process. However, our understanding of mechanisms of hair growth is far from complete. Although the pathogenesis of alopecia areata is still poorly understood, a peri- and intrabulbar accumulation of T lymphocytes[40] and aberrant expression of ICAM-1 and HLA-DR molecules on follicular keratinocytes and dermal papillae[10,41] provide evidence that an immune process is involved,[42] interfering with the hair cycle and leading to reversible hair loss. It is conceivable to assume that CD8+ T cells are of crucial importance in alopecia areata because they are able to recognize MHC-I restricted autoantigens. As a consequence, FAS- or perforin-mediated apoptosis of target cells may occur, thus leading to their destruction in alopecia areata. Hair loss may occur because proinflammatory cytokines such as IL-1 interfere with the hair cycle, leading to premature arrest of hair cycling with cessation of hair growth.[43] This concept may explain typical clinical features of alopecia areata such as a progression pattern in centrifugal waves[44] and spontaneous hair regrowth in concentric rings[45] suggesting the presence of soluble mediators within the affected

areas of the scalp. Further studies should show whether the proposed concept holds true. If so, the application of specific cytokine inhibitors would be a promising approach for the treatment of alopecia areata.

Acknowledgement

This work was supported by a grant (Ho 1598/1-3) from the 'Deutsche Forschungsgemeinschaft (DFG)'.

References

1. Safavi KH, Muller SA, Suman VJ, et al.: Incidence of alopecia areata in Olmsted Country, Minnesota, 1975 through 1989. *Mayo Clin Proc* 1995; **70**: 628–633.
2. Headington JT: The histopathology of alopecia areata. *J Invest Dermatol* 1991; **96(suppl)**: 69S.
3. Conroy JD: Alopecia areata. In: Andrews EJ, Ward BC, Altman NH (eds.). *Spontaneous Animal Models of Human Disease, Vol II*. Academic Press, New York, 1979: 30–31.
4. McElwee KJ, Boggess D, Olivry T, et al.: Comparison of alopecia areata in human and nonhuman mammalian species. *Pathobiol* 1998; **66**: 90–107.
5. Sundberg JP, Oliver RF, McElwee KF, King LE Jr: Alopecia areata in humans and other mammalian species. *J Invest Dermatol* 1995; **104(suppl)**: 32S–33S.
6. Sundberg JP, Cordy WR, King L: Alopecia areata in aging C3H/HeJ mice. *J Invest Dermatol* 1994; **102**: 847–856.
7. Tobin DJ, Orentreich N, Fenton DA, Bystryn JC: Antibodies to hair follicles in alopecia areata. *J Invest Dermatol* 1994; **102**: 721–724.
8. Tobin DJ, Sundberg JP, King LE, et al.: Autoantibodies to hair follicles in C3H/HeJ mice with alopecia areata-like hair loss. *J Invest Dermatol* 1997; **109**: 329–333.
9. Bröcker EB, Echternacht-Happle K, Hamm H, Happle R: Abnormal expression of class I and class II major histocompatibility antigens in alopecia areata: modulation by topical immunotherapy. *J Invest Dermatol* 1987; **88**: 564–568.
10. Hamm H, Klemmer S, Kreuzer I, et al.: HLA-DR and HLA-DQ antigen expression of anagen and telogen hair bulbs in long-standing alopecia areata. *Arch Dermatol Res* 1988; **280**: 179–181.
11. Khoury EL, Price VH, Greenspan BDS: HLA-DR

expression by hair follicle keratinocytes in alopecia areata: Evidence that it is secondary to the lymphoid infiltration. *J Invest Dermatol* 1988; **90**: 193–200.

12. Little JC, Westgate GE, Evans A, Granger SP: Cytokine gene expression in intact anagen rat hair follicles. *J Invest Dermatol* 1994; **103**: 715–720.

13. Gupta AK, Ellis CN, Cooper KD, et al.: Oral cyclosporine for the treatment of alopecia areata. *J Am Acad Dermatol* 1990; **22**: 242–250.

14. Gollnick H, Orfanos CE: Alopecia areata: Pathogenesis and clinical picture. In: Orfanos CE, Happle R (eds.). *Hair and Hair Diseases* Berlin, Springer-Verlag, 1990: 529–569.

15. Hoffmann R, Wenzel E, Huth A, et al.: Cytokine mRNA levels in alopecia areata before and after treatment with the contact allergen diphenylcyclopropenone. *J Invest Dermatol* 1994; **103**: 530–533.

16. Hoffmann R: Significance of cytokine patterns in alopecia areata and allergic contact dermatitis. *J Invest Dermatol* 1995; **136**: 279–280.

17. Harmon CS, Nevis TD: IL-1α inhibits human hair follicle growth and hair fiber production in whole-organ cultures. *Lymphokine Cytokine Res* 1993; **12**: 197–203.

18. Hoffmann R, Eicheler W, Huth A, et al.: Cytokines and growth factors influence hair growth in vitro: possible implications for the pathogenesis and treatment of alopecia areata. *Arch Dermatol Res* 1996; **288**: 153–156.

19. Hoffmann R, Eicheler W, Wenzel E, Happle R: IL-1β-induced inhibition of hair growth *in vitro* is mediated by cAMP. *J Invest Dermatol* 1997; **108**: 40–42.

20. Philpott MP, Sanders DA, Bowen J, Kealey T: Effects of interleukins, colony-stimulating factor and tumour necrosis factor on human hair follicle growth *in vitro*: A possible role for interleukin-1 and tumour necrosis factor-alpha in alopecia areata. *Br J Dermatol* 1996; **135**: 942–948.

21. Hull S, Nutbrown M, Pepall L, et al.: Immunohistologic and ultrastructural comparison of the dermal papilla and hair follicle bulb from 'active' and 'normal' areas of alopecia areata. *J Invest Dermatol* 1991; **96**: 673–681.

22. Philpott MP, Sanders D, Kealey T: Cultured human hair follicles and growth factors. *J Invest Dermatol* 1995; **104**: 44S–45S.

23. Hoffmann R, Happle R, Paus R: Elements of the IL-1 signalling system show hair cycle-dependent gene expression in murine skin. *Eur J Dermatol* 1998; **8**: 475–477.

24. Tarlow JK, Clay FE, Cork MJ, et al.: Severity of alopecia areata is associated with a polymorphism in the interleukin-1 receptor antagonist gene. *J Invest Dermatol* 1994; **103**: 387–390.

25. Cork MJ, Ahnini RT, Britton J, et al.: Interleukin one composite genotypes as determinants for

subtypes of alopecia areata. Third International Research Workshop on Alopecia areata, November 5, 1998, Washington. *J Invest Dermatol* 1999. In press.

26. Galbraith GM, Pandey JP: Tumor necrosis factor alpha (TNF-alpha) gene polymorphism in alopecia areata. *Hum Genet* 1995; **96**: 433–436.

27. Groves RW, Williams IR, Sarkar S, et al.: Analysis of epidermal IL-1 family members *in vivo* using transgenic mouse models. *J Invest Dermatol* 1994; **102**: 556.

28. Esche C, Sander CA, Zumdick M, et al.: Further evidence that syringolymphoid hyperplasia with alopecia is a cutaneous T-cell lymphoma. *Arch Dermatol* 1998; **34**: 753–754.

29. Merz H, Fliedner A, Orscheschek K, et al.: Cytokine expression in T-cell lymphomas and Hodgkin's disease. *Am J Pathol* 1991; **139**: 1173–1180.

30. Hsu SM, Waldron JW, Hsu PL, Hough AJ: Cytokines in malignant lymphomas: review and prospective evaluation. *Hum Pathol* 1993; **24**: 1040–1057.

31. Tron VA, Rosenthal D, Saunder DN: Epidermal interleukin-1 is increased in cutaneous T-cell lymphoma. *J Invest Dermatol* 1988; **90**: 378–381.

32. Orfanos CE, Frost PH: Seborrheic dermatitis, scalp psoriasis and hair. In: Orfanos CE, Happle R (eds.). *Hair and Hair Diseases.* Berlin, Springer-Verlag, 1990: 643–661.

33. Lee JY, Hsu ML: Alopecia syphilitica, a simulator of alopecia areata: histopathology and differential diagnosis. *J Cutan Pathol* 1991; **18**: 87–92.

34. Cuozzo DW, Benson PM, Sperling LC, Skelton HG 3rd: Essential syphilitic alopecia revisited. *J Am Acad Dermatol* 1995; **32**: 840-843.

35. Happle R, van der Steen P, Perret C: The Renbök phenomenon: an inverse Köbner reaction observed in alopecia areata. *Eur J Dermatol* 1991; **1**: 228–230.

36. Hoffmann R, Happle R: Topical immunotherapy in alopecia areata: What, how, and why? *Dermatol Clin* 1996; **14**: 739–744.

37. Hoffmann R, Wenzel E, Huth A, et al.: Growth factor mRNA-levels in alopecia areata before and after treatment with the contact allergen diphenyl-cyclopropenone. *Acta Derm Venereol (Stockh)* 1996; **76**: 17–20.

38. Happle R, Kalveram KJ, Büchner U, et al.: Contact allergy as a therapeutic tool for alopecia areata: application of squaric acid dibutylester. *Dermatologica* 1980; **161**: 289–297.

39. Freyschmidt-Paul P, Sundberg JP, Boggess D, et al.: Successful topical immunotherapy of alopecia areata-like hair loss in C3H/HeJ mice. *J Invest Dermatol* 1998; **110**: 659.

40. Perret C, Wiesner-Menzel L, Happle R: Immunohistochemical analysis of T-cell subsets in the peribul-

bar and intrabulbar infiltrates of alopecia areata. *Acta Derm Venereol (Stockh)* 1984; **64**: 26–30.

41. Nickoloff BJ, Griffiths CEM: Aberrant intercellular adhesion molecule-1 (ICAM-1) expression by hair-follicle epithelial cells and endothelial leukocyte adhesion molecule-1 (ELAM-1) by vascular cells are important adhesion-molecule alterations in alopecia areata. *J Invest Dermatol* 1991; **96**: 91S–92S.

42. Baadsgaard O: Alopecia areata: an immunologic disease? *J Invest Dermatol* 1991; **96**: 89S.

43. Hoffmann R, Happle R: Does interleukin-1 induce hair loss in vivo? *Dermatol* 1995; **191**: 273–275.

44. Eckert J, Church RE, Ebling FJ: The pathogenesis of alopecia areata. *Br J Dermatol* 1968; **80**: 203–210.

45. Rio E del: Targetoid hair regrowth in alopecia areata: the wave theory. *Arch Dermatol* 1998; **134**: 142.

18

Clinical and basic science approaches to the treatment of alopecia areata: anagen induction by contact hypersensitivity in humans and C3H mice

Kensei Katsuoka

with the collaboration of Hiromi Tsuboi, Shiro Niiyama, Takao Fujimura and Yukinori Ohta

Introduction

Since alopecia areata may be a T-cell-mediated disease or autoimmune disease,[1-3] many efforts have been made to elucidate the role of infiltrating T-lymphocytes.[4-6] In clinical practice there are many treatment options for this disease. Very severe cases can be treated by topical application of a contact allergen which is expected to bring about an immunomodulatory effect.[7-11] This treatment is effective, but many aspects regarding the working mechanism for induction of hair regrowth have still to be clarified. Therefore, to uncover the mechanism of anagen induction by contact hypersensitivity (CHS), we performed some studies on human and mice materials.

Study 1: Human hair regrowth using contact hypersensitivity (SADBE)

Human hair regrowth after squaric acid dibutylester (SADBE) treatment is observed in alopecia areata (Figure 1). Some of the materials used in this experiment were biopsy specimens before and after treatment. The patient profile is shown in Table 1—all four patients had alopecia

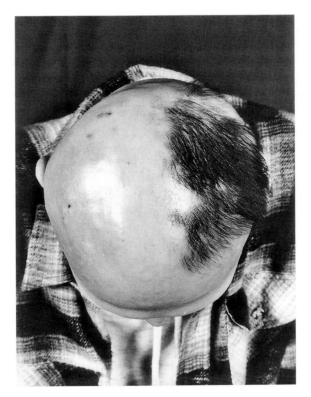

Figure 1

Hair regrowth in a patient with alopecia areata after SADBE treatment.

Table 1 Patient details. All four patients had successfully-induced hair growth following SADBE treatment.

Patient	Age	Sex	Clinical type of alopecia	Duration of disease (years)	Hair growth	Length of treatment (months)
1	47	Male	Alopecia universalis	9	Hair regrowth	1
2	20	Male	Alopecia universalis	16	Hair regrowth	1
3	19	Female	Alopecia universalis	10	Hair regrowth	1
4	14	Male	Alopecia universalis	5	Hair regrowth	1

universalis, with a duration of disease between 5 and 16 years (mean 10 years). All patients had successfully induced hair growth after SADBE treatment. Using specimens from these patients, we first evaluated the surface marker of expected infiltrating cells immuno-histochemically.

Histological and immunohistochemical findings

Approximately 1 month after SADBE treatment, anagen hair was induced. Dense infiltration of lymphocytes was noted in the upper dermis, especially around the hair follicles during hair growth induction (Figure 2). Immunohistochemistry revealed that the majority of infiltrating cells were CD3$^+$ T-lymphocytes, and that CD4$^+$ T-lymphocytes were relatively predominant.

Amplification of cDNA by reverse transcriptase-polymerase chain reaction

To characterize the infiltrating T-lymphocytes, we investigated the local production of cytokines before and after the application of contact allergen using reverse transcriptase-polymerase chain reaction (RT-PCR) from biopsied specimens.

The results of RT-PCR of the four cases are shown in Figure 3. The odd numbers show the before-treatment values, while the even numbers are those following treatment. In some material, IFN-gamma mRNA expression was weak, but the signal was detectable in all cases; this also after treatment. In contrast, IL-10 mRNA was found in only one of the four cases following treatment.

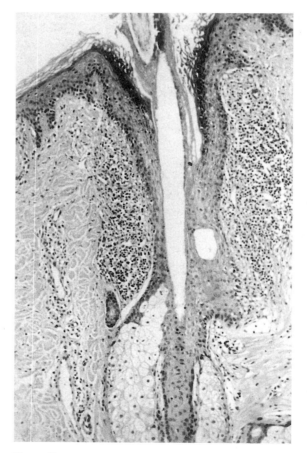

Figure 2

Dense infiltration of lymphocytes is noted around the hair follicles in the process of inducing hair growth in alopecia universalis using SADBE.

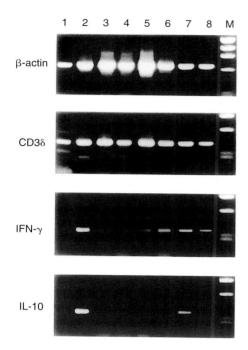

Figure 3

Expression of IFN-gamma and IL-10 mRNAs in skin biopsy specimens. The odd numbers show before-treatment values, the even numbers show after-treatment values. IFN-gamma mRNA was detectable in all cases, including after treatment.

Summary

This study was based on a similar experiment reported by Hoffman et al[6] who found that, before treatment, IFN-gamma mRNA was notably expressed, whereas after treatment IL-10 mRNA was more active, leading to decreased IFN-gamma mRNA expression. This result suggested that the 'Th-1 type of cytokine may exert some effect on the onset of alopecia areata the stage of hair regrowth, while IL-10 production may inhibit Th-1 type cytokine, leading to hair growth'. Regarding these two inflammatory cytokines, our results revealed that the development of IL-10 mRNA had no correlation with that of IFN-r mRNA, and thus we could not obtain any finding that IL-10 suppresses the emergence of

IFN-gamma, stimulating the growth of hairs. However, there were differences in the materials, contact allergens and techniques employed, which does not allow a simple comparison.

Study 2: Anagen induction by contact hypersensitivity in C3H mice

Next, using a mouse model in the telogen stage of the hair cycle, we designed the following experiment on induction of anagen by means of CHS. C3H/HeN mice have waves of hair cycling, and the second telogen phase of C3H mice occurs at 7–13 weeks of age. In this study, we attempted to elucidate the role of T cells in the phase of anagen induction during delayed hypersensitivity reaction using C3H mice whose hair cycle was in the telogen phase.

The C3H/HeN mouse used had a physiological hair cycle, with the second phase of telogen occurring at 7–13 weeks. The use of hair clippers for the removal of hairs did not affect the natural hair growth cycle in these mice. The skin in the telogen stage assumes a pinkish color. Firstly, the back of an 8-week old C3H mouse was shaved with hair clippers. Next, 0.5% dinitrofluorobenzene (DNFB) was applied to both ears of the mouse to sensitize it. After sensitization, 0.2% DNFB was topically applied once a week, three times topically to induce CHS. The control group was treated with the vehicle, acetone/olive oil in this study. Hair growth was observed daily and photographed under uniform conditions.

Three skin samples were obtained from the dorsal skin of the mice on Days 0, 8, 22 and 32.

Hair growth in C3H mice after CHS

After the second DNFB application, clinically distinct dermatitis is observed. Assuming that the day on which sensitization was performed was Day 0, the skin on Day 22 from the start of application presents a greyish color, indicating the start of hair growth. On Day 27 the start of hair growth was observed, and this was more visible on Day 32. None of the mice in the control group had any hair growth during the observation period (Figure 4).

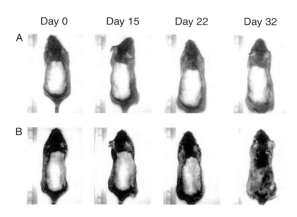

Figure 4

Hair growth stimulated in C3H mice by CHS using DNFB. A, control group; B, treated group. The skin on Day 22 appears a grayish color. Hair growth is recognized distinctly on Day 32.

The expression of IFN-gamma mRNA was increased progressively, peaking on Day 22. IFN-gamma, IL-2, IL-4 and IL-5 mRNA were expressed in none of the samples obtained from the control mice (Figure 5).

Effect of anti-mouse IFN-gamma monoclonal antibody on hair growth

Selected mice were injected with anti-IFN-gamma MoA before each elicitation. CHS reaction and hair growth were suppressed, but not completely by interaperitoneal pre-treatment of anti-mouse IFN-gamma antibody.

Histological findings

The difference in histological findings between the DNFB-applied group and the control group was apparent. In the DNFB-applied group, cell infiltration was observed in the upper dermis, particularly around the hair follicles.

Immunohistochemical findings

The immunohistochemical staining on Day 15 (after the start of application—3 days after the second application) showed the infiltration of CD3+ lymphocytes. CD4+ T-lymphocytes were dominant. CD3+ cells were not observed in the control mice (non-treated mice).

Expression of IFN-gamma and IL-2 mRNAs

We also performed RT-PCR using the mice material. In the DNFB-applied group where the hair growth was observed, the emergence of IFN-gamma mRNA and IL-2 mRNA could be detected on Day 8 (3 days after the first application), but no IL-4 mRNA or IL-5 mRNA, which are thought to be Th-2 type cytokines, were detected.

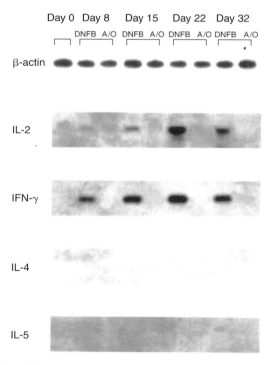

Figure 5

Local production of cytokine mRNA before and after application of DNFB in C3H mice. IFN-gamma mRNA and IL-2 mRNA could be detected in treated mice, but not IL-4 mRNA or IL-5 mRNA, which were not expressed in any of the samples obtained from control mice.

Summary

In this study, hair growth in treated C3H mice was observed on Day 27 and completed on Day 32. Hair growth ratios were gradually increased in parallel with the elicitation times (the number of times of elicitation by DNFB). The findings suggest that the CHS reaction could stimulate hair growth of telogen follicles of mice. Contact allergen-induced T cells (CD3+ T cells) may be of importance for hair regrowth. Th-1 type T cells producing IFN-gamma and IL-2 may be involved in mediating the effective phase of contact hypersensitivity. In our examination using RT-PCR methods, IFN-gamma and IL-2 mRNA expression was detected in the samples after sensitization, but IL-4 and IL-5 mRNA expression was not detected. This suggests that contact allergen-induced inflammatory Th-1 type T cells may be of importance for hair regrowth.

Discussion

In the treatment inducing the CHS reaction, the alteration from telogen to anagen hair was observed both in human alopecia areata (the disease condition) and the second telogen phase of C3H mice (the hair cycle model of mice). Before and after SADBE treatment, the expression of IFN-gamma was detected in the affected lesion of alopecia areata. In the mice study, lesional T-lymphocyte infiltration in the upper dermis may possibly lead to the induction of the anagen phase of the hair follicle. With regard to the local cytokine production, IFN-gamma was detected in the treated dorsal skin from early pre-anagen to mid-anagen phase. In the pathogenesis of alopecia areata, infiltrating T-lymphocytes producing Th-1 type cytokines, mainly IFN-gamma might affect function in the bulb portion of the hair follicle. Therefore, alopecia areata has been recognized as a T-cell-mediated/autoimmune disease. However, in our results, especially in the mice hair-cycle study, lesional T-lymphocytes infiltrating around the upper portion of the hair follicle could play a crucial role in the induction of the anagen phase. We therefore attempted to study the interaction of T cells, upper follicular cells, and epithelial cells; aiming to elucidate the role

of apoptosis in the early stage of hair regrowth. Tissue samples were taken on Day 15 after applying DNFB to a C3H mouse and then stained using the in situ apoptosis detection method (TUNNEL method). The epidermis between hair follicles presented an intensely positive, consistent image in the upper epithelial cells rather than in the basal layer, particularly in the nucleus in the granular layer. More noteworthy was that TUNNEL-positive findings were also found in the epithelial cells of the upper hair follicles immediately before transition to the anagen phase. No clear positive cells were observed on the hair follicles of the control group at the same stage. A pathway via Fas–Fas ligand is thought to exert some effect on T-cell mediated apoptosis.

Conclusion

We hypothesize that the infiltration of IFN-gamma-producing T-lymphocytes may cause apoptosis to occur in some parts of the upper follicle, thereby reactivating the entire stem cells (bulge area), thus promoting the transition to the growth stage.

References

1. Perret C, Menzel LW, Happle R: Immunohistochemical analysis of T-cell subsets in the peribulbar and intrabulbar infiltrates of alopecia areata. *Acta Derm Venereol (Stockh)* 1984; **64**: 26–30.
2. Menzel LW, Happle R: Intrabulbar and accumulation of dendritic OKT6-positive cells in alopecia areata. *Arch Dermatol Res* 1984; **276**: 333–334.
3. Bystryn JC, Tamesis J: Immunologic aspect of hair loss. *J Invest Dermatol* 1991; **96**: S88–S89.
4. Mcdonagh AJG, Messenger AG: The aetiology and pathogenesis of alopecia areata. *J Dermatol Sci* 1994; **7(Suppl)**: 125–135.
5. Shapiro J, Tan J, Ho V, Abbott F, Tron V: Treatment of chronic severe alopecia with topical diphenylcyclopropenone and 5% minoxidil: a clinical and immunopathologic evaluation. *J Am Acad Dermatol* 1993; **29**: 729–735.
6. Hoffman R, Elke W, Huth A, et al.: Cytokine mRNA levels in alopecia areata before and after treatment with the contact allergen diphenylcyclopropenone. *J Invest Dermatol* 1994; **103**: 530–533.
7. Happle R, Echternacht K: Induction of hair growth

in alopecia areata with DNCB. *Lancet* 1977; **2**: 1002–1003.

8. Daman LA, Rosenberg EW, Drake L: Treatment of alopecia areata with dinitrochlorobenzene. *Arch Dermatol* 1978; **114**: 1036–1038.

9. Happle R, Kalveram KJ, Büchner U, et al.: Contact allergy as a therapeutic tool for alopecia areata: application of squaric acid dibutylester. *Dermatologica* 1980; **161**: 289–297.

10. Van der Steen PH, Van Baar HJM, Perret CM, Happle R: Treatment of alopecia areata with diphenylcyclopropenone. *J Am Acad Dermatol* 1991; **24**: 253–257.

11. Hull SM, Pepall L, Cunliffe WJ: Alopecia areata in children: response treatment with diphencyprone. *Br J Dermatol* 1991; **125**: 164–168.

19
New therapeutic directions for alopecia areata

Jerry Shapiro

Introduction

The most significant directions for research into new therapies for alopecia areata began at the First International Alopecia Areata Research Workshop, which took place in October 1990 in Bethesda, Maryland, USA. This meeting was co-sponsored by the National Alopecia Areata Foundation (NAAF) and the National Institute of Arthritis and Musculoskeletal and Skin Diseases (NIAMS). This landmark event brought together dermatologists, immunologists, geneticists, molecular biologists, biochemists and pathologists for an historic 2-day 'think-tank' session on alopecia areata. Results of this open exchange have guided research in alopecia areata and this workshop has since been repeated twice in 1994 and 1998. The basic concepts and investigational approaches to future therapies for alopecia areata have been formulated at these workshops. The proceedings of these meetings have been published in the *Journal of Investigative Dermatology*.[1,2]

Four key areas with respect to future directions in therapy will be focused upon in this chapter: targeted immunomodulatory agents; rodent models as important research tools in understanding and implementing new therapies; phototherapy beyond psoralen + UVA light (PUVA); and gene therapy.

Targeted immunomodulatory agents

There is an overwhelming body of evidence that implicates the central role of the T cell in the pathogenesis of alopecia areata[3] (see Messenger, chapter 16 and Tobin & Bystryn, chapter 17 for further details). Immunomodulatory agents that target T cells, cytokines, specific antigens and antigen presenting cells are hypothesized to have some effect since alopecia areata is thought to be a dysregulation of the basic interactions of the T cell with antigen presenting cells around the hair follicle.

Targeting the T cell with anti-CD4 monoclonal antibodies has been shown to have some positive effects on the treatment of psoriasis[4] and it is expected that this technique will be tested on alopecia areata. Inhibitors of T-cell activation such as cyclosporine[5] or tacrolimus[6] may also have some benefit. Studies on systemic cyclosporine show some effect in alopecia areata but the side-effects resulting from marked generalized immunosuppression make this form of therapy less than practical.[5] Agents directed at specific T-cell receptors (TCR) may have some use in the autoimmune diseases using selective anti-TCR antibodies.[7] Unfortunately, because the responsible epitope for alopecia areata is unknown, the corresponding T-cell receptor has not yet been discovered. Studies have shown that there is a predisposition for certain T-cell receptor subsets or clones in alopecia areata[8,9] and this may eventually give us a clue as to what to target in the future.

Targeting cytokines involved in the T-cell antigen interaction is another therapeutic approach. Anti-TNF$_\alpha$ antibodies have already been shown to have some therapeutic benefit in those with rheumatoid arthritis.[10] IL-2-diptheria fusion antibody to the IL-2 receptor can inhibit antigen presentation and has been shown to have some value in psoriasis[11] and cutaneous T-cell lymphoma.[12] Both of these treatments may well have a role in the treatment of alopecia areata.

Tolerance that is induced to specific autoantigens may deplete responsible autoreactive

T cells. Orally induced tolerance may induce clonal T-cell depletion and has been used with some success in suppressing murine experimental autoimmune encephalomyelitis (EAE)[13] and clinical trials are underway with multiple sclerosis.[14] This has no application yet to alopecia areata until the disease-associated epitopes are discovered. A possible vaccine with the responsible epitope may be of great value for the future.

Antibodies to cell surface markers on antigen presenting cells, such as CD11a monoclonal antibodies, may also have a future role in the treatment of alopecia areata.

Rodent models

Rodent models are an important research tool for understanding, implementing and refining new therapies. The C3H/HeJ mouse,[15] discovered by John Sundberg and Lloyd King and the DEBR (Dundee Experimental Bald Rat)[16] discovered by Roy Oliver display a patchy alopecia that is clinically and histopathologically somewhat very similar to human alopecia areata. Topical sensitizers such as diphencyprone (DPCP) have been shown to be of great benefit in alopecia areata patients. The exact mechanism of action is, however, unclear. Rodent models may bring us closer to understanding how these sensitizers work since they allow us to perform several sequential biopsies. Both rodent models have been subjected to treatment with DPCP, yielding convincing hair growth on the treated portions of the animals.[17] Histopathologically, there appears to be a shift of T cells away from the follicle into the dermis during successful treatment.[17] It appears that a T cell shift away from the follicle may be important for an effective therapy agent to work. Newer immunomodulators are likely to be tested on these animal models.

Phototherapy beyond PUVA

Harnessing the photon energy of light to grow hair is certainly possible with PUVA but the side-effects may be unacceptable to many patients and physicians. Using photodynamic therapy with new topical photosensitizers, as well as new light sources may modulate the immunologic milieu around the hair follicle. Work has been initiated using delta-aminolevulinic acid (ALA) topically in human alopecia areata and the C3H/HeJ mouse model.[18] This form of therapy may have great potential.

Gene therapy

Although genetic correlates[19,20] for susceptibility and severity for alopecia areata have been identified, the exact set of genes that actually cause alopecia areata has not yet been discovered. Once these genes are discovered and the technology for gene therapy becomes more refined, appropriate gene delivery may become an important part of therapy.

Conclusion

It is hoped that these new future directions in therapy will give alopecia areata patients great benefit so that by the end of the next 10 years physicians will be able to offer either a cure or more effective therapies to patients.

References

1. Proceedings of the First International Research Workshop on Alopecia Areata. *J Invest Dermatol* 1991; **96(5):** 67S–98S.
2. Proceedings of the Second International Research Workshop on Alopecia Areata. *J Invest Dermatol* 1995; **104(5):** 2S–45S.
3. Gilhar A, Ullman Y, Berkutzki T, Assy B, Kalish RS: Autoimmune hair loss (alopecia areata) transferred by T lymphocytes to human scalp explants on SCID mice. *J Clin Invest* 1998; **101:** 62–67.
4. Bachelez H, Flageul B, Dubertret L, et al.: Treatment of recalcitrant plaque psoriasis with humanized non-depleting antibody to CD4. *J Autoimmun* 1998; **11(1):** 53–62.
5. Shapiro J, Lui H, Tron V, Ho V: Systemic cyclosporine and low-dose prednisone in the treatment of chronic severe alopecia areata: a clinical and immunopathologic evaluation. *J Am Acad Dermatol* 1997; **36:** 114–117.

6. McElwee K, Rushton D, Trachy R, Oliver R: Topical FK506: a potent immunotherapy for alopecia areata? Studies using the Dundee experimental bald rat model. *Br J Dermatol* 1997; **137(4)**: 491–497.

7. Urban J, Kumar V, Kono D, et al.: Restricted use of T-cell receptor V genes in murine autoimmune encephalomyelitis raises possibilities for antibody therapy. *Cell* 1988; **54**: 577–592.

8. Szafer F, Price V, Oksenberg J, Steinman L: T-cell receptor repertoire Vβ in alopecia areata. *J Invest Dermatol* 1995; **104(5)**: 22–26.

9. Arand C, Happle, R, Hoffman R: Expression of T-cell receptor of Vβ chains in alopecia areata. In: Van Neste D, Randall V (eds.). *Hair Research for the Next Millennium*. Amsterdam, Elsevier Science, 1996: 221–225.

10. Elliot MJ, Maini RN, Feldmann M, et al.: Treatment of rheumatoid arthritis with chimeric monoclonal antibodies to tumor necrosis factor α. *Arthr Rheum* 1993; **36**: 1681–1690.

11. Gottlieb S, Gilleaudeau P, Johnson R, et al.: Response of psoriasis to a lymphocyte-selective toxin (DAB389IL-2) suggests a primary immune, but not keratinocyte pathogenetic basis. *Nature Med* 1995; **1**: 442–447.

12. Saleh M, Le Maistre C, Kuzel T, et al.: Antitumor activity of DAB389IL-2 fusion toxin in mycosis fungoides. *J Am Acad Dermatol* 1998; **39**: 63–73.

13. Wraith D, Smilek D, Mitchell D, Steinman L, McDevitt H: Antigen recognition in autoimmune encephalomyelitis and the potential for peptide-mediated immunotherapy. *Cell* 1989; **59**: 247–255.

14. Weiner H, Mackim G, Matsui M, et al.: Double-blind pilot trial of oral toerization with myelin antigens to multiple sclerosis. *Science* 1993; **259**: 1321–1324.

15. Sundberg J, Boggess D, Montagutelli X, Hogan M, King L: C3H/HeJ mouse model for alopecia areata. *J Invest Dermatol* 1995; **104**: 16S–17S.

16. Michie HJ, Jahoda C, Oliver R, Johnson B: The DEBR rat: an animal model of human alopecia areata. *Br J Dermatol* 1991; **125**: 94–100.

17. Shapiro J, Sundberg J, McElwee K, et al.: Immunophenotypic profiles during topical immunotherapy of alopecia areata in mice and rats with diphencyprone. Presentation at the Third International Research Workshop on Alopecia Areata, Washington DC, Nov 1998. *J Invest Dermatol* [Abstract] 1999: (In press).

18. Shapiro J, Bissonnette R, McLean D, Lui H: Topical ALA in the treatment of alopecia areata. Presentation at the Americal Academy of Dermatology 1996, San Francisco.

19. Duvic M, Welsh E, Jackow C, Papadopoulos E, Reveille J, Amos C: Analysis of HLA-D local alleles in alopecia areata patients and families. *J Invest Dermatol* 1995; **104**: 5S–6S.

20. Colombe BW, Price VH, Khoury E: HLA Class II antigen associations help to define two types of alopecia areata. *J Am Acad Dermatol* 1995; **33**: 757.

20

Hair follicle innervation in alopecia areata

Maria K Hordinsky and Marna Ericson

The Peripheral Nervous System and the Hair Follicle

Myelinated nerves rising from deep in the dermis form the perifollicular plexus of nerves. Some of these fibres run parallel to the follicle, whereas other finer nerves form a net around the follicle. At the level of the bulb of small and vellus follicles and also the bulge of large follicles, nerve fibres form a stockade-like structure that encircles the hair follicle. This hair follicle nerve plexus is described as being more organized around vellus follicles compared with terminal hair follicles and is composed of an outer circular layer and an inner longitudinal layer of nerve fibres that run parallel to the hair follicle.[1,2]

The end-organs of perifollicular longitudinal nerve fibres are composed of swollen axons and non-myelinated Schwann sheaths. Axons at the mid-sebaceous gland level are in contact with the basal lamina of the follicle, whereas above and below this level, axons are usually covered by Schwann cell cytoplasm and appear detached from the hair follicle. The outer circular nerves are predominantly composed of non-myelinated axons and Schwann sheaths. Swollen axons that are free of the Schwann sheath are postulated to represent terminal bulbs or the end-organ of the outer circular nerves. It has been proposed that, given their distance from the hair follicle, these end-organs are associated with a different type of sensation, such as pain.[1]

Based on histochemical studies in animal model systems it has been presumed that the perifollicular neural plexus does not change during the hair cycle and that this nerve plexus collapses during catagen–telogen transformation and re-extends itself into its original architecture by the new, growing anagen bulb.[3,4] This dogma was recently contested when it was demonstrated the architecture of hair follicle innervation in adolescent mice changes during the hair cycle, since circular nerves increase significantly in number during the earliest stages of anagen development.[5,6]

With the development of mouse mutants with functional deletion or overexpression of genes coding for neurotrophins, neuropeptides or their receptors, and for proteins relevant to nerve sprouting, research tools are now available for establishing the significance of piloneural interactions.[6] This is particularly true in murine model systems where, in contrast to the mosaic cycling of human hair follicles, follicle cycling can be synchronized, particularly in the first months of murine post-natal life.

Both follicular neurotrophin and neuropeptide expression have been examined in several mouse model systems. Neurotrophins are a family of structurally and functionally related polypeptides that consist of four major members:

(1) Nerve growth factor (NGF);
(2) Brain-derived neurotrophic factor (BDNF);
(3) Neurotrophin-3 (NT-3); and
(4) Neurotrophin-4 (NT-4).

The tropomyosin related kinase (TrK) family of high-affinity transmembrane receptors binds neurotrophins. Neurotrophin binding to the Trk receptor causes receptor dimerization and a cellular response. The low-affinity p75 neurotrophin receptor (p75NTR) binds all neurotrophins to some degree, whereas the high-affinity binding Trk receptors are more discriminating.[7]

Neuropeptides, in contrast to the neurotrophins, are a heterogeneous group of several hundred biologically active peptides present in neurones of both the central and peripheral nervous system.[8,9] These peptides are involved with the transmission of signals not only between nerve cells but also with cells of the immune system. Similar interactions have been reported for the neurotrophins.

Neurotrophins

Each of the neurotrophins has a specific role in regulating different classes of functionally identified sensory neurones. For example, NT-3 and its receptor TrkC are required for the survival of non-nocioceptive proprioceptors, muscle afferent fibres, and cutaneous mechanoreceptors. NGF, signalling through its high-affinity receptor, TrkA, and BDNF with TrkB have distinct and non-overlapping roles in cutaneous sensory neurons. NT-4 is required for the survival of down hair (D-hair) receptors whereas BDNF supports the mechanical function of sensory afferent nerve fibres.[10]

Alterations in nerve-fibre remodelling and sprouting, as well as neurotrophin and receptor expression, occur during the murine hair cycle. During early anagen development, NT-3 overexpressing transgenic mice demonstrate precocious catagen development during the post-natal initiation of hair follicle cycling, whereas heterozygous NT-3 knock-out (+/–) mice display a significant retardation in the expression of the catagen phase of the hair cycle. In later stages of hair follicle development, TrkC mRNA, TrkC- and NT-3-immunoreactivity can be seen in the epidermis. The interfollicular dermis becomes 'hyper-innervated' and the circular nerve fibres of the hair follicle demonstrate enhanced expression of growth-associated protein (GAP-43), as well as neural cell adhesion molecules, which are indicators of active nerve-fibre remodelling and sprouting.[6,11,12] The expression of NT-3 and its high-affinity receptor, TrkC, in the skin of C57BL/6 mice is also hair cycle-dependent, with maximal transcript and protein expression occurring during the catagen phase of the hair cycle.[13]

More recently, the expression of BDNF and NT-mRNA has been found to be hair cycle dependent, peaking during catagen, whereas TrkB

mRNA and immunoreactivity are present in dermal papilla fibroblasts, epithelial strands, and the hair germ. Both NT-4 and BDNF knock-out mice have been shown to have a retarded expression of catagen, whereas mice over-expressing BDNF exhibit a shortening of hair length and accelerated catagen.[7]

Neuropeptides

Two neuropeptides that have been studied more extensively in relationship to the hair follicle are substance P (SP) and calcitonin gene-related peptide (CGRP). SP is synthesized in the dorsal root ganglia from where it migrates to the dorsal horn of the spinal cord and peripherally to nerve terminals of sensory neurones. SP, along with neurokinin A and B, belongs to the tachykinin family. The specific receptor subtypes that correspond to these three neurokinins are neurokinin 1 (NK-1) receptors for SP, neurokinin 2 (NK-2) receptors for neurokinin A and neurokinin 3 (NK-3) receptors for neurokinin B.[9,13–15]

Substance P is best known for its role in pain transmission but it has several additional functions, some of which could be involved with the pathogenesis of hair diseases such as alopecia areata. SP can induce mast cell degranulation, expression of endothelial–leukocyte adhesion molecule-1 on adjacent venular endothelial cells, enhance DNA synthesis by human peripheral blood lymphocytes, and stimulate mononuclear and polymorphonuclear leukocyte chemotaxis. More recently, SP has been described to induce hair growth in the C57BL16 mouse model.[6,9,16]

The effect of SP has been examined on the back skin of telogen mice. The neuropeptide-releasing neurotoxin, capsaicin, was either injected intradermally, or slow-release formulations of SP were implanted subcutaneously in the back skin of C57BL/6 mice with all follicles in the resting stage of the hair cycle (telogen) in order to see whether this induced hair growth. Endogenous SP skin concentrations and the activity of an SP-degrading enzyme, neutral endopeptidase (NEP), were also determined during the induced murine hair cycle by high-performance liquid chromatography (HPLC) controlled radioimmunoassay for SP levels and fluorometry for NEP levels.[16]

Both capsaicin and SP induced significant hair growth (anagen) in the back skin of telogen mice as well as substantial mast cell degranulation. The endogenous SP skin concentration showed significant, hair-cycle dependent fluctuations during the induced murine hair cycle. These were independent of the activity of NEP. The results of these studies suggest that SP may play a role in the neural control of hair growth.

CGRP is a small peptide encoded by the gene for the thyroid hormone, calcitonin. Two populations of unmyelinated sensory axons in human skin containing immunoreactivity to CGRP have been described. One population is immunoreactive to SP, whereas the other is immunoreactive to somatostatin.

CGRP, like SP, has several functions. When it is released by cutaneous nerve endings, it causes significant vasodilation of blood vessels. CGRP inhibits both mitogen-stimulated T-lymphocyte proliferation and Langerhans' cell antigen presentation; it also blocks the actions of some inflammatory mediators.[17,18] Treatment of antigen presenting cells with CGRP decreases their ability to present antigen. The addition of CGRP may also inhibit the up-regulation of CD86, as well as alter the expression of immunoregulatory cytokines.[19–21] Up-regulation of CGRP has been implicated in ultraviolet light-induced immunosuppression and CGRP is necessary for ultraviolet B-impaired induction of contact hypersensitivity.[22] Recently, it has been reported patients with alopecia areata have low serum levels of CGRP, as well as an exaggerated vasodilatory response to the local injection of CGRP.[23,24]

The peripheral nervous system and cutaneous inflammation

The peripheral nervous system is now known to modulate a variety of inflammatory and proliferative processes. Neurotrophins and their receptors, neuropeptides and their receptors, as well as neuropeptide-degrading enzymes may all interact with the immune system.[13] Therefore, it is possible that local changes in the peripheral nervous system at the level of the dermal papilla or the bulge region could be important in hair diseases, and specifically in alopecia areata,

which is a hair disease with a well-defined inflammatory component.

In animal studies, NGF has been shown to stimulate nocioception as well as increase vascular permeability via the stimulation of CGRP release from sensory nerve endings, as well as degranulation of mast cells. It is postulated that neurotrophins may play an important role in several autoimmune diseases such as rheumatoid arthritis, multiple sclerosis, lupus erythematosus, and systemic scleroderma.[25] Indeed, increases in the basal levels of NGF have been found in the synovium of patients with rheumatoid arthritis, in plasma of patients with lupus erythematosus, the cerebrospinal fluid of patients with multiple sclerosis, and in the skin of patients with systemic scleroderma. Waiting to be added to this list is a link with alopecia areata.[2,3,25,26]

Hair follicle innervation in alopecia areata

Some have postulated that alopecia areata is mediated by the nervous system. In 1886, Max Joseph produced patches of alopecia in cats by sectioning the posterior roots of the second cervical nerve peripheral to the ganglion or by ablating the ganglion itself. He concluded that the resultant alopecia was related to the nerves that had been sectioned.[27] In 1949, Gohlke and Holtschmidt demonstrated degenerative changes of the neurofibrils in the nerves to the blood vessels and sweat glands in six cases of alopecia areata.[28] Joseph's conclusions were later refuted and it was suggested that the alopecia resulted from the trauma of scratching. Moreover, pain-relieving neurosurgical procedures in which the sensory nerves supplying the scalp are cut do not routinely result in alopecia areata.

More recently, Maurer and colleagues tested the role of follicle innervation of hair follicle cycling in vivo in a mouse model system. Innervation-deficient hair follicles were generated by unilateral surgical denervation of a defined region of back skin in C57BL/6 mice; the effect of this procedure on spontaneous and induced anagen development was studied. By quantitative histomorphometry, no significant difference in spontaneous or cyclosporin A-induced anagen development could be detected between sham-operated control skin and denervated skin. Only after hair growth induction by depilation, was a discrete, marginally significant retardation of anagen development apparent in denervated hair follicles. The investigators concluded that cutaneous nerves were not essential for normal murine anagen development but that cutaneous nerves probably played some role in modulating the murine hair cycle.[29]

Despite this lack of support for the neurotrophic theory, it is still highly likely the peripheral nervous system plays a role in alopecia areata. For example, SP expression is not thought to be prominent in the scalp yet some patients with alopecia areata who express SP prominently in affected scalp skin have been

identified.[30] Patients with alopecia areata have low serum levels of CGRP.[24] Skin in alopecia areata also has an exaggerated vasodilatory response to the local injection of CGRP.[23] In the latter study, the investigators examined the possiblity that a neuropeptidergic sensory nerve disorder could be involved in alopecia areata. They measured levels of CGRP, SP, and another neuropeptide, vasoactive intestinal peptide (VIP) in pathological and healthy scalp biopsies, using radioimmunoassay (RIA). They also investigated the relationship between primay sensory neurones and scalp microvessel characteristics in patients with alopecia areata after intradermal injection of CGRP using laser-Doppler flowmetry. Tissue levels of neuropeptides such as SP and

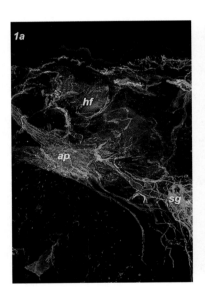 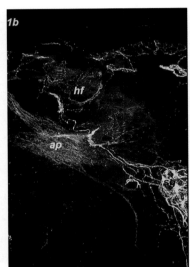 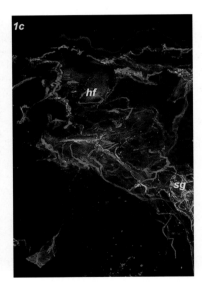

Figure 1

Vasculature, innervation, and CGRP expression in the scalp of a 13-year-old African American male with extensive alopecia areata. Each picture is a projection of a total of 46 optical sections taken at 1μ intervals. (a) UEA 1/vasculature (red) and PGP9.5/nerves (green). A small hair follicle (hf) is outlined with UEA 1. The perifollicular vasculature is less prominent compared with normal scalp vasculature. The innervation of the arrector pili muscle (ap), sweat gland (sg), and subepidermal and dermal nerves is demonstrated in green. PGP 9.5- staining nerves appear to outline the small hair follicle identified with UEA 1. Note that most cutaneous blood vessels in the scalp are not innervated. (b) PGP 9.5/nerves (green) and CGRP (red). Co-localization of PGP9.5 and the neuropeptide CGRP is depicted in yellow. The arrector pili muscle, sweat gland, and nerves in the region of the small hair follicle all stain with the antibody to PGP 9.5 (green). The majority of sweat gland (eccrine gland) nerves co-localize with CGRP (yellow) as do several nerves in the subepidermal nerve plexus. (c) UEA 1/blood vessels (red) and CGRP (green). Again, the presence of a yellow colour depicts co-localization of the vasculature with CGRP. CGRP is only rarely associated with scalp blood vessels. Fine CGRP-staining nerves surround the small hair follicle outlined by UEA 1 (red). These same CGRP-staining nerves appear to co-localize with PGP 9.5 as presented in (b). Scale bar = 100μ

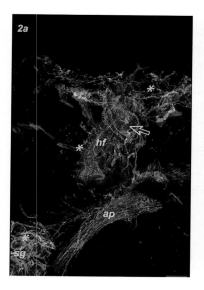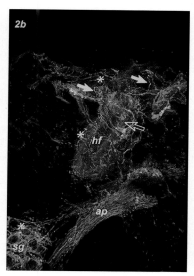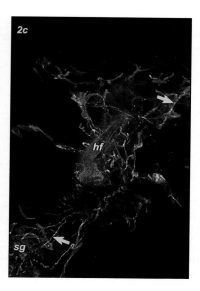

Figure 2

Vasculature, innervation, and SP expression in the scalp of a 13-year-old African American male with extensive alopecia areata. Each picture is a projection of 22 optical sections taken at 3μ intervals. (a) UEA 1/vasculature (red) and PGP 9.5/nerves (green). A small hair follicle (hf) is outlined with UEA 1 (red) as is the less-organized perifollicular vasculature. Perifollicular nerves(*) appear collapsed (green/yellow open arrow). The subepidermal nerve plexus and the innervation of the arrector pili (ap) muscle and sweat gland (sg) are highlighted in green. Co-localization of PGP 9.5 with nerves or blood vessels is demonstrated in yellow. (b) PGP 9.5/nerves (green) and SP (red). Co-localization of PGP 9.5 and the neuropeptide SP (red) is depicted in yellow. SP is present co-localizing with some of the nerves in the subepidermal nerve plexus (yellow closed arrows). SP is also prominently expressed around the lower portion of the miniaturized hair follicle. (c) UEA 1/blood vessels (red) and SP (green). SP is present within some perifollicular, sweat gland, and subepidermal blood vessel networks (yellow closed arrows). There is again an abundance of SP present around the lower portion of the miniaturized hair follicle. Scale bar = 100μ.

CGRP were found to be significantly decreased in scalp biopsies, whereas VIP levels were decreased but not significantly in alopecic biopsies; suggesting to the investigators that primary sensory innervation is affected but cholinergic innervation, which contains VIP, is not. In this same study, it was also found that an intradermal injection of CGRP induced a marked increase in blood flow in the scalp of alopecia areata patients compared to control subjects, whereas in patients affected by alopecia areata, the alopecic patch basal blood flow, measured using laser-Doppler flowmetry was significantly lower compared to the hairy scalp of control subjects, confirming some type of vascular deficiency.

Complimenting these studies is our own work in which immunohistochemical techniques and laser scanning confocal microscopy are used to analyse neuropeptide expression in relationship to perifollicular vasculature and innervation in both normal control and alopecia areata scalp samples. Using techniques standard to our laboratory, images are collected and projected generating pictures as shown in Figures 1 and 2. Sections are first examined using conventional epifluorescent microscopy and later, images are collected using laser scanning confocal microscopy (LSCM) with an MRC-1000 or MRC-1024 Confocal Imaging System (Bio-Rad, Hercules, CA). Images are collected in sequential 1-, 2-, or 3-μ serial optical sections and integrated into single in-focus images.

In long-standing (>2 years' duration) extensive alopecia areata, the perifollicular innervation is condensed and arranged in a basket-weave network around the small alopecia areata anagen follicles, rather than appearing to run parallel to the follicle. The hair follicle nerve plexus, which appears like a stockade around small miniaturized follicles, is also very prominent in some patients with long standing alopecia areata.[31] This is in contrast to previous observations that the perifollicular innervation in alopecia areata is relatively normal.[3] Whether these alterations in perifollicular innervation are a primary or secondary event in the pathophysiology of alopecia areata remains to be ascertained.

Perifollicular vasculature also appears to be decreased in alopecia areata. Moreover, many of the blood vessels identified with the lectin UEA 1 do not stain with the pan-neuronal antibody, protein gene product 9.5 (PGP 9.5). It appears as though these perifollicular blood vessels are not innervated or lack an epitope recognized by the PGP 9.5 antibody. In alopecia areata, the neuropeptides SP and CGRP surround the small follicles independently, or they co-localize with nerves or blood vessels.[2,30]

Perifollicular innervation and neuropeptide expression are altered in alopecia areata. Whether this alteration is the primary or secondary event in this disease is unknown. Nevertheless, local changes in the peripheral nervous system, either in the dermal papilla or bulge region, may be important. Finally, it has been suggested eccrine glands in alopecia areata respond abnormally to iontophoretic pilocarpine stimulation, suggesting another ectodermal derived appendage may be affected in patients with alopecia areata.[31]

Research tools are available to further study the piloneural connection in alopecia areata. The availability of mouse models to examine hair growth with agents that modulate the peripheral nervous system, as well as the availability of histochemical techniques to examine neurotrophin/neurotrophin receptor and neuropeptide/neuropeptide receptor expression are being applied to the study of the pathogenesis of alopecia areata. Moreover, since neurotrophins may initiate apoptotic signalling through p75NTR when expressed alone, investigators have suggested that tyrosine kinase C agonists and antagonists deserve systematic exploration for the management of hair growth disorders related to premature or retarded catagen.[32,33]

Capsaicin, frequently used as a topical medication to treat inflammation, excites subsets of sensory neurones associated with pain and thermoreception; it also releases SP and CGRP. All of these functions could play a role in alopecia areata. Currently, the effect of topical capsaicin on perifollicular nerves and the hair follicle in patients with extensive, long-standing alopecia areata is being examined.[34] In conclusion, it is our impression that over the next few years, the level of knowledge about the role of the peripheral nervous system in alopecia areata can only increase.

References

1. Halata Z: Sensory innervation of the hairy skin (light- and electronmicroscopic study). *J Invest Dermatol* 1993; **101**: 75S–81S.
2. Hordinsky M, Ericson ME: Relationship between follicular nerve supply and alopecia. *Dermatol Clin* 1996; **14**: 651–660.
3. Winkelmann RK, Jaffee MO: Nerve network of the hair follicle in alopecia areata. *Arch Dermatol* 1960; **82**: 142–145.
4. Winkelmann RK: Cutaneous sensory nerves. *Semin Dermatol* 1988; **7**: 236–288.
5. Botchkarev VA, Eichmuller S, Johansson O, Paus R: Hair cycle-dependent plasticity of skin and hair follicle innervation in normal murine skin. *J Comp Neurol* 1997; **386**: 379–395.
6. Paus R, Peters EMJ, Eichmuller S, Botchkarev VA: Neural mechanisms of hair growth control. *J Invest Dermatol* 1997; **2**: 61–68.
7. Botchkarev VA, Botchkareva NV, Welder P, Metz M, Lewin GR, Subramanian A: A new role for neurotrophins: involvement of brain-derived neurotrophic factor and neurotrophin-4 in hair cycle control. *FASEB J* 1999; **13**: 395–410.
8. Rossi R, Del Bianco E, Isoalni D, Baccari MC, Cappugi P: Possible involvement of neuropeptidergic sensory nerves in alopecia areata. *Clin Neurosci Neuropathol* 1997; **8**: 1135–1138.
9. Ansel JC, Armstron CA, Song IS, Quinlan KL, Olerud JE, Caughman JW: Interactions of the skin and nervous system. *J Invest Dermatol Symp Proc* 1997; **2**: 23–26.
10. Stucky CL, DeChiara T, Lindsay RM, Yancopoulos GD, Koltzenburg M: Neurotrophin 4 is required for the survival of a subclass of hair follicle receptors. *J Neurosci* 1998; **18**: 7040–7046.

11. Botchkarev VA, Welker P, Albers KM, Botchkareva NV, Metz M, Lewin G: A new role for neurotrophin-3; involvement in the regulation of hair follicle regression (catagen). *Am J Pathol* 1998; **153**: 785–799.

12. Lindsay RM: Role of neurotrophins and trk receptors in the development and maintenance of sensory neurons: an overview. *Phil Trans R Soc Lond* 1996; **351**: 365–373.

13. Botchkarev VA, Botchkareva NV, Albers KM, van der Veen C, Lewin GR, Paus R: Neurotrophin-3 involvement in the regulation of hair follicle morphogenesis. *J Invest Dermatol* 1998; **111**: 279–285.

14. Scholzen T, Armstrong CA, Bunnet NW, Luger TA, Olerud JE, Ansel JC: Neuropeptides in the skin: interactions between the neuroendocrine and the skin immune systems. *Exper Dermatol* 1997; **7**: 81–96.

15. Lotti T, Hautmann G, Pancone E: Neuropeptides in skin. *J Am Acad Dermatol* 1995; **33**: 482–496.

16. Paus R, Heinzelmann T, Klaus-Detlev S, Furkert J, Fechner K, Czarnetzki BM: Hair growth induction by Substance P. *Lab Invest* 1994; **71**: 134–140.

17. Zheng L, Fisher G, Miller RE, et al.: Induction of apoptosis in mature T cells by tumour necrosis factor. *Nature* 1996; **377**: 348–351.

18. Lambert RW, Granstein RD: Neuropeptides and Langerhans' cells. *Exper Dermatol* 1998; **7**: 73–80.

19. Hosoi J, Egan CL, Lerner EA, et al.: Regulation of Langerhans' cell function by nerves containing CGRP. *Nature* 1993; **363**: 159–163.

20. Asahini A, Hosoi J, Beissert S, Stratigos A, Granstein RD: Inhibition of the induction of delayed-type and contact hypersensitivity by calcitonin gene related peptide. *J Immunol* 1995; **154**: 3056–3061.

21. Asashina A, Moro O, Hosoi J, et al.: Specific induction of cyclic AMP in Langerhans' cells by calcitonin gene-related peptide: relevance to functional effects. *Proc Natl Acad Sci USA* 1995; **154**: 8323–8327.

22. Gillardon F, Moll I, Michel S, Benrath J, Weihe E, Zimmermann M: Calcitonin gene related protein peptide and nitric acid oxide are involved in ultraviolet radation-induced immunosuppression. *Eur J Pharmacol* 1995; **293**: 395–400.

23. Rossi R, Johansson O: Cutaneous innervation and the role of neuronal peptides in cutaneous inflammation: a mini-review. *Eur J Dermatol* 1998; **8**: 299–306.

24. Daly TJ: Alopecia areata has low plasma levels of the vasodilator/immunomodulator calcitonin gene-related protein. *Arch Dermatol* 1998; **13**: 1164–1165.

25. Aloe L, Tuveri MA: Nerve growth factor and autoimmune rheumatic diseases. *Clin Exper Dermatol* 1997; **15**: 433–438.

26. Aloe L, Bracci-Landiero L, Bonini S, Manni L: The expanding role of nerve growth factor: from neurotrophic activity to immunodiseases. *Allergy* 1997; **5**: 883–894.

27. Joseph M: Experimentelle Untersuchungen uber die Atiologie der Alopecia areata. *Monatsh Prakt Dermato* 1886; **5**: 483–489.

28. Gohlke, Holtschmidt: Neurohistologische Studien bei Alopecia Areata. *Arch Dermatol Syphilol* 1949; **191**: 527–530.

29. Maurer M, Peters EMJ, Botcharev VA, Paus R: Intact hair follicle innervation is not essential for anagen induction and development. *Arch Dermatol Res* 1998; **290**: 574–578.

30. Hordinsky M, Lorimer S, Ericson M, Worel S: Innervation and vasculature of the normal human and alopecia areata (AA) hair follicle: an immunohistochemical and laser scanning confocal microscopic study. In VanNeste D, Randall VA (eds.) *Hair Research for the Next Millennium*, Amsterdam, Elsevier, 1996: 197–202.

31. Hordinsky M, Kennedy W, Wendelschafer-Crabb G, Lewis S: Structure and function of cutaneous nerves in alopecia areata. *J Invest Dermatol* 1995; **104**: 28S–29S.

32. Botchkarev VA, Botchkareva NV, Yaar M, Gilchrest BA, Paus R: A new role for p75 neurotrophin receptor in hair follicle regression: catagen retardation in p75NTR knock-out mice and after p75NTR blockade by cyclic peptides. *J Invest Dermatol* 1999; **112**: 553.

33. Yaar M, Zhai S, Pilch PF, Doyle SM, Gilchrest BA: Design of a cyclic decapeptide to block apoptotic cell death mediated through the p75 neurotrophin receptor. *J Invest Dermatol* 1997; **108**: 568.

34. Ericson M, Binstock K, Guanche A, Hordinsky M: Differential expression of substance P in perifollicular scalp blood vessels and nerves after topical therapy with capsaicin 0.075% (Zostrix HP) in controls and patients with extensive alopecia areata. *J Invest Dermatol* 1999; **112**: 653.

21
Atypical clinical forms of alopecia areata

María José García-Hernández and Francisco M Camacho

Introduction

Alopecia areata is a common hair disorder with many clinical presentations, depending on the pattern of hair loss. A single alopecic patch on the scalp or body may be present, or there may be complete scalp and/or body hair loss.[1] Typical clinical presentations are described briefly in this chapter, and are as follows:

(1) Single patchy alopecia areata (SAA)
(2) Multiple patchy alopecia areata
    (2.1) Alopecia areata: several patches (MAA)
    (2.2) Reticular alopecia areata (RAA)
    (2.3) Ophiasic alopecia areata (OAA)
(3) Complete scalp hair loss
    (3.1) Alopecia areata totalis (AT)
    (3.2) Alopecia areata universalis (AU)
    (3.3) Alopecia totalis/alopecia universalis (AT/AU)

Typical forms of alopecia areata

Single patchy alopecia areata (SAA)

Most commonly, patients initially present with a circumscribed circular, smooth, bald patch up to several centimeters in diameter. Discrete erythema may also occur. Exclamation mark hairs may be present at the margin of the lesion and these are easily extracted, and these hairs commonly regrow white. Overall, however, the hair usually, but not always, returns to its original color. The scalp is the first affected site in almost

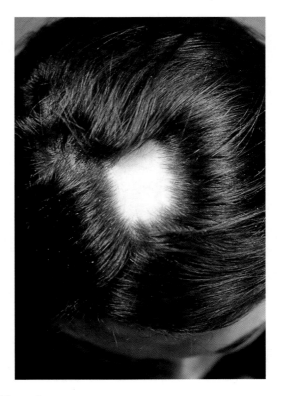

Figure 1

Alopecia areata showing a single scalp patch.

60% of cases (Figure 1). Sites other than the scalp can also be involved: the eyebrows and eyelashes are lost in many cases of alopecia areata (Figure 2); indeed, they may be the only sites affected.[2]

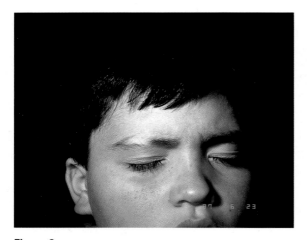

Figure 2

Single patchy alopecia areata affecting the eyebrow.

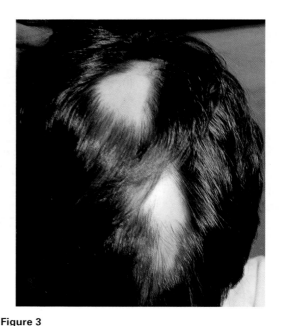

Figure 3

Two patches of alopecia areata on the scalp.

Alopecia areata in several patches (MAA)

The initial patch may regrow within a few months or further patches may appear in any place on the scalp (Figure 3). Subsequent progress is very varied. The discrete patches may become confluent owing to the diffuse loss of the remaining hair.[3]

Reticular alopecia areata (RAA)

In RAA several patches are present in various stages of disease activity.[4] Simultaneous regrowth in one region of the scalp and extension of alopecia in others leads to the development of a reticulate pattern (Figure 4). This condition has a poor prognosis.[5]

Ophiasic alopecia areata (OAA)

In greek, 'ophiasis' means serpent, and in this clinical form of alopecia areata the spread is

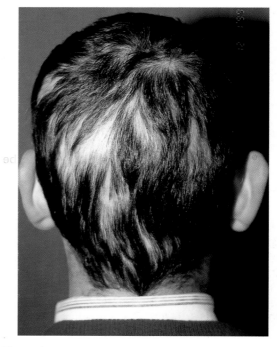

Figure 4

Reticular alopecia areata. A reticulate pattern caused by regrowth in one area and alopecia in others can be seen.

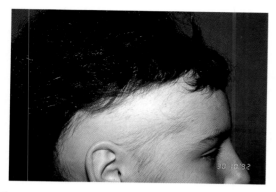

Figure 5

Ophiasic alopecia areata. This condition is usually found in children.

'serpent-like'. The extension of the alopecia localizes along the scalp margin. The initial patch starts from the occipital area and extends round the scalp edges (Figure 5). In other cases, it also can begin in the frontal zone, with hair loss in a band encircling the frontal and temporal scalp, which is easily diagnosed. Ophiasis is usually found in children and it can develop into a more severe form.[2,3]

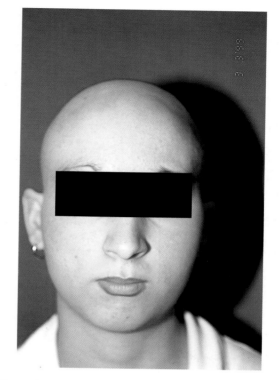

Figure 6

Alopecia areata totalis. This is the loss of all scalp hair.

Alopecia areata totalis (AT)

Extensive involvement of the scalp may result in total or almost loss of scalp hair (Figure 6), which is known as alopecia areata totalis. Onset may be acute or complete hair loss may take many years.[5]

Alopecia areata universalis (AU)

Alopecia areata universalis is the loss of all body hair (Figure 7). It may follow long-standing partial alopecia or its spread may be rapid occurring within several days.[5,6]

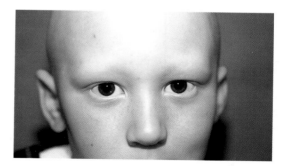

Figure 7

Alopecia areata universalis. This condition is where all body hair is lost.

Alopecia totalis/alopecia universalis (AT/AU)

According to the alopecia areata investigational assessment guidelines,[1] alopecia totalis/alopecia universalis (AT/AU) is the term now recommended to use to define AT with variable amounts of body hair loss.

Clinical associations with typical alopecia areata

Ocular changes such as cataracts and glaucoma are frequently associated with alopecia areata,[7] while nail changes, such as pitting, longitudinal ridging, irregular thickening and trachyonychia (Figure 8) occur in a high proportion of cases (cf OAA in AT/AU).[5] Other variable associations are autoimmune diseases, such as Hashimoto's thyroiditis, testicular atrophy and chromosomal alterations, especially Down's syndrome.[3]

Clinical patterns and prognosis in typical forms of alopecia areata

It is important to consider the clinical pattern in alopecia areata, for both ethical and prognostic reasons.[8,9] Poor prognosis of alopecia areata is mainly associated with childhood onset of disease, extensive alopecia, nail involvement and alopecia areata family history. Moreover, clinical studies have attempted to track the clinical course of alopecia areata in relation to a variety of factors or to determine a response to treatment. These, however, have been hampered by the lack of a method to depict clearly the type and extent of hair loss that would, in turn, facilitate pooling of data.[1]

Atypical forms of alopecia areata

Less frequent clinical forms of presentation and regrowth are possible. These are:

(1) Diffuse alopecia areata (DAA);
(2) Sisaipho;
(3) Alopecia areata type androgenetic alopecia
 — (3.1) alopecia areata type MAGA (in boys)
 — (3.2) alopecia areata type MAGA.F
 — (3.3) alopecia areata type FAGA (in girls)
 — (3.4) alopecia areata type FAGA.M;
(4) Castling phenomenon
(5) Alopecia areata type Marie-Antoinette;
(6) Perinaevoid alopecia;
(7) Targetoid hair regrowth in alopecia areata.

Diffuse alopecia areata

These patients present with a long history of slowly progressive, diffuse, non-scarring alopecia, with loss of hair density without progression to clinically recognizable alopecia areata (Figure 9).[10] A full examination and trichogram do not help in this difficult diagnosis.[3] Usually this condition appears as an advanced male or female androgenetic alopecia that is usually difficult to conceal with a change in hair style. In women, FAGA may be more difficult to diagnose than FAGA.M. In these difficult differential diagnoses, it is very useful to explore parietal and occipital areas. In contrast to MAGA or FAGA, hair loss in diffuse alopecia areata is also present in the occipital zone; this fact aids diagnosis. A scalp biopsy that shows increased miniaturized follicles and an asymmetric peribulbar lymphocytic infiltrate involving the stem cell compartment is also useful.[10]

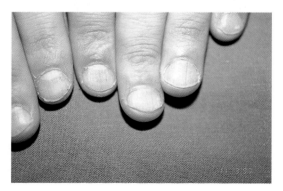

Figure 8

Trachyonychia in alopecia areata.

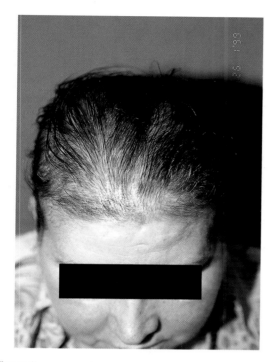

Figure 9

Diffuse alopecia areata. This condition is very difficult to diagnose.

Sisaipho

This the loss of the whole scalp hair except of the ophiasic hair line implantation. It is the opposite condition to ophiasic alopecia areata and its name is derived from the backward spelling of ophiasis. In the original paper it was described in children and adults.[11] In three patients described by Muralidhar et al,[12] their condition was associated with atopy. This rare pattern was seen by them in only 3 out of 1300 patients and they preferred to call it ophiasis inversus. The incidence in Spain is similar, being 3 cases out of 1604.[13]

The sisaipho pattern could be an evolution (Figure 10) or regrowth pattern of severe alopecia areata (Figure 11). Nevertheless, this is a form resistant to conventional treatments.[11,12]

Sisaipho may be caused by propagation of alopecia areata in centrifugal waves as postulated by Eckert et al[14] and Orecchia and Rabbiosi.[15] Tan and Delaney[16] also described marginal bands of hair regrowth during treatment of several alopecia areata patients with topical corticosteroids. This is only a hypothesis in the context of the still unknown pathogenesis of alopecia areata.

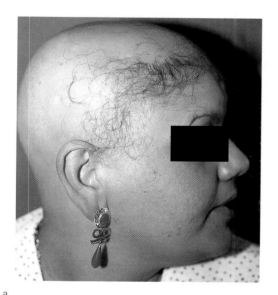

a

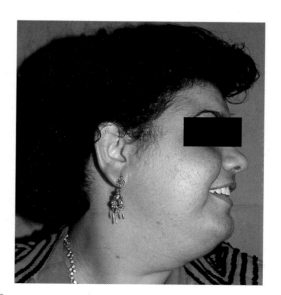

b

Figure 10

Sisaipho: **(a)** At presentation; hair is only found in the frontotemporal hair implantation line. **(b)** complete hair regrowth.

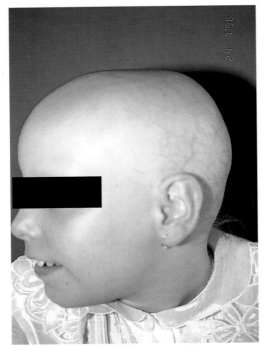

a

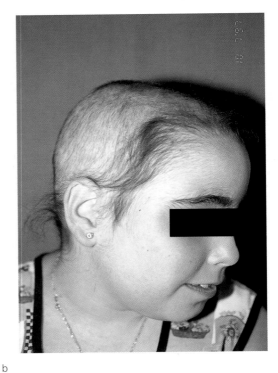

b

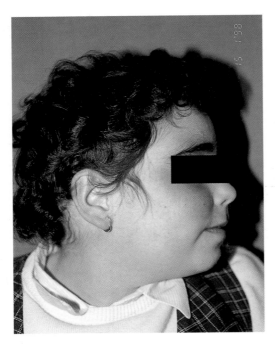

c

Figure 11

(a) Alopecia areata universalis in a 9-year-old girl. (b) Sisaipho as a regrowth form: hair is present only as a band in the hair implantation line. (c) Complete hair regrowth after 1.5 years.

Alopecia areata type MAGA

In some male alopecia areata patients, hair starts to regrow. An androgenetic alopecia (MAGA) with varying Hamilton-Ebling's scores develops, and this causes some diagnostic confusion (Figure 12). This clinical form has validity in children or teenagers with high Hamilton-grades.[3,17]

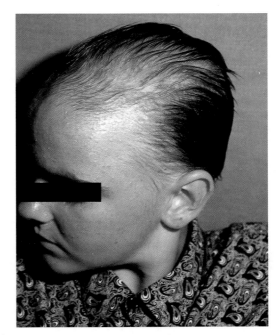

b

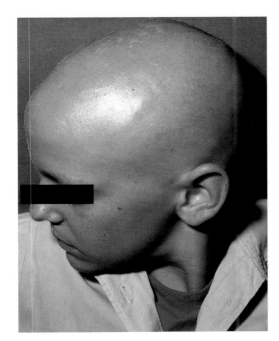

a

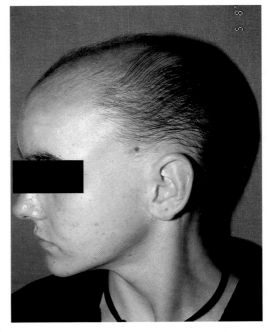

c

Figure 12

(a) Alopecia areata universalis in an 11-year-old boy. (b) Alopecia areata type MAGA: the same boy as in (a) had developed an androgenetic alopecia by the 1-year follow-up session. (c) Two years later, the same boy had advanced alopecia areata type MAGA.

Alopecia areata type MAGA.F

This pattern corresponds to some alopecia areata males whose regrowth took place with a frontovertical alopecia, keeping the frontal hair line of implantation (Figure 13). In our Department, this clinical form was interpreted as a MAGA.F type alopecia areata in only three patients, one of whom had testicular atrophy.[3]

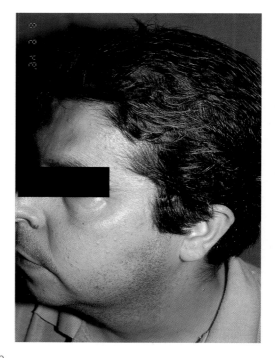

b

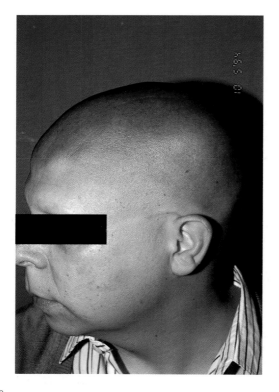

a

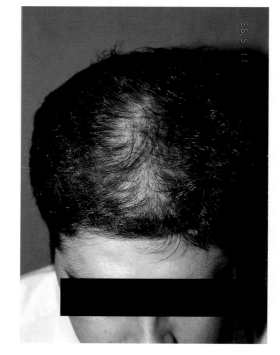

c

Figure 13

(a) Alopecia areata universalis in patient with testicular atrophy. **(b)** Complete regrowth in 4 months with corticosteroid treatment. **(c)** Alopecia areata type MAGA.F in the same patient with AA universalis whose hair regrew with a fronto-vertical alopecia.

Alopecia areata type FAGA

Women who exhibit a typical female androgenetic alopecia in their regrowth are said to have alopecia areata type FAGA. As for the male type, diagnosis is only valuable in girls (Figure 14) and female teenagers.[3] In our Department, only eight patients have been diagnosed.

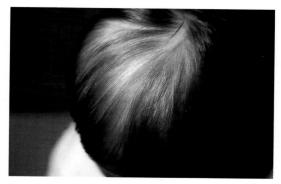

Figure 14

Alopecia areata type FAGA. This girl showed a female androgenetic alopecia in her regrowth.

Alopecia areata type FAGA.M

Some alopecia areata females underwent regrowth in a male androgenetic alopecia pattern (Figure 15). They showed frontotemporal alopecic zones. Only three patients have been seen in our Department.[17]

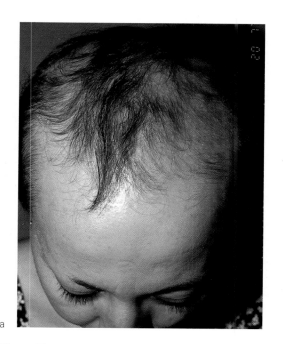

a

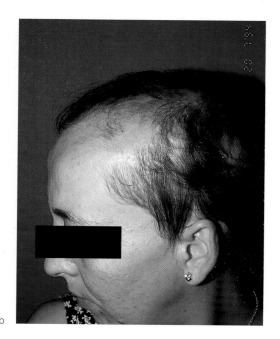

b

Figure 15

Alopecia areata type FAGA.M. This woman showed a male androgenetic alopecia in her evolution; **(a)** Frontal view; **(b)** Lateral view.

Castling phenomenon

This is the repopulation of hair in areas other than those where immunotherapy was applied.[18] This phenomenon has been described in patients treated with diphencyprone or with squaric acid dibutyl ester (SADBE).[19] Early regrowth of the eyebrows is seen in some alopecia areata universalis patients who are treated with immunotherapy only on the scalp (Figure 16).

The physiopathology of the castling phenomenon may relate to the action of the immunomodulating agent on the nerve endings of the stimulated area, with neurotransmitter released, thus explaining the remote effect.[19]

Alopecia areata type Marie-Antoinette or alopecia areata totalis for dark hair

This is a rapid whitening of all dark scalp hair.[20] This has been reported in several famous historical

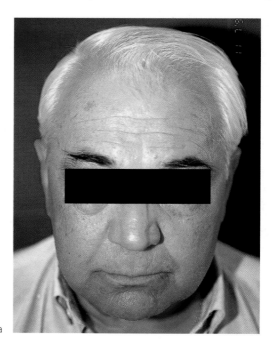

a

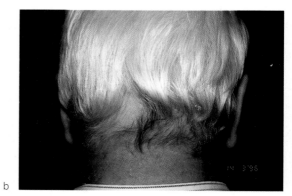

b

Figure 17

Alopecia areata totalis for dark hair. **(a)** A 60-year-old male whose scalp hair abruptly whitened but the color of his eyebrows was maintained; **(b)** The color of his back hair implantation line was preserved but there was hair loss in the ophiasic zone.

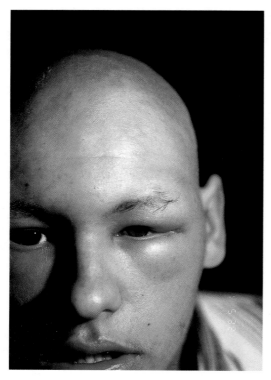

Figure 16

Castling phenomenon. This patient was treated with diphencyprone only on the scalp, but the eyebrows presented regrowth.

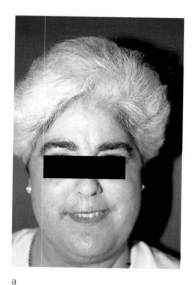
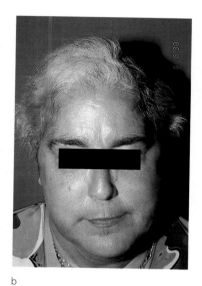
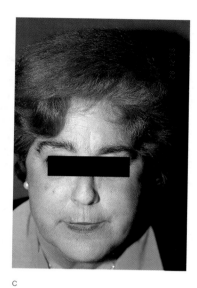

a   b   c

Figure 18

Alopecia areata type Marie-Antoinette. **(a)** 50-year-old female whose hair rapidly whitened, except for her hair implantation line, eyebrows and eyelashes; **(b)** The same patient after a second episode of hair loss; **(c)** The same patient after 6 months' treatment with biotin and zinc aspartate. This woman had dyed her hair.

personalities, such as Marie-Antoinette and Saint Thomas Moro and it was observed as a first episode of rapid whitening in the Talmud.[21] This is an exceptional form of diffuse alopecia areata with sudden telogen effluvium for dark and blond hairs. alopecia areata may selectively attack pigmented hair and cause rapid whitening. Thus, the hair appeared to 'go white' over the course of a few days;[2] indeed, the scalp hair could appear to 'turn white overnight'. Many scalp hairs are noted to 'whiten' at the same time[21] (Figures 17 and 18). The eyebrows, eyelashes and body hair were still dark, and allowed us to know the original color of the hair. Nevertheless, it is possible to observe some dark hairs in the implantation hair line (see Figures 17b and 18c). When the regrowth occurs, it is with white hairs, grey ones are lost.

McBride and Bergfeld[22] described mosaic hair color changes in two patients with extensive alopecia areata. Visually, the change is identified as patchy lightening, occasional depigmentation and whitening of existing scalp hair. They sug-gested that these changes may be the final result of localized immunological reactions against the melanocytes, thus resulting in a cytotoxic effect towards the melanocytes and the subsequent changes in color. This phenomenon may be an increase in the activity and progression of the alopecia areata.

Four patients with these features have been studied in our Department. These patients were treated with oral prednisone plus zinc aspartate and biotin. In all the cases, regrowth was observed before the end of 1 year with treatment (see Figures 17b and 18c); however, recurrence appeared immediately on discontinuing treatment (see Figure 18b).

Perinaevoid alopecia

The shedding of hair immediately surrounding a melanocytic nevus has rarely been reported but it is not very uncommon.[5,23]

Targetoid hair regrowth in alopecia areata

Several concentric hairy and alopecic circles have been seen in previously alopecic areas following therapy with intralesional cortico-steroids,[24] topical corticosteroids,[16] topical immunotherapy[15] or without treatment.[24] These cases supported the hypothesis by Eckert and co-workers[14] regarding the propagation of alopecia areata in centrifugal waves (Figure 19). This mor-phologic study of plucked hairs from concentric zones of scalp lesions has suggested that a wave of follicular damage moves centrifugally to produce expanding patches of hair loss, and that the follicles react to the damage in different ways according to the severity of stimuli. Severe damage results in the formation of exclamation-mark hair. A less severe insult may produce loss of normal club hairs at the margins of the lesions. Minimal follicular insult may result in dystropic anagen hairs, which are found at lesion margins.

This condition is thought to be more frequent than publications of its occurrence.[24]

Clinical diagnosis and treatment of atypical forms of alopecia areata

It may be important to recognize these atypical forms of presentation and regrowth because, in general, they have a poor prognosis. Diagnosis can, however, be difficult and may require a scalp biopsy because of problems with differential diag-nosis, to exclude conditions such as trichotilloma-nia, telogen effluvium, androgenetic alopecia, loose anagen syndrome, syphilis, tinea capitis, and congenital triangular temporal alopecia.[25–28]

Moreover, at first sight, atypical forms could be candidates for a more aggressive treatment, such as immunotherapy, anthralin, topical minoxidil or corticosteroids, courses of systemic corticosteroids, PUVA and oral cyclosporin A.[29] Nevertheless, they are usually resistant to these treatments, especially in children, and frequently relapse after response to treatment. Risks of long-term therapy, therefore, preclude these approaches. In some cases, therefore, a full explanation and support psychotherapy will be of far greater value.

More clinical studies of alopecia areata are needed to establish the prevalence of these atyp-ical forms of alopecia areata world-wide.

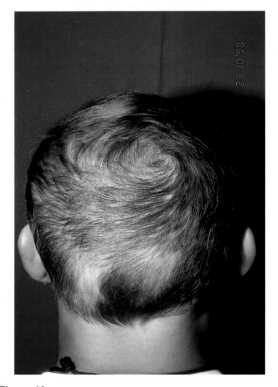

Figure 19

Targetoid hair regrowth. Concentric alopecic and hairy zones can be seen.

References

1. Olsen E, Hordinski M, McDonald-Hull S, et al.: Alopecia areata investigational assessment guide-lines. *J Am Acad Dermatol* 1999; **40**: 242–246.
2. Dawber R, Van Neste D: Alopecia areata. In: Dawber R, Van Neste D (eds.). *Hair and Scalp Disorders*. London, Martin Dunitz, 1995: 169–190.
3. Camacho F: Alopecia areata. Clinical features. Der-matopathology. In: Camacho F, Montagna W (eds.). *Trichology. Diseases of the Pilosebaceous Follicle*. Madrid, Aula Médica, 1997: 417–440.

4. Schwartz RA, Janniger CK: Alopecia areata. *Cutis* 1997; **59**: 238–241.
5. Dawber RP, Ebling FJ, Wojnarowska F: Disorders of hair. In: Champion RH, Burton JL, Ebling FJG (eds.). *Textbook of Dermatology*. London, Blackwell Scientific, 1992: 2586–2595.
6. Baden HP: Alopecia areata. In: Baden HP (ed.). *Diseases of the Hair and Nails*. Chicago, Mosby Year Book, 1987: 134–143.
7. Tosti A, Colombati S, Caponeri GM, et al.: Ocular abnormalities occurring with alopecia areata. *Dermatologica* 1985; **170**: 69–73.
8. Price VH, Colombe BW: Heritable factors distinguish two types of alopecia areata. *Dermatol Clin* 1996; **14**: 679–689.
9. García-Hernández MJ, Rodríguez-Pichardo A, Camacho F: Multivariate analysis in alopecia areata: risk factors. *Arch Dermatol* 1999; **135**: 998–999.
10. Kossard S: Diffuse alopecia with stem cell folliculitis: chronic diffuse alopecia areata or a distinct entity? *Am J Dermatopathol* 1999; **21**: 46–50.
11. Muñoz MA, Camacho F: A new form of presentation of alopecia areata. *Arch Dermatol* 1996; **132**: 1255–1256.
12. Muralidhar S, Sharma VK, Kaur S: Ophiasis inversus: a rare pattern of alopecia areata. *Pediatr Dermatol* 1998; **15**: 326–327.
13. Muñoz MA, Camacho F: Sisaipho. Why ophiasis inversus? *Pediatr Dermatol* 1999; **16**: 76.
14. Eckert J, Church RE, Ebling FJ: The pathogenesis of alopecia areata. *Br J Dermatol* 1968; **80**: 203.
15. Orecchia G, Rabbiosi G: Patterns of hair regrowth in alopecia areata. *Dermatologica* 1988; **176**: 270–272.
16. Tan RSH, Delaney TJ: Circular regrowth in alopecia areata. *Br J Dermatol* 1975; **92**: 233–234.
17. Muñoz MA, Camacho F: Regrowth of alopecia areata simulating the pattern of androgenetic alopecia. *Arch Dermatol* 1997; **133**: 114–115.
18. Van der Steen PHM, Happle R: The 'castling' phenomenon in topical immunotherapy of alopecia areata. *Eur J Dermatol* 1994; **4**: 161.
19. Cicero RL, Micali G, Sapuppo A: Paradoxical hair regrowth during the treatment of severe alopecia areata with acid dibutyl ester (SADBE). *Eur J Dermatol* 1993; **3**: 321.
20. Jelinek JE: Sudden whitening of the hair. *Bull NY Acad Med* 1972; **48**: 1003–1013.
21. Goldenhersh MA: Rapid whitening of the hair first reported in the Talmud. *Am J Dermatopathol* 1992; **14**: 367–368.
22. McBride AK, Bergfeld WF: Mosaic hair color changes in alopecia areata. *Cleve Clin J Med* 1990; **57**: 354–356.
23. Achenbach RE: Clínica de la alopecia areata. *Rev Argent Dermatol* 1996; **77**: 208–214.
24. del Rio E: Targetoid hair regrowth in alopecia areata: the wave theory. *Arch Dermatol* 1998; **134**: 1042–1043.
25. Hoss DM, Grant-Kels JM: Diagnosis: alopecia areata or not? *Semin Cut Med Surg* 1999; **18**: 84–90.
26. Elston DM, McCollough ML, Bergfeld WF, Liranzano MO, Heibel M: Eosinophils in fibrous tracts and near hair bulbs: a helpful diagnostic feature of alopecia areata. *J Am Acad Dermatol* 1997; **37**: 101–106.
27. Palacios A: Diagnóstico diferencial de la alopecia areata. *Rev Argent Dermatol* 1996; **77**: 222–223.
28. García-Hernández MJ, Rodríguez-Pichardo A, Camacho F: Congenital triangular temporal alopecia (Brauer nevus). *Pediatr Dermatol* 1995; **12**: 301–303.
29. Shapiro J, Lui H, Tron V, Ho V: Systemic cyclosporine and low-dose prednisone in the treatment of chronic severe alopecia areata: a clinical and immunopathologic evaluation. *J Am Acad Dermatol* 1997; **36**: 114–117.

Section V

SYSTEMIC DISEASE

22
Hair anomalies and syndrome recognition

Rudolf Happle

Introduction

The various hair shaft abnormalities that are inherited as mendelian phenotypes can be divided into three different groups. The first group includes hair shaft abnormalities that are not associated with defects of other organs. The second group represents hair shaft defects heralding complex syndromes. The third group comprises hair shaft abnormalities that may or may not be associated with other defects; this group is particularly large and has an important impact with regard to differential diagnosis.

Non-specific and non-diagnostic features

Trichorrhexis nodosa

Trichorrhexis nodosa is the commonest form of hair breakage. This type of breakage can be compared with that observed in green wood. It resembles two brushes put into one another (Figure 1).

It is important to be aware of the fact that any normal hair shaft may show one or multiple nodes corresponding to trichorrhexis nodosa. These nodes can be caused by twisting or rubbing the hair in the form of a tic nerveux. Conversely, many inherited hair diseases show increased breakage in the form of trichorrhexis nodosa, and no specific diagnostic conclusion can be drawn from this phenomenon. Clinicians should refrain from a diagnosis such as 'trichorrhexis nodosa congenita', for the simple reason that such entity does not exist. The presence of many lesions of trichorrhexis nodosa should

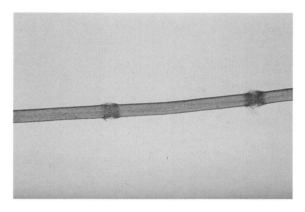

Figure 1

Trichorrhexis nodosa: a common type of hair breakage without diagnostic significance.

stimulate the search for a specific diagnosis that may be an acquired or hereditary disorder.

Isolated hair shaft abnormalities

Monilethrix

Definition
Monilethrix is a structural anomaly of the hair shaft characterized by regular 'nodes' of normal thickness and 'internodes' of abnormal thinning (Figure 2).

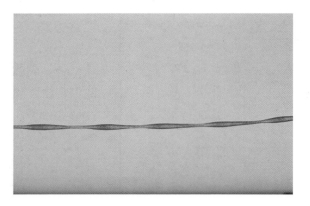

Figure 2

Monilethrix.

Differential diagnosis
The trait should not be confused with pseudo-monilethrix (see later text).

Course and prognosis
In many cases, the increased fragility of the hair shafts tends to improve with age. Adults who take care not to traumatize too much of their hair by combing and grooming may show scalp hair of almost normal appearance. In other patients, however, this trait remains visible throughout life.

Prevention
From a physician's view, the trait appears too mild to justify prenatal diagnosis. Nevertheless, there was a severely affected woman who decided to refrain from reproduction because of the psychosocial burden of this disease. She took this decision after having been informed on the mendelian mode of transmission of this trait.

Pseudo-monilethrix

Definition
This disease is quite different from monilethrix. The affected hair shafts vaguely resemble monilethrix but show 'nodes' in an irregular distribution. A common feature of pseudo-monilethrix is increased brittleness.

Etiology
The disease is inherited as an autosomal dominant trait. The underlying gene has been mapped to chromosome 12q11-q13. Various mutations within a keratin gene (hHb6, hHb1) have been elucidated. Zlotogorski et al.[1] described a family in which both parents had monilethrix and three of their children were severely affected because they were homozygous for an hHb6 mutation.

Clinical features
The hair in monilethrix is abnormally brittle. The occipital region is particularly affected, and follicular hyperkeratosis and inflammation is often present in this area.[2]

Laboratory examination
To establish the diagnosis, it is important to cut the abnormally short hair shafts, and not to pluck them. Light microscopical examination shows the typical regular nodes and internodes. Breakage occurs always in the internode regions.

Diagnostic clue
When a family is examined, it should be borne in mind that, in adults, the scalp hair may look completely normal, both macroscopically and microscopically. Notwithstanding, a careful examination of body hair using a magnifying glass may reveal some typical beaded hair shafts.[3]

Etiology
According to the report of Bentley-Philipps and Bayles,[4] pseudo-monilethrix is inherited as an autosomal dominant trait.

Clinical features
Affected individuals complain of increased 'weathering' and brittleness of hair. On microscopical examination, the hair shafts show irregular 'nodes' or indentations. In contrast to monilethrix, the nodes of pseudo-monilethrix are caused by mechanical trauma.

Laboratory examination
It is important that every single hair shaft is mounted separately on a microscope slide. If a multitude of irregular 'nodes' is seen, a diagnosis of pseudo-monilethrix should be considered. If several hair shafts have been mounted on a microscope slide and covered with a coverslip, the finding of several 'nodes' is non-diagnostic,

because the 'nodes' result from crossing of normal hair shafts.

Diagnostic clue
In patients with increased brittleness of hair, the physician should not perform a hair pluck but should cut an abnormally short hair shaft.

Differential diagnosis
The irregular pattern of pseudo-monilethrix can easily be distinguished from the regular nodes and internodes of monilethrix.

Treatment
Individuals affected with pseudo-monilethrix should be informed that their hair shafts are particularly weak and that, for this reason, any trauma by aggressive combing or hair dressing should be avoided. When this advice is followed, the appearance of the hair will improve.

Pili annulati

Definition
Pili annulati are characterized by regular bright and dark bands, giving the hair a characteristic spangled sheen.

Etiology
This is an autosomal dominant trait.

Clinical features
When viewed by reflected light the hair looks spangled.

Laboratory examination
Light microscopical examination of hair shafts shows bands of dark and bright areas (Figure 3). Electron microscopical studies have shown that the bright bands represent areas containing abnormal cavities filled with air.[5]

Treatment
No treatment is needed for this innocuous abnormality.

Pili bifurcati

Definition
Pili bifurcati are hair shafts that show ramifications forming two separate shafts with a complete circumferential cuticula. Such bifurcations run a short distance and then the rami fuse again.

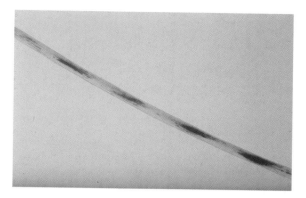

Figure 3

Microscopical appearance of pili anulati.

Etiology
The mendelian basis of the trait is so far unclear. The author has observed two siblings with unaffected parents. It appears too early to draw any conclusion regarding the mode of transmission.

Clinical features
The hair may be abnormally brittle.

Laboratory examination
Many hair shafts should be examined under the microscope. In addition to the typical bifurcations, many lesions of trichorrhexis nodosa may be observed outside the regions of bifurcation, indicating that the increased brittleness cannot be explained by the bifurcations alone.

Diagnostic clue
Pili bifurcati are often overlooked. Clinicians should bear this rare hair defect in mind.

Hair shaft abnormalities heralding a syndrome

Trichorrhexis invaginata

Definition
In trichorrhexis invaginata, which is also called bamboo hair, the characteristic nodes are composed of two parts. The proximal part forms a

tulip-like socket, and the distal part shows a ball-shaped end compressed into this socket.

Etiology
Trichorrhexis invaginata is a sign of Comèl-Netherton syndrome, which is transmitted as an autosomal recessive trait.[6]

Clinical features
The hair is abnormally brittle. Newborn patients may show congenital ichthyosiform erythroderma, while infants may show failure to thrive and may die during the first year of life. Surviving children develop either a diffuse ichthyosis or a peculiar skin disorder, which is characterized by linear scaling lesions in the form of ichthyosis linearis circumflexa. Characteristically, the patients show signs and symptoms similar to atopy, with increased levels of IgE. A typical feature is intolerance to nuts.

Laboratory examinations
In patients with ichthyosiform erythroderma, a routine examination of hair shafts should be performed. Such hair shafts should not be plucked but shaved.

Diagnostic clue
In some patients, the scalp hair may appear completely normal, but careful examination of the eyebrows using a magnifying glass may show some nodes. When these hair shafts are cut, the characteristic bamboo hair is found (Figure 4).

Differential diagnosis
The microscopical abnormality of the hair shaft is pathognomonic, excluding all other diagnostic possibilities. However, without a hair shaft examination, many patients with Comèl-Netherton syndrome are erroneously taken as having therapy-resistant atopic eczema.

Course and prognosis
When the diagnosis is established in a newborn, the prognosis is somber because one-half of the children will die from an unclassifiable failure to thrive. When the children have completed their first year of life, life-expectancy appears to be almost normal; however, most patients are severely handicapped by this disorder.

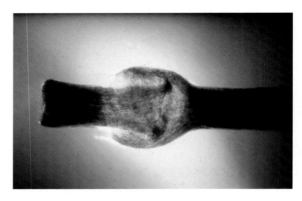

Figure 4

The characteristic bamboo hair of trichorrhexis invaginata as found in an eyebrow hair.

Treatment
The skin should be treated with smoothening creams. For the hair defect, no specific treatment is known.

Prevention
Appropriate genetic counseling should be given to the parents of an affected child.

Trichothiodystrophy

Definition
Trichothiodystrophy is a term applied to sulfur-deficient brittle hair showing characteristic microscopical features.

Etiology
This hair shaft abnormality is a sign of various autosomal recessive syndromes.[7]

Clinical features
The scalp hair is abnormally fine, scarce and brittle. Patients are mentally retarded and may show other abnormalities such as short stature, abnormal facial appearance, ichthyosis, increased proneness to infections, or hypogonadism (see differential diagnosis).

Laboratory examinations
On routine microscopical examination, the hair shafts show an undulating contour and folding

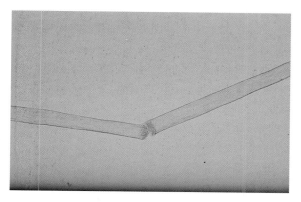

Figure 5

Trichothiodystrophy. The hair shaft shows an undulating contour and trichoschisis.

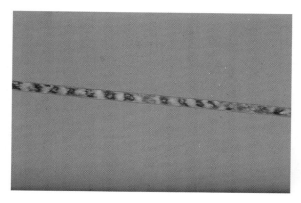

Figure 6

Trichothiodystrophy. When examined between polarizing filters, alternating bright and dark regions are seen.

along their axis. A very characteristic feature is trichoschisis representing clean transverse fractures that are dissimilar from common trichorrhexis nodosa (Figure 5). When examined between polarizing filters, the hair shafts show characteristic alternating bright and dark regions that change when the filters are moved (Figure 6). Scanning electron microscopy reveals a flat, ribbon-like hair shaft. The structure of the cuticula appears to be abnormal. Biochemical analysis of hair shafts shows a decreased amount of sulfur-containing amino acids such as cysteine and proline.

Diagnostic clue
In children showing brittle hair and mental retardation, microscopical examination of hair shafts by use of polarizing filters should be performed.

Differential diagnosis
Trichothiodystrophy is a sign of several different autosomal recessive syndromes such as Amish brittle hair syndrome (BIDS = Brittle hair, Intellectual impairment, Decreased fertility, Short stature); Tay syndrome (similar features plus congenital ichthyosis); and PIBIDS syndrome (Photosensitivity and Ichthyosis associated with the features of BIDS syndrome).[6]

Hair shaft abnormalities that may or may not be associated with other features

Uncombable hair

Unruly and uncombable hair is observed in several different monogenic disorders such as spun glass hair (pili trianguli et canaliculi), hypotrichosis of Marie Unna, AEC syndrome and EEC syndrome (see later text for definition of AEC and EEC).

Pili trianguli et canaliculi (spun glass hair)

Definition
This isolated hair shaft abnormality is characterized by irregular twisting of hair that is impossible to comb in a given direction.[8]

Etiology
The abnormality is presumably inherited as an autosomal dominant trait.

Clinical features
Usually, the mother complains that the hair of her child is unruly and impossible to comb. Clinical examination shows that the frizzy appearance

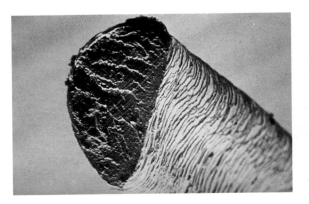

Figure 7

Pili trianguli et canaliculi (spun glass hair).

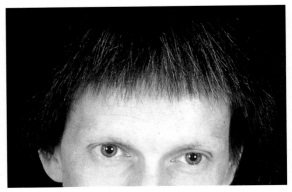

Figure 8

Hypotrichosis congenita of Marie Unna: children and adolescents show uncombable hair reminiscent of an ill-fitting wig.

is caused by the fact that the hair shafts change the direction at irregular intervals along their axis.

Laboratory examination
When examined between polarizing filters, the irregular changes of the hair shafts can be seen. Cross-sections of hair shafts show triangular or kidney-shaped configurations (Figure 7).

Differential diagnosis
It should be borne in mind that there are other forms of uncombable hair (see later text).

Course and prognosis
The trait tends to improve and to disappear with age. This explains why the abnormality is described almost exclusively in children.

Treatment
No treatment is needed for this innocuous abnormality. The parents should be informed that the hair tends to become normal after puberty.

Hypotrichosis congenita of Marie Unna

Definition
This is a particular form of uncombable hair associated with progressive alopecia.

Etiology
The disorder is transmitted as an autosomal dominant trait.[9]

Clinical features
In affected children, the scalp hair is unruly and uncombable, resulting in an appearance suggesting an ill-fitting wig (Figure 8). After puberty, alopecia develops at the crown of the head and may result, over years, in complete hairlessness.

Laboratory examination
Knotting of a hair shaft results in a characteristic wire-like microscopical appearance. On scanning electron microscopic examination, the hair shafts show flattening and irregular twisting.

Diagnostic clue
Paradoxically, affected children show a particularly thick and strong-looking scalp hair. Within a given family, this is an important diagnostic sign.[10]

AEC syndrome

Definition
The abbreviation AEC means Ankyloblepharon, Ectodermal dysplasia, and Cleft palate.[11]

Etiology
The disorder is inherited as an autosomal dominant trait.

Clinical features
A typical facial appearance with a small nose and low-set ears is present. During early infancy and early childhood, affected individuals show scalp hair of unruly, wiry texture. During the first months or years of life, periods of non-infectious inflammation involve the scalp and result in irreversible hair loss (Figure 9). The cleft palate may be associated with a cleft lip. It is important to know that the ankyloblepharon filiforme adnatum may go unnoticed because the bridging tissue between the upper and lower eyelid is usually separated already in the delivery room. AEC syndrome is an ectodermal dysplasia of the hypohidrotic type, and this explains why the skin is rather dry. Absence of the lacrimal puncta results in chronic inflammation of the eyelids.

Laboratory examination
The microscopical abnormalities of the hair shafts are non-specific.

Diagnostic clue
The diagnosis should be established on the basis of a characteristic combination of cutaneous and extracutaneous features.

Differential diagnosis
Some authors believe that the Rapp-Hodgkin syndrome is a different phenotype. However, the only distinguishing feature is absence of ankyloblepharon, and this trait is, therefore, most likely identical to the AEC syndrome. In contrast, AEC syndrome should be distinguished from EEC syndrome (see below).

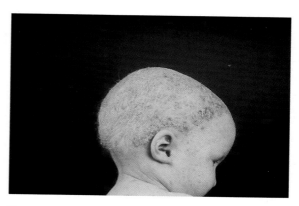

Figure 9

AEC syndrome. The uncombable hair is lost during periods of non-infectious inflammation involving the scalp.

Clinical features
The hair is unruly, scanty and hypopigmented. The disorder resembles AEC syndrome but can be distinguished by the presence of lobster claw deformities of the hands or feet.

Laboratory findings
The hair shaft deformities are non-specific and not diagnostic.

Differential diagnosis
The EEC syndrome should be distinguished from the AEC syndrome. It is important to bear in mind that in some affected members of a family with the EEC syndrome, the characteristic ectrodactyly may be absent.[12]

EEC syndrome

Definition
The abbreviation EEC means Ectrodactyly, Ectodermal dysplasia, and Cleft lip and palate.

Etiology
The syndrome is transmitted as an autosomal dominant trait.

Curly hair

Curly or woolly hair may occur as an isolated abnormality or as part of a syndrome.

Woolly hair as an isolated abnormality

Definition
The occurrence in Caucasians of curly hair similar to that observed in black Africans is called woolly hair.

Etiology
Reported pedigrees suggest inheritance as an autosomal dominant trait.[13]

Clinical features
The hair has a characteristic woolly appearance.

Laboratory examination
No diagnostic measures are necessary.

Differential diagnosis
Curly and woolly hair should be distinguished from pili trianguli et canaliculi.

Treatment
No treatment is indicated because woolly hair is not a disorder but a trait within normal human variability.

Cardiofaciocutaneous syndrome (Noonan's syndrome)

Definition
The disorder is characterized by Noonan-like facial appearance, woolly hair, keratosis pilaris, multiple melanocytic nevi, cardiac defects, and mental retardation.[14]

Etiology
The syndrome is inherited as an autosomal dominant trait.

Clinical features
The scalp hair is tightly curled, and the face shows keratosis pilaris atrophicans, which also involves the eyebrows in the form of 'ulerythema ophryogenes'. The lips are unusually thick resulting in a 'Noonan-like' appearance. Multiple melanocytic nevi may involve the trunk and the limbs. Among the associated cardiac anomalies, stenosis of the pulmonary artery branch is especially frequent.

Laboratory examination
Microscopic examination of hair shafts does not show any specific abnormality. A careful search for cardiac defects should, however, be performed.

Differential diagnosis
In the past, Noonan's syndrome and cardiofaciocutaneous syndrome have been taken as separate entities; however, a comparison of clinical reports suggests that these traits are identical.

CHANDS

Definition
The term CHANDS stands for Curly Hair, Ankyloblepharon, and Nail Dysplasia Syndrome.

Etiology
Baughman[15] suggested autosomal dominant inheritance, but a re-evaluation of CHANDS indicated that autosomal recessive inheritance is far more likely.[16]

Clinical features
Affected individuals show rather mildly curled hair, as well as mildly hypoplastic fingernails. At birth, the eyelids are fused by adhesions.

Laboratory findings
Microscopical examination of the curly hair shafts does not reveal specific abnormalities.

Differential diagnosis
With the exception of curly hair, the clinical features observed in cardiofaciocutaneous syndrome are different.

Pili torti

Pili torti are characterized by tight twisting of the hair shaft resulting in a corkscrew appearance (Figure 10). It should be noted that some irregular twists are not sufficient to establish a diagnosis of pili torti. When this definition is applied, pili torti will turn out to be a very rare abnormality.

Isolated pili torti

Definition
This trait is characterized by unruly hair showing a corkscrew-like appearance on microscopical examination.[17]

Etiology
The mendelian background is not quite clear. Both autosomal dominant and recessive inheritance has been suggested.

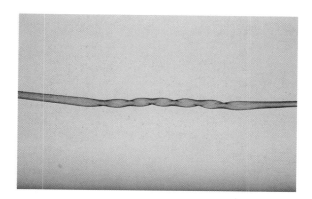

Figure 10

Typical tight twisting of pili torti in a case of Menkes' syndrome.

Clinical features
The hair is brittle and short. Bilateral neurosensory deafness is present.

Laboratory findings
Light microscopy and scanning electron microscopy show twisting and torsions of ribbon-like hair shafts. Remarkably, a report by Voigtländer[18] does not show the abnormalities of true pili torti.

Diagnostic clue
An appropriate examination of hair shafts may help to establish a rare syndrome characterized by hearing loss.

Differential diagnosis
Trichothiodystrophy can be ruled out by microscopical examination of hair shafts with the use of polarizing filters.

Menkes' syndrome

Definition
Menkes' syndrome is caused by a defect in copper metabolism and characterized by severe mental and physical retardation.[19] It is also referred to as Menkes' disease; this is discussed more extensively by Díaz-Pérez in Chapter 26.

Etiology
The disorder is an X-linked recessive trait occurring almost exclusively in boys. Female carriers may be very mildly affected. The underlying gene has been mapped to Xq13. The disease is caused by a defect of an ATPase responsible for $Cu^{(2+)}$ transport.

Clinical features
Affected male infants show scarce, brittle and kinky hair. They suffer from severe mental retardation, epileptic seizures, hypothermia and bone defects and usually die during the first years of life. Recently a treatment for this fatal disease has been proposed (see *Treatment*).

Laboratory findings
Microscopical examination of hair shafts may help to establish the diagnosis. Irregular kinking, numerous fractures, and the typical tight twisting of pili torti (see Figure 10) are found. In the past, the twisting has erroneously been described in

Laboratory examination
Microscopical examination shows flattened, regularly twisted hair shafts.

Differential diagnosis
From the literature one gains the impression that pili torti have been overdiagnosed in the past. In fact, many cases may simply represent examples of pili trianguli et canaliculi. Furthermore, an unexperienced physician may confuse pili torti with monilethrix, but careful examination will show the difference between twisting and the nodes and internodes of monilethrix.

Treatment
Since affected individuals may have especially brittle hair, they should be advised to avoid aggressive combing or grooming.

Bjørnstad syndrome

Definition
The disorder is characterized by the association of pili torti with neurosensory deafness.

Etiology
Bjørnstad syndrome is inherited as an autosomal recessive trait.

several textbooks as 'monilethrix', but monilethrix never occurs in Menkes' syndrome. Other diagnostic measures, such as evaluation of copper metabolism, are a task of the pediatrician.

Differential diagnosis
Trichothiodystrophy can be distinguished easily by examination of hair shafts. In clinical practice, isolated pili torti will not constitute a problem of differential diagnosis.

Treatment
Recently, a therapeutic approach in the form of a particular diet has been proposed, but the long-term results appear to be disappointing.

References

1. Zlotogorski A, Harev L, Glaser B: Monilethrix: A keratin hHb6 mutation is co-dominant with variable expression. *Exper Dermatol* 1998; **7**: 268–272.
2. Bentley-Phillips B: Monilethrix and pseudomonilethrix. In: Orfanos CE, Happle R (eds.). *Hair and Hair Diseases.* Berlin, Springer Verlag, 1990: 423–441.
3. Hamm H, Echternacht-Happle K, Happle R: Monilethrix: ausschließlicher Befall der Körperbehaarung. *Z Hautkr* 1984; **59**: 1177–1178.
4. Bentley-Phillips B, Bayles MAH: Pseudomonilethrix. *Br J Dermatol* 1975; **92**: 113–115.
5. Price VH, Thomas RS, Jones FT: Pseudopili annulati. An unusual variant of normal hair. *Arch Dermatol* 1970; **102**: 354–358.
6. Traupe H: The Ichthyoses. *A Guide to Clinical Diagnosis, Genetic Counseling, and Therapy.* Berlin, Springer, 1989: 168–178.
7. Happle R, Traupe H, Gröbe H, Bonsmann G: The Tay syndrome (congenital ichthyosis with trichothiodystrophy). *Eur J Pediatr* 1984; **141**: 147–152.
8. Dupré A, Bonafé JL, Litoux F, Victor M: Le syndrome des cheveux incoiffables: pili trianguli et canaliculi. *Ann Dermatol Venereol* 1978; **105**: 627–630.
9. Spiegl B, Hundeiker M: Hypotrichosis congenita hereditaria: Autosomal dominante generalisierte Hypotrichose mit Pili torti (Hypotrichosis congenita hereditaria Marie Unna). *Fortschr Med* 1979; **97**: 2018–2022.
10. Happle R: Genetic defects involving the hair. In: Orfanos CE, Happle R (eds.). *Hair and Hair Diseases.* Berlin, Springer, 1990: 325–362.
11. Hay RJ, Wells RS: The syndrome of ankyloblepharon, ectodermal defects and cleft lip and palate: an autosomal dominant condition. *Br J Dermatol* 1976; **94**: 277–289.
12. Küster W, Majewski F, Meinecke P: EEC syndrome without ectrodactyly? Report of eight cases. *Clin Genet* 1985; **28**: 130–135.
13. Hutchinson PE, Cairns RJ, Wells RS: Woolly hair: clinical and general aspects. *Trans St Johns Hosp Dermatol Soc* 1974; **60**: 160–177.
14. Neild VA, Pegum JS, Wells RS: The association of keratosis pilaris atrophicans and woolly hair, with and without Noonan's syndrome. *Br J Dermatol* 1984; **110**: 357–362.
15. Baughman FA: CHANDS: the curly hair-ankyloblepharon-nail dysplasia syndrome. *Birth Defects* 1971; **7/8**: 100–102.
16. Toriello HV, Lindstrom JA, Waterman DF, Baughman FA: Re-evaluation of CHANDS. *J Med Genet* 1979; **16**: 316–317.
17. Ronchese F: Twisted hairs (pili torti). *Arch Dermatol Syphilol (Chicago)* 1932; **26**: 98–109.
18. Voigtländer V: Pili torti with deafness (Bjørnstad syndrome): report of a family. *Dermatologica* 1979; **159**: 50–54.
19. Menkes JH: Kinky hair disease. *Pediatrics* 1972; **50**: 181–183.

23
New genetic diseases characterized by hypotrichosis

Ramon Grimalt

Introduction

Most of the congenital and hereditary hair shaft abnormalities were well described many years ago in terms of clinical and microscopic characteristics. The past knowledge and current traits identified for specific hair abnormalities facilitate targeted topical selective gene therapy being developed for hair follicle faults. Substantial progress has been made in our knowledge of genes that control normal and abnormal development, and the search is on to define the genes implicated in hair diseases. It is not the purpose of this chapter to cover all hypotrichotic syndromes. Most classified abnormalities are included; and with regard to new research we have specifically selected those hair disorders with new undescribed aspects to be developed.

Classification

There have been numerous attempts to classify the conditions characterised by congenital alopecia or hypotrichosis. The classification proposed by Bonnet in 1892[1] has been used widely and was said to be based on embryological principles. Bonnet proposed three main groups:

(1) Congenital absence of hair, with associated defects of teeth and nails;
(2) Congenital absence of hair with normal teeth and nails;
(3) Congenital absence of hair with partial or complete recovery at puberty.

In 1922 Cockayne[2] attempting a more critical analysis proposed a working classification that allowed the known syndromes to be identified, and provided a provisional status for those not yet characterised. Cockayne's classification was modified by Muller in 1973[3] as follows:

(1) Congenital alopecia or hypotrichosis without associated defects;
(2) Congenital alopecia or hypotrichosis as a major feature of well-defined hereditary syndromes;
(3) Congenital alopecia or hypotrichosis as a major feature of uncharacterised hereditary syndromes;
(4) Congenital alopecia or hypotrichosis as a minor or inconstant feature of hereditary syndromes.

In 1981, after the Berlin Congress, Sâlamon[4] proposed a classification for the global problem of hair loss that probably has been considered one of the most useful for the study of congenital hypotrichosis. He divided them into four groups (Table 1).

In this chapter, we follow the practical classification based on clinical observation proposed by Camacho[5] (Table 2). Since the clinical manifestations present in most groups of congenital hypotrichosis are much too complex and manifold to fit into the rigid framework of a classification, any classification of congenital and hereditary alopecia must be tentative and its value largely didactic.

It is not the purpose of this chapter to cover all hypotrichotic syndromes. We will classify most of them, and based on the new literature references, we selected some of them to be described.

Table 1   Sâlamon classification of hypotrichosis and alopecia.[4]

(1)   Genetically determined hypotrichosis of hair loss as main symptom
    1.1   Without associated symptoms
        (a)   Autosomal dominant phenotypes
              Total hypotrichosis of Pajtas
              Numerous families described by Abraham, Petersen et al.
              Some cases of alopecia areata
        (b)   Autosomal recessive phenotypes
              Numerous families described by Henckel, Tillmann, Baer
              Dyskeratosis of the hair shaft (Porter)
        (c)   Probably multifactorial determination
              Androgenetic alopecia
    1.2   Without associated symptoms
        (a)   Autosomal dominant phenotype
              Hydrotic type of ectodermal dysplasia
        (b)   X-Chromosomal recessive phenotype
              Anhydrotic ectodermal dysplasia
        (c)   In-between cases
        (d)   Complex abnormalities in isolated cases with hypotrichosis

(2)   Genetically determined syndromes with changes of physical or chemical properties of hair and hypotrichosis or hair loss, as the only or main symptom
    2.1   Autosomal dominant
            Monilethrix
            Alopecia with curly hair (Touraine and Lambergeon)
            Marie Unna syndrome
    2.2   Autosomal recessive
            Netherton syndrome
            Hypotrichosis with curly hair and other disorders (Sâlamon)
            Trichorrhexis congenita (Wolf et al.)
            Hypotrichosis, hair disorders, scars of scalp, and cornea, congenital cardiac anomaly etc. (Lazovic et al.)
    2.3   Autosomal dominant or autosomal recessive
            Pili torti

(3)   Hypotrichosis or alopecia in genodermatoses
    3.1   Autosomal dominant:
            Pachionychia congenita syndrome
            Milia hypotrichosis syndrome
            Congenital ectodermal dysplasia with cataract
            Aplasia cutis congenital capillitii
    3.2   Autosomal recessive
            Acrodermatitis enteropathica
            Erythrodermia ichthyosiformis congenita sicca
            Psoriasiform ichthyosis
            Erythrodermia ichthyosiformis congenital, deaf, mutism, hypotrichosis, and hydrosis (Sâlamon et al.)
            Rothmund syndrome
            Progeria
            Werner syndrome
            Epidermolysis bullosa polyplastica
            Hypotrichosis nail and other anomalies (Sâlamon et al.)
            Typhus maculatus of bullous hereditary dystrophy (Mendes da Costa)
    2.3   X-Chromosomal recessive
            Keratosis follicularis spinulosa decalvans
    2.4   X-Chromosomal with lethality of hemizygotes
            Bloch-Sulzberger syndrome
            Focal dermal hypoplasia (Golz)

(4)   Hypotrichosis or alopecia in other genetically determined syndromes
    4.1   Autosomal dominant
            Oculo dental digital syndrome
            Popliteal web syndrome
            Ullmo syndrome
    4.2   X-chromosomal dominant
            Orofacial digital syndrome

4.3   Autosomal recessive syndromes

4.4   X-chromosomal recessive

Genodermatoses with non-scarring hypotrichosis

With alterations to the skeleton

Trichorhinophalangeal syndrome type I

Trichorhinophalangeal syndrome (TRPS) comprises a distinctive combination of hair, facial and bony abnormalities, with variable expression. It is characterised clinically by the presence of a variable hypotrichosis, bulbous nose, coniform epiphyses, prognatia and mandibular hypoplasia (Figure 1).

The hair alterations consist of a diffuse alopecia with a broad forehead and a partial alopecia of the external third of the eyelashes. Scanning electronmicroscopic studies of the hair reveal flattened hair with an elliptical pattern on transverse section. The mechanical behaviour of the hair might also be abnormal, with a significant increase in the viscous parameter, indicating a decreased intermolecular bridging within the keratin matrix.[6]

Trichorhinophalangeal syndrome type II (Langer-Giedion syndrome)

Patients with trichorhinophalangeal syndrome type II (Langer-Giedion syndrome) usually present with hypotrichosis of the scalp hair, an abnormally bulbous nose and redundant skin as the type I, plus multiple cartilaginous exostoses. In a recent article by Lu et al.[7] associated alterations to this syndrome, including aplasia of the

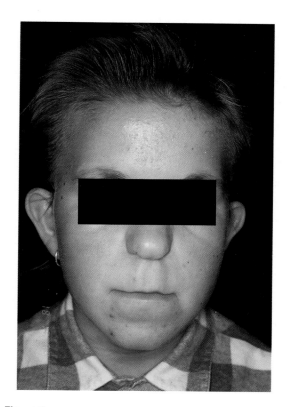

Figure 1

Trichorhinophalangeal syndrome: hypotrichosis, bulbous nose, prognatia and mandibular hypoplasia.

Table 2   Camacho's classification of alopecia and hypotrichosis.[5]

(1)   Genodermatoses with non-scarring hypotrichosis
    1.1   With alterations to the skeleton
        1.1.1   McKusich disease or chondrodysplasia
        1.1.2   Moynahan disease (hypotrichosis, syndactyly, retinitis)
        1.1.3   Trichorhinophalangeal syndrome (Langer-Giedion disease)
        1.1.4   Pierre-Robin syndrome
        1.1.5   Cardiofacial cutaneous syndrome
        1.1.6   ACD syndrome with mental retardation
        1.1.7   Oculo-dental-digital syndrome
        1.1.8   Dubowitz syndrome
        1.1.9   Noonan's syndrome
    1.2   With ectodermal alterations
        Ectodermal dysplasias
    1.3   With neuroectodermal alterations
        Trichothiodystrophy
    1.4   With chromosomal alterations
        Down's syndrome
        Klinefelter's syndrome
        Turner's syndrome
    1.5   With alterations in amino acid metabolism
        Citrulinaemia
        Hartnup disease
        Homocystinuria
        Phenylketonuria
        Tyrosinaemia I and II
    1.6   Other genodermatoses with hypotrichosis
        1.6.1   Progeria
                   Werner syndrome or pangeria
                   Hutchinson-Gilford or childhood progeria
                   Variot-Cailleau syndrome or childhood gerodermia
                   Other progerias
        1.6.2   Pityriasis rubra pilaris
        1.6.3   Congenital ichthyosiform erythrodermia
                   Netherton syndrome
                   Tay syndrome
                   Rud syndrome
                   KID syndrome
                   Rothmund-Thomson disease
                   PARC syndrome
                   Zinsser-Cole-Engman disease
                   Kallin syndrome or epidermolysis bullosa simplex
    1.7   Genodermatosis with hypotrichosis and tumours
        1.7.1   Rombo syndrome
        1.7.2   Bazex-Dupré-Christol syndrome
(2)   Genodermatosis with non-scarring hypotrichosis
        2.1   Darier disease
        2.1   Ichthyosis X
        2.3   Dystrophic epidermolysis bullosa
        2.4   Incontinentia pigmenti
        2.5   Poliostotic fibrous dysplasia
        2.6   Conradi syndrome

epiglottis and non-Finnish type congenital nephrotic syndrome are described. The same authors[7] believe that these associated alterations have never previously been reported and that they could be new associations in this disease; this would support the concept of contiguous gene syndrome in patients with trichorhinophalangeal syndrome. In their patient, an interstitial deletion of chromosome 8 with karyotype 46, XY, del (8) (q24.11→q24.13) was found.

Trichorhinophalangeal syndrome type III

Trichorhinophalangeal syndrome type III is a newly defined clinical entity.[8] This complex entity is inherited as an autosomal dominant trait and characterised clinically by growth retardation, craniofacial abnormalities, severe brachydactyly and sparse hair. In addition, absence of mental retardation and cartilaginous exostoses are required for the diagnosis of TRPS III. Other associated abnormalities include a short stature, a thin upper lip and a prominent lower lip, a pear-shaped nose, stubby fingers and toes with cone-shaped epiphyses and sparse scalp hair.

Dubowitz syndrome

This syndrome described by Dubowitz in 1965[9] is characterised by a peculiar facies, infantile eczema, small stature and mild microcephaly. The dermatological abnormalities consist mostly of eczematous eruption on the face and flexural areas starting during the first months of life and lasting until 3–4 years of age. Hair is sparse and brittle and typically affects the lateral eyebrows.

Patients affected by Dubowitz syndrome have a moderate mental deficiency with a tendency toward hyperactivity, short attention span, stubbornness and shyness. They have also been characterised by their high-pitched weak cry.

The peculiar facies consist of mild microcephaly, small face, shallow supraorbital ridge with nasal bridge, short palpebral fissures with lateral telecanthus and hypertelorism, variable ptosis and blepharophimosis and micrognathia.

With ectodermal alterations

We will follow the classification proposed by Freire-Maia[10] for the ectodermal dysplasias as follows:

Ectodermal dysplasias

The term ectodermal dysplasia was originally applied to anhydrotic ectodermal dysplasia in which hair, teeth, nails and sweat glands are defective. As increasingly more syndromes have been described, their nomenclature has become

Table 3 Classification of ectodermal dysplasia by Solomon and Keuer.[11]

Subgroups 1, 2, 3 and 4: Hair, teeth, nails and sweating defects
  Anhydrotic ectodermal dysplasia
  Rapp-Hodgkin syndrome
  EEC syndrome (see text for description)
  Popliteal web syndrome
  Xeroderma, talipes and enamel defect (XTE) syndrome

Subgroups 1, 2 and 3: Hair, teeth and nail defects
  Clouston dysplasia
  Trichodento-osseous syndrome
  Ellis-van Creveld syndrome
  Ankyloblepharon, ectodermal dysplasia, cleft lip and palate (AEC) syndrome
  Basan syndrome
  Tooth-nail syndrome

Subgroup 1, 3 and 4: Hair, nails and sweating defects
  Freire-Maia syndrome

Subgroups 1 and 2: Hair and teeth defects
  Orofaciodigital syndrome I
  Sensenbrenner syndrome
  Trichodental syndrome

Subgroups 1 and 3: Hair and nail defects
  Curly hair, ankyloblepharon and dysplastic nails (CHAND) syndrome
  Onychotrichodysplasia with neutropenia

Subgroup 1: Hair defects
  Trichorhinophalangeal syndromes I and II
  Dubowitz syndrome
  Moynahan syndrome

confused and complex and ectodermal dysplasia has been applied loosely and inconsistently to a wide variety of states. The classification proposed by Freire-Maia[10] in 1977 was based on the ectodermal conditions that show a primary defect. Conditions in which the ectodermal changes are secondary, as in xeroderma pigmentosum, are thus excluded from the ectodermal dysplasias. According to Freire-Maia's classification: subgroup 1 is a hair dysplasia; subgroup 2 a dental dysplasia; subgroup 3 a nail dysplasia; subgroup 4 a sweat gland defect; and subgroup 5 a defect of other ectodermal structures. A case of anhydrotic ectodermal dysplasia would fall in the subgroups 1, 2, 3 and 4, and a case of hydrotic ectodermal dysplasia only in the subgroups 1, 2 and 3. If a syndrome affects only hair it would have to be included only in the subgroup 1.

In 1980 Solomon and Keuer[11] defined more precisely the effect on hair in ectodermal dysplasia as shown in Table 3.

Anhydrotic ectodermal dysplasia (Christ-Siemens-Touraine syndrome)

In this X-linked syndrome, sweat glands and other skin 'appendages' are absent or few in number (Figure 2). The full syndrome only occurs in males. Scalp hair is short, fine and very sparse and often light in colour, but may increase in quantity after puberty. Eyebrows and eyelashes may also be sparse or absent but may be relatively little affected. Body hair may be sparse or absent. The prominent square forehead, saddle nose, the thick lower lip and the pointed chin produce a distinctive facies. The skin around the eyes is finely wrinkled and may be pigmented. The teeth may be absent or few in number, characteristically the canines and incisors are conical (Figure 3). The absent or reduced sweating leads to heat intolerance, and unexplained pyrexia may be the presenting symptom in infancy. Carrier females may be clinically normal but may show, to some degree, one or more of the features of the syndrome such as the conical teeth, hypotrichosis or heat intolerance. Otherwise apparently normal carriers may show dermatoglyphic abnormalities, the presence of which may help in diagnosis.[11]

EEC syndrome (ectrodactyly, ectodermal dysplasia and cleft lip and palate)

The association of ectrodactyly (lobster-claw deformity), ectodermal dysplasia, and cleft lip and palate is a well-defined autosomal dominant syndrome known as the EEC syndrome.[12] Nevertheless, the expressivity of the gene is very variable and there are numerous reported cases of pedigrees of complex syndromes that are probably genetically distinct but which show some of the main features of the EEC syndrome. All cases in which ectrodactyly (Figure 4) or syndactyly and/or cleft lip or palate are associated with an ectodermal defect are worthy of full investigation so that the genetic pattern of these syndromes may be elucidated.

Cases reported as EEC syndrome show sparse hair, malformed teeth with early caries, ectrodactyly, cleft lip and/or palate, lachrymal duct stenosis and renal anomalies; however, not all defects are present in all affected individuals within a single family. Other cases are reported

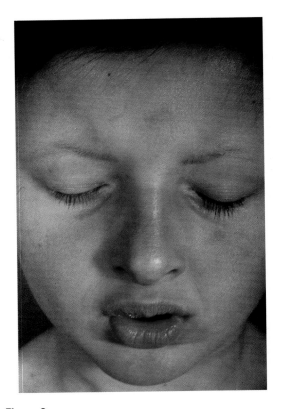

Figure 2

Christ-Siemens-Touraine syndrome: prominent forehead, sparse eyebrows, thick lower lip.

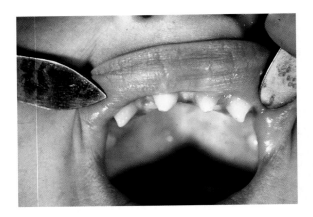

Figure 3

Christ-Siemens-Touraine syndrome: conical canines and incisors.

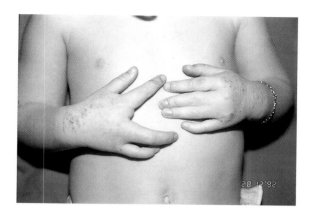

Figure 4

EEC syndrome: ectrodactyly.

in which hypotrichosis as one manifestation of ectodermal dysplasia is associated with cleft lip or palate and a variety of other defects. The presence of such an association should suggest the need of a search of the rapidly growing genetic literature in which such syndromes are gradually being characterised.

'Pure' hair–nail ectodermal dysplasia

'Pure' ectodermal dysplasias are developmental disorders affecting only tissues of ectodermal origin. Two different pure ectodermal dysplasias involving only hair and nails have been described to date. In a recent article Barbareschi et al.[13] describe congenital nail dystrophy and hypotrichosis associated with folliculitis decalvans in a family suggesting autosomal dominant transmission. In their report, the authors document peculiar clinical and ultrastructural hair findings that fit poorly into previously described conditions. They suggest that the patients reported could represent a new type of pure ectodermal dysplasia.

Familial juvenile macular dystrophy with congenital hypotrichosis capitis

In 1998, Becker et al.[14] described two sisters of a family of consanguineous parents with the com-
bination of hypotrichosis of the head and macular dystrophy in the context of a trichoocular malformation of an ectodermal dysplasia. They studied two 13- and 17-year-old sisters with reduced visual acuity because of symmetrical central changes of the retinal pigment epithelium and chorioatrophic scars of macular dystrophy combined with hypotrichosis capitis. The 13-year-old patient exhibited central changes of the retinal pigment epithelium leading to a relative central scotoma for Goldmann 1/4 during fundus perimetry in both eyes (with visual acuity of 0.125 and 0.4). In the 17-year-old sister they found central chorioatrophic scars, followed by absolute central scotomas, with unstable fixation in the upper retinal hemisphere with reduced visual acuity scores of 0.16 and 0.2. The authors concluded that there are few descriptions of the association of macular dystrophy and hypotrichosis. The combination of hypotrichosis and macular dystrophy could make genetic analysis easier. Mutational analysis of the TIMP-3 gene that has previously been associated with Sorsby fundus dystrophy did not reveal any disease-causing mutations in their patients.

Other genodermatoses with hypotrichosis

KID syndrome

The KID (keratitis, ichthyosis, deafness) syndrome is a congenital disorder of ectoderm that affects not only the epidermis but also other ectodermal tissues such as the corneal epithelium and the inner ear. In a recent review of the literature,[15] 61 patients fulfilling the criteria for this syndrome were identified. All had cutaneous and auditory abnormalities, and 95% also had ophthalmological defects. The most frequent clinical features were neurosensory deafness (90%), erythrokeratoderma (89%), vascularising keratitis (79%), alopecia (79%), and reticulated hyperkeratosis of the palms and soles (41%). All of these findings constitute the major criteria for the diagnosis. In the same article, the authors state that the KID acronym does not define accurately this entity since the disorder is not an ichthyosis, as scaling is not the main cutaneous feature, neither do all patients have keratitis early in the course. They suggest that this syndrome should be included under the general heading of congenital ectodermal defects as a keratodermatous ectodermal dysplasia (KED).

Genodermatoses with hypotrichosis and tumours

Rombo syndrome

Rombo syndrome was described by Michaëlson in 1981.[16] This autosomal dominant disease consists of hypotrichosis affecting the eyelashes, with yellowish papules (sometimes follicular) affecting part of the face. They also present cyanotic lips, hand and feet where they show multiple tricoepitheliomata and basal cell carcinomata.[17]

Bazex-Dupré-Christol syndrome

Bazex-Dupré-Christol syndrome (BDCS) is an X-linked dominant disorder of the hair follicle that is characterised by follicular atrophoderma, multiple basal cell carcinomas, hypotrichosis, milia, and localised hypohydrosis.[18] Follicular atrophoderma (FA) are follicular tunnel-shaped depressions, 'ice pick marks', seen most commonly on the dorsum of the hands. In a recent article, Kidd et al.[19] describe the first known Scottish family with this syndrome, with five affected members spanning three generations. These patients had hypohydrosis confined to the face, coarse hair, dry skin, milia, and follicular atrophoderma. All the adults had a history of multiple basal cell carcinomas. None of them had any skeletal features suggestive of Gorlin's syndrome. The authors[19] suggest that the BDCS should be considered as a differential diagnosis in patients with early onset or familial basal cell carcinomas.

In 1994, Goeteyn et al.[20] described a large family in which 20 people across four generations presented with typical features of the Bazex-Dupré-Christol syndrome. The clinical picture in this family, however, differs with regard to gender and age. Male subjects have a uniformly severe disease, whereas female subjects exhibit a range of severity of the syndrome. The most striking difference between male and female subjects is provided by hypotrichosis. In male subjects, hypotrichosis is diffuse and affects all scalp hairs. Conversely, female subjects do not have hypotrichosis but normal hairs are intermingled with abnormal hairs. In infancy and childhood, multiple milia are present, whereas in adults only a few milia are observed. The same authors conclude that the family pedigree seems to be consistent with an X-linked inheritance, since male-to-male transmission does not occur. Moreover, further evidence of an X-linked dominant mode of inheritance could be derived from the observation of gender differences that can be attributed to the lyonization phenomenon in female subjects. From a clinical and morphological point of view, the Bazex-Dupré- Christol syndrome seems to be a disorder of the hair follicle.

Localized congenital hypotrichosis

Congenital triangular alopecia (CTA, Brauer naevus)

Congenital triangular alopecia (CTA) is manifested at 3 to 5 years of age by unilateral or, less frequently, bilateral patches of alopecia in the frontotemporal region (Figure 5).[21] At this age, the differential diagnosis is important, particularly with regard to alopecia areata and sebaceous naevus. Only about 47 cases of CTA have been reported, probably because the lesion is benign and non-progressive. A frequency of 0.11% is reported by García Hernández et al.[22] Males affected by CTA do not require treatment because of the later development of androgenic alopecia, but women might receive benefit from surgical treatment.

Adams-Oliver syndrome (aplasia cutis congenita and terminal digital anomalies)

Adams-Oliver syndrome is characterised by the association of aplasia cutis with terminal digital abnormalities, namely shortening of fingers and

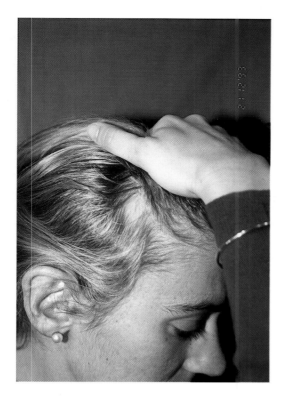

Figure 5

Congenital triangular alopecia in frontotemporal region.

toes, absence of phalanges or, more rarely, the absence of the entire hand or foot.

In 1995 Zapata et al.[23] described two patients with Adams-Oliver syndrome and congenital cardiac malformations. A review of the literature revealed a 13.4% occurrence of congenital cardiac malformations in individuals with Adams-Oliver syndrome, suggesting that cardiac anomalies are a frequent manifestation of this syndrome. All patients with Adams-Oliver syndrome should thus be evaluated for cardiac anomalies.

Alopecia areata

Alopecia areata is not a congenital disorder, thus it is generally assumed that alopecia areata is acquired only postnatally, and its presence at birth virtually excludes its diagnosis. Recently de Viragh et al.[24] documented a case of alopecia areata in a premature new-born infant.

Recently described syndromes (non-classified disorders)

More recently, some unclassified new hypotrichotic syndromes have appeared subtitled 'A new genodermatosis?' or 'A new syndrome?'. These will be discussed briefly.

Congenital ichthyosis with follicular atrophoderma

In a recent article, Lestringant et al.[25] describe five Emirati sibs (three girls and two boys), aged 4–18 years old, with normal stature, diffuse congenital ichthyosis, patchy follicular atrophoderma, generalised and diffuse non-scarring hypotrichosis, and marked hypohydrosis. Steroid sulphatase activity, assessed in the two boys, was found to be normal. Electron microscopic studies of ichthyotic skin did not show any specific abnormality. The association of congenital diffuse ichthyosis with follicular atrophoderma and hypotrichosis, which has not been reported before, was emphasised. The patients were reminiscent of Bazex syndrome; however, ichthyosis is not a component of Bazex syndrome. The authors conclude that congenital ichthyosis with follicular atrophoderma represents a new autosomal recessive genodermatosis.

Hypotrichosis, hair structure defects, hypercysteine hair and glucosuria

Structural hair changes may be the expression of a genetic disorder affecting hair growth, part of a congenital syndrome with accompanying hair malformations, or a marker for an underlying metabolic disorder. Blume-Peytavi et al.[26] report upon a 22-month-old Turkish girl and her 10-month-old brother, whose scalp hair become fragile and sparse at about 6–7 months of age. Glucosuria, without diabetes or kidney disease, was detected 3–4 months later. Clinical examination revealed normal physical and mental development, and an analysis of plucked hairs showed dysplastic and broken hair shafts. Polarising microscopy and scanning electron microscopic studies revealed torsion, together with irregularities and impressions of the hair shaft, as seen in pili torti, trichorrhexis nodosa and pseudomonilethrix. Analysis of the amino acid composition of the hair demonstrated a significant reduction of sulphonic cysteic acid and an elevated cysteine and lanthionine content in the girl, and elevated lanthionine levels in her brother. Electrophoretic analysis of the girl's hair proteins revealed a normal composition but a high extractability of hair proteins. The authors concluded that the triad of hypotrichosis, structural hair shaft defects and abnormal amino acid composition, accompanied by glucosuria without diabetes, may represent a new genetic syndrome.

Congenital atrichia, palmoplantar hyperkeratosis, mental retardation and early loss of teeth

Steijlen et al.[27] reported four siblings with a syndrome consisting of congenital atrichia, palmoplantar hyperkeratosis, mental retardation and early loss of teeth. The pedigree in that family was suggestive of either an autosomal recessive mode of inheritance or the inheritance of a (small) chromosomal translocation. This combination of findings has not been reported previously and is therefore considered to be a new genetic entity.

Aplasia cutis congenita, high myopia and cone–rod dysfunction

Recently Gershoni-Baruch et al.[28] reported a peculiar association of a brother and a sister with congenital nystagmus, cone–rod dysfunction, high myopia, and aplasia cutis congenita on the midline of the scalp vertex. The authors believe that this familial oculocutaneous condition, transmitted as an autosomal recessive trait, has not been reported previously and should be considered a new autosomal recessive disorder.

Keratoderma, hypotrichosis and leukonychia totalis

Basaran et al.[29] report three members of a family with congenital hypotrichosis, characterised by trichorrhexis nodosa and trichoptilosis, dry skin, keratosis pilaris and leukonychia totalis. The patients also developed a progressive transgrediens type of palmoplantar keratoderma, and hyperkeratotic lesions on the knees, elbows and perianal region. According to the authors, this combination of clinical features has not been described previously, so they suggest that it could be considered a new entity.

Alopecia and mental retardation syndrome associated with convulsions and hypergonadotrophic hypogonadism

Devriendt et al.[30] reported two brothers with congenital total alopecia, mental retardation, childhood convulsions and hypergonadotrophic hypogonadism. The authors believe that this association has not previously been reported and probably represents a new autosomal recessive condition.

'Universal congenital alopecia'

Recently, the publication of two separate articles[31,32] on a gene for universal congenital alopecia has attracted general interest. The world press has come to the erroneous conclusion that this particular type of atrichia could be a form of alopecia areata.

Complete or partial congenital absence of hair may occur either in isolation or with associated defects. Most family members with isolated congenital alopecia follow an autosomal recessive mode of inheritance. As yet, no gene has been linked to isolated congenital alopecia, nor has linkage to a specific region of the genome been established. In an attempt to map the gene for the autosomal recessive form of the disorder, Nothen et al.[31] performed genetic linkage analysis on a large inbred Pakistani family in which affected persons show complete absence of hair development and they used the term 'universal congenital alopecia'. They analysed individuals of this family using over 175 microsatellite polymorphic markers of the human genome. A maximum LOD score of 7.90 at a recombination fraction of 0 was obtained at the locus D8S258. Haplotype analysis of recombination events localised the disease to a 15-cM region between marker loci D8S261 and D8S1771. They have thus mapped the gene for this hereditary form of isolated congenital alopecia (alopecia universalis congenitalis, ALUNC) to a locus on chromosome 8p21-22.

In a more recent article[32] the same group of investigators reported the cloning and characterisation of the human homologue of the mouse hairless gene and showed that it is located in the critical region on chromosome 8p21-22. Determining the exon-intron structure allowed detailed mutational analysis of DNA samples of patients with universal congenital alopecia. They detected a homozygous missense mutation in the Pakistani family and a homozygous splice donor mutation in a family from Oman. In addition, they showed that the human hairless gene undergoes alternative splicing and that at least two isoforms generated by alternative usage of exon 17 are found in human tissues. Interestingly, the isoform containing exon 17 is the predominantly expressed isoform in all tissues but skin, where exclusive expression of the shorter isoform was observed. They speculate that this tissue-specific difference in the proportion of hairless transcripts lacking exon 17 sequences could contribute to the tissue-specific disease phenotype observed in individuals with this type of isolated congenital alopecia.

Hallermann-Streiff syndrome

Hallermann-Streiff syndrome is a rare, congenital anomaly characterised by a peculiar bird facies, mandibular and maxillary hypoplasia, dyscephaly, congenital cataracts, microphthalmia, hypotrichosis, skin atrophy and short stature.[33] Dental abnormalities are present in 80% of cases;[34] these include malocclusion, crowding, severe caries, supernumerary and neonatal teeth, enamel hypoplasia, hypodontia, premature eruption of primary dentition, agenesis of permanent teeth, and anterior displacement or absence of condyles.

Congenital hypotrichosis and milia

Patients with congenital hypotrichosis and milia have coarse, sparse hair and multiple milia on the face, chest, axillae and pubic regions. There are no abnormalities of the teeth and nails. Polarising light microscopy shows an increased diameter of the hair shaft. Rapelanoro et al.[35] reported a large family of four generations in which individuals had congenital hypotrichosis and multiple milia, which disappeared by adolescence. The pedigree in this family was compatible with an autosomal or an X-linked dominant mode of inheritance.

Happle syndrome

Gobello et al.[36] described a 13-year-old girl suffering from chondrodysplasia punctata, which was associated with ichthyosis arranged along Blaschko's lines, follicular atrophoderma, cicatricial alopecia and coarse, lustreless hair. The patient also showed a congenital cataract of the right eye, dysplastic facial appearance and symmetrical shortening of the tubular bones. The pathogenetic concept of functional X-chromosome mosaicism introduced by Happle is used to denominate this syndrome. The recent results obtained by molecular research have failed, so far, to solve the problem of regional assignment of the underlying X-linked gene.

References

1. Bonnet R: Ueber Hypotrichosis congenital universalis. *Anatomishe Hefte* 1892; **1**: 233.
2. Cockayne AE: *Inherited Abnormalities of the Skin and its Appendages*. Oxford University Press; 1933: 229.
3. Muller SA: Alopecia: syndromes of genetic significance. *J Invest Dermatol* 1973; **60**: 475.
4. Sâlamon T: Hypotrichosis and alopecia in cases of Genodermatosis. In: Orfanos CE, Montagna W, Stüttgen G (eds.). *Hair Research Status and Future Aspects*. Berlin, Springer-Verlag, 1981: 396–407.
5. Camacho F: Genodermatosis con Hipotricosis. In: Camacho F, Montagna W (eds.). *Tricologia*. Madrid, Aula Médica, 1996: 219–236.
6. Boni R, Boni RH, Tsambaos D, Spycher MA, Trueb RM: Trichorhinophalangeal syndrome. *Dermatol* 1995; **190**: 152–155.
7. Lu FL, Hou JW, Tsai WS, et al.: Tricho-rhinophalangeal syndrome type II associated with epiglotic aplasia and congenital nephrotic syndrome. *J Formos Med Assoc* 1997; **96**: 217–221.
8. Itin PH, Bohn S, Mathys D, Guggenheim R, Richard G: Trichorhinophalangeal syndrome type III. *Dermatol* 1996; **193**: 349–352.
9. Paradis M, Angelo C, Conti G, et al.: Dubowitz syndrome with keloidal lesions. *Clin Exp Dermatol* 1994; **19**: 425–427.
10. Freire-Maia N: Ectodermal dysplasia revisited. *Acta Genetico Medico e Gemellologia* 1977; **26**: 121.
11. Solomon LM, Keuer EJ: The ectodermal dysplasias. *Arch Dermatol* 1980; **116**: 1295.
12. Jones EM, Hersh JH, Yusk JW: Aplasia cutis congenita, cleft palate, epidermolysis bullosa and ectrodactyly: a new syndrome? *Pediatr Dermatol* 1992; **9**: 293–297.
13. Barbareschi M, Cambiaghi S, Crupi AC, Tadini G: Family with 'pure' hair-nail ectodermal dysplasia. *Am J Med Genet* 1997; **72**: 91–93.
14. Becker M, Rohrschneider K, Tilgen W, Weber BH, Volcker HE: Familial juvenile macular dystrophy with congenital hypotrichosis capitis. *Ophthalmologe* 1998; **95**: 233–240.
15. Caceres-Rios H, Tamayo-Sanchez L, Duran-Mckinster C, de la Luz Orozco M, Ruiz-Maldonado R: Keratitis, ichthyosis, and deafness (KID syndrome): review of the literature and proposal of a new terminology. *Pediatr Dermatol* 1996; **13**: 105–113.
16. Camacho F: Genodermatosis con Hipotricosis. In: Camacho F, Montagna W (eds.). *Tricología*. Madrid, Aula Médica, 1996: 232.
17. Ashinoff R, Jacobson M, Belsito DV: Rombo syndrome: a second case report and review. *J Am Acad Dermatol* 1993; **28**: 1011–1014.
18. Lacombe D, Taieb A: Overlap between the Bazex syndrome and congenital hypotrichosis and milia. *Am J Med Genet* 1995; **56**: 423–424.
19. Kidd A, Carson L, Gregory DW, et al.: A Scottish family with Bazex-Dupré-Christol syndrome: follicular atrophoderma, congenital hypotrichosis, and basal cell carcinoma. *J Med Genet* 1996; **33**: 493–497.
20. Goeteyn M, Geerts ML, Kint A, De Weert J: The Bazex-Dupré-Christol syndrome. *Arch Dermatol* 1994; **130**: 337–342.
21. Armstrong DK, Burrows D: Congenital triangular alopecia. *Pediatr Dermatol* 1996; **13**: 394–396.
22. García-Hernández MJ, Rodriguez-Pichardo A, Camacho F: Congenital triangular alopecia (Brauer nevus). *Pediatr Dermatol* 1995; **12**: 301–303.
23. Zapata HH, Sletten LJ, Pierpont ME: Congenital cardiac malformations in Adams-Oliver syndrome. *Clin Genet* 1995; **47**: 80–84.
24. de Viragh PA, Gianadda B, Levy ML: Congenital alopecia areata. *Dermatol* 1997; **195**: 96–98.
25. Lestringant GG, Kuster W, Frossard PM, Happle R: Congenital ichthyosis, follicular atrophoderma, hypotrichosis, and hypohidrosis: a new genodermatosis? *Am J Med Genet* 1998; **75**: 186–189.
26. Blume-Peytavi U, Fohles J, Schulz R, Wortmann G, Gollnick H, Orfanos CE: Hypotrichosis, hair structure defects, hypercysteine hair and glucosuria: a new genetic syndrome? *Br J Dermatol* 1996; **134**: 319–324.
27. Steijlen PM, Neumann HA, der Kinderen DJ, et al.: Congenital atrichia, palmoplantar hyperkeratosis, mental retardation, and early loss of teeth in four siblings: a new syndrome? *J Am Acad Dermatol* 1994; **30**: 893–898.
28. Gershoni-Baruch R, Leiby R: Aplasia cutis congenita, high myopia, and cone-rod dysfunction in two sibs: a new autosomal recessive disorder. *Am J Med Genet* 1996; **61**: 42–44.
29. Basaran E, Yilmaz E, Alpsoy E, Yilmaz GG: Keratoderma, hypotrichosis and leukonychia totalis: a new syndrome? *Br J Dermatol* 1995; **133**: 636–638.
30. Devriendt K, Van den Berghe H, Fryns JP: Alopecia-mental retardation syndrome associated with convulsions and hypergonadotropic hypogonadism. *Clin Genet* 1996; **49**: 6–9.
31. Nothen MM, Cichon S, Vogt IR, et al.: A gene for universal congenital alopecia maps to chromosome 8p21-22. *Am J Hum Genet* 1998; **62**: 386–390.
32. Cichon S, Anker M, Vogt IR, et al.: Cloning, genomic organisation, alternative transcripts and mutational analysis of the gene responsible for autosomal recessive universal congenital alopecia. *Hum Mol Genet* 1998; **7**: 1671–1679.
33. Vadiadas G, Oulis C, Tsianos E, Mavridou S: A

typical Hallermann-Streiff syndrome in a 3-year-old child. *J Clin Pediatr Dent* 1995; **20**: 63–86.

34. da Fonesca MA, Mueller WA: Hallerman-Streiff syndrome: case report and recommendations for dental care. *ASDC J Dent Child* 1994; **61**: 334–337.

35. Rapelanoro R, Taieb A, Lacombe D: Congenital hypotrichosis and milia: report of a large family suggesting X-linked dominant inheritance. *Am J Med Genet* 1994; **52**: 487–490.

36. Gobello T, Mazzanti C, Fileccia P, et al.: X-linked dominant chondrodysplasia punctata (Happle syndrome) with uncommon symmetrical shortening of the tubular bones. *Dermatol* 1995; **191**: 323–327.

24
Congenital hypertrichosis

Antonella Tosti and Bianca Maria Piraccini

Introduction

The term hypertrichosis describes the presence of an excessive amount of hair in non-androgen dependent areas. Congenital hypertrichosis can be localized or generalized, and in either it can be an isolated symptom or occur in association with other developmental abnormalities. Hypertrichosis may also be a feature of several genetic syndromes.[1-4]

Localized hypertrichosis

Conditions associated with localized hypertrichosis are listed in Table 1.

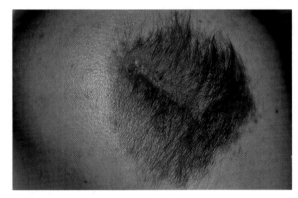

Figure 1

Terminal hairs associated with congenital melanocytic nevus.

Congenital melanocytic nevi

Large, coarse, terminal hairs are present in up to 95% of congenital giant melanocytic nevi (Figure 1). The presence of hair is not an indicator of possible malignant transformation.

Table 1 Localized congenital hypertrichosis.

Congenital melanocytic nevi
Becker's nevus
Hypertrichosis cubiti (hairy elbows syndrome)
Cervical hypertrichosis
   Anterior
   Posterior
Faun tail (lumbosacral hypertrichosis)
Hairy pinnae
Hairy palms and soles
Polythelia pilosa (hairy polythelia)
Nevoid hypertrichosis

Becker's nevus

Becker's nevus is an epidermal nevus characterized by irregular macular pigmentation with hypertrichosis.[5] The pigmentation, which is light brown in color, usually develops in childhood or at puberty, most commonly involving the trunk or the upper arm. The pigmented patch may reach the size of 10–15 cm. Becker's nevus may occasionally be bilateral. In patients with Becker's nevus, the hypertrichosis (Figure 2) always appears after puberty, and usually 2–3 years after the onset of the pigmentation in about 50% of cases. Nevertheless, the extent of the hypertrichosis may considerably vary from case to case; i.e. folliculitis and acneiform lesions may also be observed.

Although Becker's nevus is reported to occur much more frequently in males than in females (with a ratio of 10:1), some believe that Becker's

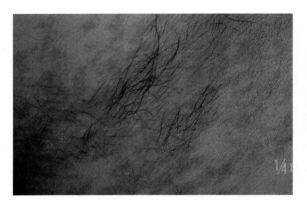

Figure 2

Becker's nevus.

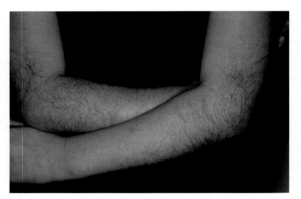

Figure 3

Hypertrichosis cubiti.

nevus in females is often undiagnosed since it is unassociated with hypertrichosis. Hypertrichosis of Becker's nevus appears to be androgen-dependent and androgen receptors have been found in the nevus.

Although Becker's nevus is usually an isolated defect, some associated abnormalities have been reported, especially in women. These include ipsilateral breast and areolar hypoplasia, ipsilateral hypoplasia of a limb, pectus carenatum, spina bifidaocculta, accessory scrotum and morfea.

Hypertrichosis cubiti (hairy elbows syndrome)

Hypertrichosis cubiti is characterized by the presence of lanugo hair on the extensor surface of the elbows extending from mid humerus to mid forearm.[6] This condition is usually autosomal dominant but may be genetically heterogeneous. It is typically bilateral (Figure 3) and is usually present at birth or develops in the first months of life, being more evident during childhood and often disappearing in adult life. A possible association between hypertrichosis cubiti and short stature has been reported more recently.[7-8]

Cervical hypertrichosis

Two types of cervical hypertrichosis exist: that localized in the anterior and that localized in the

posterior side of the neck. This condition is present at birth.

Anterior cervical hypertrichosis

In anterior cervical hypertrichosis, a tuft of terminal hair is present 1–4 cm above the sternal notch (Figure 4). The mode of inheritance is possibly autosomal recessive. Anterior cervical hypertrichosis has been reported in association with peripheral neuropathy and retinal changes.[9-10]

Posterior cervical hypertrichosis

A tuft of terminal hair is present over the cervical vertebrae (Figure 5). Both an X-linked recessive

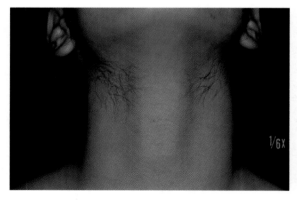

Figure 4

Anterior cervical hypertrichosis.

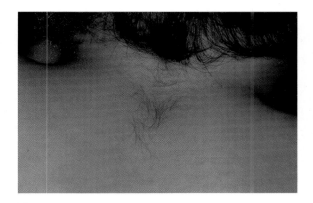

Figure 5

Posterior cervical hypertrichosis.

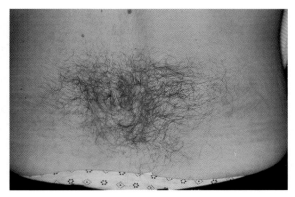

Figure 6

Faun tail.

as well as an autosomal dominant inheritance have been reported. In one family, posterior cervical hypertrichosis was associated with kyphoscoliosis.[11]

Faun tail (lumbosacral hypertrichosis)

Faun tail is the presence of a patch of long terminal hair on the lumbosacral region (Figure 6). This condition is usually evident at birth or soon afterwards. Faun tail is an important clinical sign since it is frequently associated with underlying neurological defects, including spina bifida occulta, spina bifida, traction bands, diastematomyelia, myelomeningocele and dermal sinus trait.[12] Since prompt diagnosis of the neurological abnormalities is essential for preventing definitive damage of the nerves, a full neurological and radiological workup is mandatory in all children with faun tail.

Hairy pinnae

The presence of coarse terminal hair on the pinnae (Figure 7) is a genetic trait that is more frequently observed in South Indians but has

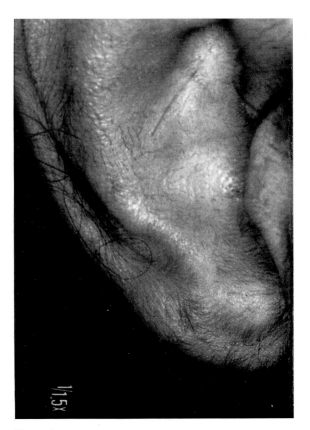

Figure 7

Terminal hair on the ear pinna.

also been reported in Italians and in other Mediterranean populations. Hairy ears usually become evident after the age of 18 years and almost exclusively affect men. The mode of inheritance is still unknown but it is possible that it may be an autosomal dominant sex-limited trait.[13]

Hairy palms and soles

It this hereditary condition, patches of hairs are present on areas of the palms and soles that are normally devoid of hair follicles.[14]

Polythelia pilosa (hairy polythelia)

This is a form of aberrant mammary tissue. Single or multiple tufts of hair occur along the mammary line on the chest and abdomen (Figure 8). The patches of hairs are neither associated with skin pigmentation nor structures of areola or nipple.[15] The condition may be symmetrical.

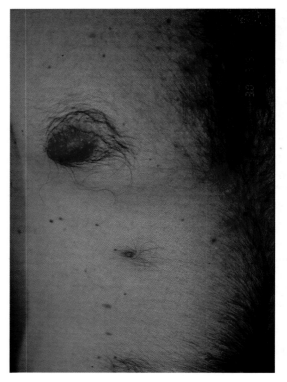

Figure 8

Hairy polythelia. Multiple tufts or hair along the mammary line (courtesy of Prof. F Camacho Martinez).

Nevoid hypertrichosis

Nevoid hypertrichosis[16,17] is an uncommon form of congenital hypertrichosis characterized by single or multiple patches of terminal hair on apparently normal skin. The scalp may also be involved. An underlying cutaneous meningioma may also be present.[18] Hypertrichosis may disappear spontaneously.[19]

Generalized hypertrichosis

Hypertrichosis universalis

This variety of hypertrichosis is common in men from the Mediterranean areas. Hair distribution is normal but the density and length of the hair is above the normal range (Figure 9).

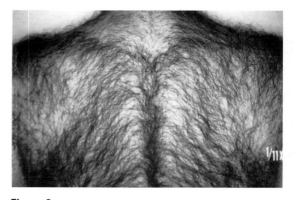

Figure 9

Hypertrichosis universalis.

Hypertrichosis lanuginosa

Hypertrichosis lanuginosa (Mendelian Inheritance in Man (MIM): 145700, 307150) is an extremely rare disorder that is most commonly transmitted by an autosomal dominant trait.[20] Hypertrichosis is present at birth and affects all the skin surfaces except for the palms, soles, lips, glans penis and distal phalanges. The abnormal hairs, that may be blond to black in color, are lanugo-type hairs that continue to grow and may reach the length of 5–10 cm. In some families, the hairs are lost in childhood, while in others they persist into adult life.

Hypertrichosis associated with gingival hyperplasia represents a different condition (MIM: 135400) even though the distribution and appearance of the hypertrichosis is similar to that of hypertrichosis lanuginosa. Gingival hyperplasia appears in early childhood and progresses to completely obscure the teeth.[21]

Primary diffuse focal hypertrichosis

This new form of hypertrichosis has recently been reported by García-Hernández et al.[22] in two members of a Spanish family. From birth patients had long body hairs on the upper part of the trunk, back and arms (Figure 10).

According to the authors, this type of hypertrichosis has characteristics similar to generalized and localized hypertrichosis.

Hereditary syndromes associated with hypertrichosis

Hypertrichosis may be prominent or a minor feature of several genetic syndromes and these are listed in Table 2.[23]

Congenital erythropoietic porphyria

In congenital erythropoietic porphyria (also known as Gunter's disease; MIM: 263700), hypertrichosis is not present at birth but gradually develops in infancy on sun-exposed areas. It is characterized by blond lanugo hairs over the face and extremities.

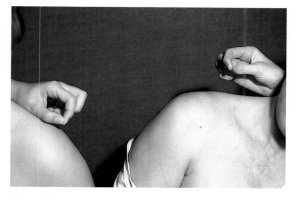

Figure 10

Diffuse focal hypertrichosis showing the presence of long hairs on the shoulders. (Courtesy of Professor F Camacho Martinez).

Table 2 Hereditary syndromes associated with hypertrichosis.

Byars-Jurkiewicz syndrome
Congenital erythropoietic porphyria (Gunter's disease; MIM: 263700)
Congenital generalized lipodystrophy (MIM: 269700, 272500)
Cornelia de Lange syndrome (MIM: 122470)
Cowden disease (MIM: 158350)
Crouzon craniofacial dysostosis (MIM: 123500)
Labaud syndrome (MIM: 135500)
Leprechaunism (MIM: 246200)
Mucopolysaccaridosis
Oliver MacFarlane syndrome
Rubinstein-Taybi syndrome
Schinzel-Gideon syndrome (MIM: 269150)
Stiff skin (MIM: 184900, 260530)
Trisomy 18 (Edward's syndrome)
Winchester's syndrome (MIM: 277950)

Congenital generalized lipodystrophy

In congenital generalized lipodystrophy (MIM: 269700, 272500), hypertrichosis of both body and face is typical. It is present since birth and tends to become more evident with ageing. Patients also present thick, curly scalp hair with a low frontal hairline.

Cornelia de Lange syndrome

Patients with Cornelia de Lange syndrome (MIM: 112470) show diffuse hypertrichosis, as well as overgrowth of the eyebrows and eyelashes. In addition, a low hair implantation line both on the forehead (Figure 11) and on the neck is an associated feature.

Leprechaunism

Generalized hypertrichosis is a prominent feature in leprechaunism (MIM: 246200). At birth, children are covered by fine lanugo-like hairs, which are particularly prominent over the face. In a patient who survived until the age of 10 years, long, pigmented terminal hairs were present over the back and limbs.[24]

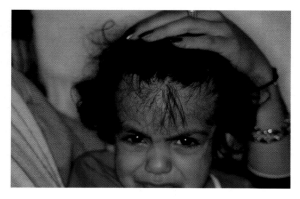

Figure 11

Low hair implantation line on the forehead in a child affected by Cornelia de Lange syndrome.

Mucopolysaccharidosis

Diffuse hypertrichosis occurs in mucopolysaccharidosis, especially in the Sanfilippo's syndrome (MPS 3). Lanugo-type hair diffusively covers the trunk and the extremities.

Oliver–MacFarlane syndrome

In Oliver–MacFarlane syndrome,[25] abnormally long eyelashes and eyebrows, which may even require a periodical cut, are present since birth. Hypertrichosis of the scalp may also be an associated finding.

Rubinstein-Taybi syndrome

In this condition hypertrichosis of the face, trunk and extremities occurs in 64% of patients.

Trisomy 18

In trisomy 18 (Edwards' syndrome), hypertrichosis of the forehead and back has been reported.

References

1. Camacho C: Hypertrichosis. In: Camacho F, Montagna W (eds.). *Trichology.* Madrid, Aula Medica Group: 1997.
2. Happle R: Genetic defects involving the hair. In: Orfanos CE, Happle R (eds.), *Hair and Hair Diseases.* Berlin, Springer-Verlag: 1989.
3. Barth JH: Hypertrichosis. In: Dawber R (ed) *Diseases of the Hair and Scalp,* 3rd edn. Oxford, Blackwell Scientific Publications: 1997.
4. Bayliss Mallory S, Leal-Khouri S: *An Illustrated Dictionary of Dermatologic Syndromes.* London, The Parthenon Publishing Group: 1994.
5. Happle R, Koopman RS: Becker nevus syndrome. *Am J Med Genet* 1997; **68**: 357–361.
6. Escalouilla P, Aguilar A, Gallego M, et al.: A new case of hairy elbows syndrome (Hypertrichosis cubiti). *Pediatr Dermatol* 1996; **13**: 303–305.

7. Cambiaghi S, Tadini G, Gelmetti C: Hairy elbows. *J Dermatol* 1998; **37**: 317–318.
8. Di Lernia V, Neri I, Trevisi P, Patrizi A: Hypertrichosis cubiti. *Arch Dermatol* 1996; **132**: 589.
9. Garty BZ, Snir M, Kreener I, et al.: Retinal changes in familial peripheral sensory and motor neuropathy associated with anterior cervical hypertrichosis. *J Pediatr Ophthalmol Strabismus* 1997; **34**: 309–312.
10. Trattner A, Hodak E, Sagie-Lermorn T, et al.: Familial congenital anterior cervical hypertrichosis associated with peripheral, sensory and motor neuropathy – a new syndrome? *J Am Acad Dermatol* 1991; **25**: 767–770.
11. Reed OM, Mellette JR Jr, Fitzpatrick JE: Familiar cervical hypertrichosis with underlying kyphoscoliosis. *J Am Acad Dermatol* 1989; **20**: 1069–1072.
12. Davis DA, Cohen PR, George RE: Cutaneous stigmata of occult spinal dysraphism. *J Am Acad Dermatol* 1994; **31**: 892–896.
13. Kamalam A, Thambiah AS: Genetics of hairy ears in South Indians. *Clin Exp Dermatol* 1990; **15**: 192–194.
14. Jackson CE, Callies QC, Krull EA, Mehsegan A: Hairy cutaneous malformations of palms and soles. *Arch Dermatol* 1975; **111**: 1146–1149.
15. Camacho F, Gonzalez-Campora R: Polythelia pilosa: a particular form of accessory mammary tissue. *Dermatology* 1998; **196**: 295–298.
16. Taskapan O, Dogan B, Cekmen S, et al.: Nevoid hypertrichosis associated with duplication of the right thumb. *J Am Acad Dermatol* 1998; **39**: 114–115.
17. Chang SN, Hong SE, Kim DK, Park WH: A case of multiple nevoid hypertrichosis. *J Dermatol* 1977; **24**: 337–341.
18. Peñas PF, Jones-Caballero M, Amigo A, et al.: Cutaneous meningioma underlying congenital localized hypertrichosis. *J Am Acad Dermatol* 1994; **30**: 363–366.
19. Dudding TE, Rogers M, Roddick LG, et al.: Nevoid hypertrichosis with multiple patches of hair that underwent almost complete spontaneous resolution. *Am J Med Genet* 1998; **79**: 195–196.
20. Marcias-Flores MA, Garcia-Cruz D, Rivera H, et al.: A new form of hypertrichosis inherited as an X-linked dominant trait. *Human Genet* 1984; **66**: 66–70.
21. Cuestas-Carnero R, Bornancini CA: Hereditary generalized gingival fibromatosis associated with hypertrichosis: report of five cases in one family. *J Oral Maxillofac Surg* 1998; **46**: 415–420.
22. García-Hernández MJ, Rodríguez-Pichardo A, Camacho FM: Primary diffuse focal hypertrichosis. II *Intercontinental Meeting of Hair Research Societies, Washington DC, 5–7 November 1998.*
23. Sibert VP: Genetic Skin Disorders. Oxford, Oxford University Press: 1997.
24. Barba A, Chieregato C, Scheda D, et al.: Leprechaunism. *J Eur Dermatol* 1995; **5**: 185–190.
25. Zaun H, Stenger D, Zabronsky S, Zanke M: Das Syndrom der Langer Wimpern ('Trichomegalie Syndrom' Oliver-MacFarlane). *Hautarzt* 1984; **35**: 162–165.

25
Metabolic disorders involving the hair

Christoph C Geilen, Ulrike Blume-Peytavi and Constantin E Orfanos

Introduction

Apart from particular entities that cause hair diseases, changes of the hair may be seen as a marker for genetic disorders, internal malignancy, drug abuse, environmental damage, metabolic disorders and nutritional deficiencies. The hair cycle involves, and depends on, the growth and differentiation of different cellular components of the hair follicle and the perifollicular dermis. The formation of a follicle and the production of a hair is closely associated to the biosynthesis of proteins such as different keratins and extracellular matrix proteins, glycosaminoglycans, nucleic acids and lipid membranes. The loss of up to 80–100 hairs/day and the hair growth of 0.3 mm/day of the remaining 100–200 000 follicles implicates a high rate of biosynthetic activity. Matrix cells of anagen hair follicles are some of the most active cells in humans. It is not surprising, therefore, that this finely tuned, well-balanced process of hair growth and differentiation is very sensitive not only to toxic or hormonal effects but also to alterations in the supply of amino acids, vitamins, trace elements and other nutritional components.[1,2] Hair changes can be observed clinically in a broad spectrum of metabolic disorders. These disorders can be divided into primary and secondary metabolic failures, the latter including metabolic diseases and nutritional deficiencies.

Primary metabolic disorders

Primary metabolic disorders are hereditary diseases involving the uptake and/or metabolism of amino acids, proteins and trace elements. Menkes' disease, trichothiodystrophy, homocysteinuria, argininosuccinic aciduria or citrullinemia represent such genotrichoses with an underlying metabolic dysfunction. Since most of these genotrichoses are described in more detail in other chapters of this book, only a brief summary shall be given for Menkes' disease and trichothiodystrophy.

Menkes' disease

Menkes' disease (trichopoliodystrophy or kinky hair syndrome) is an X-linked recessive disorder of copper metabolism resulting in markedly decreased copper levels of the serum, brain and liver of affected males. A copper ATPase was demonstrated to be affected and the gene locus was mapped to Xq13.3.[3] Careful analysis of hair reveals accumulation of copper in the hair. Patients may develop normally until the onset of symptoms, usually between the age of 5 weeks and 5 months. They show characteristic white, brittle, steely hair and serious neurological symptoms, such as seizures, delayed development and muscular hypotony. The facial appearance is characteristic, with pale skin and plump cheeks, a bowed upper lip and broken, twisted eyebrows.[4] A patient with typical clinical manifestations of Menkes' disease is demonstrated in Figure 1. The syndrome will be also described in more detail in Chapter 26.

Trichothiodystrophy

This genohypotrichosis is characterized by ruptures of the hair with trichoschisis resulting from the low sulfur content of the cortex and the cuticle. Trichothiodystrophy represents a group

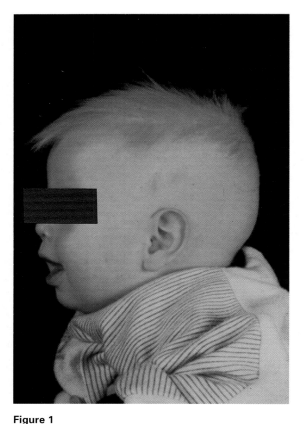

Figure 1

Clinical appearance in Menkes' disease.

xeroderma pigmentosum and Cockayne's syndrome, with a defect in the nucleotide excision repair system, especially of components of the transcriptional factor TFIIH.[7–9] TFIIH has two different functions, DNA repair and DNA transcription. It is suggested, therefore, that in trichothiodystrophy the transcriptional function is affected, whereas in xeroderma pigmentosum and in Cockayne's syndrome the DNA repair function is defective. This concept fits well with the absence of increased skin neoplasms in trichothiodystrophy.

Microscopic examination of the hair involved shows trichoschisis, irregularly formed hair shafts and trichorrhexis nodosa-like fractures. Under polarizing light, the hair shafts reveal typical alternating light and dark bands, the so called 'tiger-tail pattern'. Scanning electron microscopy reveals severe cuticular and secondary cortical degeneration along almost the entire hair shaft, with reduced or absent cuticular pattern and abnormal ridging and fluting.[10] Amino-acid analysis reveals a reduced cysteine, proline, threonine and serine content. Analysis of hair proteins indicates a deficient synthesis of the usual high-sulfur and ultra-high-sulfur proteins with appearance of new low-molecular-mass proteins.[11]

of rare, autosomal recessive neuroectodermal disorders with heterogenic clinical appearance.[5,6] Fragile hair is the single common symptom in all patients and is therefore an important clinical marker for diagnosis. Hair characteristics are key diagnostic factors in these patients with defects in synthesis of high-sulfur proteins. Scalp hair, eyebrows, and eyelashes are all brittle, short, uneven, and sparse. Patients involved have a similar facial appearance with receding chin, protruding ears, and slightly aged appearance. The voice may be raspy. Sulfur-deficient brittle hair serves as an important clinical marker for the constellation of neuroectodermal syndromes. Photosensitivity has been reported in 50% of the cases. It has been shown that trichothiodystrophy belongs to a group of disorders such as

Secondary metabolic disorders

As already indicated, secondary metabolic disorders may be classified into: alterations of hair growth resulting from metabolic diseases, and nutritional deficiencies.

Metabolic diseases

Changes of hair growth, color, distribution, density and/or texture of hair shafts are seen clinically in diseases of the liver, kidneys, in endocrinopathies, in malignant diseases or after severe, feverish infections.

Hepatic and renal dysfunction

Alterations in hair growth can be seen in five types of porphyrias, including two erythropoietic

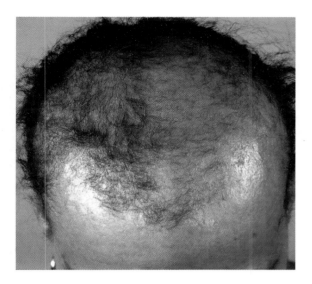

Figure 2

Diffuse alopecia in a patient with porphyria cutanea tarda.

porphyrias—erythropoietic porphyria (Günther's disease) and erythropoietic protoporphyria—and also in three different types of hepatic porphyrias—porphyria cutanea tarda, porphyria variegata and hepatoerythropoietic porphyria. In all these types of porphyria, dysfunction in the biosynthesis of haem and hypertrichosis occurs, together with other systemic abnormalities and skin manifestations. The mechanisms underlying the phenomenon of hypertrichosis in these metabolic disorders are unknown. In some cases of hepatic porphyria, diffuse effluvium occurred, as seen in Figure 2, which shows a patient with porphyria cutanea tarda and diffuse alopecia. Furthermore, in patients with severe liver dysfunction (e.g. in hepatic cirrhosis) loss of axillary and pubic hair, as well as of the hair on the scalp is reported frequently. This is often accompanied by gynecomastia. Metabolic disorders underlying these alterations are primary dysfunctions of both amino acids and steroid hormone metabolism.[12]

In chronic kidney disease the scalp hair is fragile, and dry and diffuse hair loss may be observed; diffuse hypertrichosis of the extremities and the trunk has also been reported in patients undergoing haemodialysis.[13]

Endocrine disease

Endocrine disorders can be associated with alterations of the hair through several different mechanisms. Hypothyroidism and hyperthyroidism are frequently associated with changes in the skin and its appendages. Head and body hair is typically dry, brittle, and tends to fall out, resulting in diffuse, partial alopecia. In addition, decreased growth rate of the hair can be observed.[14] It has been demonstrated that the anagen/ telogen ratio is reduced and the secretion of the sebaceous glands is decreased. These changes are normalized with restoration of the euthyroid state. In patients with pituitary insufficiency, clinical signs are sparse body, pubic and axillary hair.[15] In these patients, combined therapy with testosterone and growth hormone is sufficient. In conclusion, alterations of hair growth and structure described are reversible after adequate supplementary therapy.[16]

In polycystic ovarian syndrome, hypertrichosis due to peripheral hyperandrogenemia may occur, and this may be one of the first clinical signs indicating the underlying disorder. Polycystic ovarian syndrome is one of the most common reproductive endocrinopathies of women, having a prevalence of 2–20%.[17,18]

Malignant disease

Malignant diseases disturb the metabolic homeostasis and may reduce the synthesis of keratin, the delivery of energy substrates and finally the growth of hair. Therefore, in many cases a diffuse effluvium is recognized in patients with malignant tumors. In most cases, the hair of the scalp is affected and, more rarely, also the hair of other areas of the body. Conversely, hypertrichosis occurs in patients with metastatic renal adenocarcinoma and paraneoplastic hypertrichosis lanuginosa.[19]

Nutritional deficiencies

The regulation of hair growth is closely associated with the hormonal and nutritional state of an individual.[20,21] A study of more than 4000 preschool children in Zaire indicated that changes of the hair were related to their nutritional state. In children with normal weight-to-age ratio, hair signs were associated with the presence of clinical muscle wasting, indicating deficient intake of amino acids.[22]

Administration of home parenteral nutrition to patients with intestinal failure may also result in insufficient serum levels of copper, zinc, selenium, manganese and vitamins. In these patients hair changes were also observed.[23]

Amino acids

Normal uptake, transport and supply of amino acids is of fundamental importance in tissues with high biosynthetic activity. Deficiency of essential amino acids particularly influences the growth and differentiation of hair since 27% of the protein content of human hair comprises essential amino acids such as phenylalanine, isoleucine, tryptophan, methionine, leucine, valine, lysine and threonine. A reduced availability of protein leads, in all age groups, to thin and slow-growing hair, and finally, to diffuse alopecia. Histologic studies revealed that most hair bulbs are in telogen, with many broken-off hair shafts within the follicles.[24]

Trace elements and minerals

The main nutritional deficiencies in trace elements and minerals include zinc, copper, iron and selenium deficiencies.

Zinc is a well-known factor for hair growth and development; it plays a crucial role in the synthesis of testosterone, the function of steroid receptors, and also synthesis of nucleic acids and functional proteins, such as cellular retinoid binding protein (CRBP). In Figure 3 the typical clinical presentation of a patient with zinc deficiency is presented. Zinc is involved in the function of more than 100 enzymes, where zinc is a co-factor or covalently linked to the protein moiety. Zinc has also been shown to be a stabilizer of cellular membranes. A further important function is the formation of so-called 'zinc fingers'. These finger motifs are protein structures interacting with nucleic acids such as those in steroid hormone receptors.

Copper is an essential trace element and necessary for several metabolic processes. In copper deficiency, decreased activity of ATP synthetase and enzymes of the cytochrome oxidase

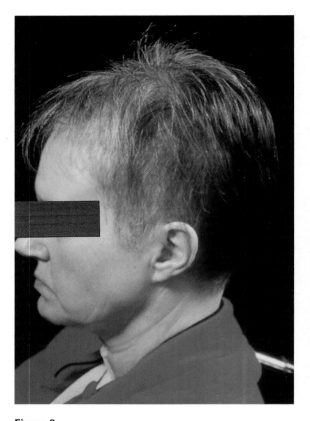

Figure 3

Typical clinical appearance of a patient with zinc deficiency.

system has been reported. Dysfunction of copper metabolism is present in hereditary disorders, for example in Menkes' disease and Wilson's disease.[25]

Iron, besides its role in heme synthesis, is a co-factor for several enzymes, for example monamine oxidase, succinate dehydrogenase and α-glycerophosphate oxidase. Iron deficiency may trigger a wide range of mucocutaneous alterations, although the mechanism underlying these alterations remains unknown. The influence of iron deficiency on hair growth has been described by Sato.[26]

The trace element *selenium* is involved in many antioxidant processes; it can be covalently bound to cysteine, thereby substituting sulfur in

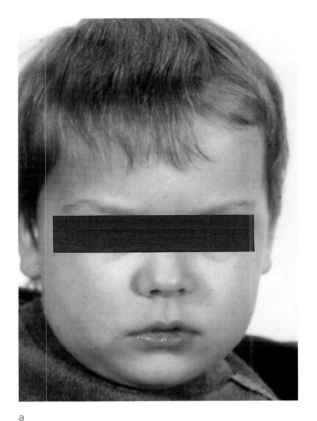

a

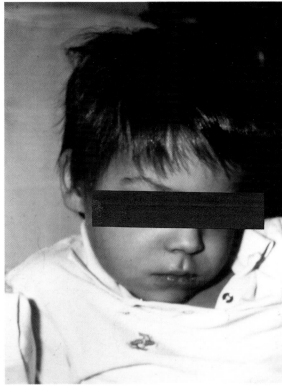

b

Figure 4

(a) Hypopigmented hair in selenium deficiency; **(b)** The effect of selenium supplementation in the same patient.

the sulfhydryl groups. An example is the glutathione peroxidase, where the covalently bound selenium atom acts as an electron acceptor and is regenerated by glutathione. The bioavailability of selenium is high, because of its good enteral absorption, but in cases with unbalanced parenteral substitution selenium deficiency may occur. Clinical symptoms are myopathy, retarded growth and pseudoalbinism. In Figure 4, a young boy with selenium deficiency after necrosis of the small intestine and after long-term parenteral nutrition without selenium supplementation, developed a switch from his dark hair to light hair accompanied by myopathy. After parenteral substitution of selenium, the hair pigmented again and myopathy disappeared.

Vitamins

With respect to the involvement of vitamins in hair growth and pigmentation, the roles of biotin, vitamin C, vitamin B_{12} and niacin will be discussed in more detail.

Biotin is a water-soluble vitamin, representing an essential co-factor for four carboxylating enzymes of intermediary metabolism: acetyl-CoA-carboxylase, 3-methyl-crotonyl-CoA-carboxylase, pyruvate carboxylase and propionyl-CoA-carboxylase. Under normal dietary conditions, nutritional biotin deficiency is unusual because biotin will be synthesized by intestinal bacteria in adequate amounts. Deficiency may occur after, however, raw egg intake or when the gut flora is altered. Nevertheless, human

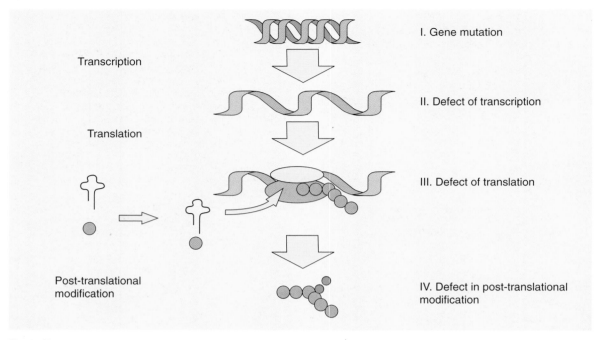

Figure 5

Subcellular targets of metabolic disorders involving the hair.

requirements for biotin remain uncertain and controversial.[27] Two forms of hereditary biotin deficiency have been described:

(1) holocarboxylase synthetase deficiency; and
(2) a defect of biotinidase.[28]

Hair changes caused by biotin deficiency are diffuse alopecia and depigmentation of the hair.[29]

Vitamin C (ascorbic acid) is a co-factor of several enzymes; however, most mucocutaneous alterations of vitamin C deficiency, or scurvy, are related to the role of vitamin C in collagen biosynthesis. Vitamin C is a co-factor of the enzyme proline hydroxylase, which is necessary for the post-translational modification of collagen molecules eventually leading to mature collagen triple helices. Dermatological features include follicular hyperkeratosis with 'corkscrew' hairs, perifollicular hemorrhages, and gingival hypertrophy. Alterations to the hair are related to

a decreased cross-linkage of hair keratin resulting from the decreased number of reduced disulfide bonds. The mechanism underlying the curling of the follicles is considered to be a result of altered perifollicular connective tissue.[20]

Vitamin B_{12} (cyanocobalamin) is involved in methyl group transfer. In vitamin B_{12} deficiency, altered pigmentation of the hair was found, and the hair reverted to normal following vitamin B_{12} supplementation.[30]

Niacin also plays an important role in the intermediary metabolism as a component of NADH and NADPH. In particular, NADH connects the citric acid cycle to the process of oxidative phosphorylation, which is important for the generation of ATP and, thereby, for energy supply. NADPH also plays a crucial role in the metabolism of steroids, for example in androgen biosynthesis at the level of the 5α-reductase, and also in fatty acid biosynthesis. Niacin deficiency is the cause of pellagra, which still occurs in areas of

Asia, Africa and India where maize and millet form the main diet. Sporadic cases of pellagra have also been reported in individuals with increased alcohol intake and in others with inadequate dietary intake, in patients with Crohn's disease, gastroenterostomy or jejunoileitis with impaired absorption of niacin. Hair changes seen in pellagra are the inhibition of hair growth, which may lead to diffuse alopecia.

Conclusion

Metabolic failures may involve disturbances in transcription (e.g. zinc deficiency), translation (e.g. deficiency of essential amino acids) or the post-translational modification (e.g. vitamin C deficiency). Figure 5 summarizes the main steps in protein biosynthesis and the possible defects. Most changes to the hair are non-specific to an underlying metabolic disorder, but are important premonitory clinical signs and markers. The distribution, thickness, density and color of the hair may provide the first indications for an underlying metabolic disorder or nutritional deficiency. The therapeutic approach depends on the type of disorder. In primary metabolic disorders such as genotrichoses for example, dietary or substitution therapy may be helpful. The benefit of novel approaches such as gene therapy targeting defective genes remains to be elucidated. In secondary metabolic disorders resulting from metabolic diseases such as diabetes mellitus, the first approach is the treatment of the underlying disease; additional dietary management will also be helpful. In nutritional deficiencies, an adequate supplementation and/or a change of dietary behavior is, in most cases, successful.

References

1. Comaish JS: Allgemeinzustand, Stoffwechsel und Haarkrankheiten. In: Orfanos CE (ed.). *Haar und Haarkrankheiten*, 2nd edn. Stuttgart, New York, Fischer Verlag, 1991: 321–342.
2. Geilen CC: Vitaminabhängige Veränderungen an Haut, Haaren und Nägeln. *Vitaminspur* 1995; **10**: 143–145.
3. Tumer Z, Horn N: Menkes disease: underlying genetic defect and new diagnostic possibilities. *J Inherit Metab Dis* 1998; **21**: 604–612.
4. Blume-Peytavi U, Völger S, Föhles J, Phan KH, Götte G, Orfanos CE: The hair: a diagnostic clue in Menkes' syndrome. In: Randall VA, Van Neste DJJ (eds.). *Hair Research for the Next Millennium*. Amsterdam, Elsevier Science, 1996: 27–30.
5. Price VH, Odom RB, Ward WH, Jones FT: Trichothiodystrophy: sulfur-deficient brittle hair as a marker for a neuroectodermal symptom complex. *Arch Dermatol* 1980; **116**: 1375–1384.
6. Itin PH, Pittelkow MR: Trichothiodystrophy with chronic neutropenia and mild mental retardation. *J Am Acad Dermatol* 1990; **24**: 356–358.
7. Hoeijmakers JHJ: Human nucleotide excision repair syndromes: molecular clues to unexpected intricacies. *Eur J Cancer* 1994; **30A**: 1912–1921.
8. Jaspers NG: Multiple involvement of nucleotide excision repair enzymes: clinical manifestations of molecular intricacies. *Cytokines Mol Ther* 1996; **2**: 115–119.
9. Auerbach AD, Verlander PC: Disorders of DNA replication and repair. *Curr Opin Pediatr* 1997; **9**: 600–616.
10. Blume-Peytavi U, Mandt N: Hair shaft abnormalities. In: Hordinsky M, Sawaya M, Scher R (eds.). *Atlas of Hair and Nails*. Philadelphia, WB Saunders, 1999: [In press].
11. Gillespie JM, Marshall RC, Rogers M: Trichothiodystrophy—biochemical and clinical studies. *Aust J Dermatol* 1988; **29**: 85–93.
12. Berchtold B: Skin manifestations in liver disease. *Ther Umsch* 1995; **52**: 226–229.
13. Lubach D: Dermatologische Veränderungen bei Patienten mit Langzeithämodialyse. *Hautarzt* 1980; **31**: 82–85.
14. Freinkel RK, Freinkel N: Hair growth and alopecia in hypothyroidism. *Arch Dermatol* 1972; **106**: 349–352.
15. Zaun H: Haarsymptome bei Endokrinopathien. *Z Hautkr* 1981; **9**: 555–560.
16. Feingold KR, Elias PM: Endocrine-skin interactions. *J Am Acad Dermatol* 1987; **17**: 921–940.
17. Ben-Chetrit A, Greenblatt EM: Recurrent maternal virilization during pregnancy associated with polycystic ovarian syndrome: a case report and review of the literature. *Hum Reprod* 1995; **10**: 3057–3060.
18. Knochenhauer ES, Key TJ, Kahsar-Miller M, Waggoner W, Boots LR, Azziz R: Prevalence of the polycystic ovary syndrome in unselected black and white women of the southeastern United States: a prospective study. *J Clin Endocrinol Metab* 1998; **83**: 3078–3082.
19. Velez A, Kindelan JM, Garcia-Herola A, Garcia-Lazaro M, Sanchez-Guijo P: Acquired trichomegaly and hypertrichosis in metastatic adenocarcinoma. *Clin Exper Dermatol* 1995; **20**: 237–239.

20. Miller SJ: Nutritional deficiency and the skin. *J Am Acad Dermatol* 1989; **21**: 1–30.

21. Galbraith H: Nutritional and hormonal regulation of hair follicle growth and development. *Proc Nutr Soc* 1998; **57**: 195–205.

22. Van den Biggelaar I, Van den Broeck J: Nutrition-related hair signs in Zairian preschool children and associations with anthropometry. *Trop Geogr Med* 1995; **47**: 248–251.

23. Forbes GM, Forbes A: Micronutrient status in patients receiving home parenteral nutrition. *Nutrition* 1997; **13**: 941–944.

24. McLaren DS: Skin in protein energy malnutrition. *Arch Dermatol* 1987; **123**: 1674–1676.

25. Nath R: Copper deficiency and heart disease: molecular basis, recent advances and current concepts. *Int J Biochem Cell Biol* 1997; **29**: 1245–1254.

26. Sato S: Iron deficiency: structural and microchemical changes in hair, nails, and skin. *Semin Dermatology* 1991; **10**: 313–319.

27. Mock DM: Biotin status: which are valid indicators and how do we know? *J Nutr* [Suppl] 1999; **129**: 498–503.

28. Nyhan WL: Inborn errors of biotin metabolism. *Arch Dermatol* 1987; **123**: 1696–1698.

29. Mock DM: Skin manifestations of biotin deficiency. *Semin Dermatol* 1991; **10**: 296–302.

30. Carmel R: Hair and fingernail changes in acquired and congenital pernicious anemia. *Arch Intern Med* 1985; **145**: 484–485.

26
Menkes' disease

José Luis Díaz-Pérez

with the collaboration of R Zabala Echenagusía, L Díaz Ramón, N Agesta Sanchez, A Sanchez Díez

Introduction

Menkes' disease, also known as kinky hair disease and trichopoliodystrophy, is a multisystem lethal disorder, first described by Menkes in 1962.[1] It is a rare disorder and estimates of its incidence range between 1 in 100 000 and 1 in 250 000.

In 1972 Danks et al.[2] found low serum levels of copper and ceruloplasmin in patients with this condition. The abnormal copper metabolism in Menkes' disease explains most of the clinical features and pathologic findings of this process. Numerous enzymes, such as lysil oxidase, cytochrome c oxidase, dopamine(-beta) hydroxylase and superoxide dismutase are all copper-dependent, and its deficiency can explain the connective tissue alterations, as well as neurodegenerative changes and hair and skin manifestations.[3]

Although this X-linked disease is detectable at birth, or even during intrauterine life, the first clinical manifestations become apparent in the first 6 months of life. The more remarkable clinical features at onset are: seizures; sparse, coarse, brittle hair in a child with hypotony; and delayed psychomotor and somatic development.

Localization of the Menkes' locus and isolation of the responsible gene have linked Menkes' disease to the occipital horn syndrome (OHS). Mild cases of Menkes' disease of late onset do not usually follow the aggressive lethal course found in cases of early onset.

Pathogenesis of Menkes' disease

Changes in copper metabolism can explain many if not all the clinical findings of Menkes' disease. The impaired intestinal absorption of copper accounts for the low levels of copper in blood, and subsequently in brain and liver. Paradoxically, accumulation of copper appears in most tissues (e.g. pancreas, spleen, kidney, muscles, fibroblast, lymphocytes, etc.). The alterations in copper metabolism begin with its impaired intestinal absorption and continue with failed utilization in other cells and tissues.

Numerous enzymes are copper-dependent. (Table 1). Most clinical findings in Menkes' disease are clearly linked to deficient activity of specific copper-dependent enzymes. Defective lysil oxidase and tyroxinase activity account for alterations in collagen and elasticity, also hypopigmented hair and skin. The neurologic and other tissue dysfunctions can also be explained on the base of other enzyme alterations (see Table 1).

Clinical features of Menkes' disease

As expected in an X-linked disease, Menkes' disease occurs in male infants. At birth, the clinical changes are usually unremarkable; however, retrospective studies of clinical histories of these patients from birth have shown that these children may have cephalohematomas (Figure 1) premature delivery, hypotermia, jaundice, inguinal and umbilical hernias (Figure 2), and pectum excavatum. Sparse, hypopigmented hair may also be present at birth but this is a common finding in many normal neonates.[4]

At the age of 2–3 months, the disease becomes evident. The first alarming sign is usually an episode of seizures or clonic convulsions (see

Table 1   Copper-dependent enzymes.

Enzyme	Function	Effects of deficient activity
Cytochrome c oxidase	Electron transport	Myopathy, muscle weakness, ataxia, seizures
Lysyl oxidase	Collagen and elastin sintexis	Vascular elastic tissue abnormalities, vessel tortuositi, bladder diverticulae, osseos abnormalities, loose skin and joints
Superoxide dismutase	Free-radical neutralization	Myelin degeneration, spasticity seizures
Dopamine β-hydroxylase	Catecholamine production	Temperature instability, hypothermia, hypotension, hypoglycemia, dehydration, eyelid ptosis, pupillary constriction, somnolence
Peptidylyglycine alpha-amidating mono-oxygenase (PAM)		Reduced gastrin cholecystokinin, vasoactive intestinal polypeptide (VIP), corticotrophin-releasing hormone, bioactivity of neuroendocrine peptides, thyrotrophin-releasing hormone, calcitonin, vasopressin, melanocyte-stimulating hormone
Diamine oxidases	Histamine metabolism Tyrosinase production	Reduced histamine degradation Skin and hair hypopigmentation
Cross-linkase	Cross-linking of keratin	Brittle hair, eczema
Ceruloplasmin	Copper metabolism?	Decreased circulating copper levels

Other enzymes
  Ascorbate oxidase
  Urate oxidase
  Galactose oxidase
  Hexose oxidase		

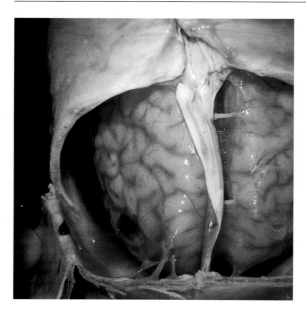

Figure 1

Large cephalohematoma (Case 1, Table 1).

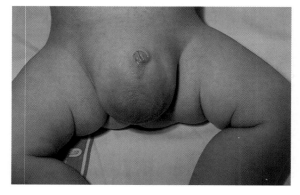

Figure 2

Inguinal hernia (Case 2, Table 1).

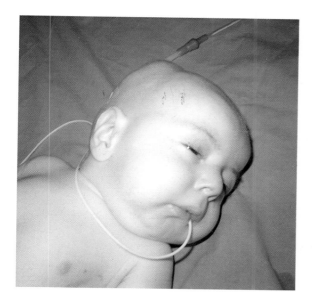

Figure 3

Palor, round, puffy cheek (Case 1).

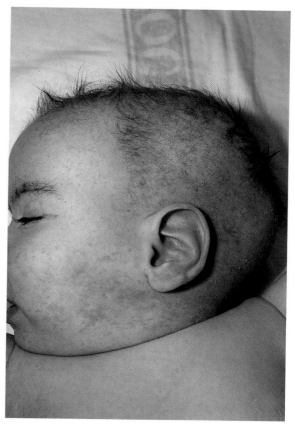

a

Table 1). At this time, electroencephalographic changes are frequently evident. The patient may also have failure to thrive, hypotony, palor and hypotermia. The hair is hypopigmented, sparse, brittle, and shorter than in most children of this age. On the sides and posterior scalp, the hair is less abundant and shorter than on the top. The eyebrows may have the same changes, although these are not so prominent as in the scalp.

These children usually have a characteristic facies. The palate is highly arched, and the micrognatia, together with puffy, sagging cheeks, gives them a peculiar aspect that has been called 'piggy face' (Figures 3 and 4).

The skin is pale, and appears loose and redundant on the trunk and folds. Inguinal or umbilical herniations may also be present (Figure 2). Signs of neurological involvement are prominent. Profound hypotony with diminished motility and strength is also present. Deep tendon reflexes may be hyper-reactive. Somatic development may appear normal early after birth but, later, children usually fail to gain weight despite the linear grow being normal.

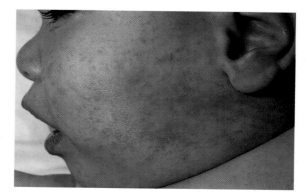

b

Figure 4

(a) Puffy cheek, seborrheic-like dermatitis, and sparse, short hair (Case 2); (b) Shown in close-up photograph.

Hair changes in Menkes' disease

The hair anomalies that are always present become more clinically apparent with evolution of the disease. In most cases, the hair is studied when the patient is hospitalized because of an episode of seizures, which is frequently the first alarming manifestation. On microscopic examination, the hair shows diagnostic alterations. Twisted hairs (pili torti) are the more prominent and frequent finding. Pili torti can be detected on low-power (×40) examination using the regular light microscope or by stereoscopic microscopy, although these changes may be more evident using higher magnifications or polarized light (Figures 5 and 6). Apart from twisted hair, several other anomalies can also been seen; for example, trichoschisis (fractures with a paint-brush appearance); trichosclasis (transverse fractures); and trichoptilosis (longitudinal splitting of the hair shaft).[5] Thickenings and narrowings (pseudo-monilethrix-like changes), without the regularity found in true monilethrix can also be found (see Figure 6).

Cuticular anomalies may be moderate or absent, but they can also be very intense. In one patient we observed profound cuticular indentations that simulated saw teeth; this alteration was more prominent on examination using a scanning electron microscope. (Figure 7).

Seizing the opportunity to study the hair changes in two patients since birth we detected diagnostic pili torti changes preceeding the electroencephalographic changes, and the episodes of seizures. In both cases, pili torti was evident at the age of 1 month (Table 2, Cases 4 and 5) several months earlier than the first episode of seizures.

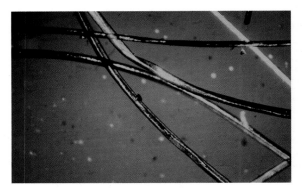

Figure 5

Twisted kinky hairs shown under polarized light (×40 magnification).

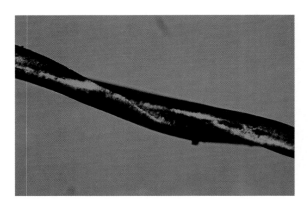

Figure 6

Twisted hair shown under polarized light (×200 magnification).

Analytical studies

Hypocupremia and hypoceruloplasminemia are the more consistent and frequent analytical changes found in patients with Menkes' disease. These, together with pili torti, are the basic diagnostic criteria. Hypocupremia and hypoceruloplasminemia are not present at birth, but usually became apparent at 2 months of age and are a consistent finding throughout evolution of Menkes' disease (Table 3). Plasma levels of catecholamines are usually low from birth, and this change is a more reliable indicator for early diagnosis, than hypocuremia or hypoceruloplasminemia, which may not be found at birth and which can also be low in normal neonates.[6] Increased alkaline phosphatase, anemia, increased sedimentation rate, and other changes are variable and thus are unhelpful during diagnosis.

With the exception of liver, brain, and hair, all other organs and tissues have increased amounts of copper (see Table 3).

Anatomopathologic changes in Menkes' disease

The defective function of copper-dependent enzymes accounts for the cutaneous, osseous, and neurologic changes of this disease. The pathological changes in the collagen and elastic tissue of the dermis, although present, are not evident on morphological grounds, either by routine microscopic studies or by electron microscopy. By contrast, medium- and large-size vessels have prominent morphological changes that are easily visualized using conventional microscopy. Defective elastin synthesis is the cause of the tortuosities of the intracranial, and other visceral vessels. Changes in the vessels in autopsy tissue from two children with Menkes'

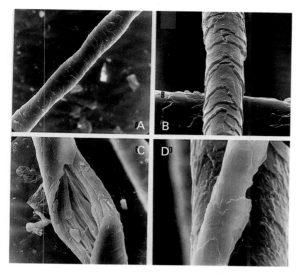

Figure 7

(A) Twisted hair with longitudinal splitting; **(B)** Twisted hair mimicking the appearance of pseudo monilethrix; **(C)** Cuticular defects; **(D)** Cuticular changes with appearance of saw-teeth.

Table 2 Clinical cases of Menkes' disease.

Case	Age at diagnosis (months)	Changes	Plasma copper levels (70–165 µgr/dl)	Plasma ceruloplasmin levels (20–60 mg/dl)	Age at death (months)
1	3	Seizures Hypothermia Hypotonia Bone fractures Cephalohematoma	25	25	4
2	6	Seizures Anemia Respir. infections Seborrheic derm.	12	17	9
3	2	Seizures Hypothermia Anemia	29	4	7
4	1	Seizures Hypothermia Anemia Respir. infections Seborrheic derm.	31	4	28
5	1	Seizures Hypothermia Plaquetopenia	20	4	24
6	2.5	Seizures Hypothermia Hypotonia	22	0.2	32

Table 3   Plasma copper concentration in Menkes' disease.

Anatomical site	Fetus	Neonate	Infant
Serum Skin	Normal or increased	Normal or increased	Decreased
Liver Brain	Decreased	Decreased	Decreased
Kidney Spleen Pancreas Duodenum Fibroblasts	Increased	Increased	Increased

disease[7] showed duplication of the internal elastic lamina in arteries, fenestrations and multiple fracture points in the elastic layers of arteries and veins and these are frequent findings in large- and medium-sized vessels (Figures 8–13).

Arteries and veins have a high requirement for new elastic tissue because of their rapid growth in infancy. Two morphologically different types of elastic tissue can be observed. The elastic tissue synthesized during fetal life has a normal appearance, while the new elastic tissue synthesized in the vessels under hypocupremic conditions has a basophilic irregular appearance and it is randomly deposited between the normal-appearing elastic tissue synthesized during fetal life (Figures 9, 11 and 12). Using electron microscopy, there are important differences between the fetal and the newly synthesized elastic tissue (Figures 14 and 15). In our study it became apparent that the elastic tissue of arteries with faster growth requirements became earlier and more intensively affected than arteries without important growth requirements at that age. For example, epididimal or testicular arteries had elastic tissue of normal appearance because it was synthesized during fetal life in conditions of normal serum copper levels.

Image studies

Regular radiographic studies may reveal abnormalities on the skull (wormian bones), subdural hematomas, long bone and rib fractures, meta-

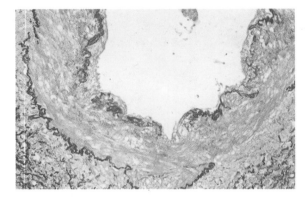

Figure 8

Fenestration seen in multiple breaking points of elastic layers of a branch of the arteria cerebri media.

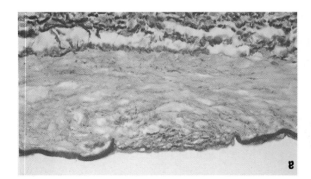

Figure 9

Arteria coronaria showing fenestration of the internal elastic lamina. The elastic tissue is attempting to restore the defect of the internal elastic lamina.

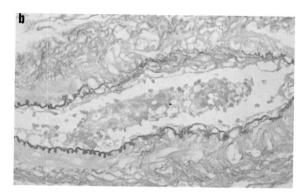

Figure 10

Branch of arteria pulmonalis showing splitting of the internal elastic lamina.

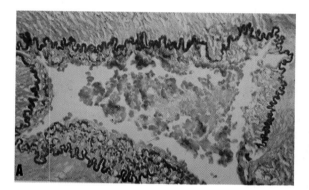

Figure 11

Arteria lingualis with ectopic elastic tissue below the internal elastic lamina, mimicking arteriosclerotic changes.

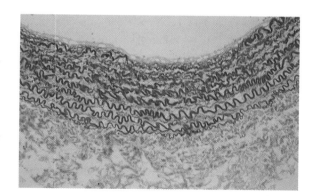

Figure 12

Arteria pulmonalis with similar changes to that shown in Figure 11. This artery, however, is not arteriosclerotic.

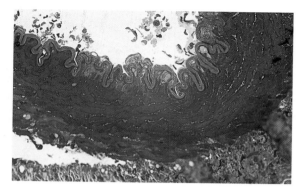

Figure 13

Semi-thin section of a branch of the arteria cerebri media, showing two zones of duplication of the internal elastic lamina.

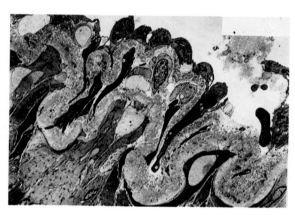

Figure 14

Widening of the subendothelial space, with elongated muscular cells migrating through the internal elastic lamina (detail of Figure 13, ×5200 magnification).

physeal spurring and hypodense (ricket-like) bones.[4] Angiographic studies may reveal the corkscrew appearance of cerebral vessels (Figure 16). Cystography or pelvic ultrasound can be used to show diverticula of the urinary bladder. Magnetic resonance imaging (MRI) of the brain may show evidence of white-matter anomalies (mainly diffuse atrophy), impaired myelinization, ventriculomegaly and tortuosity of the cerebral

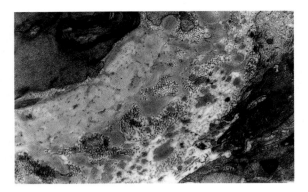

Figure 15

Homogeneous, normal-appearing, internal elastic lamina, underlying abnormal more electron dense elastic tissue (×13 200 magnification).

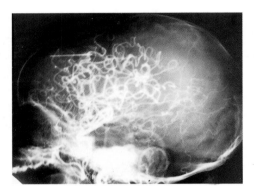

Figure 16

Carotid arteriography showing arterial tortuosities.

blood vessels. Electroencephalographic (EEG) studies are usually normal in the first few months of life but disclose moderate to severe abnormalities later in life.[8]

Prenatal diagnosis and neonatal signs in Menkes' disease

Cells from amniocentesis and chorionic villus sampling cells have an elevated content of copper, and there is also a reduced copper egress from cultured amniocytes and chorionic cells. These facts form the basis for the prenatal diagnosis of Menkes' disease. This testing is indicated in pregnancies of known or suspected female carriers.[8–13]

Following the diagnosis of Menkes' disease in a son, the risk recurrence in future pregnancies has been estimated to be 25%. Suspected carriers are the mother, sisters and daughters of a woman with a son diagnosed with Menkes' disease.[14] Carrier women experience minimal effects of Menkes' disease, including pili torti, which can be also found in 50% of obligate Menkes' heterozygotes.

The clinical manifestations of Menkes' disease in neonates are minimal or subtle and usually not diagnosed at birth. Nevertheless cephalohematomas, inguinal or umbilical hernias and pectum excavatum are frequently present at birth in children later diagnosed as having Menkes' disease. Premature labor and delivery, hypothermia and hypoglucaemia can also indicate the presence of Menkes' disease. Hypopigmented sparse hair can also be present at birth but microscopic findings of pili torti can be found only after the first month of life. The phenotypic appearance of the face is rather characteristic (e.g. micrognathia, puffy cheeks) (see Figures 3 and 4), but a high degree of experience and suspicion is necessary to indicate diagnosis on these grounds.

The occipital horn syndrome and late-onset Menkes' disease

In the occipital horn syndrome (X-linked cutis laxa), the occipital calcification within the trapezius and the sternocleidomastoid muscles, gives a radiographic horn appearance. This protuberance can be palpated in some patients but is easily visualized using conventional radiography, computerized tomography or MRI. Patients with the occipital horn syndrome may also have radiographic abnormalities in long bones and clavicles. Other clinical findings include lax skin and joints, vascular tortuosity, abdominal hernias, bladder diverticula and low intelligence; these are also common findings in Menkes' disease.

The analytical changes are less intense than in Menkes' disease, but low copper and ceruloplasmin levels can also be detected in some patients with the occipital horn syndrome. Copper egress in cultured fibroblasts is impaired as it is in classical Menkes' disease and the activity of the lysyl oxidase in fibroblasts is also markedly reduced.

A variable spectrum of severity exists in patients with Menkes' disease. There are several reported cases of mild late-onset Menkes' disease.[8–13,15–20] All of them had pili torti, and they may share features of both Menkes' disease and the occipital horn syndrome (X-linked cutis laxa). They may have low copper and ceruloplasmin levels, abnormal plasma catecholamines, mental retardation, neuromuscular weakness and joint abnormalities. Seizures may start late in childhood and not in the first year of life as usually happens in the early-onset of classical Menkes' disease.

The Menkes' gene

Menkes' disease is known to have X-linked inheritance from the earliest descriptions.[1,2] Linkage studies on families with Menkes' diseases and an additional chromosomal rearrangement described in a Menkes' patient support an Xq13 location for the Menkes' defect.[17,18]

In 1993 the Menkes' disease gene was physically mapped, and subsequent cloning of the gene revealed a 1500 amino acid protein very similar to a bacterial copper-transporting ATPase. This study demonstrated that the Menkes' gene was expressed in almost all human tissues tested (except in liver) and was also physiologically consistent with the biochemical defect of Menkes' disease. This ATPase is essential for the copper transport across the gastrointestinal tract, blood–brain barrier and placenta, and its absence or dysfunction results in the clinical features of this disorder.

In recent immunocytochemical studies, the Menkes' copper transport protein (ATP7A) has been located at the trans-Golgi network (one of the three functional subcompartments of the Golgi complex) of all cells. It is known that the increase in cellular copper concentration results in trafficking of these ATPases from the trans-Golgi network to a cytoplasmatic vesicular compartment, prior to transcytoplasmic membrane elimination. The exact biochemical change that blocks the transport of copper to the outside of the cells in Menkes' disease is not yet well understood, although a functional defect of this ATPase is probably implicated.[19–20]

Treatment of Menkes' disease

Oral administration of copper or copper derivatives is not useful because the absorption of this metal is blocked at the intestinal level. Parenteral administration of copper may, however, restore the circulating copper and ceruloplasmin to normal levels. Hepatic storage of copper is quickly replenished by parenteral therapy; however, the levels of copper in the brain may either not increase at all or increase very slowly.[21] Copper histidine has been the parenteral treatment more frequently used. When used very early on, the most severe neurological problems may occasionally be partially prevented. Some modest clinical benefit, including decreased seizure frequency and reduced irritability, have been reported.[10,22–24] Proximal renal tubular damage is a well-known side-effect of copper overloading. The copper replacement treatment deserves a stronger consideration in the very few cases in which the diagnosis has been made prior to the onset of the neurological damage. Vitamins E and C have also been suggested as therapy because of their antioxidant properties that may enhance copper uptake by cells.

Gene therapy for Menkes' disease is a theoretical possibility, although this requires targeting specific organs and Menkes' disease affects most tissues in the body. Genetic counselling may also be offered, since, as an X-linked recessive disease, the gene is transmitted by female asymptomatic carriers to 50% of their male offspring, who will suffer Menkes' disease, and also to 50% of their female offspring, who will be carriers. Female relatives of a gene carrier should be offered genetic counselling, carrier testing, and when positive if pregnant, prenatal diagnosis.

References

1. Menkes JH, Alter M, Steigleder GK, Weakley DR, Sung JH: A sex-linked recessive disorder with retardation for growth, peculiar hair, and focal cerebral and cerebellar degeneration. *Pediatrics* 1962; **29**: 764.

2. Danks DM, Stevens BJ, Campbell PE, et al.: Menkes' kinky hair syndrome; an inherited defect in intestinal copper absorption with widespread consequences. *Lancet* 1972; **1**: 1100.

3. Danks DM, Cartwright E, Stevens BJ, Townley RRW: Menkes' kinky hair disease: further definition of defect in copper transport. *Science* 1973; **179**: 1140.

4. Wesemberg RL, Gwinn JL, Barnes GR: Radiological findings in the kinky hair syndrome. *Radiology* 1969; **92**: 500.

5. Horn N, Mikkelsen M, Heydorn K, Damsgaard B, Tysgrup I: Copper and steely hair. *Lancet* 1975; **1**: 1236.

6. Gokat J, Stevenson RE, Hefferan PM, Rodney Howell R: Menkes' disease: biochemical abnormality in cultured human fibroblast. *Proc Natl Acad Sci* 1976; **73**: 604.

7. Díaz-Pérez, JL, Rua MJ, Prats JM, Bilbao FJ, Rivera JM: Enfermedad de Menkes: estudio anatomoclínico. *Med Cut ILA* 1980; **8**: 23.

8. Stephen G, Kaler MD: Menkes' disease. *Adv Pediatr* 1994; **41**: 263–304.

9. Tumer Z, Horn N: Menkes' disease: underlying genetic defect and new diagnostic possibilities. *J Inherit Metab Dis* 1998; **21**: 604.

10. Christodoulou J, Danks DM, Sarkar B, et al.: Early treatment of Menkes' disease with parenteral copper-histidine: long-term follow-up of four treated patients. *Am J Med Genet* 1998; **76(2)**: 154.

11. Tumer Z, Horn N: Menkes' disease: recent advances and new aspects. *J Med Genet* 1997; **34(4)**: 265.

12. Ramos Fernández JM, Lorenzo G, Aparicio Meix JM, Briones P, Fernández Toral J, Martínez Pardo M: Menkes' disease with normal cytochrome oxidase activity in fibroblast: report of a case and an update. *An Esp Pediatr* 1998; **49**: 85.

13. Tümer Z, Horn N: Menkes' disease: recent advances and new insights into copper metabolism. *Ann Med* 1996; **28**: 121.

14. Horn N: Menkes' X-linked disease: prenatal diagnosis and carrier detection. *J Inherited Metab Dis* 1983; **6(Suppl 1)**: 59.

15. Horn N, Tonnesen T, Tümer Z: Variability in clinical expression of X-linked copper disturbance, Menkes' disease. In: Sarkar B (ed.). *Metals and Genetics*. New York, Marcel and Dekker, 1995: 285

16. Yang H-M, Lund T, Niebuhr E, Norby S, Schwartz M, Shen L: Exclusion mapping of 12 X-linked disease loci and 10 DNA probes from long arm of the X-chromosome. *Clin Genet* 1990; **38**: 94.

17. Verga V, Hall BK, Wang S, Johnson S, Higgings JV, Glover TW: Localization and translocation breakpoint in a female with Menkes' syndrome to Xq13.2-q13.3 proximal to PGK-1. *Am J Hum Genet* 1991; **48**: 1133.

18. Tommerup N, Tümer Z, Tonnesen T, Horn NA: Cytogenetic survey in Menkes' disease: implications of chromosomal rearrangements in X-linked disorders. *J Med Genet* 1993; **30**: 314.

19. Harrinson MD, Dameron CT: Molecular mechanisms of copper metabolism and the role of the Menkes' disease protein. *J Biochem Mol Toxicol* 1999; **13**: 93.

20. Harris ED, Qian Y, Reddy MC: Genes regulating copper metabolism. *Mol Cell Biochem* 1998; **188(1–2)**: 57.

21. Garnica AD: The failure of parenteral copper therapy in Menkes' kinky hair syndrome. *Eur J Pediatr* 1984; **142**: 98.

22. Nadal D, Baerlocher K: Menkes' disease: long-term treatment with copper and D-penicillamine. *Eur J Pediatr* 1988; **147**: 621.

23. Sherwood G, Sarkar B, Sass-Kortsak A: Copper histidine therapy in Menkes' disease. Prevention of progressive neurodegeneration. *J Inherited Metab Dis* 1989; **12 (Suppl 2)**: 393.

24. Kaler SG, Gahl WA: Early copper histidine therapy in Menkes' disease. *Pediatr Res* 1992; **31**: 186A/1101.

Section VI

HAIR SHAFT ABNORMALITIES

27
Office diagnosis of hair shaft abnormalities

David A Whiting

Introduction

Most hair shaft abnormalities can be diagnosed in the office by any interested clinician. The important requirements here are a good clinical history of the complaint, a careful examination of the hair and scalp, and evaluation of affected hair shafts under the light microscope. It is important to take representative hairs showing the abnormality from different areas of the scalp.

Hair shaft defects can be inherited or acquired and are sometimes useful indicators of underlying disease. Some defects are associated with increased fragility of the hair causing damage and patchy hair loss, and others have no functional significance.[1–5]

It is sometimes possible to detect hair damage with the naked eye; usually, however, examination under an adequate light microscope is required, either with normal transmitted light or with polarized light. Hairs can be examined dry between two glass slides; they are seen better and under higher magnification if a mounting medium is used, with the hairs placed side by side on the slide without overlap under the cover slip. This provides a permanent preparation that is free of optical distortion. Hairs can also be examined quickly when applied to slides coated with clear double-sided sticky tape. Scanning or transmission electron microscopes are rarely necessary for a clinical diagnosis of a hair shaft abnormality, although they have great value as research tools.[3]

Before making the diagnosis of a hair shaft abnormality, it is important to have a thorough knowledge of the variations in normal hairs. It should be remembered that normal hairs differ considerably in length, diameter, cross-section, color and cuticular pattern even in the same patient. Most hair shaft abnormalities can be seen sporadically in normal hair so need to be found consistently in different areas of the scalp to be of diagnostic importance.[6]

Remember that a normal hair varies in structure and may be straight, wavy, curly, woolly or peppercorn.[7] Asiatic hair is rounded in cross-section and is usually straight. Caucasian hair is oval in cross-section and may be straight, wavy or curly. Negroid hair is usually elliptical or flattened in cross-section and is either woolly or peppercorn in form.

The normal hair shaft maintains a fairly constant diameter throughout its length.[8,9] The shaft may or may not have a central medullary cavity with loosely keratinized cells and pigment. Surrounding the cavity is the keratinized cortex, which provides most of the tensile strength of the hair. Melanin granules are aligned longitudinally in cortical cells and delicate air spaces may exist between the cortical cells. The cortex consists of many parallel, elongated cortical cells aligned along the long axis of the shaft. These provide most of the tensile strength of the hair. The cortex is covered by a single layer of imbricated cuticular cells, which overlap to form a layer six to ten cells thick. This cohesive keratinized exoskeleton binds the inner cortical fibers together, providing support and protection for the hair shaft.

Another factor to remember is that hair undergoes periods of growth and rest and therefore undergoes changes that distinguish anagen from catagen and telogen hair and these phases should be recognized.[10]

Weathering

Weathering is the 'wear-and-tear' that affects the free end of both normal and abnormal hairs.[11] It is an important phenomenon and extremely common. Weathering causes damage to cuticle and cortex. Abnormal hairs with inherited weaknesses are particularly susceptible to weathering, nevertheless weathering can occur in normal hair, particularly hair that is left to grow long.[12] Weathering is exaggerated by sun, wind, swimming, washing, friction and excessive hair styling. Various physical and chemical factors, both environmental and cosmetic, can damage the hair cuticle in a progressive manner. Cuticular cells are gradually eroded and broken away, especially in the distal shaft where they are less adherent.[13] The cuticle is often totally lost at the free end of the hair exposing the underlying cortical fibers. These fray and split. It is a good idea when evaluating hair shaft abnormalities to examine the proximal 1–2 cm of the affected shaft adjacent to the scalp to exclude the effects of weathering.

Classification of hair shaft defect

For easy office diagnosis, a microscopic classification of hair shaft abnormalities is most useful. The precise diagnosis of the hair shaft defect often depends on its appearance under the light microscope, and nearly all known abnormalities can be recognized in this way. Even the longitudinal grooves present in uncombable hair can usually be seen by careful manipulation of the substage condenser and judicious use of the polarizer.

With light microscopy hair shaft abnormalities can be divided into four categories, these include:

(1) fractures of the hair shaft;
(2) irregularities of the hair shaft;
(3) hair shaft coiling and twisting; and
(4) extraneous matter on the hair shaft.[1,3]

The abnormalities in this classification are detailed in Table 1, where an association with hair fragility[2] is also indicated.

Fractures of the hair shaft

Transverse fractures

Trichorrhexis nodosa

Trichorrhexis nodosa is one of the most common defects of the hair shaft. It appears along the hair shaft as beaded swellings associated with a loss of cuticle.[9,14,15] This exposes the underlying cortical fibers which separate and fray, producing a nodular swelling that resembles two paint brushes thrust into one another. If there is a complete breakage at this point, a typical expanded fracture results. Clinically, the nodes are seen as pale specks fixed to the proximal or distal hair shaft. The basic cause of trichorrhexis nodosa is mechanical or chemical trauma.[14,16] A contributory factor here is underlying weakness of the hair shaft. Trauma includes excessive weathering, backcombing, stressed hair styles, head rolling and banging, habit tics, trichotillomania, scratching, perming and dyeing of hair. The condition is aggravated if the hair is already brittle such as in pili torti, monilethrix, pseudomonilethrix, trichorrhexis invaginata, trichothiodystrophy,[17] argininosuccinic aciduria,[18,19] citrullinemia[20] or Menkes' disease.[21] Trichorrhexis nodosa can be congenital or acquired. Congenital trichorrhexis nodosa is rare[22] but may occur as an isolated entity or it may occur with a metabolic abnormality such as argininosuccinic aciduria,[23] citrullinemia,[20,24] Menkes' disease[21] or trichothiodystrophy.[17,25] Acquired trichorrhexis nodosa resulting from excessive hair straightening, styling or brushing is much more common. The proximal form is common in black populations and the distal form of trichorrhexis nodosa occurs in white or Oriental populations as a rule.[22] A microscopic demonstration of the typical expanded fractures resulting from loss of cuticle and fraying of cortical fibers is diagnostic.

Trichoclasis

Trichoclasis is the common greenstick fracture of the hair shaft.[26] It consists of a transverse fracture of the shaft, which is splinted in part by an intact cuticle. This is usually a sporadic defect and it is caused by physical and chemical trauma. There is no constant abnormality of

Table 1   Classification of hair-shaft abnormalities.*

Fractures of the hair shaft	Transverse	**Trichorrhexis nodosa
		Trichoclasis
		**Trichoschisis
		**Trichorrhexis invaginata
	Oblique	**Tapered fracture
	Longitudinal	Trichoptilosis
Irregularities of the hair shaft		Longitudinal ridging and grooving
		Uncombable hair or pili trianguli et canaliculi or spun glass hair, including straight hair nevus
		Loose anagen syndrome
		Pili multigemini and pili bifurcati
		Trichostasis spinulosa
		Pili annulati
		Pseudopili annulati
		**Monilethrix
		**Pseudomonilethrix
		**Tapered hairs, including Pohl-Pinkus mark, bayonet hairs, tapered newly growing anagen hairs, and trichomalacia
		Bubble hairs
		**Intermittent hair follicle dystrophy
Hair shaft coiling and twisting		**Pili torti, including corkscrew hair and Menkes' syndrome
		Woolly hair, including acquired progressive kinking, acquired non-progressive kinking, and whisker hair
		Trichonodosis (knotted hair)
		Circle hairs
Extracutaneous matter on the hair shaft	Fungi	Tinea capitis
		Piedra
	Bacteria	Trichomycosis axillaris
	Pediculosis	Nits
	Peripilar casts	Pseudonits
	Deposits	Lacquer, paint, glue

* After Whiting DA: Structural abnormalities of the hair shaft. *J Am Acad Dermatol* 1987; **16:** 1–25.
** Associated with hair fragility.

cuticle, cortex or sulfur content. Trichoclasis can be associated with congenital hair shaft abnormalities such as pili torti and pseudomonilethrix in which the cuticles remain intact, or it can occur in normal hair. It is caused by physical trauma such as excessive hair care or chemical trauma from perms and dyes. It is usually patchy rather than widespread.

Trichoschisis

Trichoschisis is a clean, transverse fracture across the hair shaft. It is associated with a localized absence of cuticle cells.[27] It is caused by trauma and can occur sporadically but is usually seen in the congenitally brittle hair of tricho-

thiodystrophy.[17] In this condition, the hair sulfur content is 50% lower than normal. The affected hair shafts are often ribbon-like, with flattening and folding. Most fractures show the clean breaks of trichoschisis but others can show the appearance of trichorrhexis nodosa. The diagnostic features here are the alternating bright and dark bands, or tiger or zebra stripes, which are seen in the hair shaft under polarized light (Figure 1). Severe alopecia occurs in scalp, eyebrows and eyelashes. The hairs are dry and coarse and break off near the skin surface. Trichothiodystrophy can be associated with many other conditions such as intellectual impairment,[28] decreased fertility,[29] short statue,[30] ichthyosis,[31] photosensitivity,[32] and other abnormalities.[33]

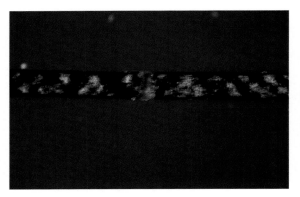

Figure 1

Trichothiodystrophy. Trichoschisis and alternating bright and dark bands are shown using polarized light.

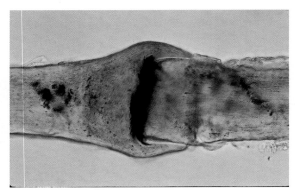

Figure 2

Trichorrhexis invaginata. Netherton's syndrome, bamboo hair.

The use of polarizing sheets and the office microscope demonstrates the banded hairs and, in conjunction with the clinical findings, confirms the diagnosis.

Trichorrhexis invaginata or bamboo hair

Trichorrhexis invaginata is characterized by a nodular expansion of the hair shaft in which a ball-and-socket joint is formed.[34] Many small nodules are seen at irregular intervals along affected hairs. The hair is usually brittle, thin and short.[35] This abnormality is seen scattered around the scalp in Netherton's syndrome.[36] This is characterized by the presence of ichthyosis – normally usually ichthyosis linearis circumflexa – which is a migrating, annular, red, scaly dermatosis.[37] Sometimes it is characterized by lamellar ichthyosis or congenital ichthyosiform erythroderma;[35] it is also frequently associated with atopy and episodes of erythroderma can occur, following any infection.[38]

Under the light microscope the ball-and-socket joint of trichorrhexis nodosa is distinctive (Figure 2). However pili torti and trichorrhexis nodosa are sometimes seen in Netherton's syndrome. The combination of these two defects causes torsion nodes.[34] A fracture through the ball-and-socket joint leaving the proximal cup-shaped segment intact results in the so-called 'golf tee hairs' of Netherton's syndrome.[39] These are all easily recognized under the light microscope but are often sparse and hard to find among many normal hairs. The ball-and-socket fractures are diagnostic of the condition.

Oblique fractures

Tapered fracture

Tapered fractures resembling pencil points are caused by inhibition of nucleic acid and protein synthesis in the hair root.[26] Progressive narrowing of the emerging hair shaft may lead to a fracture near the skin surface. This results in a detached hair with a tapered, proximal end. This sort of appearance is common in anagen effluvium caused by a cytostatic drug. Once the drug is removed, hair growth renews and the newly growing anagen hair has the pencil pointing in reverse, with the hair shaft gradually thickening up back to a normal appearance. Tapered hairs can also be seen in localized areas following radiotherapy and they can also occur in a more generalized fashion in severe protein calorie malnutrition, such as seen in marasmus or kwashiorkor. They can also be seen in dystrophic anagen hairs in alopecia areata, their tapered tips contrasting with the nodular trichorrexis nodosa-like fracture found at the top of the classical telogen exclamation point hairs of alopecia areata.[40]

Longitudinal fracture

Trichoptilosis

Trichoptilosis is the longitudinal splitting of the distal end of the hair.[26] This results from weathering of the cuticle exposing cortical fibers, which separate like the frayed ends of a rope. Sometimes, however, central trichoptilosis is seen where the longitudinal split does not involve the free end of hair.[41]

Trichoptilosis is a common fracture and is often seen in normal hair from excessive weathering, causing the so-called 'frizzies'.[22] The damage may be caused or aggravated by trichotillomania, pruritic dermatoses or excessive hair styling. It is quite frequently seen in congenitally brittle hair such as seen in monilethrix, trichothiodystrophy, trichorrhexis invaginata and pili torti. The splitting is obvious on light microscopy.

Irregularities of the hair shaft

According to the classification in Table 1, a variety of conditions may be described as irregularities of the hair shaft.

Longitudinal ridging and grooving

Longitudinal ridges and grooves may occur along the hair shaft. They are usually covered by intact cuticle. Longitudinal grooving is probably the most common hair shaft irregularity and is frequently seen in normal hair.[42] It is a sporadic phenomenon as a rule but is more significant if it occurs diffusely. Widespread grooving is seen in congenital hypotrichosis of various types including that of the Marie-Unna type[43] but is also seen in many related syndromes and in various forms of ectodermal dysplasia. It has also been seen in pili torti,[44] pili bifurcati,[45] uncombable hair syndrome,[46] acquired progressive kinking[47] and trichothiodystrophy.[17] It is present around the hair root in loose anagen syndrome;[48] whereas,

fine fluting can occur in pili annulati;[49] and vertical grooving of the internodes may be present in monilethrix.[9] Nevertheless, longitudinal ridging and grooving is such a common abnormality that it cannot be used as a specific sign of any particular syndrome.

It is not always easy to see vertical grooving under the light microscope but careful use of the substage condenser and the polarizing sheets will usually reveal it.

Uncombable hair syndrome

Uncombable hair is characterized by hair shafts that are traversed by several longitudinal grooves, resulting in a triangular or kidney-shaped cross-section.[46,50–52] The hair usually is silvery blond in color and glitters as a result of reflection and refraction of incident light on the differently shaped hairs. It is usually noticed at about 3 years of age and spontaneous improvement may occur later on. This condition is sometimes difficult to diagnose under the light microscope and hairs should then be embedded in epon and cut transversely in order to review the triangular or reniform shape of the shaft in cross-section (Figure 3).

Loose anagen syndrome

This is a relatively common condition. It is usually seen in fair-haired girls of 3–5 years of

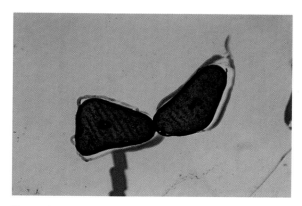

Figure 3

Uncombable hair. Hairs are triangular in cross-section, embedded in epon.

age but is often found in other members of the family, such as parents or siblings or aunts or uncles.[48,53,54] There is usually weakness in the root sheath permitting anagen hairs to be extracted easily and painlessly. The condition may improve spontaneously in later life.

Under the microscope many anagen hairs are seen and they lack inner and outer root sheaths. There is usually a ruffled cuticle present on the hair shaft and longitudinal grooving may be seen.

Pili multigemini

In pili multigemini between two and eight hair papillae and matrices with separate and complete root sheaths form compound hairs that emerge from one follicular canal.[4,55] These hairs generally emerge as a tuft of individual hairs but re-adhesion may occur. They are flattened and triangular in cross-section and may show longitudinal grooving. In adults, pili multigemini is usually found in the beard area but in children it is usually reported on the scalp. Pili bifurcati has also been described in a 3-year-old boy in whom hairs arose from a single papilla and then divided into two separate shafts, each invested by its own cuticle.[45] These shafts subsequently reunited.

Pili bifurcati may occur as an isolated defect in normal follicles and presumably represents a restricted form of pili multigemini.[4] These conditions are easily recognizable under the light microscope.[4]

Trichostasis spinulosa

Trichostasis spinulosa is another condition in which multiple hairs may be present on one follicle.[5] Anything from 5–50 normal, clubbed, vellus hairs are embedded in a large comedo with one hair matrix and papilla. It is a fairly frequent phenomenon and is presumably caused by the retention of telogen hairs extruded into sebaceous follicles.[56] It occurs at all ages, and is seen mainly on the chest and back.[57] Multiple vellus hairs embedded in a comedo are diagnostic.

Pili annulati

Pili annulati, or ringed hairs, have characteristic alternating light and dark bands in the hair shaft, causing an attractive appearance.[58] These can be seen clinically and under the light microscope. The colors of these bands are reversed when viewed by reflected light. This condition is usually more detectable in blond or lightly pigmented hair. Although fine fluting of the affected hair shaft may be seen by scanning electron microscopy,[49] it does not usually result in any hair fragility and is therefore more of cosmetic than of pathological importance. It may be present at birth or appear during infancy. It is usually familial and is easily recognized under the light microscope.

Pseudopili annulati

In pseudopili annulati, light and dark bands are found in hair shafts under reflected light. The hair cortex is normal. The appearance is caused by a flattened hair shaft, elliptical in cross-section, that is partially twisted every few millimeters. The flattened surfaces on the shaft act as mirrors and reflect light as periodic bright bands, highlighting the hair.[59]

Monilethrix

Monilethrix is a genetic condition that usually results from autosomal dominance. Currently several gene studies are under way in families with monilethrix. The hair shows a regular beaded appearance.[60] This is caused by elliptical expansions of the hair shaft at approximate 1 mm intervals with internodes in between where the shaft is fragile and easily breaks.

The characteristic regular beading with internodes of the hair is visible under the light microscope and frequently can be seen by the naked eye, and is diagnostic of the condition.

Variations in the beading configuration also exist;[61] these include a cortical defect,[62] where there is a loss of cuticle cells over the nodes from weathering and there is no medullary cavity in the internodes. The hairs will break off at the internode. This condition usually appears in early childhood on the occiput and nape of the neck but can affect the entire scalp and even the facial or body hairs. The beaded hairs emerge from keratotic follicular papules. They rarely grow longer than 1–2 cm and cause obvious baldness. It is common for this condition to improve spontaneously with age later in life. It can be associated with physical retardation, juvenile cataracts and abnormalities of the nails and teeth.

Pseudomonilethrix

In pseudomonilethrix irregular beading is present along the hair shaft in contrast to the regularity seen with monilethrix. The beaded appearance is actually produced by expansion of the normal hair shaft as a result of indentation and flattening.[3] The cuticle cells are intact over the nodes and internodes and no longitudinal grooves are present over the internodes, as seen in monilethrix. Pseudomonilethrix is now considered to be artifactual in that nodes are produced by trauma of various kinds such as compression by tweezers, forceps or other overlapping hairs between glass slides.[63] This condition was originally reported in several different families with fragile hair damaged by overzealous hair care,[64] but responded to gentle grooming and unstressed hair styles.

Tapered hairs

Tapered hairs may occur with other structural abnormalities of the hair shaft such as woolly hair nevus.[1] They can also arise from temporary inhibition of cell division in the matrix cells of the hair bulb, leading to progressive constriction of the hair shaft.[26] If the adverse influence is removed before a fracture occurs, the hair thickens again, producing a dumb-bell constriction in the emerging shaft. Pohl-Pinkus described constrictions of this type following severe illness or operation.[5] These zones have been likened to Beau's lines in the fingernails.[65]

Bayonet hairs show 2–3 mm spindle-shaped expansions of the hair cortex just proximal to a tapered tip.[26] Bayonet hairs occur in various conditions treated with radiotherapy or cytostatic drugs.

Tapered newly growing anagen hairs

Short, tapered, newly-growing anagen hairs can be seen in large numbers in patches of trichotillomania[66] or acquired progressive kinking,[67] or as new growth in areas of alopecia areata or traumatic alopecia. All the tapered hairs described above can be identified by light microscopy.

Trichomalacia

Trichomalacia, which comprises the twisted, deformed and fragmented hair partially avulsed in trichotillomania,[5] is best seen in histological sections of scalp biopsies.

Bubble hairs

Bubble hairs contain rows of easily visible and characteristic air bubbles.[68,69] They are caused by excessive heat from a hair dryer, which is either switched up too high or is defective and overheats.[70] The heat literally boils the hairs, especially when they are wet. Droplets of moisture in the hair shaft swell up and cause bubbles. This leads to localized areas of hair breakage and hair loss. The diagnosis is easily made by light microscopy of affected hairs (Figure 4).

Intermittent hair follicle dystrophy

Hair shafts in intermittent hair follicle dystrophy are brittle and break off.[71] The condition was described in a 6-year-old girl with extensive hair loss and periods of partial remission. Hair shafts showed irregular loss of cuticle with longitudinal ridges and transverse and longitudinal cracks.

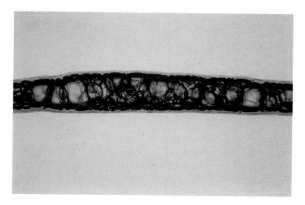

Figure 4

Bubble hair. This is caused by overheating the hair.

Hair shaft coiling and twisting

Coiling and twisting of the hair shaft can be inherited or acquired and is often due to physical or chemical trauma.

Pili torti, including corkscrew hair and Menkes' disease

In pili torti the hair shaft is flattened and twisted from 90–360° on its own axis. Four or five twists are found at irregular intervals along the hair shaft. Although the cuticle cells are often intact, the hairs are brittle and usually fracture within the twists.[72] Classical pili torti is found in association with thin, blond hairs and occurs in early childhood.[73] Normal scalp hairs are replaced by spangled hairs, usually on the occipital and temporal regions and sometimes on eyebrows and eyelashes. The hairs are brittle and alopecia may persist. The condition may improve after puberty but it can also persist into adulthood. Pili forti is associated with dental abnormalities, nail dystrophy, corneal opacities, sensorineural deafness, keratosis pilaris and ichthyosis, and it occurs predominantly in females. The association of pili torti and deafness has been reported enough to justify recommending hearing tests in children with pili torti.[74,75]

In addition to the classical presentation, there is a postpubertal form of pili torti associated with mental retardation that affects both sexes.[76] Familial pili torti can occur with acne conglobata and cataracts.[77] Other causes of pili torti have been described in association with hypogonadism[78] or with mental retardation.[28] Pili torti has also been reported in association with trichothiodystrophy,[17] anhidrotic ectodermal dysplasia,[5] Basex's syndrome[5] and citrullinemia.[79] There is a unique type of pili torti in which many hairs are twisted in a double spiral that has been described as corkscrew hair. It occurs in association with widely spaced teeth and syndactyly of fingers and toes,[80] and is a form of ectodermal dysplasia.

The kinky hairs that occur in Menkes' disease show changes that are typical of pili torti.[21] Note that pili torti can also be acquired following physical or chemical trauma, or in cicatricial alopecia,[81,82] or after taking etretinate or isotretinoin.[83]

Woolly hair

Woolly hairs are similar to the common Negroid hair form and are tightly coiled with an average curl diameter of 0.5 cm.[74] They are usually abnormal in non-Negroid people.[5] Woolly hair may be hereditary, with rare associated abnormalities,[84–88] familial and sporadic, or may occur as a woolly hair nevus. The hair shafts show a variable number of 180° axial twists. Usually the hairs are ovoid in cross-section but show no other abnormalities. In woolly hair nevus the hairs may show irregularities of the hair shaft, with tapering and loss of cuticle.[1] In woolly hair nevus, 50% of cases are associated with linear nevus on the neck or arms and ocular abnormalities may be present.[86,89]

Acquired progressive kinking

This usually appears in the late teenage years or in the early twenties.[67,90] It produces a gradual symmetric curling and darkening of the hair in the frontal, temporal, and auricular areas but sometimes can occur in other parts of the scalp. Some cases may progress to androgenetic alopecia,[47] while others may improve spontaneously.[91] The affected hairs show a kinked or wavy appearance in contrast to the normal hairs which are usually straight (Figure 5). Acquired progressive kinking can be induced by etretinate and radiotherapy.[3]

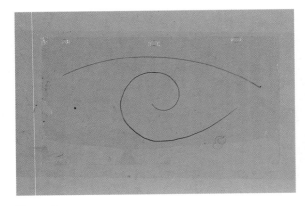

Figure 5

Acquired progressive kinking. Normal straight hair compared with kinked and curled hair from the same patient.

Whisker hair

This is the short, curly, dark hair sometimes seen around the ears in young men who may be destined to develop androgenetic alopecia.[92,93] It resembles beard hair and is bilateral, symmetric and common. Some regard it as a variant of acquired, progressive kinking.[47]

Trichonodosis

Trichonodosis is knotting of the hair shaft and can manifest as single (Figure 6) or double knots. Secondary changes from the knotting include cuticular loss with possible fractures in the shaft. Knotting in the hair can be caused by trauma and traction from cosmetic procedures or friction from pillows. It nearly always occurs in short, curly hair and does not usually involve straight hair.[94] It usually affects scalp hair but can involve pubic or other body hair.

Circle hairs

Circle and spiral hairs are commonly found on the back, abdomen and thighs of middle-aged men, perhaps associated with dry skin. They represent an unusual form of ingrown hair and appear as small dark circles next to hair follicles which appear otherwise normal. The hair is tightly coiled, lies just below the stratum corneum, and is easily extracted. It can be stretched into a hair some 2–5 cm long but retains its recoil ability.[95] The black color leads to

concern about early melanoma in some patients. However, the diagnosis is easily made by extracting the hair, which is easily distinguished from the rolled hairs of keratosis pilaris or the looped 'corkscrew' hairs of scurvy.

Extraneous matter on the shaft

Extraneous matter around hair shafts can arise from fungal and bacterial infections, louse infestation, detached hair root sheath and from deposits of lacquer, paint, glue and other chemicals

Fungi

Dermatophytes and black and white piedra can affect and damage hair shafts. Endothrix infection from Trichophyton tonsurans (Figure 7) or T. violaceum are becoming more common around the world.[96] These are negative on Wood's light. These hairs are abnormally brittle and will break off flush with the scalp resulting in the characteristic black dot appearance. Microscopic examination using a potassium hydroxide stain will reveal the fungal spores inside the hair shaft. Ectothrix infections usually result from Microsporum audouinii or M. canis and here the hairs are

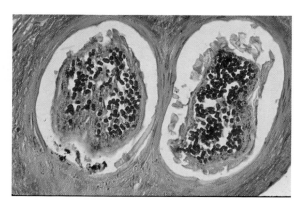

Figure 7

Endothrix tinea capitis. Trichophyton tonsurans spores and hyphae inside hair shaft. A PAS stain is used on this horizontal section of a scalp biopsy.

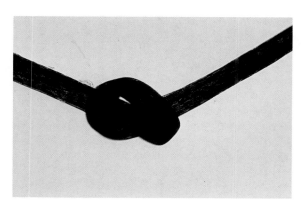

Figure 6

Trichonodosis. A single knot is shown.

less brittle and are broken off a millimeter or so away from the scalp and are surrounded by a whitish material that fluoresces green with a Wood's light.[97] Again, examination with potassium hydroxide will establish the diagnosis here with the spores being present outside of the hair shaft. Favic invasion caused by Trichophyton schoenleinii is an endothrix infection that is characterized by air spaces in the hair shaft and is rarely seen today.

Black piedra is caused by Piedraia hortai, which penetrates the hair cuticle and proliferates in the cortex and subsequently encircles the hair shaft to form adherent black nodules.[98] This is seen on scalp hair and mustache hair and even body hair. Fractures can occur in the affected hair shaft. This is easy to diagnose under the light microscope.

White piedra is caused by Trichosporon beigelii, which also invades and fractures the hair shaft. Whitish nodules develop on the hair shaft and are easily detachable.[99] The diagnosis is confirmed by microscopic examination of the hairs (Figure 8) and by fungal cultures.

Bacteria

Trichomycosis axillaris is caused by Corynebacterium tenuis, which forms adherent, yellow or orange nodules around axillary or pubic hairs.[100,101] These hairs become brittle and fracture easily.[102] The diagnosis is easily confirmed using light microscopy.

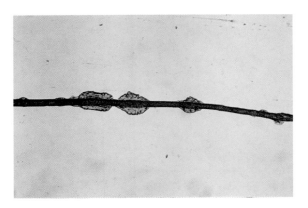

Figure 8

White piedra. Pale nodules are seen on the hair shaft.

Pediculosis capitis

In pediculosis capitis the nits are often easier to find than the adult lice. On the scalp, both nits and lice are most numerous on the occiput and behind the ears.[98] The nit is oval and is attached securely to the hair and lies to one side of it. It cannot be slid along the hair shaft like a peripilar cast. The free distal end of the nit points towards the hair tip and is covered by an operculum while the nit is inside but this is detached when the young louse emerges from the egg case. Nits are easy to recognize under the light microscope since they are attached securely to the shaft by an enveloping capsule, which surrounds the nit and the hair shaft leaving the free end pointing outwards but separated from the hair shaft itself.

Peripilar casts or pseudonits

Peripilar casts are common and are commonly found in normal hair, especially in female children. They are whitish or yellowish in color and they are easily moved along the hair shaft, which pierces the cast centrally. True peripilar keratin casts are usually composed of external root sheath only, but rarely of internal root sheath and sometimes of both.[103]

Deposits

Deposits of lacquer, paint, glue and other chemicals may be deposited on hair shafts. These can cause diagnostic difficulty; however, it helps to remember that deposits are localized to the areas of contact.

Conclusions

Abnormalities of the hair shaft are easily recognizable under the light microscope as fractures, irregularities, hair shaft coiling and twisting, and extraneous matter on hair shafts. These microscopic appearances taken in conjunction with the history and examination should generally allow a diagnosis to be made. Sometimes the cause is obscure and sometimes further examination may be necessary under the scanning electron microscope or transmission electron microscope, but this is rarely the case. Many hair shaft abnormalities are caused by or are aggravated by weathering.

References

1. Whiting DA: Structural abnormalities of the hair shaft. *J Am Acad Dermatol* 1987; **16**: 1–25.
2. Price VH: Structural anomalies of the hair shaft. In: Orfanos CE, Happle R (eds.). *Hair and Hair Diseases*. Berlin, Springer-Verlag, 1990: 363–422.
3. Whiting DA: Hair shaft defects. In: Olsen EA (ed.). *Disorders of Hair Growth: Diagnosis and Treatment*. New York, McGraw-Hill, 1994: 91–137.
4. Camacho F, Whiting D, Ferrando J, Price V: Hair shaft dysplasias. Genodermatosis with hypotrichosis. In: Camacho F, Montagna W (eds.). *Trichology. Diseases of the Pilosebaceus Follicle*. Madrid, Aula Medica, 1997: 179–242.
5. de Berker D, Sinclair R: Defects of the hair shaft. In: Dawber RPR (ed.). *Diseases of the Hair and Scalp, 3rd edn*. Oxford, Blackwell Science, 1997: 239–298.
6. Montagna W, Parakkal PF: *The Structure and Function of Skin. 3rd edn*. New York, Academic Press, 1974: 172–182.
7. Hardy D: Quantitative hair form variation in seven populations. *Am J Phys Anthropol* 1973; **39**: 7–18.
8. Rook A, Dawber R: *Diseases of the Hair and Scalp*. Oxford, Blackwell Scientific, 1982: 29–40.
9. Dawber R, Comaish S: Scanning electron microscopy of normal and abnormal hair shafts. *Arch Dermatol* 1970; **101**: 316–322.
10. Kligman AM: The human hair cycle. *J Invest Dermatol* 1959; **33**: 307–316.
11. Rook A: Review: The clinical importance of 'weathering' in human hair. *Br J Dermatol* 1976; **95**: 111–112.
12. Dawber RPR: Weathering of hair in some genetic hair dystrophies. In: Brown AC, Crounse RG (eds.). *Hair, Trace Elements and Human Illness*. New York, Praeger, 1980: 273–280.
13. Swift JS, Brown AC: Scanning electron microscopy observation of human hair weathering. In: Brown AC (ed.). *The First Human Hair Symposium*. New York, Medcom Press, 1974: 332–345.
14. Chernosky ME, Owens DW: Trichorrhexis nodosa. Clinical investigative studies. *Arch Dermatol* 1966; **94**: 577–585.
15. Papa CM, Mills OH, Hanshaw W: Seasonal trichorrhexis nodosa. Role of cumulative damage in frayed hair. *Arch Dermatol* 1972; **106**: 888–892.
16. Owens DW, Chernosky ME: Trichorrhexis nodosa. In vitro reproduction. *Arch Dermatol* 1966; **94**: 586–588.
17. Price VH, Odom RB, Ward WH, Jones FT: Trichothiodystrophy. Sulfur-deficient brittle hair as a marker for a neuroectodermal symptom complex. *Arch Dermatol* 1980; **116**: 1375–1384.
18. Allan JD, Cusworth DE, Dent CE, Wilson VK: A disease, probably hereditary, characterized by severe mental deficiency and a constant gross abnormality of amino acid metabolism. *Lancet* 1985; **i**: 182–187.
19. Levin B, Mackay HMM, Oberholzer VG: Argininosuccinic aciduria: an inborn error of amino acid metabolism. *Arch Dis Child* 1961; **36**: 622–632.
20. Goldblum OM, Brusilow SW, Maldonado YA, Farmer ER: Neonatal citrullinemia associated with cutaneous manifestations and arginine deficiency. *J Am Acad Dermatol* 1986; **14**: 321–326.
21. Menkes JH, Alter M, Steigleder GK, et al.: A sex-linked recessive disorder with retardation of growth, peculiar hair and focal cerebral and cerebellar degeneration. *Pediatrics* 1962; **29**: 764–779.
22. Price VH: Office diagnosis of structural hair anomalies. *Cutis* 1975; **15**: 231–240.
23. Brenton DP, Cusworth DC, Hartley S, et al.: Argininosuccinic aciduria: clinical, metabolic and dietary study. *J Ment Defic Res* 1974; **18**: 1–13.
24. Danks DM, Tippett P, Zentner G: Severe neonatal citrullinemia. *Arch Dis Child* 1974; **49**: 579–581.
25. Leonard JN, Gummer CL, Dawber RPR: Generalized trichorrhexis nodosa. *Br J Dermatol* 1980; **103**: 85–90.
26. Brown AC: Congenital hair defects. In: Bergsma D (ed.). *Birth Defects, Original Article Series* [Skin, hair and nails, Part XII.] Baltimore, Williams & Wilkins, The National Foundation – March of Dimes, 1972: 52–68.
27. Brown AC, Belser RB, Crounse RG, Wehr RF: A congenital hair defect: trichoschisis and alternating birefringence and low sulfur content. *J Invest Dermatol* 1970; **54**: 496–509.
28. Pollitt RJ, Jenner FA, Davies M: Sibs with mental and physical retardation and trichorrhexis nodosa with abnormal amino acid composition of the hair. *Arch Dis Child* 1968; **43**: 211–216.
29. Jorizzo JL, Atherton DJ, Crounse RG, Wells RS: Ichthyosis, brittle hair, impaired intelligence, decreased fertility and short stature (IBIDS syndrome). *Br J Dermatol* 1982; **106**: 705–710.
30. Jackson CE, Weiss L, Watson JHL: 'Brittle' hair with short stature, intellectual impairment and decreased fertility: an autosomal recessive syndrome in an Amish kindred. *Pediatrics* 1974; **54**: 201–207.
31. Jorizzo JL, Crounse RG, Wheeler CE Jr: Lamellar ichthyosis, dwarfism, mental retardation, and hair shaft abnormalities. *J Am Acad Dermatol* 1980; **2**: 309–317.
32. Crovato F, Rebora A: PIBI(D)S syndrome. A new entity with defects of the deoxyribonucleic acid excision repair system. *J Am Acad Dermatol* 1985; **13**: 683–685.
33. Itin PH, Pittelkow MR: Trichothiodystrophy.

Review of sulfur-deficient brittle hair syndromes and association with ectodermal dysplasias. *J Am Acad Dermatol* 1990; **22**: 705–717.

34. Ito M, Ito K, Hashimoto K: Pathogenesis in trichorrhexis invaginata (bamboo hair). *J Invest Dermatol* 1984; **83**: 1–6.

35. Brodin MB, Porter PS: Netherton's syndrome. *Cutis* 1980; **26**: 185–191.

36. Netherton EW. A unique case of trichorrhexis nodosa – 'bamboo hairs'. *Arch Dermatol* 1958; **78**: 483–487.

37. Altman J, Stroud J: Netherton's syndrome and ichthyosis linearis circumflexa: psoriasiform ichthyosis. *Arch Dermatol* 1969; **100**: 550–558.

38. Krafchik BR: Netherton syndrome. *Pediatr Dermatol* 1992; **9**: 158–160.

39. de Berker D, Paige D, Harper J, Dawber RPR: Golf tee hairs: a new sign in Netherton's syndrome. *Br J Dermatol* 1992; **127(suppl 40)**: 30.

40. Eckert J, Church RE, Ebling FJ: The pathogenesis of alopecia areata. *Br J Dermatol* 1968; **80**: 203–210.

41. Burkhart CG, Huttner JJ, Bruner J: Central trichoptilosis. *J Am Acad Dermatol* 1981; **5**: 703–705. [Letter to Editor].

42. Aguiar A, Sobrinto-Simóes MM, Finseth I, et al.: Uncombable hair. *Arch Dis Child* 1984; **59**: 92–93.

43. Peachey RDG, Wells RS: Hereditary hypotrichosis (Marie Unna type). *Trans St. John's Hosp Dermatol Soc* 1971; **57**: 157–166.

44. Robinson GC, Johnston MM: Pili torti and sensory neural hearing loss. *J Pediatr* 1967; **70**: 621–623.

45. Weary P, Hendricks AA, Warner F, Ajkaonkar G: Pili bifurcati. A new anomaly of hair growth. *Arch Dermatol* 1973; **108**: 403–407.

46. Shelley WB, Shelley ED: Uncombable hair syndrome: observation in response to biotin and occurrence in siblings with ectodermal dysplasia. *J Am Acad Dermatol* 1985; **13**: 97–102.

47. Mortimer PS, Gummer C, English J, Dawber RPR: Acquired progressive kinking of hair. Report of six cases and review of literature. *Arch Dermatol* 1985; **121**: 1031–1033.

48. Price VH, Gummer CL: Loose anagen syndrome. *J Am Acad Dermatol* 1989; **20**: 249–256.

49. Gummer CL, Dawber RPR: Pili annulati: electron histochemical studies on affected hairs. *Br J Dermatol* 1981; **105**: 303–309.

50. Larralde de Luna MM, Rubinson R, Gelman de Kohan ZB: Pili triranguli canaliculi: uncombable hair syndrome in a family with apparent autosomal dominant inheritance. *Pediatr Dermatol* 1985; **2**: 324–327.

51. Stroud JD, Mehregan AH: 'Spun glass' hair. A clinicopathologic study of an unusual hair defect. In: Brown AC (ed.). *The First Human Hair Symposium.* New York, Medcom Press, 1974: 103–107.

52. Stroud JD: Complementation of the inner root sheath of human hair. In: Brown AC, Crounse RD (eds.). *Hair, Trace Elements and Human Illness.* New York, Praeger, 1980: 163–168.

53. Hamm H, Traupe H: Loose anagen hair of childhood: the phenomenon of easily pluckable hair. *J Am Acad Dermatol* 1989; **20**: 242–248.

54. Li VW, Baden HP, Kvedar JC: Loose anagen syndrome and loose anagen hair. In: Whiting DA (ed.). *Update on Hair Disorders: Dermatologic Clinics.* Philadelphia, WB Saunders, 1996: 745–751.

55. Mehregan AH, Thompson WS: Pili multigemini. Report of a case in association with cleidocranial dysostosis. *Br J Dermatol* 1979; **100**: 315–322.

56. Goldschmidt H, Hoyjo-Tomoka MT, Kligman AM: Trichostasis spinulosa: a common inapparent follicular disorder of the aged. In: Brown AC (ed.). *The First Human Hair Symposium.* New York, Medcom Press, 1974: 50–60.

57. Young MC, Jorizzo JL, Sanchez RL, et al.: Trichostasis spinulosa. *Int J Dermatol* 1985; **24**: 575–580.

58. Price VH, Thomas RS, Jones FT: Pili annulati. Optical and electron microscopic studies. *Arch Dermatol* 1968; **98**: 640–647.

59. Price VH, Thomas RS, Jones FT: Pseudopili annulati. An unusual variant of normal hair. *Arch Dermatol* 1970; **102**: 354–358.

60. de Berker DAR, Dawber RPR: Monilethrix. Clinical and microscopic findings in 21 cases. *Br J Dermatol* 1991; **125(suppl 38)**: 24.

61. de Berker DAR, Dawber RPR: Variations in beading configuration in monilethrix. *Pediatr Dermatol* 1992; **9**: 19–21.

62. de Berker DAR, Ferguson DJP, Dawber RPR: Monilethrix: a clinicopathological demonstration of a cortical defect. *Br J Dermatol* 1993; **128**: 327–331.

63. Zitelli JA: Pseudomonilethrix: an artifact. *Arch Dermatol* 1986; **122**: 688–690.

64. Bentley-Phillips B, Bayles MAH: Pseudomonilethrix. *Br J Dermatol* 1975; **92**: 113–115.

65. Sims RT: 'Beau's lines' in hair. Reduction of hair shaft diameter associated with illness. *Br J Dermatol* 1967; **79**: 43–49.

66. Steck WD: Telogen effluvium. A clinically useful concept, with traction alopecia as an example. *Cutis* 1978; **21**: 543–548.

67. Coupe RL, Johnston MM: Acquired progressive kinking of the hair. Structural changes and growth dynamics of affected hairs. *Arch Dermatol* 1969; **100**: 191–195.

68. Brown VM, Crounse RG, Abele DC: An unusual new hair shaft abnormality: 'Bubble hair'. *J Am Acad Dermatol* 1986; **15**: 1113–1117.

69. Elston DM, Bergfeld WF, Whiting DA, et al.: Bubble hair. *J Cutan Pathol* 1992; **19**: 439–444.

70. Detwiler SP, Carson JL, Woolsey JT, et al.: Bubble Hair: case caused by an overheating hair dryer and reproducibility in normal hair with heat. *J Am Acad Dermatol* 1994; **30(1)**: 54–60.

71. Birnbaum PS, Baden HP, Bronstein BR, et al.: Intermittent hair follicle dystrophy: report of a new disorder. *J Am Acad Dermatol* 1986; **15**: 54–56.

72. Dawber RPR: Weathering of hair in monilethrix and pili torti. *Clin Exp Dermatol* 1977; **2**: 271–277.

73. Ronchese F: Twisted hairs (pili torti). *Arch Dermatol Syph* 1932; **26**: 98–109.

74. Reed WB, Stone VM, Boder E, Ziprkowski L: Hereditary syndromes with auditory and dermatological manifestations. *Arch Dermatol* 1967; **95**: 456–461.

75. Robinson GC, Johnston MM: Pili torti and sensory hair loss. *J Pediatr* 1967; **70**: 621–623.

76. Beare JM: Congenital pilar defect showing features of pili torti. *Br J Dermatol* 1952: **64**: 366–372.

77. Gold SC, Delaney TJ: Familial acne conglobata, hidradenitis suppurativa, pili torti and cataracts. *Br J Dermatol* 1974; **91(suppl 10)**: 54–57.

78. Crandall BG, Samec L, Sparkes RS, Wright SW: A familial syndrome of deafness, alopecia and hypogonadism. *J Pediatr* 1973; **82**: 462–465.

79. Patel HP, Unis ME: Pili torti in association with citrullinemia. *J Am Acad Dermatol* 1985; **12**: 203–206.

80. Whiting DA, Jenkins T, Whitcomb MJ: Corkscrew hair – a unique type of congenital alopecia in pili torti. In: Brown AC, Crounse RG (eds.). *Hair, Trace Elements, and Human Illness.* New York, Praeger, 1980: 228–239.

81. Kurwa AR, Abdel-Aziaz AM: Pili torti–congenital and acquired. *Acta Derm Venereol (Stockh)* 1973; **53**: 385–392.

82. Scott OLS: Localized pili torti. *Proc Roy Soc Med* 1950; **43**: 68.

83. Hays SB, Camisa C: Acquired pili torti in two patients treated with synthetic retinoids. *Cutis* 1985; **35**: 466–468.

84. Hutchinson PE, Cairns RJ, Wells RS: Woolly hair. Clinical and genetic aspects. *Trans St. Johns Hosp Dermatol Soc* 1974; **60**: 160–177.

85. Robinson GC, Miller JR. Hereditary enamel hypoplasia: its association with characteristic hair structure. *Pediatrics* 1966; **37**: 498–502.

86. Jacobsen KU, Lowes M: Woolly hair nevus with ocular involvement. Report of a case. *Dermatologica* 1975; **151**: 249–252.

87. Verbov J: Woolly hair – study of a family. *Dermatologica* 1978; **157**: 42–47.

88. Neild VS, Pegum JS, Wells RS: The association of keratosis pilaris atrophicans and woolly hair, with and without Noonan's syndrome. *Br J Dermatol* 1984; **110**: 357–362.

89. Grant PW: A case of woolly hair nevus. *Arch Dis Child* 1960; **35**: 512–514.

90. Wise F, Sulzberger MB: Acquired progressive kinking of the scalp hair accompanied by changes in its pigmentation. *Arch Dermatol Syph* 1932; **25**: 99–110.

91. Coupe RL: Acquired progressive kinking of the hair. *Arch Dermatol* 1986; **122**: 133.

92. Norwood OT: Whisker hair. *Arch Dermatol* 1979; **115**: 930–931.

93. Norwood OT: Whisker hair – an update. *Cutis* 1981; **27**: 651–652.

94. Dawber RPR: Knotting of scalp hair. *Br J Dermatol* 1974; **91**: 169–173.

95. Levit F, Scott MJ Jr: Circle hairs. *J Am Acad Dermatol* 1983; **8**: 423–425.

96. Lee JY, Hsu ML: Pathogenesis of hair infection and black dots in tinea capitis caused by Trichophyton violaceum: a histopathological study. *J Cutan Pathol* 1992; **19**: 54–58.

97. Kligman AM. Tinea capitis due to M. audouinni and M. canis. *Arch Dermatol* 1955; **71**: 313–357.

98. Dawber RPR, Fenton DA. Infections and infestations. In: Dawber RPR (ed.). *Diseases of the Hair and Scalp, 3rd edn.* Oxford, Blackwell Scientific, 1997: 418–460.

99. Kalter DC, Tshcen JA, Cernoch PL, et al.: Genital white piedra: epidemiology, microbiology, and therapy. *J Am Acad Dermatol* 1986; **14**: 982–983.

100. Freeman RG, McBride ME, Knox JM: Pathogenesis of trichomycosis axillaris. *Arch Dermatol* 1969; **100**: 90–95.

101. White SW, Smith J: Trichomycosis pubis. *Arch Dermatol* 1979; **115**: 444–445.

102. Orfanos CE, Schloesser E, Mahrle G: Hair-destroying growth of Corynebacterium tenuis in the so-called trichomycosis axillaris. *Arch Dermatol* 1971; **103**: 632–639.

103. Scott MJ, Roenigk HH Jr: Hair casts: classification, staining characteristics, and differential diagnosis. *J Am Acad Dermatol* 1983; **8**: 27–32.

28
Acquired hair kinking

Juan Ferrando

Introduction

Acquired hair kinking (AHK) is characterized by the presence of curly hairs on the scalp with irregular twisting of the hair shaft, of late onset. Usually there are localized flat hairs that follow a diffuse pattern depending on different conditions. The following types can be distinguished:

- Circle hairs (rolled hairs);
- Acquired pili torti (including corkscrew hair);
- Acquired woolly hairs (pseudowoolly hair)
    - Localized forms: whisker hair (symmetrical circumscribed allotrichia)
    - Diffuse forms: acquired progressive kinking of hair
    Diffuse partial woolly hair
    Drug induced curling of hair;
- Trichonodosis.

Circle hairs (rolled hairs)

Circle hairs occur in middle-aged men and appear as black dots on the trunk, abdomen and thighs, corresponding to a spiral pattern of ingrowing body hair. Circle hairs are frequent, especially in obese men and elderly individuals.[1] They can be familial or acquired and are sometimes associated with atopic dermatitis or steroid treatment.[2] Circle hairs are not associated with follicular abnormalities but are placed just under the stratum corneum, and as such are easily removed. Scanning electron microscopy (SEM) studies show a normal cuticle appearance. At present, it is accepted that circle hairs may represent the result of abnormal keratinization of the distal part of the hair follicle. Some authors differentiate circle hairs from rolled hairs (RH), mostly through the association of the latter condition with hyperkeratotic disorders[1] such as keratin plugging, keratosis pilaris, xerosis or palmoplantar keratoderma.[3] Rolled hairs should be of normal hair diameter and form irregular circles, in contrast to circle hairs, which are perfect circles of small diameter hair that are unable to penetrate the stratum corneum.[1] Itin and co-workers[4] described a peculiar type of rolled hairs associated with multiple large knots. Using SEM, they demonstrated multiple hairs that originated from different hair follicles and rolled and stuck together centrally. The authors concluded that it may represent a minor variant of body hair matting or felting.

Acquired pili torti

Pili torti (PT) is a hair shaft in which the hair is twisted up to 360° on its own axis. Clinically, a particular regular reflection of light is observed through the hair, especially if the patient moves his or her head (Figure 1). The classic type of pili torti is congenital and is associated with various syndromes:[5]

- Ronchese type: PT + hair fragility (patchy alopecia);
- Beare type: PT + patchy alopecia + mental retardation;
- Björnstad type: PT + sensorineural deafness;
- Crandall type: PT + sensorineural deafness + secondary hypogonadism.

Images of pili torti have been also found in Bazex syndrome, citrullinemia, anhidrotic ectodermal dysplasia, trichothiodystrophy, Salamon syndrome, Rapp-Hodgkin syndrome and Menkes

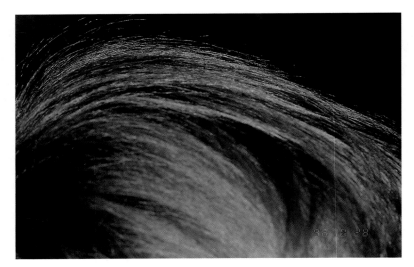

Figure 1

Pili torti. Clinical aspects: peculiar reflection of the light through the hair.

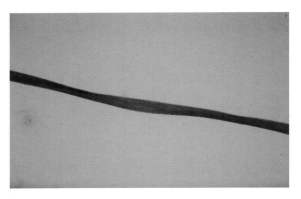

a

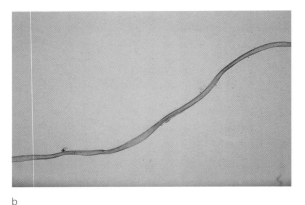

b

Figure 2

Pili torti. **(a)** Classical—regular—pili torti; **(b)** Acquired—irregular—pili torti.

syndrome (atypical PT (kinky hair) including atypical monilethrix and trichorrhexis nodosa plus cerebral degeneration, nerve deafness and retarded growth).[5,6]

Acquired pili torti (also known as pseudopili torti) can be defined as an irregular twisting of the hair (Figure 2). It is a non-hereditary form of PT that is restricted to areas of scarring alopecia induced by lupus erythematosus, scleroderma, porphyria or infection of the scalp. Local trauma

can also produce acquired PT. Most likely, it is the result of residual perifollicular fibrosis secondary to any of the above mentioned conditions.

Acquired PT has recently been observed in girls who had suffered from anorexia nervosa. Lurie and co-workers[7] demonstrated that 14 out of 17 teenage girls with anorexia nervosa had pili torti, whereas 15 girls without the disease did not. Significant increases in levels of serum carotene, retinol and retinoic acid, all caused by

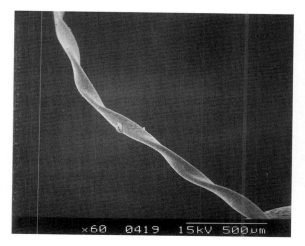

Figure 3

Corkscrew hair. This scanning electron micrograph is of a hair taken from a patient with pili torti.

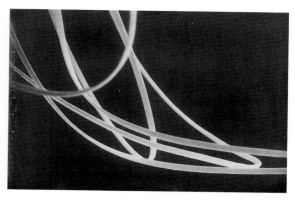

Figure 4

Woolly hair. Characteristic thin flat and curly hairs can be seen on SEM.

increased yellow vegetable intake, and malnutrition, could be involved in this hair shaft dysplasia.

Corkscrew hair

Corkscrew hair can be defined as atypical acquired pili torti (Figure 3). Clinically thick, dark, scalp hairs that are coiled into a unique double spiral characterize this rare condition. Corkscrew hair may be associated with ordinary pili torti or its occurrence may be an isolated finding. A woman with congenital hypotrichosis, spaced teeth and syndactily has been reported to have corkscrew hair.[7,8]

Acquired woolly hair (pseudowoolly hair)

Woolly hair (WH) is defined as a flat, thin and curly hair (Figure 4). It is a rare congenital con-

dition that has been classified by Hutchinson and colleagues[9] into three types:

(1) Hereditary woolly hair: is an autosomal dominant trait in which a variable degree of tight curling is present in all hairs throughout the scalp.
(2) Familial woolly hair: is an autosomal recessive form that is characterized by abnormal, tightly-curled, fine, white or blond hair that tends to be short and is present from birth.
(3) Woolly hair nevus: in this condition, affected hair is within a well-demarcated area, is curly, lighter than the normal hair, and has a reduced diameter.[10]

Irrespective of the classical definition of Hutchinson, the term 'acquired curling of hair' seems to be more appropriate for designating clinical conditions characterized by the presence of non-congenital curly or wavy hair. Both localized (whisker hair) and diffuse forms (acquired progressive hair kinking, diffuse partial woolly hair and drug-induced curling of hair) are recognized.

Whisker hair (symmetrical circumscribed allotrichia)

This disorder is characterized by short, curly and dark hair that is symmetrically located around the ears but later grows and extends above the temples towards the occipital region. It affects young men before the onset of severe androgenetic alopecia[8] but disappears in older individuals after entering common baldness. An androgen-dependent mechanism might be involved.

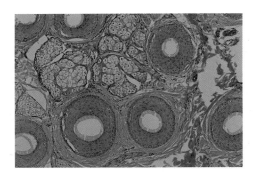

a

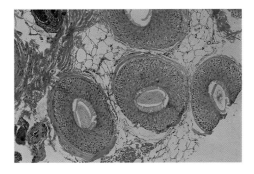

b

Acquired progressive kinking of hair

Acquired progressive kinking of hair (APKH) is a gradual symmetrical curling and darkening of the hair that appears around puberty, occurring mainly in men and involving frontal, temporal and occipital areas without sharply defined margins.[11] APKH was first described by Wise and

Figure 6

Acquired progressive kinking of hair. **(a)** Normal areas **(b)** Abnormal areas. Histological studies confirmed the presence of intrafollicular flattened hair shafts in (b).[13]

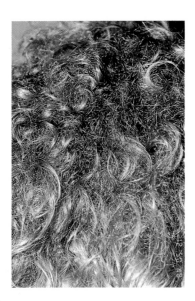

Figure 5

Acquired progressive kinking of hair. This girl had sharply demarcated areas of curly alternating with normal hair.

Sulzberger in 1932[12] and a few cases have been reported so far. It is a condition that only exceptionally affects girls[13] (Figure 5).

Histological studies confirm the presence of intrafollicular flattened hair shafts in the affected areas[13] (Figure 6). APKH appears fine, short, curly, and of the woolly hair type. SEM reveals flat hairs with kinks and half twists (Figure 7). The condition may also progress to androgenetic alopecia. A girl who was affected from trichorrhinophalangeal syndrome type I presented a transitional acquired kinking of hair in the occipital area (Figure 8) (unpublished data).

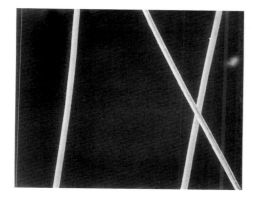

a

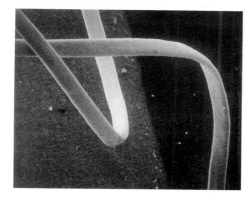

b

Figure 7

Acquired progressive kinking of hair. SEM studies reveal **(a)** normal aspects of unaffected hairs and **(b)** thin flattened hairs with kinks in the affected areas.

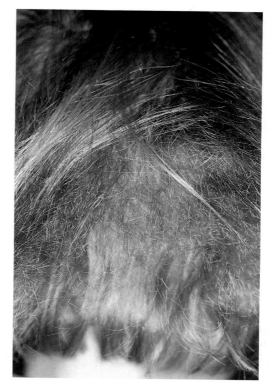

Figure 8

Acquired transitional kinking of hair. This girl suffers from trichorrhinophalangeal syndrome type I.

Diffuse partial woolly hair

Diffuse partial woolly hair (DPWH) is an acquired type of woolly (curling) hair that also appears at puberty. Mostly affecting females, it is characterized by the presence of two different populations of hairs—fine, curly or wavy and short hairs— and these appear intermingled with normal hair (Figure 9). The condition can be familial or sporadic and only three reports have been published so far. Hair loss, kinky hair that is easily pluckable, and a chronic and progressive course of the

disease are the main Ormerod's criteria. Scanning electron microscopy (SEM) reveals fine flattened wavy hairs with an oval-shaped section, some single torsions and some canalicular formations. Cuticular weathering is also present.[15] DPWH may represent a prior state to APKH with familial predisposition in some cases. A weathering or styling-induced form of DPWH was recently described as acquired partial curly hair (APCH).[16] This new type of acquired hair kinking is also characterized by the presence of two different populations of hairs on the scalp—normal straight hair intermingled with thinner curled hair. APCH differs from DPHW in that the patients do not complain of hair loss, kinky hair is not easily pluckable and the condition improves spontaneously. The most important

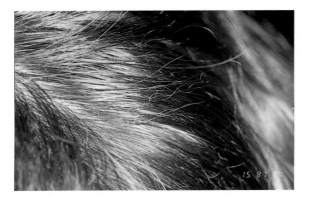

Figure 9

Diffuse partial woolly hair. The presence of thin curly hairs intermingled with the straight normal hair population can be seen.

differential criterion, however, is that in acquired partial curly hair only the distal portion of the hair shaft is affected (Figure 10), a condition that may be explained by the fact that the distal hair shaft is thinner and more prone to weathering and cuticular damage that is induced by cosmetic procedures. In this case cuticular weathering is found in both affected hairs and also in the normal hair population (Figure 11).

Drug induced hair curling

Synthetic retinoids have been described as possible causes of drug-induced woolly hair. Etretinate may produce alopecia, hair discoloration,[17] and a diffuse, curly and kinky hair disorder.[18] This

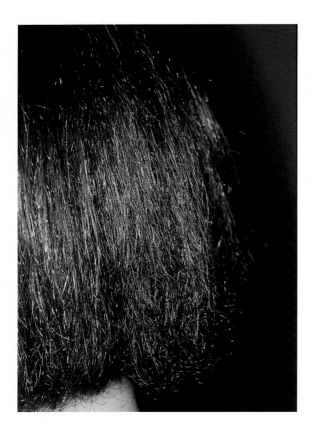

a

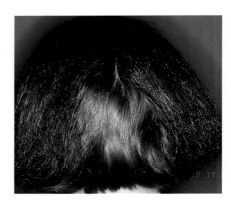

b

Figure 10

Acquired partial curly hair. In this new condition the curly aspect of some hairs is only observed in the distal part of the hair shaft **(a)** General view of the hair with curled isolated hairs intermingled between normal, straight hairs. **(b)** The proximal atlas of the hairs are unaffected.

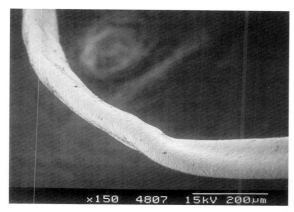

a

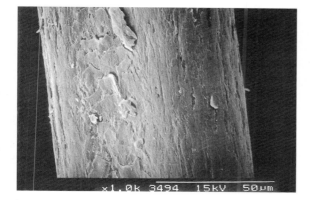

b

Figure 11

Acquired partial curly hair. In this SEM, **(a)** flat and thin hair with a single twist and cuticular weathering and **(b)** severe cuticular weathering in a straight normal hair can be seen.

Trichonodosis (hair knotting)

Trichonodosis is not a rare condition but is difficult to find and reports of trichonodosis are uncommon (Figure 12). Trichonodosis affects scalp, body or pubic hair and seems to be more frequent in caucasoid or negroid hair types.[21] Local trauma, rubbing with a pillow, especially in

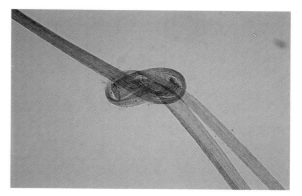

Figure 12

Trichonodosis. Knotting of the hair with trichopthylosis emerging from the knot is shown.

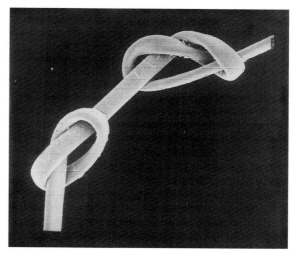

Figure 13

Trichonodosis. A double knot in a pubic hair of a patient with acarophobia is shown.

situation has been reported in patients with psoriasis and ichthyosis who are undergoing treatment. Isotretinoin has also been described as a drug inducer of thin hair kinking in patients with acne and systemic sclerosis.[19] It has been suggested that isotretinoin affects sheath-shaft interactions.[20] This condition reverts itself when the implied drug is withdrawn.

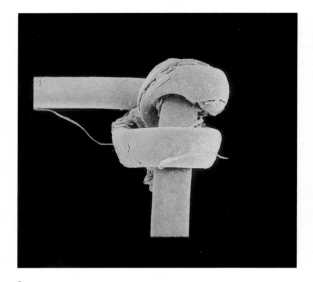
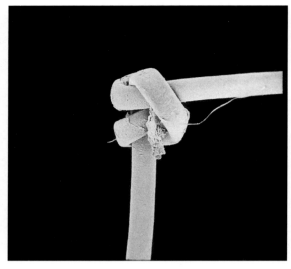

a   b

Figure 14

Trichonodosis. This 'tie knot' type shows the **(a)** anverse and **(b)** reverse image after 180°.

young people and newborns, scratching and cosmetic procedures may all be causative factors. Trichonodosis may be suspected if a hair abruptly changes its direction due to a knot causing hair shaft angulation. Trichonodosis has been found in 9 out of 80 normal females[22] and in 36 out of 134 patients with complaints of different cutaneous diseases.[23] A patient with pubic trichonodosis associated with local acarophobia that induced scratching is shown in Figure 13. Trichonodosis associated with *pediculus pubis* in the same hair is exceptional.[24]

Trichonodosis affects one or more hairs and a varying number of knots may be found in a single hair. The knot can be single, double or complex ('tie knot', 'sailor's knot') (Figure 14). SEM studies reveal that hair knotting is usually associated with trichophylosis and cuticular damage.

References

1. Smith JB, Hogan DJ: Circle hairs are not rolled hairs. *J Am Acad Dermatol* 1996; **35**: 634–635.

2. Fergusson AG, Derblay PR: Rolled hairs, a possible complication of corticosteroid therapy. *Arch Dermatol* 1963; **87**: 311–314.

3. Ortonne JP, Juhlin L, El Baze P, Pautrat G: Familial rolled and spiral hairs with palmoplantar keratoderma. *Acta Derm Venereol (Stockh)* 1985; **65**: 250–254.

4. Itin PH, Bircher AJ, Lautenschlager S, Zuberbühler E, Guggenheim R: A new clinical disorder of twisted and rolled body hairs with multiple, large knots. *J Am Acad Dermatol* 1994; **30**: 31–35.

5. Kurwa AR, Abdel-Aziz AHM: Pili torti—congenital and acquired. *Acta Derm Venereol (Stockh)* 1973; **53**: 385–392.

6. Camacho F, Montagna W: *Trichology, diseases of the pilosebaceus follicle.* Aula Médica, Madrid, 1997.

7. Lurie R, Danziger Y, Kaplan Y, Sulkes J, Abramson E, Mimouni M: Acquired pili torti—a structural hair shaft defect in anorexia nervosa. *Cutis* 1996; **57**: 151–156.

8. Whiting DA: Structural abnormalities of the hair shaft: continuing medical education. *J Am Acad Dermatol* 1987; **16**: 1–25.

9. Hutchinson PE, Cairns RD, Wells RS: Woolly hair. *Trans St John's Hosp Dermatol Soc* 1974; **60**: 160–167.

10. Ferrando J, Gratacós MR, Fontarnau R: Woolly hair. Estudio histológico y ultraestructural en

cuatro casos. *Actas Dermosifiliogr* 1979; **70**: 203–214.

11. Cullen ST, Fulghum DD: Acquired progressive kinking of the hair. *Arch Dermatol* 1989; **125**: 252–255.

12. Wise F, Sulzberger MB: Acquired progressive kinking of the scalp hair accompanied by changes in its pigmentation. Correlation of an unidentified group of cases presenting circumscribed areas of kinky hair. *Arch Dermatol* 1932; **25**: 99–100.

13. Ferrando J, Salas J, Vicente A, Hausmann R, Navarra R, Barriga A: Ensortijamiento adquirido y progresivo del cabello: una forma adquirida de cabello lanoso. *Actas Dermosifiliogr* 1993; **84**: 235–240.

14. Ormerod AD, Main RA, Ryder ML, Gregory DW: A family with diffuse partial woolly hair. *Br J Dermatol* 1987; **116**: 401–405.

15. Lalevic-Vasic BM, Nikolic MM, Polic DJ, Radosavljevic B: Diffuse partial woolly hair. *Dermatology* 1993; **187**: 243–247.

16. Ferrando J, Grimalt R: Acquired partial curly hair:

17. Nanda A, Alsaleh QA: Hair discoloration caused by etretinate. *Dermatology* 1994; **188**: 172.

18. Schauder A, Tsambaos D, Nikiforidis G: Curling and kinking of hair caused by etretinate. *Hautarzt* 1992; **43**: 509–513.

19. Bunker CB, Maurice PDL, Dowd PM: Isotretinoin and curly hair. *Clin Exper Dermatol* 1990; **15**: 143–145.

20. Williams D, Siock P, Stenn K: 13-*cis*-retinoic acid affects sheath-shaft interactions of equine hair follicles in vitro. *J Invest Dermatol* 1996; **106**: 356–361.

21. Zhu WY, Xia MY: Trichonodosis. *Pediatr Dermatol* 1993; **10**: 392–393.

22. Dawber RPR: Knotting of scalp hair. *Br J Dermatol* 1974; **91**: 169.

23. Trüeb RM: Trichonodosis neurotic and familial trichonodosis. *J Am Acad Dermatol* 1994; **31**: 1077–1078.

24. Scott MJ: Trichonodosis. Report of a case. *Arch Dermatol Syph* 1951; **63**: 769.

Report of six cases *Eur J Dermatol* 1999 (In press).

29
Loose anagen hair syndrome

Rachel Reynolds and Howard P Baden

History

Loose anagen hair syndrome (LAHS) was first described by Zaun in 1984 at The First Congress of the European Society for Pediatric Dermatology.[1] A similar syndrome was presented by Price in 1986 at the 106th Annual Meeting of the American Dermatological Association.[2] Nodl et al.[3] were the first to publish their findings on LAHS in 1986, followed by Hamm and Traupe,[4] and Price and Gummer[5] in 1989. The histological and ultrastructural aspects of the syndrome were then further elucidated by Lalevic-Vasic et al.[6] in 1990 and Baden et al.[7] in 1992. The latter authors also described three families with the syndrome, and were the first to suggest an autosomal dominant mode of inheritance. Since its initial description, at least 80 cases and 9 familial cases of LAHS have been cited in the international literature.[3–21]

Clinical presentation

Loose anagen hair syndrome usually presents in early childhood in healthy children aged 6 months–9 years. It may also be diagnosed in a smaller proportion of adults who either had symptoms since childhood[5,20] or whose symptoms began in adulthood.[21] This syndrome appears to be more common in females and typically presents in those with blonde to light-brown hair.[5,7] Parents often state that the child requires few, if any, haircuts, and that the hair is difficult to manage. The history is further characterized by the painless, easy plucking of hair, often experienced during grooming or play.

The clinical findings are characterized by sparse hair of uneven length that may be unmanageable, dry and lustreless. Some authors have noted occipital hair that is rough, sticky and matted.[5–7] There may be frank alopecia in ill-defined patches, diffuse hair thinning, or fine hair of normal density but of uneven length (Figure 1). Hair color tends to be lighter than that of

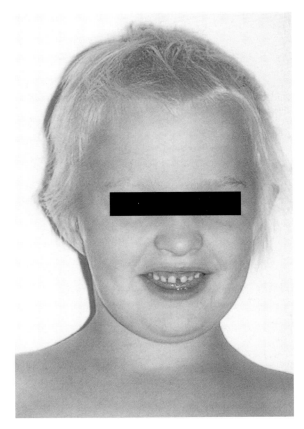

Figure 1

Loose anagen hair syndrome. Photograph of a child with hair of uneven length.

other family members, but the color tends to darken with the spontaneous improvement in the appearance of the hair that occurs with aging. Even as hair thickens and darkens, anagen hairs may still be pulled out easily; these have similar microscopic findings as in earlier, more severe disease[5] but the overall number is reduced.[21] There is no inflammation or scarring of the scalp, and there is no involvement of the teeth or nails. In general, eyebrows, eyelashes and body hair are normal. There is one report, however, of a 21-year-old male who also had loose hairs of the eyebrows, trunk and limbs.[20] Although overall hair growth is abnormal, this is probably the result of a shortened anagen phase rather than an actual decrease in rate of growth.[5] In our experience, the condition improves after puberty and the hair acquires a normal appearance.

Several diseases have been reported in association with LAHS. Sadick[11] described two adult patients infected with the human immunodeficiency virus (HIV) who also had characteristics of LAH, including hair thinning and easily pluckable hairs, 90% of which were in the anagen phase with absent external root sheaths. Loose anagen hairs are also found in the peeling skin syndrome, a disadhesive epithelial disorder of unclear etiology.[22] Two cases of Noonan's syndrome with features of LAHS have also been cited[8,21] as have cases of alopecia areata,[21] ocular colombata,[16] hypohidrotic epidermal dysplasia[19] and ectrodactyly ectodermal dysplasia cleft lip palate syndrome.[15] No true genetic linkage was identified in these cases, and therefore these associations were thought to be coincidental.

Light microscopy of pulled hairs

The 'pull test' is an extremely helpful diagnostic aid in evaluating a patient for loose anagen hair. To test for loose hairs, a group of hairs is grasped firmly with the fingers and slow, steady traction applied. Normally, only a few hairs are extracted easily, and these are generally in the telogen phase. In LAH, a few anagen hairs are extracted painlessly with each pull. Under light microscopy, the trichogram reveals the presence of 97–100% anagen hairs and none to very few

telogen hairs.[4,5,7,21] In unaffected children, the representation of telogen hairs is normally 1–10%, whereas in adults the percentage increases to 4–25%.[13] The loose anagen hairs are identified by a moist, pigmented, distorted hair bulb that is devoid of cuticle and inner and outer root sheaths (Figure 2). Staining with cinnimaldehyde has confirmed the absence of the normally red-staining, citrulline-rich inner root sheath on the affected hairs.[7,8] Just distal to the bulb, the cuticle has a characteristic ruffled appearance. Although normal anagen hairs that are forcibly plucked from the scalp may have a similar appearance, the hallmark of LAH is that these hairs are extracted painlessly and with little effort.[5]

Light microscopy of the hair shafts can demonstrate longitudinal grooving and twisting along the long axis. Examination using the shrinking tube technique has demonstrated abnormal cross-sectional shapes of hairs including oval, triangular, quadrangular, trapezoid, kidney-shaped and heart-shaped hairs.[4] Other cross-sectional

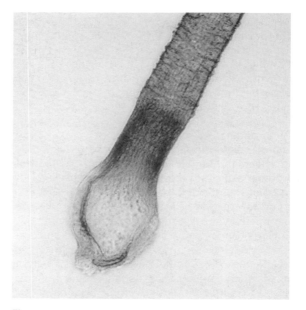

Figure 2

LAHS. Typical appearance of the hair shaft devoid of cuticle and inner and outer root sheaths.

techniques have confirmed similar abnormalities in the hair shaft.[6,7,18] Examination with polarized light has revealed a variable appearance, including light and dark patches in speckled, mosaic or parallel band arrays.[4,6]

Electron microscopy of pulled hairs

Examination of loose anagen hairs under scanning electron microscopy has confirmed the ultrastructural findings seen by light microscopy and has further delineated the abnormalities of the shaft. These include a distorted bulb end with absent root sheaths and cuticle, rippling of the cuticle just distal to this region as shown by a rolled-back appearance of the scales, and a normal cuticle appearing distally along the shaft in the cornified region. Hair distal to the level of the scalp demonstrates significant grooving and ridging and occasional absence of cuticular cells.[4–7,13,16,18,19]

More detailed examination of follicles in LAHS by transmission electron microscopy has revealed abnormalities of all layers. The most significantly affected layer is the outer root sheath, which, at the level of the lower portion of the follicle, demonstrates cellular disadhesion as shown by prominent cytoplasmic processes and fewer desmosomal attachments. The cells of the outer root sheath demonstrate nuclear variability, dysmaturation, and immaturity of the chromatin pattern. In addition, these cells maintain a round shape instead of flattening as they approach the center of the follicle, and do not produce a distinct marginal band at the level of complete keratinization of Henle's layer.[7]

Further cytological abnormalities may be identified in the inner root sheath and the hair cuticle, for example cytoplasmic vacuolation, nuclear degeneration and absence of the exocuticle of the hair cuticle. The hair cortex may also be affected as degenerative changes and diminished keratin filament production is seen. The distal portion of the follicle and hair shaft starting at the level of complete keratinization of the inner root sheath tends to be more normal.[7]

Histology

Scalp biopsies of patients with LAHS may also be helpful in diagnosis. Two common findings in all reports are the complete lack of either an inflammatory infiltrate or evidence of scarring. Although Price and Gummer[5] reported an increased number of small, vellus sized follicles, most authors report no abnormalities in number or size of follicles.[4,6,7,21] Only some follicles may be abnormal; this may indicate a variable expression of the disease.[7] Typically, there may be empty follicles, or follicles that contain irregularly shaped hairs.[4,6,7] Although clefting between the hair shaft and inner root sheath may also be seen, this finding is difficult to distinguish from fixation artifact.[4,21] Baden et al.[7] described separation between the hair cortex and hair cuticle as well as between the hair cuticle and the inner root sheath cuticle (Figure 3). Furthermore, they described separation of the bulbar outer root sheath from both the vitreous layer and the inner root sheath as well as focal disadhesion of the bulb.[21] One distinct finding of LAHS, however, is the early presence of trichohyaline granules and premature keratinization of the inner root sheath at the inferior portion of the hair bulb.[5–7]

Pathogenesis of LAHS

The exact molecular mechanisms responsible for the LAHS phenotype remain to be elucidated. To date, nine families have been reported to be affected by LAHS.[5,7,16,21] This observation, taken together with the variability in expression of the disease, suggests that some cases may be inherited in an autosomal dominant manner.[7,23]

Several theories have been proposed to explain the molecular defects in the LAHS follicle. Normally, the shaft cuticle cells and the inner root sheath cuticle cells interlock in a shingle-like fashion to secure the shaft in the follicle and to allow the two structures to move as one as growth of the hair takes place.[24,25] Price and Gummer have suggested that the premature keratinization of the inner root sheath could interfere with this mechanical relationship and thus lead to abnormal anchoring of anagen hairs.[5]

Another therapy implicates faulty desmosomes as a cause for loose anagen hairs. Mils et

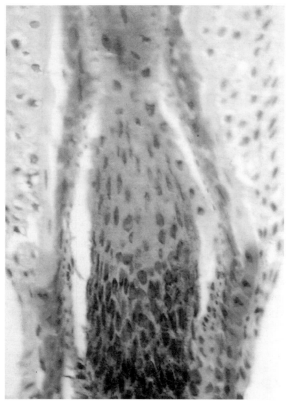

Figure 3

Histology of LAHS. Separation between various layers of the hair can be seen.

al.[26] have used indirect immunofluorescence to identify the location of desmosomes and corneodesmosomes in the hair follicle. They found that desmosomes are present in the matrix, hair shaft, inner root sheath and outer root sheath. In the shaft and inner root sheath they persist only until the level of the keratogenous zone, whereas the outer root sheath continues to express desmogleins until it reaches the isthmus. Corneodesmosomes are present exclusively in the inner root sheath and are expressed until the level of the isthmus. Nevertheless, the authors also reported that there are no functional corneodesmosomes between the cuticles of the shaft and inner root sheath. They suggested that desmosomes disappear during cell differentiation and are replaced by alternate cell–cell junc-

tions. This line of thought suggests that the premature keratinization of the inner root sheath in LAHS may correlate with the loss of functional desmosomes or corneodesmosomes, resulting in poorly anchored hairs.

Recently, Commo and Bernard[27] have described the presence of $\alpha 2 \beta 1$ and $\alpha 3 \beta 1$ integrins along the inferior portion of the outer root sheath possibly linked to the presence of the vitreous membrane. The location of these integrins could correlate with the site of the outer root sheath abnormalities described by Baden et al.[7] Moreover, Fujita et al.[28] have also identified E (epithelial) cadherin and P (placental) cadherin in the hair follicle, where the expression of P–cadherin appears to be restricted to the proliferating cells of the matrix and outer root sheath, and where E–cadherin is found throughout. It is possible that abnormalities of any of these adhesion molecules could lead to the disadhesion of multiple follicular layers and the expression of loose anagen hairs.

Other theories proposed by Baden et al.[7] and Li et al.[23] include:

(1) An abnormality of intercellular signalling occurring early in follicle development within the inner root sheath;

(2) An abnormality of mesenchymal–epithelial interactions resulting in faulty keratinization and expression of cellular adhesion molecules; and

(3) An alteration in normal mechanical cell signalling triggered by the structural effect of the misshapen, rounded, dysmature outer root sheath cells on the integrated cytoskeleton.[7,23]

No studies to date have investigated the role of cell signalling, cell adhesion molecules, epithelial–mesenchymal interactions or abnormal keratinization in LAHS.

Differential diagnosis of LAHS

The differential diagnosis of LAHS includes alopecia areata, trichotillomania, telogen effluvium and anagen effluvium. Alopecia areata may be distinguished from LAHS by its well-defined, discrete areas of hair loss, with its exclamation point hairs and the presence of an inflammatory infiltrate on histological examination. Trichotillomania is identified by broken hairs in the areas of alopecia, a normal hair pluck and a characteristic histopathology. Telogen effluvium is generally preceded by an acute illness, and reveals an increased number of telogen hairs on a hair pull. Anagen effluvium presents acutely most commonly following chemotherapy, with a copious loss of anagen hairs that have dystrophic, tapered ends.

Treatment and prognosis

No specific treatment exists for LAHS. Gentle care and avoidance of grabbing and pulling the hair can minimize loss. Fortunately, a normal appearance of the hair occurs after puberty in most patients; however, the ability of hair to be pulled easily and painlessly from the scalp persists.

References

1. Zaun H: Differential diagnosis of alopecia in children. In: Happle R, Grosshans E (eds.) *Pediatric Dermatology* Berlin, Springer-Verlag, 1987: 157–166.
2. Price VH: The short anagen syndrome [Abstract]. 106th Annual Meeting of the American Dermatological Association, Greenbrier, West Virginia, 1986; **18**.
3. Nodl F, Zaun H, Zinn KH: Gesteigerte Epilierbarkeit von Anagenhaaren bei Kindern als Folge eines Reifungsdefekts der Follikel mit gestorter Verhaftung von Haarschaft und Wurzelscheiden. Das Phanomen der leicht ausziehbaren Haare. *Aktuelle Dermatologie* 1986; **12**: 55–57.
4. Hamm H, Traupe H: Loose anagen hair of childhood: the phenomenon of easily pluckable hair. *J Am Acad Dermatol* 1989; **20**: 242–248.
5. Price VH, Gummer CL: Loose anagen syndrome. *J Am Acad Dermatol* 1989; **20**: 249–256.
6. Lalevic-Vasic B, Polic DJ, Milinkovic R: Le syndrome des cheveux anagenes caducs. *Ann Dermatol Venereol* 1990; **127**: 701–707.
7. Baden HP, Kvedar JC, Magro CM: Loose anagen hair as a cause of hereditary hair loss in children. *Arch Dermatol* 1992; **128**: 1349–1353.
8. Tosti A, Misciali C, Borrello P, et al.: Loose anagen hair in a child with Noonan's syndrome. *Dermatologica* 1991; **182**: 247–249.
9. O'Donnell BP, Sperling LC, James WD: Loose anagen hair syndrome. *Int J Dermatol* 1992; **31**: 107–108.
10. Trueb RM, Burg G: Loses Anagen-Haar. *Hautarzt* 1992; **43**: 505–508.
11. Sadick NS: Clinical and laboratory evaluation of AIDS trichopathy. *Int J Dermatol* 1993; **32**: 33–38.
12. Thomas L, Robart S, Balme B, Moulin G: Syndrome des cheveux anagenes caducs. *Ann Dermatol Venereol* 1993; **120**: 535–537.
13. Martinez JA, Velasco JJ, Vilata E, et al.: Loose anagen syndrome: a new case [letter]. *Acta Derm Venereol (Stockh)* 1994; **74**: 473.
14. Haskett M: Loose anagen syndrome. *Australas J Dermatol* 1995; **36**: 35–36.
15. Camacho FM, Gata I: Hypotrichosis and loose anagen hair in EEC (ectrodactyl, ectodermal dysplasia, cleft lip palate) syndrome. *Eur J Dermatol* 1995; **5**: 300–302.
16. Murphy MF, McGinnity FG, Allen GE: New familial association between ocular coloboma and loose anagen syndrome. *Clin Genet* 1995; **47**: 214–216.
17. Pride HB, Tunnessen WW: Picture of the month. *Arch Pediatr Adolesc Med* 1995; **149**: 819–820.
18. Boyer JD, Cobb MW, Sperling LC, Rushin JM: Loose anagen hair syndrome mimicking the uncombable hair syndrome. *Cutis* 1996; **57**: 111–112.
19. Azon-Masoliver A, Ferrando J: Loose anagen hair in hypohidrotic ecodermal dysplasia. *Pediatr Dermatol* 1996; **13**: 29–32.
20. Chapman DM, Miller RA: An objective measurement of the anchoring strength of anagen hair in an adult with the loose anagen hair syndrome. *J Cutan Pathol* 1996; **23**: 288–292.
21. Tosti A, Peluso AM, Misciali C, et al.: Loose anagen hair. *Arch Dermatol* 1997; **133**: 1089–1093.
22. Levy SB, Goldsmith LA: The peeling skin syndrome. *J Am Acad Dermatol* 1982; **7**: 606–613.
23. Li VW, Baden HP, Kvedar JC: Loose anagen syndrome and loose anagen hair. *Dermatol Clin* 1996; **14**: 745–751.
24. Hashimoto K: The structure of human hair. *Clin Dermatol* 1988; **6**: 7–21.
25. McKee PH: *Pathology of the Skin*. Barcelona, Mosby-Wolfe, 1996: 1–20.
26. Mils VM, Vincent C, Croute F, Serre G: The expression of desmosomal and corneodesmosomal antigens shows specific variation during the terminal differentiation of epidermis and hair follicle epithelia. *J Histochem Cytochem* 1992; **40**: 1329–1337.

27. Commo S, Bernard BA: The distribution of alpha 2 beta 1, alpha 3 beta 1 and alpha 6 beta 4 integrins identifies distinct subpopulations of basal keratinocytes in the outer root sheath of the human anagen hair follicle. *Cell Mol Life Sci* 1997; **53**: 466–471.

28. Fujita M, Furukawa F, Fujii K, et al.: Expression of caherin cell adhesion molecules during human skin development: morphogenesis of epidermis, hair follicles and eccrine sweat ducts. *Arch Dermatol Res* 1992; **284**: 159–166.

30
Shaft effects from cosmetics and styling

Ramon Grimalt and Juan Ferrando

Introduction

During the last three decades, scanning electron microscopy (SEM) studies have shown that from root to tip the shaft degenerates progressively (weathering) as a result of factors such as ultraviolet radiation, brushing and combing, and a variety of cosmetic treatments.[1]

Cosmetic products are used by the consumer for the primary purpose of cleansing and beautification of the skin, hair and nails. Since these keratinizing structures continue to grow and are influenced by endogenous and exogenous environmental changes, the cosmetic products employed for beautification are used repetitively and frequently to maintain the desired appearance.

Hair care products represent one of the most important classes of cosmetics that are used by the consumers. These products can be divided into categories according to their chemical formulations and also according to their action, for example cleansing, increased manageability, softening, thickening, curling, straightening and adding or removing colors. Since these cosmetic products employ both chemical formulations and physical modalities there is, at anytime, potential for temporary adverse effects on hair fibers and scalp skin. These adverse effects appear primarily on the hair cuticle.[2]

The 'straighteners' are usually based on thioglycollic acid and rearrange sulphide bonds to produce a permanent straightening of the hair. When these products are used incorrectly or over-used, they may produce different degrees of morphological changes on the hair surface, leading, in severe cases, to a partial alopecia.[3]

External weathering factors including humidity, wind, sea salt, dust, and pollution also contribute to the cuticular hair damage, especially in previously (cosmetically) damaged hair or in particular hair alterations such as those seen in dysplastic hair.[4]

Developments in hair care products aim to reduce these damaging environmental influences, and to compensate for effects of the environment; beyond this, in a cosmetic sense, they aim to make the hair more attractive. These effects of hair care products have both positive and negative aspects. Until now dermatologists have dealt mainly with the negative aspect and emphasized intolerance to these products. In this chapter the different effects that hair care products may produce in our hair shaft will be analysed.

Racial variations in hair morphology

Morphologically, hair can be classified according to racial lines, although phenotypic variation may occur within groups. Three main categories exist: Mongoloid, Caucasoid and Negroid (Table 1).

(1) **Mongoloid** or Oriental hair is straight, round in cross-section, eumelanin-rich and greater in diameter than the hair of other population groups;

(2) **Caucasoid** hair is usually straight, wavy, or helical, shows a mixture of eumelanine and phaeomelanin and is round to oval in cross-section;

(3) **Negroid** hair is tightly coiled, helical or spiraled, eumelanin-rich, and elliptic or flattened in cross-section.

Table 1 Racial variations in hair morphology.

Type of hair	Cross-section	Shape	Diameter	Color	Melanin	Biochemical differences
Mongoloid	Round	Straight	Greater (80 μm)	Black	Eumelanin-rich	Normal ratio of SCM fibrous/SCM matrix protein
Caucasoid	Oval	Wavy	Normal (70 μm)	Brown/ blond	Eumelanin/ phaeomelanin mixture	Normal ratio of SCM fibrous/SCM matrix protein
Negroid	Elliptic/flattened	Curly	Lesser (60 μm)	Black	Eumelanin-rich	Lower ratio of SCM fibrous/SCM matrix protein

SCM, S-carboxymethylated

Although this division is extremely academic, mixtures within the three different groups commonly occur such that, in a 'standard' population, it might be quite difficult to obtain 'pure' hair types.[5]

Despite the obvious differences in phenotype, there are few biochemical differences found to date to explain the differences between the hair of different racial groups in general. Pioneering the field were Rutherford and Hawk in 1907[6] who ran a comparative study of hair of different racial origins and found little difference in their chemical character. Similarly, no relation could be demonstrated by Wilson and Lewis in 1927.[7] Clay in 1940[8] claimed that male hair contained slightly more cystine than female hair but this data was not confirmed. Recent progress in techniques of amino acid analysis and improvement in methods for protein characterization have, however, led to the generation of the wealth of information indispensable for the study of keratinization and thorough product evaluation.[9]

The most commonly used method for keratin fiber analysis uses hydrochloric acid, which degrades tryptophan and partially decomposes cystine, threonine, tyrosine, phenylalanine, and arginine during the process. There are no significant differences in low-sulfur protein composition between the groups when using two-dimensional electrophoresis, acrylamide gel electrophoresis, stress-strain, or X-ray diffraction analysis. Deiko and Jidio[10,11] examined the differential centrifugration of S-carboxymethylated (SCM) fibrous protein derivatives compared with SCM matrix protein derivatives. Solubilization by

S-carboxymethylation breaks disulfide bonds by reduction into low-sulfur and high-sulfur groups, with the high-sulfur proteins predominantly found in the matrix and the low-sulfur proteins in the filamentous proteins. Negroid hair has a lower ratio of SCM fibrous protein to SCM matrix protein than Mongoloid hair or Caucasoid hair. Thus, the differential expression of low-sulfur protein to high-sulfur protein may be involved in phenotypic racial variations.

A better understanding of the Negroid hair follicle has been gained through the work of Lindelof and co-workers[12] who showed that the pilary

Table 2 Hair cosmetics currently available.

Cleansing products
- Shampoos
- '2-in-1' shampoos

Increasing manageability products
- Conditioners

Styling hair
- Setting agents
- Perms
- Relaxers
- Straighteners
- Hot-combing

Color additives (hair dyes)
- Temporary hair colorants
- Hair color restorers
- Natural hair colorants
- Semi-permanent hair colorants
- Permanent hair colorants

Color removers (bleachers)

canal in African Americans is actually spiral in shape. A three-dimensional computerized reconstruction of hair follicle morphology showed that the shape of the hair conformed to the shape of the follicle in all three major racial hair types. The physical characteristics of shape and degree of kink and curl, then, are probable reflections of cross-links in the cortex that develop during the molding of the hair shaft.

Negroid hair is typically very dry, and the cuticle weathers more readily than that of other racial hair phenotypes. Most published data suggest that Negroids produce more sebum than Caucasians, and that most of the hair lipids are derived from the scalp lipids. However, because of the extreme curliness of Negroid hair, the natural oils may not be distributed along the hair shaft.[13]

There is an enormous variety in cosmetic hair products; to unify their effect they have been divided according to categories listed in Table 2.

Cleansing products

Shampoos

Shampoos containing anionic agents are particularly drying to the hair as is sodium lauryl sulfate. The sodium laureth sulfate-containing shampoos are not so harsh, but damaged hair needs shampoos that contain humectants and milder cleansing agents, such as amphoteric and non-ionic blends. Anti-dandruff and anti-seborrheic shampoos are especially harsh on weathered hair. Selenium sulfide shampoos, in particular, make the hair very dry and brittle. If there are no alternatives to using these medicated shampoos, it is best to limit their use to the scalp and to shampoo the hair with a milder agent followed by an effective moisturizer.

'2-in-1' shampoos

'2-in-1' shampoos contain both cleansing agents and high levels of conditioning agents. These shampoos are everyday products now but they created considerable debate when they were first introduced in the 1980s.[14] Today all the major manufacturers produce '2-in-1' formulations, and over 20% of the shampoos sold are of this type.[15]

They basically rely on silicones, which are positively charged molecules derived from natural substances, to achieve conditioning. There is no question of conditioning agents building upon the hair if these shampoos are used repeatedly. Shampooing always removes the conditioning agents that were applied previously. Cosmetical damage from '2-in-1' shampoos is minimal.

Increasing manageability products

Conditioners

Hair conditioners are defined as any product that enhances the appearance, manageability and growth of the hair. A conditioner may be simply an emollient or a very complex mixture of proteins, quaternary ammonium compounds, oils, gums, and humectants. The type of conditioning agent needed will depend on the hair phenotype and the type of chemical or other styling aids used. Non-chemically treated hair may be conditioned simply by using a good moisturizer. Hot-pressed hair may require an agent that contains proteins and quaternary ammonium compounds, such as stearyl benzyl dimethyl ammonium chloride, the quaternized cellulose polymers of dimethyl diallyl ammonium chloride plus acrylamide. These agents have to prevent breakage by adding a protective coating to the hair, as well by creating ionic attractions to the negatively charged fibers. Chemically relaxed hair would benefit from the same type of conditioner or one that is relatively rich in proteins. Curled or waved hair is kept conditioned by moisturizers and activators or by combination products.

Styling hair

Styling hair means temporarily or permanently altering its shape.

Setting hair

Setting is different from perming in that there is no chemical reaction in the hair. All that happens is that some of the weak hydrogen bonds are broken by water and they re-form in the newly positioned hair as the water evaporates. A curl can be produced by setting hair on a former such as a curler or roller, that is, allowing wet hair to dry while being twisted round the former. Fixing wet hair into pin curls has a similar effect. After the curlers or rollers have been removed, the hair holds its shape until it gets wet again. Most people would use a hair dryer in this process. Heat is a great enemy to hair, however, and that means that dryers must always be used with great care and at a moderate setting. A hair dryer on its hottest setting will reach temperatures well above that at which water boils, and this can have a disastrous effect on the hair. Using 'hot oil' has a protective effect; so too do hair mousses, which contain especially formulated resins.

Curls that are produced by setting are tight when they are first formed but they can be brushed out into a lighter style. Using setting lotions or hair sprays gives a firmer effect, and helps to hold the temporary curl in for longer.

Softer, looser styles can be created by brushing and blow drying only, without using rollers. The principle is exactly the same as that of the setting process. The only difference is that the hydrogen bonds re-connect to form the style that has been shaped by the brush.

All hair gradually absorbs moisture from the air, and as the hydrogen bonds break it will in time lose its style, especially in damp weather.

Hair cuticular damage from setting is minimal. Hair cuticles tend to lift after water exposure and brushing can more easily damage hair especially when brushed upwards. Hair dryers applied on wet hair at high temperatures may also provoke the well-known phenomenon of 'bubble hair' (Figures 1 and 2).[16]

Perming hair

A permanent wave is a process that creates a curl in the hair shaft by altering its internal chemical structure. The curl cannot be destroyed except by further chemical treatment. The curl or wave process is a two-step procedure requiring that the chemically unaltered new growth be straightened first with a rearranger, straightener, or pre-softening gel and then set on rollers with a booster. Both the rearranger and booster are based on thioglycolates, the latter being of a lower concentration than the former.

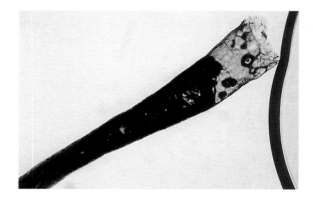

Figure 1

Bubble hair: optical microscope image.

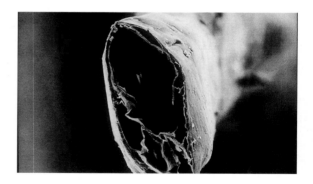

Figure 2

Bubble hair: scanning electron microscopy aspect.

Today's 'cold' permanent wave lotions contain reducing agents in an alkaline solution. The reducing agent most often used is ammonium thioglycollate. It will act on the keratin in the hair, breaking the disulfide linkages that join the pairs of cysteine units together. The result is that the keratin softens and swells. The softened hair is then put into its new shape. As the hair is manipulated the cysteine linkages slip past each other and realign themselves with new cysteine partners.

Neutralizing lotion is then applied. The hair is

saturated with this oxidizing agent, (neutralizer), usually sodium bromate or hydrogen peroxide, which is also used in hair bleaches. This process is repeated every 2–3 months and is very harsh on the hair. Structural bonds are impaired, and the hair loses much of its water-retaining capacity.

Oxidizing agents work in the opposite way to reducing agents. They make the cysteine units link together into pairs again, hardening the hair and giving it its new, permanent shape.

In hair that has been permed repeatedly, the original disulfide cross-links may have been broken and re-formed so many times that hardly any remain.

Once the perming solution has been put on, the hair is in a very vulnerable condition. The keratin is softened and greatly swollen (particularly during rinsing), the cortex is in the process of being chemically changed, and the cuticle may have been slightly damaged. At this point every possible care is needed to protect the hair from any unwanted change in conditions. A sudden temperature change can damage the softened keratin to such an extent that the hair may break down completely.

Damage can also result from either the reduction step (rearranger and booster) or the oxidation step (neutralizer). Curls and waves, like relaxers, can cause severe hair breakage; the breakage will usually be more widespread and limited to the distal ends of the hair shafts. With curls and waves, the entire hair shaft is treated with the booster each time the hair is styled, which can lead to severe damage to the hair shaft. Managing hair breakage from curls or waves is the same as that for chemical relaxers, with one notable exception—the hair must be kept hydrated because curled or waved hair is stronger when wet, as opposed to chemically relaxed hair, which is stronger when dry. With curled hair, products with high concentrations of protein should be avoided because they cause absorption of moisture by the hair.[13]

Relaxing hair

Relaxing or straightening hair is the opposite of perming. It is traditionally used by people with Afro-Caribbean hair to straighten the hair. Hair alterations from cosmetics procedures in African Americans has been studied widely by Wilborn.[13] Relaxing is popular because it makes hair easier to manage. The chemistry of the relaxing process is identical to that of perming, with the breakage of disulfide linkages and re-forming of the hair shape (in a straighter arrangement this time, rather than in curls), followed by the re-making of linkages.

The oval-elliptical shape and natural crimp of Afro-Caribbean hair, however, makes it difficult to straighten without damage. The chemical treatment can weaken the hair structure, and breakage after relaxation treatment is common. Contributing factors include incorrect concentrations of relaxing solution, mistakes in timing of the application and incomplete rinsing. Often the hair breakage is seen at the back of the neck. In addition, straightening leaves the hair fibers in a high degree of torsional stress and a slightly wavy look. This makes them liable to a rapid weathering, with the cuticle wearing down at the ends of the cross-sectional ellipse and showing a characteristic lengthwise splitting.

Two types of relaxers currently dominate the market: sodium hydroxide and guanidine hydroxide. Potassium and lithium hydroxide relaxers also exist; ammonium bisulfite has also been used in commercial relaxers but is relatively ineffective as a straightening agent. Hair that is more Caucasoid than Negroid in texture responds best to these agents. The bisulfites work best at a pH close to 7 and have a similar, yet less harsh, effect on hair than the thioglycolates. Ammonium bisulfite relaxers usually require heat to accelerate the relaxing process, an alkali to decompose the formed thiosulfates, and a neutralization step. One major advantage of the bisulfate relaxers is that potentially one could perform a curl on bisulfite-treated hair: which cannot be performed using the caustic alkali relaxers.

Mild caustic burns of the scalp and neck secondary to relaxers are relatively common, especially with the alkali relaxers, but usually not severe enough to require medical attention. More severe burns may result in blistering; however, scarring rarely occurs and palliative treatment is usually all that is required. Permanent hair loss is highly unlikely with hair restructuring chemicals because the burns are generally only superficial and do not destroy the follicular unit. Residual post-inflammatory hyperpigmentation is the only long-lasting sequel to even the most severe burns.

Hair breakage is the most common side-effect from chemical relaxers. Factors that influence the degree of breakage include the strength of the relaxer, the speed of application, the effectiveness of its removal, and the phenotype of the hair. Hair breakage is most common in the nape area, with the anterior scalp margin being next in frequency. The prime location of damage is related to where the hair stylist first applies the relaxer and, hence to the duration of exposure to the relaxer. A 'touch-up' is the application of the relaxer to the new hair growth that has developed since the first treatment. Some women have a 'touch-up' every 3–4 weeks. This is too frequent since, with only a small amount of new growth, the relaxer will invariably overlap onto previously treated hair, causing resultant irreparable damage to the hair shaft and subsequent breakage. A depilatory effect may occur from improper use of a chemical relaxer. Since there are no stringent standards for these hair restructuring agents, lack of quality control is also a significant problem and may contribute to hair damage.

Chemically relaxed hair should be handled very gently when wet because it is more susceptible to breakage when wet than dry. Combing, brushing and styling must be kept to a minimum. In general, hair that has been damaged by relaxers will benefit from a protein, gum, or cationic gum conditioner. If the damage is more distal, simply cutting off the damaged portion of the hair is an excellent remedy.[13]

Hot-combing

Hair-pressing, as it is also called, employs the use of an emollient followed by the combing of the hair with a hot metal comb. The temperature may at times exceed 400°F. Petrolatum, or an oil that tends to emit little smoke when heated, is used most commonly. The treated hair subsequently remains straight until moisture causes reversion. Pomades are applied as required to help prevent this reversion and to add sheen to the shaft. Later, the hair may be set either onto rollers or with a hot curling iron.

This process can damage both the hair and scalp: scalp burns are frequent, and burns on the face and other areas are sometimes seen if the iron is accidentally dropped. Another sequel of this process is hot-comb alopecia,[17] which has

been recently termed 'the follicular degeneration syndrome'.[18]

Color additives

Hair dyes

The last few years have been seen considerable controversy concerning the safety of hair dyes, mostly concerning the increased risk of cancer from the use of hair dyes containing 2,4-diaminoanisole, 2-nitro-p-phenylenediamine, 4-amino-2-nitrophenol, 2,4-diamino-toluene, and 4-chloro-o-phenylenediamine.[19]

In this chapter hair dyes are divided into five types:

(1) Temporary hair colorants;
(2) Hair color restorers;
(3) Natural hair colorants;
(4) Semi-permanent hair colorants;
(5) Permanent hair colorants.

Temporary hair colorants

Temporary hair colorants, as the name implies, produce a coloration that is removed when the hair is shampooed. To accomplish this, it is necessary to employ high-molecular-weight dyes that do not diffuse through the cuticle. Accordingly, it is customary to use water-soluble textile dyes in an aqueous base, which may also include a setting resin. Among them, triphenylmethane and anthraquinones are the most commonly used. Hepatocarcinomas have been produced when these substances have been fed to rats but the absorption of these molecules during temporary hair dyes has not been proven.[19]

Allergic reactions to temporary hair dyes are very rare since they are probably unable to diffuse through the stratum corneum.

Hair color restorers

The hair color restorers, or gradual hair colorants, are essentially aqueous solutions of lead acetate or bismuth citrate that contain small amounts of glycerol and suspended sulfur. When applied to the hair, small amounts of lead or bismuth ions are absorbed and slowly converted to the dark-colored oxides and sulfides. Their major advantage is the apparent absence of allergic reaction and the ease of application. There are, however, a very limited range of shades and these products tend to produce a coated feel to the hair.

Natural hair colorants

Most natural hair colorants are plant-derived dyes such as henna, camomile, indigo and logwood. Although these dyes are relatively safe, allergic reactions to henna have been described.[20]

Semi-permanent hair colorants

This type of dye requires from four to six shampoos before losing its color. These colorants are based on low-molecular-weight dyes that are derivatives of nitrophenylenediamines, anthroquinones and nitroaminophenols. These dyes diffuse into the cortex during the 20–30 min coloring process.[21]

While dermatological effects from semi-permanent dyes are rare, there have been a few reports of allergic reactions.[19]

Permanent hair colorants

Oxidizers or permanent hair colorants represent the major segment of the hair color market. This can be explained by their extreme versatility in respect of color effect afforded. These products achieve their coloring effect by the oxidation of mixtures of aromatic para-diamines and aminophenols in the presence of meta-diamines, aminophenols and dihydroxybenzenes, with the consequent production of indodyes.[21] Allergic potential of permanent hair dyes is well-known, although it is less than patch testing with p-phenylenediamine or p-toluenediamine in petrolatum might suggest. True allergic reactions on patch testing with permanent hair colorants may be as low as 1 per million units sold.[22]

The controversy concerning permanent hair dyes has, however, centered around their mutagenicity and carcinogenicity. Nevertheless, the safety of hair dyes under the conditions of use has been supported by numerous series of chronic animal tests involving topical applications of hair dyes. The relevance of 'maximal tolerated dose' feeding studies in rodents to the safety of hair dyes is questionable, especially if the dose can be shown to produce acute toxicity in the target organs. Even when feeding study data is assumed to be valid, conservative risk assessment gives lifetime risks of 1 in several million.[22] Human experience appears to support the absence of chronic effects from the use of hair dyes.

Hair cosmetics

Color removers

Hair is made lighter by changing part or all of the melanin pigment in the cortex into a colorless substance. The melanin is not washed out of the hair, it is changed chemically and this change is irreversible. The chemical solutions used are called **bleaches** and contain oxidizing agents like those in neutralizing lotions for perms, in an alkaline solution. The bleach most commonly used is hydrogen peroxide. Hydrogen peroxide can be used alone to lighten dark hair, or together with a coloring agent. Red and blond hair contain more phaeomelanin than eumelanin. Conversely, dark hair contains more eumelanin than phaeomelanin. Of the two kinds of melanin in hair, eumelanin is the more easily removed from the cortex by bleaches. This is why bleached dark hair tends to look reddish: the eumelanin has been decolorized, and what is left is mostly phaeomelanin. Further bleaching also removes the phaeomelanin. This is why red hair is harder to bleach than dark hair.

Strongly bleached hair looks yellowish, because keratin itself is naturally pale yellow. This natural color is the reason why an elderly person's white hair looks slightly yellow at the roots. It also explains why repeatedly bleached hair looks the color of nicotine-stained skin. The hair needs to be tinted as well as bleached if it is to be turned white or to a 'platinum' blond color.

The commonest problems during the bleaching process include the following:

(1) Raising the scales of the cuticle for penetration by the bleach is in itself a potentially risky process;

(2) Repeated bleaching can leave permanently raised scales and upset the moisture content of the hair;

(3) Bleaching increases the porosity of the hair, and this makes further bleaching more difficult; very porous hair bleaches badly, with uneven shading;

(4) Repeated bleaching leaves weak, brittle hairs, which have little shine or luster, and which weather rapidly;

(5) Additional cosmetic procedures such as perming simply make things worse.

Bleaching is not the only effect of treating hair with oxidizing agents. Side-reactions often happen, such as breakage of some of the strong disulfide bonds of the hair. Re-bleaching, which means treating the whole length of the hair rather than just the roots, is certain to break more of these. The cuticle is especially easily weakened in that way; as a result it becomes extremely easy to strip it away from the cortex, even during routine hair care. Wet combing, for instance, becomes more difficult and causes additional damage. Back-combing is especially damaging because it can remove large amounts of cuticle with a single sweep of the comb.

Bleached hair being porous swells more readily when it is wet, and its wet strength is reduced still further.

Damage from hair cosmetics

Shampooing should not in itself damage the hair, since modern shampoos do not lift the cuticle. In the past, when harsh shampoos were used, acute and irreversible tangling or matting sometimes followed shampooing. The culprits were usually antiseptic shampoos, which could turn hair into a mass that looked more like sheep's wool than human hair. This kind of matting is seldom seen today since most modern shampoos contain conditioning agents that help to protect hair. Small amounts of tangling and occasionally matting are still quite common, however, especially in long, weathered hair. Usually small locks of hair or even a few adjacent hairs are affected. Matting may be the result of wetting and drying hair without shampoo, since friction is higher in wet hair than in dry; it

can also occur when the hair is piled up on top of the head during shampooing.

Of the common cosmetic procedures, permanent waving, bleaching and dyeing all damage the hair to some extent. Permanent waving, by its nature, disrupts the structure of the hair; indeed, it has to do so for the 'perm' to be successful. In order to change the shape of the hair, permanent waving agents first break the disulfide bonds that give the hair shaft its structure. The hair is then put into its new shape and neutralized. Neutralization is the name given to the re-forming of the chemical bonds in their new positions, a process that fixes the hair permanently into its new shape. The amount of cuticular damage provoked by permanent waving depends on the manufacturer's formulation of the product, and the stylist's expertise in applying the neutralizing lotion after just the right length of time.

Bleaching and dyeing also change hair structure because the dyes and bleaches used must penetrate the cuticle as they exert their effect in the cortex. Some degree of chemical damage is thus unavoidable.

Cosmetic procedures do not damage the hair follicle within the scalp, neither do they cause hair loss. Only a serious chemical burn to the skin of the scalp that destroys the follicle cells can do so. Burns like this can follow indiscriminate overuse of permanent waving or relaxing solutions, and therefore these solutions must be handled carefully at all times.

Damage from hair cutting and styling

Cutting hair with blunt scissors results in a cut with a long, jagged edge, at which the cuticle scales will be especially vulnerable to further damage. It is even possible to tell whether a stylist chose to use scissors or a razor by looking at the record of the hair: razor cutting produces long, tapering sections of cuticle which weather quickly and even peel back.

Some stylists prefer to cut hair when it is dry, in the belief that this will save the hair from heavy brushing when it is damp and vulnerable to damage. A circular or semicircular brush is probably the least damaging to hair.

Scanning electron microscopy studies on damage from hair cosmetics

In a study of retrospective microscopic changes caused by hair cosmetics, using scanning electron microscopy, alterations in most cases were found to be predominantly cuticular and varied from minimal changes to severe damage, including the total loss of the cuticle.[4] In increasing order of severity the alterations were: cuticular detachment; saw margins of the cuticular cells; fissuring of cuticular cells; depressions; decreased number of cuticular layers (on transversal sections); orifices of different sizes on the cuticular cell body; and total loss of the cuticular layer (Figures 3–9).

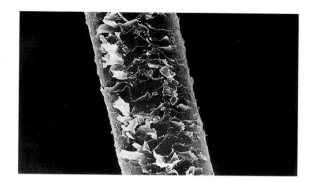

Figure 4

Cuticular hair damage grade II: adhered material.

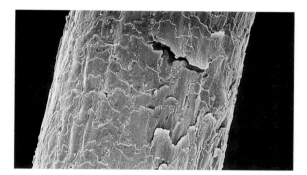

Figure 5

Cuticular hair damage grade II: initial fissuring on the cuticular layers.

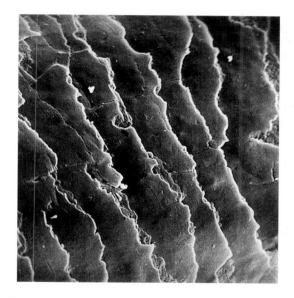

Figure 3

Cuticular hair damage grade I: saw margins of the cuticular cells.

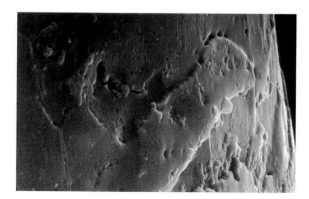

Figure 6

Cuticular hair damage grade III: orifices on the cuticular cell body.

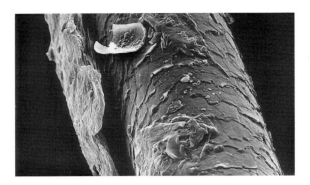

Figure 7

Cuticular hair damage grade III: partial decuticulation.

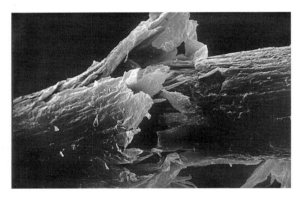

Figure 8

Cuticular hair damage grade III: partial decuticulation.

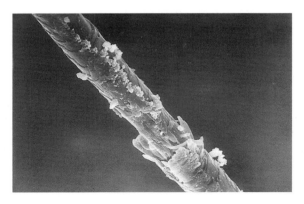

Figure 9

Cuticular hair damage grade IV: total loss of the cuticular layer.

The alterations found in this study lead us to propose a classification for cuticular hair damage.

- **Grade I**: Saw-margins of the cuticular cells or cuticular detachment; initial fissuring of the cuticular cells.
- **Grade II**: Fissuring and depressions of the cuticular cells; decreased number of cuticular layers (transverse section).
- **Grade III**: Orifices of different sizes in the cuticular cell body and partial decuticulation.
- **Grade IV**: Total loss of the cuticular layer with exposed hair shaft.

Relaxers and straighteners are caustic substances, with their pH strictly regulated, and all commercial products carry specific instructions for application. These state that the procedure should be performed no more than once in 8 weeks, and for a maximum of 20 min, and only to new hair growth. The reasons for such strict regulations are that the ultrastructural rearrangement increases the fragility of the hair shaft, and that the caustic nature of the agents will cause damage to the scalp.

Despite the precise instructions that all these products carry, they are frequently ignored by the users. Therefore, so long as individuals desire to conform with the dictates of fashion, the misuse of these chemical agents will continue. The abuse and malpractice of physicochemical hair treatments for cosmetic purposes induce mostly cuticular changes, which leave the cortex unprotected and exposed. These changes are similar to those seen in states of malnutrition, hypotricosis congenita, dysplastic syndromes,[23] and changes provoked by weathering factors.

Nevertheless, all scalp fibers undergo some degree of cuticular and secondary cortical breakdown from root to tip, the rough imbricated cuticular surface having a high coefficient of friction. The more frequent the brushing and combing and cosmetic procedures, such as permanent waving and bleaching, the greater the tendency to enhance the process. Particularly in women who undergo these cosmetic procedures too frequently, the enhanced breakdown may give rise to the fissuring and fracturing.

Special thanks

We would like to thank Procter & Gamble for supporting part of this study.

References

1. Dawber RPR: Weathering of hair in monilethrix and pili torti. *Clin Exper Dermatol* 1977; **2**: 271–277.
2. Bergfeld WF: The side-effects of products on the scalp and hair. In: Orfanos CE, Montagna W, Stüttgen G (eds.). *Hair Research*. Springer-Verlag, Berlin, 1981: 507–511.
3. Nicholson AG, Harland CC, Bull RH, Mortimer PS, Cook MG: Chemically induced cosmetic alopecia. *Br J Dermatol* 1993; **128**: 537–541.
4. Grimalt R, Ferrando J, Fontarnau R, Capdevila JM, Mascaró JM: Scanning electron microscopy changes induced by hair cosmetic procedures. In: Van Neste D, Randall VA (eds.). *Hair Research for the Next Millennium*. Amsterdam, Elsevier, 1996: 113–116.
5. Steggerda M, Seiber HC: Size and shape of head hairs form six racial groups. *J Hered* 1942; **32**: 315–318.
6. Rutherford TA, Hawk PB: A study of the comparative chemical composition of the hair in different races. *J Biol Chem* 1907; **3**: 459–489.
7. Wilson RH, Lewis HB: Cystine content of hair and other epidermal tissues. *J Biol Chem* 1927; **73**: 543–553.
8. Clay RC, Cook K, Routh JI: Studies in composition of human hair. *J Am Chem Soc* 1940; **62**: 2709–2710.
9. Gold RJM, Schriver CR: The amino acid composition of hair from different racial origins. *Clin Chim Acta* 1971; **33**: 465–466.
10. Deiko S, Jidio J: Hair low-sulfur protein composition does not differ electrophoretically among races. *J Dermatol* 1988; **15**: 393–396.
11. Deiko S, Jidio J: Amounts of fibrous proteins and matrix substances in hairs of different races. *J Dermatol* 1990; **17**: 62–64.
12. Lindelof B, Forslind B, Hedblad M, Kaveos U: Human hair form: morphology revealed by light and scanning electron microscopy and computer aided three-dimensional reconstruction. *Arch Dermatol* 1988; **124**: 1359–1363.
13. Wilborn WS: Disorders of hair growth in African Americans. In: Olsen EA (ed.). *Disorders in hair growth: Diagnosis and Treatment* 2nd Edn. McGraw Hill Publishing, 1999: 389–407.
14. Rushton H, Gummer CL, Flasch H: '2-in-1' shampoo technology: state-of-art shampoo and conditioner in one. *Skin Pharmacol* 1994; **7**: 78–83.
15. Gray J: *The World of Hair: A Scientific Companion*. London, Jarrolds, 1997.
16. Ferrando J, Solé T, Grimalt R, Dominguez A: Scanning electron microscopy changes in bubble hair. In: Van Neste D, Randall VA (eds.). *Hair Research for the Next Millennium*. Amsterdam, Elsevier, 1996: 113–116.
17. LoPresti P, Papa CM, Kligman AM: Hot comb alopecia. *Arch Dermatol* 1968; **98**: 234.
18. Sperling LC, Sau P: The follicular degeneration syndrome in black patients: 'hot comb alopecia' revisited and revised. *Arch Dermatol* 1992; **128**: 68–74.
19. Corbett JF: Hair dye toxicity. In: Orfanos CE, Montagna W, Stüttgen G (eds.). *Hair Research: Status and future aspects*. Berlin, Springer-Verlag, 1981: 529–535.
20. Abdulla KA, Davidson NM: A woman who collapsed after painting her soles. *Lancet* 1996; **348**: 658.
21. Brown K, Corbett J: The role of meta difunctional benzenes in oxidative hair dyeing. *J Soc Cosm Chem* 1979; **30**: 191.
22. Corbett J, Menkart J: Hair coloring. *Cutis* 1973; **12**: 190.
23. Ferrando J, Fontarnau R, Mascaró JM: Aplicación de la microscopía electrónica de barrido al estudio y diagnóstico de las distrofias pilosas. In: Camacho F, Montagna W (eds.). *Tricología, Trichology, Trichologie*. Madrid, Egraf Ed, 1982: 105–122.

Section VII

HYPERTRICHOSIS AND HIRSUTISM

31
Observations on the clinical features of hypertrichosis

Rodney D Sinclair

Introduction

Hypertrichosis is defined as excessive growth of hair on skin that is not normally hairy. The word *growth* is emphasized, since the number of hair follicles present is not altered. Hypertrichosis indicates a difference in the quality and length of the hair that is produced from the follicle. While the word *excessive* is subject to cultural and racial influences and personal preferences, most cases are self-evident. The pathogenesis of hypertrichosis predominantly involves elongation of the anagen phase. While some degree of hair follicle and hair fibre enlargement may be seen, it is commonly not pronounced.

Hirsutes, in contrast, is androgen-driven excessive hair growth in a female in a pattern that mimics hair growth in males. It preferentially affects the body sites where the hair follicles are sensitive to androgens, while sparing areas where the hair follicles are insensitive to androgens (Figure 1). Hirsutes begins after puberty and, while most cases appear to be caused by end-organ hypersensitivity, it can be the hallmark of an endocrinological disorder producing systemic androgen excess. The pathogenesis includes elongation of the anagen phase of the hair cycle, and consequently hair length, together with enlargement of the hair follicle, and consequently hair fibre diameter, which transforms the vellus hairs into terminal hairs.

The desire to distinguish hypertrichosis from hirsutes is based on practical considerations. Since hypertrichosis is not androgen-dependent, it is not associated with androgen excess and it does not respond to anti-androgen therapy. Unfortunately, the distinction between hypertrichosis and hirsutes is not absolute and the two conditions may co-exist, since hypertrichosis

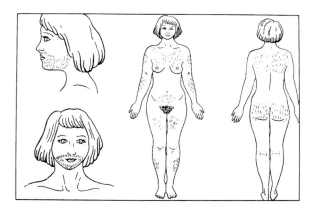

Figure 1

Androgen sensitive sites.

may occur anywhere on the skin and androgen sensitivity is a relative phenomenon.

Embryology of the hair follicle and pathogenesis of hypertrichosis

The pathogenesis of hypertrichosis and hirsutes are better understood in the context of the embryological development of the hair follicle. Human hair growth is cyclical, with each follicle producing many distinct hairs during a lifetime. The hair follicles first form on the eyebrow, upper lip and chin at between 9 and 12 weeks' gestation and, at birth, the full complement of hair follicles is present. There are approximately 5 million hair follicles on the body, of which, on average, only 100 000 are on the scalp. There is some variation in the number of scalp follicles ranging from about 70 000–150 000.

Hair growth rate is relatively constant at about 1 cm per month. Hair follicle formation occurs in a frontal to occipital wave on the scalp and a cephalocaudal wave on the body, reaching the feet at about 22 weeks. The first hair grows from the follicle between Weeks 16 and 22. The hair grows for about 10–12 weeks to a length of 2–3 cm, and covers the entire body from head to toe. These fine and non-pigmented hairs are known as lanugo hairs.

The growth then terminates in similar fronto-occipital and cephalocaudal waves, with the follicles traversing through the involutional catagen phase to enter the dormant telogen phase. Telogen terminates with the development of the second hair bud forming at the base of the bulb. This results in shedding of the first coat of hair between Weeks 32 and 36.

The second hair produced by the follicle is different to the first. Site variation is introduced, with the growth phase of the scalp hairs progressively elongating and the body hairs shortening to the point where most of the hairs are shorter than the first and grow for about 4–8 weeks, reaching a length of about 1 cm uniformly over the body. The second coat is shed during the first 3–4 months of life, as the second set of hairs pass through telogen and are replaced by the third set.

On the body, the third hair type is smaller than the second hair type and many no longer protrude from the pore, or do so only as fine light vellus hairs. In contrast, scalp hair follicles enlarge and produce thicker and pigmented hairs known as terminal hairs.

This site specificity of hair follicle development mirrors how follicles react to pubertal androgens. Scalp hairs miniaturize in response to androgens while body hairs enlarge. The degree of enlargement is highly variable, with pubic and axillary hair being most sensitive and capable of enlarging in response to physiological levels of adrenal androgens. Facial, chest, thigh, abdominal and buttock hair require at least physiological levels of gonadal androgens, but are more likely to appear in women with abnormally high levels of either adrenal or ovarian androgens. There is enormous person-to-person variation in the response of follicles to circulating androgens, which is influenced by a variety of genetic and metabolic factors.

The fourth and subsequent hairs from scalp follicles continue to enlarge and elongate until a steady state is achieved. The average duration of anagen is about 3 years, producing hairs that will grow to a final length of 36 cm; however, the range is large, with some women having prolonged anagen phases of up to 7 years and these women are thus able to grow their hair longer. By late adolescence, the anagen duration tends to be fixed and will remain constant unless an acquired disorder, such as androgenetic alopecia, supervenes.

In addition, the synchrony of neonatal hair growth is progressively lost and the wave of hair growth and shedding from the frontal to occipital scalp is disturbed. Apparently random shedding tends to occur thereafter, so that, in contrast to our mammalian counterparts who have a seasonal molt, adult humans tend to only shed a few hairs each day. Some seasonal fluctuation in the number of hairs shed daily exists, suggesting a mosaic pattern persists rather than true asynchrony.

Hair follicle physiology

The type and pattern of hair growth on the adult body is dynamic. Terminal hairs on the scalp have the potential to miniaturize into vellus hairs, as found in androgenetic alopecia, and vellus hairs can enlarge into long, thick terminal hairs, which, on the beard area of men, may grow to 30 cm long. Every follicle retains the potential to produce vellus, terminal or even lanugo hairs as found in the rare syndrome of acquired hypertrichosis lanuginosa.

Apes have relatively uniform hair growth. In comparison with humans, the so-called 'naked apes', the scalp hair is elongated and the body hair significantly diminished. In parallel with these equal and opposite phylogenetic shifts in hair growth, is an equal and opposite response of these hairs to physiological androgens. There is a paradoxical induction by dihydrotestosterone of androgenetic alopecia on the scalp and hirsutes on the face and trunk. This corresponds to the equal and opposite response of these hair follicles to anti-androgen therapy. The effect of androgens on hair follicle is discussed in Chapter 5 by Randall.

Sawaya and Price[1] have evaluated a mechanism for the sequence of hair loss that occurs in the scalp in androgenetic alopecia, with the more sensitive areas of the scalp displaying more 5-α reductase, less aromatase and more androgen receptors. However, this neither explains the postreceptor events that determine whether the follicle will respond to dihydrotestosterone by miniaturizing or enlarging, nor does it shed light on the factors that regulate the expression of these enzymes and receptors. The crucial determinants of when and how hairs will respond to androgens are programmed into the follicles early in life. This has been demonstrated conclusively by work by Orentreich, who transplanted hair follicles both on the scalp and also on the forearm, and established the principle of donor dominance.[2]

Androgen interactions with hair follicles

The window of opportunity for vellus to terminal hair transformation, and vice versa, is small.[3] Once growing hairs have emerged from the follicular ostium (stage VI anagen hairs) they do not change calibre.[4] Thus any change must occur either during catagen, telogen or early anagen (stage I–V), with the latter being the most likely. It is not known how changes in hair calibre relate to the concurrent alteration in the duration of the anagen phase, which is a crucial co-factor in the pathogenesis of both hypertrichosis and hirsutes (as well as androgenetic alopecia).

It has been demonstrated that hair fibre diameter is related to the size of the dermal papilla.[5] However, by contrasting the large dermal papilla size of eyebrows and beard hair follicles to the smaller papilla of scalp hair follicles it can be seen that the duration of anagen is not solely dependent on dermal papilla size.

Since the window of opportunity is small for follicle enlargement in hirsutes, the process is slow. Hairs have to grow for the full duration of anagen, involute and remain dormant for the full duration of telogen before re-emerging as an enlarged new anagen hair.

If the follicle is already producing an elongated hair as a result of concurrent hypertrichosis, the development of hirsutes will require fewer hair cycles and the final hair will have a greater maximum potential. This is seen post puberty in prepubertal hypertrichosis.

The classification of hairs as either androgen-dependent follicles or androgen-independent follicles is overstated. In androgenetic alopecia, even the hairs on the occiput will eventually be lost, while, in hirsutes of the body even the back hairs will eventually enlarge in susceptible people. Thus these follicles are not androgen-insensitive but relatively less sensitive. The relative sensitivity of hairs on the body to androgens is probably mediated by similar factors that mediate the relative sensitivity to androgens on the scalp (e.g. local dihydrotestosterone (DHT) production, aromatase production and androgen receptor expression); however, the cause of this relative sensitivity is unknown, although it is likely to be genetically pre-programmed.

Observations on normal hair patterns in men and women

Since hirsutes has been defined as 'androgen-driven excessive hair growth in a female in a pattern that mimics normal hair growth in males', it is useful to reflect on the so-called normal patterns of hair growth.

Regional variations in hair pattern are related to age (Table 1), genetic constitution and endocrine status.[6] In addition, dark-haired people have both an increased amount and also more noticeable body hair than their fair-haired counterparts. While eunuchs do not develop secondary body hair, and castration or hypogonadism in men results in a loss of body hair, there is not a direct relationship between the volume of body hair and the level of circulating free testosterone. This indicates the significance of the inherent follicle factors that determine the relative sensitivity of hair follicles to androgens.

Hair patterns in women are materially different from men, highlighting the importance of androgens. Table 1 indicates that virtually every hair on the body is, to some degree, androgen-

Table 1   Presence (%) of terminal hair at different sites in women (from Ferriman and Gallwey).[6]

Area	15–24	25–34	35–44
Upper lip	29	39	53
Chin	2	11	16
Chest	7	14	24
Upper back	1	0	0
Lower back	14	12	14
Upper abdomen	0	0	1
Lower abdomen	28	21	23
Arm	26	23	7
Thigh	43	32	29
Forearm	88	86	60
Leg	95	97	91

sensitive, even in those sites traditionally stated to be insensitive.

Further classification of hypertrichosis

Hypertrichosis may be generalized or localized, and can occur as an isolated phenomenon or as a part of a syndrome. Localized and syndromic hypertrichosis have been discussed in Chapter 24 on congenital hypertrichosis by Antonella Tosti and Bianca Maria Piraccini and will not be discussed further.

Prepubertal hypertrichosis, drug-induced hypertrichosis and acquired hypertrichosis lanuginosa are all acquired forms of generalized hypertrichosis. Further discussion of these will be illustrated by case reports that highlight a particular aspect of each condition.

Acquired hypertrichosis lanuginosa

This rare condition is characterized by the rapid growth of long, fine, downy lanugo hairs particularly over the face, but also on the body.[7] It is a paraneoplastic phenomenon often seen late in the course of an internal malignancy, a so-called 'malignant down'. The importance of this condition is that it may be the presenting sign of the malignancy and can appear up to 2 years prior to other manifestations. A hair growth factor produced by the tumour has been postulated but not identified.

Acquired hypertrichosis lanuginosa has an age range of 19–69, with a female predominance of 3:1. The extent and degree of lanuginose transformation varies considerably. In early cases, the growth of down on the forehead and temples is the only abnormality. In others, the striking feature is the rapidity with which obvious hypertrichosis develops. Hair appears on the forehead, eyelids, nose, ears (Figure 2) and torso (Figure 3) giving the patient a simian appearance. The palms, soles, pubic regions and scalp tend to be spared. Balding scalps are rejuvenated by a dense growth of hair, albeit lighter and finer than the neighbouring hair. Hairs may grow as fast as 2.5 cm/week and achieve a length of 15 cm but are more commonly found to be about 1 cm long.

Other cutaneous abnormalities that may co-exist include hyperkeratotic lesions on the palms, soles and limbs, glossitis, acquired ichthyosis and acanthosis nigricans with tripe palms. The malignancies most often associated with this condition are carcinoma of the lung, colon and uterus, and also lymphoma.

This condition illustrates that both the terminal and vellus human hair follicles retain the ability to produce lanugo hairs.

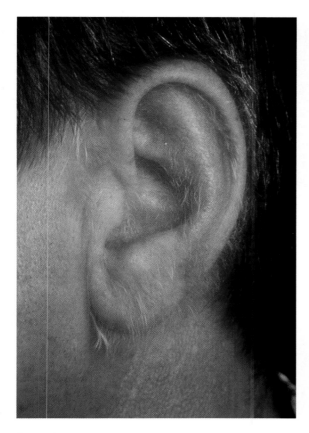

Figure 2

Acquired hypertrichosis lanuginosa showing excessive hair growth on the ears.

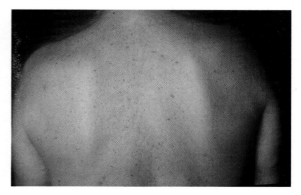

Figure 3

Acquired hypertrichosis lanuginosa showing excessive hair growth on the back.

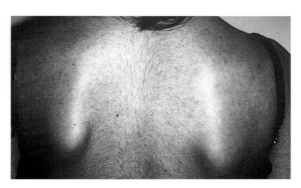

Figure 4

Prepubertal hypertrichosis in a post-pubertal girl showing dark, downy hair evenly distributed over the upper back.

Prepubertal hypertrichosis

This is a non-familial hypertrichosis, present at or near birth, that increases steadily during early childhood.[7] Since it occurs equally in people of Asian and European descent, the term 'racial hypertrichosis' is inappropriate. There is growth of terminal hairs on the temples, spreading across the forehead, bushy eyebrows and marked growth on the upper back and proximal limbs. In contrast to the synchronized growth of congenital hypertrichosis lanuginosa, hair growth in this condition is unsynchronized.

The patient shown in Figures 4 and 5 is an 18 year old female, born in Australia of Indian parentage who presented with long-standing generalized hypertrichosis, that had been present since early childhood. Interestingly, the condition had remained stable until puberty when, in addition to the diffuse hypertrichosis, she developed an accentuation of hair growth in the inner

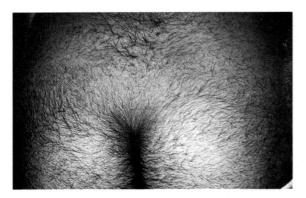

Figure 5

Prepubertal hypertrichosis in a post-pubertal girl showing accentuation of the hair over the buttocks.

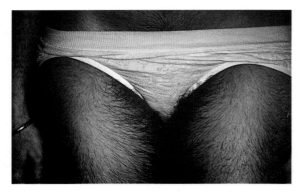

Figure 6

Accentuation of thigh hair following puberty in a post-pubertal girl with prepubertal hypertrichosis.

thighs (Figure 6) and escutcheon, as well as the nipples.

Neither parent had hypertrichosis. One sister was similarly affected, while another sister was unaffected. There was no associated acne, scalp hair loss or male habitus. Investigations demonstrated a normal serum testosterone, sex hormone binding globulin and dihydroepiandrosterone.

This case illustrates that hairs enlarged by preexisting hypertrichosis maintain the potential to further enlarge when exposed to pubertal androgens.

Drug-induced hypertrichosis[7]

Minoxidil, diazoxide, phenytoin, cyclosporin A photochemotherapy, prednisolone, streptomycin, acetazolamide, benoxaprofen, penicillamine and fenoterol have all been reported to induce hypertrichosis in some users. The mechanism of hair induction is unknown and the same mechanism is not involved in all cases.

Minoxidil and diazoxide are vasodilators that produce hypertrichosis in 80% of recipients, predominantly over the face, shoulders (Figure 7), arms and legs. The hair falls out several months after cessation of therapy. Minoxidil is also active topically and has been used to treat androgenetic alopecia. The resultant hairs that appear on the scalp after oral minoxidil are often fine, poorly pigmented indeterminate-type hairs of marginal cosmetic significance.

Cyclosporin A, an immune modulator, may induce a switch from telogen to anagen in hair follicles. In humans, it produces a diffuse growth of hair across the shoulders, back, upper extremities, face, scalp, eyebrows and earlobes (Figure 8). It begins within a few weeks of taking cyclosporin in more than 60% of recipients. Hypertrichosis is more common in childhood and adolescence and reverses about 1 month after stopping treatment.

In about 10% of people receiving phenytoin an excessive growth of hair develops after 1–2 months across the extensor aspects of the limbs, and subsequently on the face and trunk. It remits within 1 year of cessation of therapy. This hypertrichosis does not appear to be related to dose or duration of therapy.

Prolonged administration of cortisone can induce hypertrichosis that is most marked on the forehead, the temples and the sides of the cheeks. It also occurs on the back and the extensor surface of the arms. Steroid-induced acne may be associated.

PUVA induces hair in exposed sites, as does benoxaprofen following the induction of drug-induced photosensitivity. The mechanism may be similar to the hypertrichosis seen in porphyria cutanea tarda.

Penicillamine tends to produce lengthening and coarsening of hair on the trunk and limbs.

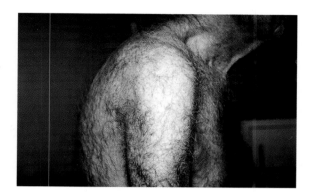

Figure 7

Minoxidil-induced hypertrichosis.

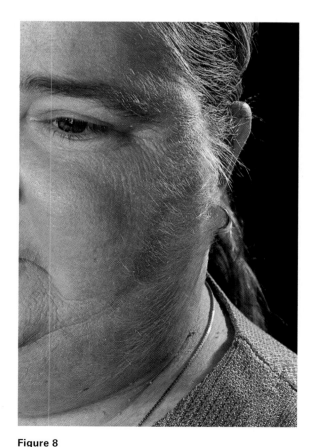

Figure 8

Cyclosporin-A-induced hypertrichosis.

Conclusion

The clinical presentation of hypertrichosis is distinctive, and easily differentiated from hirsutes. This distinction is important since the natural history, prognosis and response to treatment of these two conditions is different. Nevertheless, the pathophysiology of these two conditions is poorly understood and it is important to acknowledge that there are overlap cases where both conditions occur.

The normal hair patterns seen in men, but not women, indicate that almost all hairs on the body have the ability to transform from vellus to terminal hairs in the presence of sufficient androgens. In contrast, only the scalp hairs respond to androgens by reverting from terminal to vellus-like hairs. Prepubertal hypertrichosis indicates that body hairs can also enlarge as a result of stimuli other than androgens, albeit to a lesser degree. In addition, the case illustrated shows that these separate pathways are not mutually exclusive and may contribute to produce an additive enlargement of the hair follicles. Drug-induced hypertrichosis indicates that there are at least several additional possible mechanisms of stimulating hair growth.

The condition of acquired hypertrichosis lanuginosa highlights the fact that human hair follicles retain, throughout life, not only the ability to produce either terminal or vellus hairs, but also the ability to produce lanugo hairs.

It appears that there are several independent and interdependent controls on hair length and hair thickness, as well as hair type. In hypertrichosis, the predominant alteration appears to be an increase in the hair length, with a lesser increase in thickness, while in hirsutes there appears to be a predominant increase in hair thickness with a secondary increase in hair length. This is entirely consistent with observations made the additive effects of minoxidil and finasteride in the treatment of androgenetic alopecia in the stump-tail macaque monkey (see Chapter 11 by Uno et al). The separate consideration of these two characteristics of enlarged hairs may facilitate investigation into the pathogenesis of these two disorders.

References

1. Sawaya ME, Price VE: Different levels of 5α-reductase type I and II, aromatase, and androgen receptors in hair follicles of men and women with androgenetic alopecia. *J Invest Dermatol* 1997; **109**: 296–300.

2. Orentreich D, Orentreich N: Androgenetic alopecia and its treatment, a historical view. In: Unger WP (ed.). *Hair Transplantation 3rd ed.* New York, Marcel Dekker, 1995.

3. Sinclair R: Male pattern androgenetic alopecia. *Br Med J* 1998; **317**: 865–869.

4. Hutchinson PE, Thompson JR: The cross-sectional size and shape of human terminal scalp hair. *Br J Dermatol* 1997; **136**: 159–165.

5. Oliver RF, Jahoda CAB: The dermal papilla and the maintenance of hair growth. In: Rogers GA, Reis PR, Ward KA, et al. (eds.). *The Biology of Wool and Hair.* London, Chapman and Hall, 1989: 51–67.

6. Ferriman D, Gallwey W: Clinical assessment of body hair growth in women. *J Clin Endocrinol* 1961; **21**: 1440–1447.

7. Sinclair RD, Banfield C, Dawber RPR: *Handbook of Diseases of the Hair and Scalp.* Oxford, Blackwell Science, 1999.

32

Pathogenesis of hirsutism

Dimitris Rigopoulos and Sofia Georgala

Introduction

Hirsutism is a term to describe the condition in women in whom the pattern of terminal hair growth follows a similar mode to that which develops in men after puberty, in other words, in androgen-dependent sites. So, hirsutism, by definition, refers only to females.[1] The androgen-dependent sites include cheeks, the upper lip, chin, chest, lower abdomen, inner aspects of the thighs, the back and the legs. In females, only vellus hair is normally found at these sites.

Hirsutism should be differentiated from hypertrichosis, which is defined as a diffuse hair growth over the entire body surface. Hypertrichosis thus affects sites that are not androgen-dependent. Moreover, in hypertrichosis, the hair shaft tends to be fine, soft and lies flat against the skin in contrast to hirsutism, where hair shafts are coarse, often curly and tend to rise above the skin surface.

Hirsutism may be present with or without other features of virilization, for example, hypertrophy of the clitoris, acne, deepening of the voice, breast atrophy, muscle hypertrophy, oligamenorrhea or even amenorrhea and thinning of the scalp.

Pathogenesis

Hirsutism may be the result of an increased androgen production or caused by an enhanced sensitivity of the hair follicle in sexual areas, to normal levels of circulating androgens.[2]

Circulating androgen levels in females depend upon direct secretion by the ovaries and the adrenal glands, upon peripheral conversion of androgen precursors and also on the metabolic clearance rate, which is related to androgen production.

The most important androgens, in decreasing order of potency, are: 5α-dihydrotestosterone (DHT), which is 2–3-fold more potent than testosterone; testosterone (T), which is 5–10-fold more potent than adrostenedione and 20 times than dihydroepiandrosterone; androstenedione (A); dihydroepiandrosterone (DHEA) and dihydroepiandrosterone–sulfate (DHEA-S).

More than 98% of circulating testosterone in non-pregnant women is bound to specific plasma proteins, such as sex hormone binding globulin (SHBG; 78%), cortisol binding globulin (CBG; 1%) and albumin (20%). Thus only 1% of testosterone circulates freely in an unbound state.[3]

Intracellularly, testosterone is reduced to 5α-DHT (dihydrotestosterone), via the enzyme 5α-reductase.

The target cells of androgens are the dermal papilla cells, the follicular keratinocytes, the melanocytes and the endothelial cells. The response of hair follicles to androgens requires the presence of a specific androgen receptor, which resides in the dermal papilla cells, since these cells control hair growth. The post-binding mechanism of androgen action is currently under investigation. The action of androgens on the hair follicle is discussed by Randall in Chapter 5.

In patients with hirsutism, the conversion rate of testosterone to 5α-DHT is increased significantly, almost reaching male levels. Moreover, interleukin-1 may also be implicated. Interleukin (IL)-1 seems to control the hair cycle, among other factors, as it is an inhibitor of hair follicle growth, in vitro and in vivo. Furthermore, at concentrations as low as 0.01 mg.ml^{-1} IL-1a has already been shown in vitro to lengthen both the hair shaft and the outer root shaft, to degrade the hair bulb and to produce an outward growing of the follicle that 'squeezes' the dermal papilla out of the bulb.

The exact role of IL-1 in hirsutism, if any, is yet

to be determined. The roles of cytokines and growth factors in hair growth are discussed in Chapter 8 by Philpott and Chapter 7 by Blume-Peytavi and Mandt.

Classification of disorders causing hirsutism

Hirsutism can result from excessive androgen production (from the ovaries, adrenal glands or by ectopic production), increased concentration of free testosterone, increased 5α-reductase activity or increased sensitivity of the hair follicles to normal levels of androgens. These conditions all lead to the conversion of vellus to terminal hair, in sex hormone-responsive follicles.[4] The causes of hirsutism are listed in Table 1.

Idiopathic hirsutism

'Idiopathic' or 'endogenous' hirsutism also used to be called 'constitutional' or 'dermatological' hirsutism and this will be discussed further in Chapter 34. This seems to be the most common cause of hirsutism, although, latterly, the number of females that are believed to constitute this group is getting less because of more sensitive and accurate diagnostic techniques.

Idiopathic hirsutism is probably the result of hypersensitivity of hair follicles to androgens, decreased SHBG or increased activity of 5α-reductase. Decreased SHBG results in

Table 1   Causes of hirsutism.

Idiopathic
Ovarian causes
    Polycystic ovary syndrome
    Ovarian tumors
Adrenal causes
    Congenital adrenal hyperplasia
    Adrenal tumors
Prolactinoma
Iatrogenic causes
Pregnancy
Post-menopausal causes

increased levels of free testosterone which becomes available for peripheral conversion.

Females with idiopathic hirsutism usually have no apparent underlying endocrine disorder. The onset of hirsutism is usually noted at puberty and, in most cases, there is a positive family history. It is common in certain ethnic groups, probably due to genetic factors that determine both the number and the sensitivity of hair follicles.[5]

Ovarian causes of hirsutism

Polycystic ovary syndrome

The pathogenesis of polycystic ovary syndrome (PCOs) remains a challenging enigma. It is hypothesized that there are two genetic defects, caused by a single gene defect that is inherited in an autosomal dominant manner. These genetic defects result in both an increase in luteinizing hormone (LH) by the pituitary gland (where the cause is unknown) and an increase in insulin levels. These two defects seem to have a synergistic action on the ovaries, enhancing ovarian growth, androgen secretion and probably ovarian cyst formation. Further studies are, however, needed to confirm this hypothesis.[6]

Patients with PCOs present (usually just before or at the time of puberty) with hirsutism, acne, dysfunctional uterine bleeding or amenorrhea, infertility and obesity. Obesity results in reduced levels of SHBG and increased levels of insulin. Increased circulating insulin leads to decreased production of the insulin like growth factor binding protein-1 (ILGF-1); this is because insulin has the ability to attach to ILGF-1 receptors, whose structure is very similar to that of the insulin receptors. Thus, if the receptors are occupied or decreased, as happens in a hyperinsulinemic state, insulin attaches to the ILGF-1 receptors which then become activated. This activation results in overproduction of ovarian androgens.

Elevation of LH and mild elevation of testosterone and/or androstenedione are the more frequent laboratory findings. A variant of PCOs is the HAIR-AN syndrome consisting of hyperandrogenism, insulin resistance and acanthosis nigricans.[7] The pathogenesis of acanthosis nigricans (which is present in 5–10% of females with PCOs syndrome and normal weight and in 50% of obese females with PCOs syndrome) is unclear. It is probable that high concentrations of insulin stimulate the growth of keratinocytes and/or dermal fibroblasts, resulting in the development of the characteristic skin lesions of this condition. It is also probable that other unknown factors contribute to the development of the disease and that insulin resistance is not the only factor involved.

Ovarian tumors

Functional ovarian tumors represent less than 1% of all ovarian tumors. The most common ovarian tumors that are detected in these cases are arrenoblastomas, luteomas, hilar cell tumors, microadenomas and granular-type thecal cell tumors.

Hirsutism usually has a sudden onset between the ages of 20–40 years with a rapid progression. Virilization is a common finding and patients sometimes complain of abdominal pain (due to ovarian torsion). Elevated levels of testosterone and androstenedione are common laboratory findings.

Adrenal causes of hirsutism

Congenital adrenal hyperplasia

Three types of congenital adrenal hyperplasia (CAH) exist:

(1) The severe form (with masculinization of the female infant at the time of birth);
(2) The less severe form (masculinization at childhood with girls being very tall at an early age but with comparatively diminished height later, due to closure of the bone-growing centers); and
(3) The late-onset form (onset after puberty or after pregnancy). In clinical practise, two forms of the disease are recognized, the severe one (with virilization of female infant at birth), and the less severe form (with virilization at late ages).

In CAH the most common deficiency (in 95% of all cases) is that of 21-hydroxylase. In the case of partial deficiency of 21-hydroxylase, there is an increased production rate of all steroid precursors (e.g. progesterone, 17-hydroxyprogesterone, androstenedione and DHEA), while increased levels of testosterone result from peripheral conversion of androstenedione. In the case of complete deficiency of 21-hydroxylase, decrease of aldosterone is also present and the salt-losing form of CAH ensues.

Deficiency of 11-β hydroxylase is much less common than 21-hydroxylase deficiency. In 11β-hydroxylase deficiency there is accumulation of 11-deoxycorticosterone (with salt-retaining properties), which results in hypertension. In addition, there is abnormal build-up of 17-hydroxyprogesterone, which is shunted into the synthesis of androgens, particularly androstenedione. The major difference between 21-hydroxylase and 11β-hydroxylase deficiency is the presence of hypertension that is only found in the 11-β type.[8]

Adrenal tumors

Virilizing adrenal tumors are a rare cause of hirsutism. They can appear at any age but usually occur before puberty or after the menopause. Symptoms usually arise suddenly and have a rapid progression. Plasma levels of testosterone and DHEA are increased. In patients with Cushing's syndrome, 25% are reported to have both hirsutism and hypertrichosis due to hypercortisolemia.

Prolactinoma

Hyperprolactinemia is another cause of hirsutism, although the exact relationship between prolactin and hirsuties is unclear. Hyperprolactinemia can result from pituitary adenoma, hypothalamic disease or hypothyroidism. It is reported that prolactin might have a direct effect on androgen production from the adrenals.

Iatrogenic causes of hirsutism

Hirsutism can result as a side-effect of systemic administration of various compounds, such as testosterone, danazol (its androgenic action is evident only with the highest doses of 800 mg/24 h), oral contraceptives (in less than 5% of the cases), synthetic glucocorticosteroids, ACTH (which can stimulate adrenal androgen production), phenothiazines (due to stimulation of the adrenal androgen production), minoxidil, metyrapone (which is an adrenal hormone antagonist), cyclosporin, etc.

Hirsutism can be also the result of ectopic hormone production caused by choriocarcinoma, metastatic lung cancer and carcinoid tumor located in the stomach or ileum.

Pregnancy

Hirsutism can also be a symptom in pregnant females. Hirsutism in pregnancy has been rarely reported until now. It may result from the development of PCO or virilizing tumors. PCO with virilization has been reported to present in the 1st or 3rd trimester and may regress post-partum.

Virilization of the female fetus may also be apparent, since androgens freely cross the placenta.

Post-menopausal causes of hirsutism

Hirsutism in post-menopausal non-hirsute women is poorly understood. In women over 50 years old, body hair gradually decreases, probably because of the involution of androgen-secreting ovarian tissue. The growth of hair on the face, continues, however, probably because of prolonged stimulation by normal adrenal androgens. Ovarian and adrenal tumors continue to develop after menopause, while some post-menopausal women develop hyperthecosis (iso-lated islands of luteinized theca cells within the stroma with excess androgen production) or hypertrophy of the ovarian stroma, probably in response to stimulation by the high concentration of gonadotropins.

Conclusions

Hirsutism is a multifactorial disorder of the hair follicle. Understanding the causes of this disorder may help treatment and prevent serious complications associated with the probable underlying diseases or, even in the absence of these, it may help to prevent psychological distress to affected females.

References

1. Barth J: How hairy are hirsute women? *Clin Endocrinol* 1997; **47**: 255–260.
2. Barth J: Investigations in the assessment and management of patients with hirsutism. *Curr Opin Obst Gynecol* 1997; **10**: 187–192.
3. Leung A, Robson WL: Hirsutism. *Int J Dermatol* 1993; **32**: 773–777.
4. Barth J: How robust is the methodology for trials of therapy in hirsute women? *Clin Endocrinol* 1996; **45**: 379–380.
5. Brechwoldt M, et al.: Hirsutism, its pathogenesis. *Hum Reprod* 1989; **4**: 601–604.
6. Jacobs HS: Polycystic ovary syndrome: aetiology and management. *Curr Opin Obst Gynecol* 1995; **7**: 203–208.
7. Camacho F: Hirsutism. In: Camacho F, Montagna W (eds.). *Trichology. Diseases of the Pilo-Sebaceous Follicle*, Madrid, Aula Medica 1997: 265–298.
8. Simpson N, Barth J: Hirsuties. In: *Diseases of the Hair and Scalp*, Dawber R (ed.), 3rd ed. London, Blackwell, 1997; 71–101.

33

Clinical features of hirsutism: variations with age and race

David de Berker

Introduction

There are qualitative and quantitative definitions of hirsutism. The first usually describes aspects of expectation, such as gender and distribution of the hair; for example 'excess terminal hair in a woman in a distribution characteristic of male gender'. This definition will cover a wide range of appearances, some where there will be a difference between the opinion of the doctor and the woman. In some instances, the diagnosis may be hypertrichosis, rather than hirsutism, where hypertrichosis is characterized by hair in a distribution unrelated to gender and is usually vellus (non-pigmented and of narrow bore).

In a clinical setting, a woman with a subjective complaint of hirsutism does not mind whether she fills medical criteria for the condition—she wants treatment. Nevertheless, quantitative definitions of hirsutism have developed through a range of anthropological and medical studies.[1-3] These are valuable to the clinician in that they can be employed in clinical trials as a commonly understood standard, and allow the clinician to judge whether the treatment under trial is useful. Quantitative measures also allow accurate record-keeping in patients' notes and longitudinal assessment of the clinical state.

Quantitative clinical measures of hirsutism

The most commonly used scale of hirsutism is that devised by Ferriman and Gallwey in 1961,[1] which in turn was based on a study by Garn.[2]

They examined 430 women (aged 15–43 years) attending a hospital outpatient department for conditions unrelated to hair growth. Body hair was assessed at 11 sites and scored between 0 and 4 depending on presence, thickness and confluence of hair, where an F and G score of '4' represents a heavy confluent growth (Table 1). This work provided a useful description of what was 'normal' and a profile of the changes in distribution of body hair with age. Their conclusion was that hair growth on the forearm and on the leg below the knee was not hormone-dependent and that a composite score of the other nine sites gave a useful indicator of hirsutism. At these nine sites, a total score of greater than 10 was found in 1.2%, and greater than 7 in 4.3% (Figure 1).

In clinical practice, certain body sites have more significance than others. In particular, women will seek advice about facial hirsutism where the chin and upper lip are the main focus. A high F and G score at these sites indicates dense hair that meets in the midline; a few pigmented hairs at the lateral extremes is common. In a study of 400 women students in a Welsh university, 36 assessed themselves as hirsute.[4] Examination revealed that over 80% of these 36 women had terminal hair on the face in comparison with 28% of the remaining 364. A similar comparison was revealed for abdominal hair. About 60% had hair on the chest compared with less than 20% of the larger group.

These findings illustrate the areas requiring close assessment; namely the lip and chin, the abdomen between pubes and umbilicus, and the chest. Hair around the breast areolae is common but hair on the sternum causes particular distress and is relatively rare in the normal population. Hair across the upper back is also rare and can be a marker of substantial hirsutism.

Table 1   Ferriman and Gallwey scoring system of hirsutism.[1]

Site	Grade	Definition
1. Upper lip	1	A few hairs at outer margin
	2	A small moustache at outer margin
	3	A moustache extending half way from outer margin
	4	A moustache extending across midline
2. Chin	1	A few scattered hairs
	2	Scattered hairs with small concentrations
	3 & 4	Complete cover, light and heavy
3. Chest	1	Circumareolar hairs
	2	Circumareolar hairs with midline hair in addition
	3	Fusion of these areas with three-quarter cover
	4	Complete cover
4. Upper back	1	A few scattered hairs
	2	Rather more, still scattered hairs
	3 & 4	Complete cover, light and heavy
5. Lower back	1	A sacral tuft of hair
	2	A sacral tuft of hair with some lateral extension
	3	Three-quarter cover
	4	Complete cover
6. Upper abdomen	1	A few midline hairs
	2	Rather more, midline hairs
	3 & 4	Half and full cover
7. Lower abdomen	1	A few midline hairs
	2	A midline streak of hair
	3	A midline band of hair
	4	An inverted V-shaped growth
8. Arm	1	Sparse growth affecting not more than a one-quarter of the limb surface
	2	More than the above: cover still incomplete
	3 & 4	Complete cover, light and heavy
9. Forearm	1, 2, 3, 4	Complete cover of dorsal surface, two grades of light and two grades of heavy growth
10. Thigh	1, 2, 3, 4	As for forearm
11. Leg	1, 2, 3, 4	As for forearm

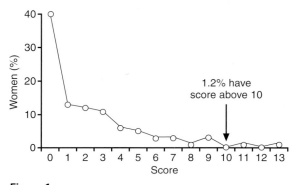

Figure 1

F and G score for 161 females: 18–38 years.[1]

Change in body hair with age

On a descriptive level, data from many publications allow us to make generalizations concerning how body hair changes with age. At some sites, such as the axilla and pubic regions, similar changes are seen in men and women.[5] The sexes may also have similarities with respect to hair on the legs and face,[6,7] but these changes carry particular significance in women. Ferriman and Gallwey described the gradual reduction of hair on the legs of women:[1] 93% of women in the 25–34 year age group have more than a sparse covering on the leg in comparison with only 2% after the age of 65 years. Conversely, between the ages of 15 and 24 years, only 10% of women have more than a few hairs at the outer margin of the upper lip. This figure rises to 42% after the age of 65 years. It is paradoxical that, at the age when facial hair is of greatest concern to women, it is usually at its least. The pattern of loss of hair from the legs and an increase on the face has been noted in several other studies.[7,8]

Changes of body hair with race

True comparisons between multiple different racial groups are not available. General observations allow an impression of the natural level of pilosity in different races, where mongoloids such as the Chinese and Japanese have very little body hair and Northern Europeans have more. Groups termed 'Euroamericans' were compared with East Asians by Ewing, confirming this generalization in both sexes. Sex-matched androgen estimations were the same, and consistent with an end-organ difference.[10]

Even when different ethnic groups have the same underlying diagnosis, their levels of hirsutism may differ. Only one out of nine Japanese with polycystic ovarian syndrome (PCOS) were found to have hirsutism[11] compared with 63% of Northern Europeans[12] with the same diagnosis. When 25 Japanese women with PCOS were compared with 25 Italian and 25 Hispanic American women with the same disease, the Japanese were significantly less hirsute and less obese.[13]

Afro-Caribbeans are usually considered to have less body hair than Northern Europeans; however, a detailed study reveals little information. A report from the United States Health Examination Survey commented that Afro-Carribeans developed secondary sexual hair earlier than their white counterparts but no comparison of hair distribution was made.[14] When facial hair was examined in adult white and black Americans, it was commented that no difference was found until the age of 40 years. At that point the hair on the face of white Americans continued to increase, whereas that on black Americans levelled off[15] (Figure 2).

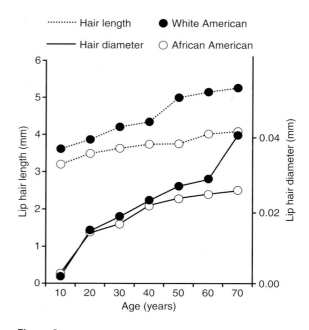

Figure 2

Comparison of lip hair characteristics in American women of African and Caucasian origin.[13]

Comparisons between Europeans were made in de-mobilized soldiers after World War I.[16] Current statistical methods and ethnic categories were not used at that time and the results allow the observation that 'Russian Jews' and those 'from Italian provinces' had a high proportion of men considered of high pilosity, compared with 'English and German protestants'.

Additional clinical features associated with hirsutism

Lorenzo[3] formulated a scoring system for hirsutism, combining the density of terminal hair at five 'unusual' sites (i.e. upper lip, chin, thighs, abdomen, forearms) with additional features. These features included rating any of four pathological patterns of menstruation, acne, frontal baldness and clitoromegaly. Scores were unable

Table 2 Comparative features of androgenization and virilization in women.

Androgenization	Virilization
Hirsutism	Clitoromegaly
Acne	Increase in muscle bulk
Alopecia	Male habitus
Oily skin	Deep voice

Additional features of polycystic ovary syndrome
Acanthosis nigricans
Menstrual disturbance
Infertility
Central obesity
Hyperinsulinaemia
Diabetes mellitus
Dyslipidaemia

to distinguish between the proposed aetiologies of the hirsutism, namely ovarian, adrenal and idiopathic. In all these categories androgenization could be seen, where androgenization is described as the effects of androgens on the skin (Table 2).

Causes of hirsutism

When considering the investigation and treatment of hirsutism, it is useful to think in terms of

the possible causes (Table 3). These are divided into ovarian and adrenal, although there are additional categories where there is pituitary pathology or a drug cause.

Ovarian disease

Polycystic ovary syndrome (PCOS) is the proposed diagnosis in 33–91% of hirsute women.[17,18] The diagnostic criteria for PCOS vary slightly. The central definition of cystic ovaries is reliant not only on the ultrasonographer, but also the ultrasonographic method (transvaginal versus abdominal) and the specified ultrasonographic criteria. Where polycystic ovaries exist a range of other clinical and endocrine features may also be present.[19] In one survey of 556 patients with polycystic ovaries, the spectrum of skin changes included hirsutism, acne, alopecia and acanthosis nigricans. In the majority, fertility had not been tested and so was not a helpful criterion. Menstruation was normal in 25%.

Obesity is a further important feature of PCOS. The significance of obesity arises from the relationship between hyperinsulinaemia, insulin resistance, ovarian stimulation by excess insulin and androgenization.[20] In some instances, PCOS can be interpreted as an endocrinopathy, where obesity, particularly truncal obesity,[21] combines

Table 3 Causes of hirsutism and their associated features.

Adrenal causes	Frequency	Age of onset	History	Menses
LO-CAH	1–9%	Early adulthood	Medium	Variable
21-hydroxylase deficiency				
11-hydroxylase deficiency				
3β hydroxysteroid dehydrogenase deficiency				
Carcinoma	0.7%	Any age	Short	Usually absent
Cushing's syndrome	<1%	Any age	Short	Usually absent
Combined ovarian and adrenal causes				
'Idiopathic'—*includes increased androgen sensitivity*	5–35%	Near menarche	Long	Normal
Ovarian				
PCOS (includes HAIR AN)	60–90%	Near menarche	Long	Variable
Androgen-secreting neoplasms	1%			
Arrhenoblastoma	Rare	Menarche onwards	Short	Absent
Hilar cell tumour	Rare	Near menopause	Short	Absent
Krukenberg and Leydig cell	Rare	Adulthood onwards	Short	Absent
Luteoma of pregnancy	Very rare	During pregnancy	Short	Absent

with the PCOS disposition to contribute to insulin resistance and consequent hyperinsulinaemia. There is an additional group of women who have hyperinsulinaemia but they are not obese; thus it has been proposed that a defect in insulin receptor-signalling represents the unifying mechanism.[22] Pathological levels of insulin act upon the adrenals, ovaries and liver to produce inter-related changes resulting in the PCOS phenotype. Some of these are endocrine and manifested through an increase of androgens, causing menstrual disturbance, infertility and hirsutism. Others are metabolic, with glucose intolerance, hypertension and dyslipidaemias. The metabolic features justify screening of PCOS patients for diabetes mellitus and altered blood lipids. An impaired glucose tolerance test may be found in 8% of those with PCOS.[23] Where diabetes mellitus presents in PCOS it is commonly found in the third and fourth decade, rather than the sixth and seventh decade.

Obesity is not only a marker for diagnosis, but it is also a handle for treatment. There is a direct relationship between body mass index and hirsutism in younger women.[24] In a study of 20 obese amenorrhoeic hirsute women, a mean of 9.7 kg weight loss achieved over a mean period of 8.6 months resulted in reduction of hirsutism in over one-half of women.[25] When the long-term health dividends of weight loss are considered in this group, it must be advocated as a central element of therapy.

Where PCOS demonstrates the full range of features associated with hyperinsulinaemia, it is called the HAIR-AN syndrome, although it is debatable whether this additional classification is really helpful. The acronym stands for Hyper-Androgenism, Insulin Resistance and Acanthosis Nigricans.[26]

The ovarian pathology may be caused by stromal hyperthecosis. This condition is not limited to premenopausal women and, when presenting in older women, it may mimic an adrenal or ovarian tumour.[27]

Androgen-secreting tumours

Androgenization is the term given to the physical attributes seen in PCOS with or without obesity. The onset of these attributes is gradual but usually occurs in early adulthood. Virilization, conversely, is a more extreme process, comprising clitoromegaly, increased muscle bulk, male habitus and deepening voice (see Table 2). These features are sometimes found in subjects with an androgen-secreting tumour and their onset may be at any time during life, often in addition to the initial androgenization. Androgen-secreting tumours are a rare cause of hirsutism. Although all clinicians should be aware of the potential diagnosis, routine investigation of androgenization does not require imaging or complex biochemistry with a malignancy in mind. In 1050 women presenting with hirsutism in six studies five women (0.5%) had carcinoma of the adrenal gland or ovary[16,17,25, 28–30] (Table 4).

Derksen reported on 14 patients presenting with hirsutism attributable to an adrenal tumour,[31] 12 of which were carcinomas in women of mean age 42 years, where the

Table 4   The range of conditions revealed as underlying causes of hirsutism in six separate studies.[17,18,26,28–30]

	Gatee[28] UAE	Mithal[29] India	Moran[18] Mexico	Erkkola[17] Finland	O'Driscoll[30] England	Barbieri[26] USA	Totals
n	102	60	250	229	309	100	**1050**
% PCOS	91	75	53	33	60	78	**58**
Idiopathic	5	17	25	38	38	15	**28**
LO-CAH	2	8	2	22	1.5	3	**6**
Ovarian tumour	2	—	0.8	—	0.25	1	**0.6**
Adrenal tumour	—	—	—	—	0.25	—	**0.1**
Obesity	—	—	18	7	—	—	**6**
Other	—	—	0.4	—	0.5	3	**0.7**

prodrome was between 4 and 24 months (geometric mean 18 months) in all but two women. Hirsutism was not universally severe, with three women having an F and G score of less than 10. Most women had baldness, while three had clitoromegaly and half had the clinical features of Cushing's syndrome (central obesity, moon face, hypertension). In the single case of adrenal neoplasm reported in the study by O'Driscoll and coworkers,[30] there was marked hirsutism and clitoromegaly, with acne, weight loss and an abdominal mass. An abdominal mass is a relatively common finding,[32] indicating the advanced state of the pathology at diagnosis.

An estimated 1% of ovarian tumours secrete androgens[33] and so may present with androgenization but not Cushing's syndrome. In one series of seven women with such tumours, the mean duration of the history was again 18 months, alopecia was present in all and clitoromegaly in four out of seven women.[34]

Other causes of hirsutism

Adrenal carcinoma

Adrenal carcinoma may present as Cushing's disease but this may also be the end point of more benign tumours or of long-term medication, where truncal obesity and hirsutism are features. Hyperprolactinaemia may result from a pituitary adenoma but is also a physiological response in some conditions where hirsutism may be a manifestation.

Late-onset congenital adrenal hyperplasia

Late onset congenital adrenal hyperplasia (LO-CAH) has been described over the last 20 years as a cause of hirsutism.[28,35,36] In many instances, it is probably incorporated into the diagnosis of idiopathic hirsutism or benign hyperandrogenism. Metabolically, it represents a partial deficiency of any one of at least three of the enzymes in the adrenal corticosteroid pathway. Metabolic compensation within the adrenal leads to the overproduction of androgenic steroid with androgenic features. In true congenital adrenal hyperplasia, there is the potential for a 'salt-losing crisis' when under physiological stress.

No such crisis has been described in LO-CAH. In both the late-onset and congenital form, oral corticosteroid therapy will reverse the adrenal overcompensation and largely correct the androgenic features. While this is justifiable in the congenital form to avoid dangerous crises, the situation is less clear in LO-CAH.[35] Chronic corticosteroid therapy carries considerable risk of physical and metabolic side-effects and there is no precise way of judging the correct dose. Moreover, Spritzer and co-workers have shown that ethinyl oestradiol combined with cyproterone acetate is more effective than steroid replacement.[35] Although the diagnosis of LO-CAH may be useful as a means of excluding other pathology, it does not present with features that distinguish it from other causes of hirsutism and does not require specific treatment.

Iatrogenic causes

Hypertrichosis is the most common change in hair growth associated with chronic immunosuppression with cyclosporin, although hirsutism has also been reported. Where minoxidil is used either systemically or topically, excess facial hair has been reported as a side-effect. While this is normally described as hypertrichosis, the distinction between hypertrichosis and hirsutism is not always easy at this site.

References

1. Ferriman D, Gallwey JD: Clinical assessment of body hair growth in women. *J Clin Endocrinol Metab* 1961; **24**: 1440–1447.
2. Garn SM: Types and distribution of the hair in man. *Ann NY Acad Sci* 1950–1951; **53**: 498–507.
3. Lorenzo EM: Familial study of hirsutism. *J Clin Endocrinol Metab* 1970; **31**: 556–564.
4. McKnight E: The prevalence of hirsutism in young women. *Lancet* 1964; **I**: 410–413.
5. Hamilton JB: Quantitative measurement of a secondary sex character, axillary hair. *Ann NY Acad Sci* 1950–1951; **53**: 585–599.
6. Kynaston Thomas P, Ferriman DG: Variation in facial and pubic hair growth in white women. *Am J Phys Anthropol* 1957; **15**: 171–180.
7. Melick R, Taft HP: Observations on body hair in old people. *J Clin Endocrinol Metab* 1959; **19**: 1597–1607.
8. Beek CH: A study on extension and distribution of

the human body hair. *Dermatologica (Basel)* 1950; **101**: 317–331.

9. Lunde O: A study of body hair density and distribution in normal women. *Am J Phys Anthropol* 1984; **64**: 179–184.

10. Ewing JA, Rouse B: Hirsutism, race and testosterone levels: comparison of east Asians and Euroamericans. *Hum Biol* 1978; **50**: 209–215.

11. Kurachi K, Mizutani MS, Matsumoto K: Plasma testosterone and urinary steroids in Japanese women with polycystic ovaries. *Acta Endocrinol* 1971; **68**: 293–302.

12. Conway GS, Honour JW, Jacobs HS: Heterogeneity of the polycystic ovary syndrome: clinical, endocrine and ultrasound features in 556 patients. *Clin Endocrinol* 1989; **30**: 459–470.

13. Carmina E, Koyama T, Chang L, Stanczyk FZ, Lobo RA: Does ethnicity influence the prevalence of adrenal hyperandrogenism and insulin resistance in polycystic ovary syndrome? *Am J Obstet Gynaecol* 1992; **167**:1807–1812.

14. Harlan WR, Harlan EA, Grillo GP: Secondary sex characteristics of girls 12 to 17 years of age: the US Health Examination Survey. *J Pediatrics* 1980; **96**: 1074–1078.

15. Trotter M: A study of facial hair on the white and negro races. *St Louis Missouri Washington University Studies Series* 1922; **9**: 273–279.

16. Danforth CH, Trotter M: The distribution of body hair in white subjects. *Am J Phys Anthropol* 1922; **5**: 259–265.

17. Erkkola R, Ruutiainen K. Hirsutism: definitions and etiology. *Ann Med* 1990; **22**: 98–103.

18. Moran C, Tapi MDC, Hernandez E, et al.: Etiological review of hirsutism in 250 patients. *Arch Med Res* 1994; **25**: 311–314.

19. Hopkinson ZEC, Sattar N, Fleming R, Greer IA: Polycystic ovarian syndrome: the metabolic syndrome comes to gynaecology. *Br Med J* 1998; **317**: 329–332.

20. Dunaif A: Insulin resistance and the polycystic ovary syndrome: mechanisms and implications for pathogenesis. *Endocrinol Rev* 1997; **18**: 774–800.

21. Evans DJ, Barth JH, Burke CW: Body fat topography in women with androgen excess. *Int J Obesity* 1988; **12**: 157–162.

22. Dunaif A: Hyperandrogenic anovulation (PCOS): a unique disorder of insulin action associated with an increased risk of non-insulin-dependent diabetes mellitus. *Am J Med* 1995; **98 (Suppl 1A)**: 1A-33S–1A-39S.

23. Conway GS, Jacobs HS. Clinical implications of hyperinsulinaemia in women. *Clin Endocrinol* 1993; **39**: 623–632.

24. Ruutiainen K, Erkkola R, Grönroos MA, Irjala K: Influence of body mass index and age on the grade of hair growth in hirsute women of reproductive ages. *Fertil Steril* 1988; **50**: 260–265.

25. Pasquali R, Antenucci D, Casimirri F, et al.: Clinical and hormonal characteristics of obese amenorrhoeic hyperandrogenic women before and after weight loss. *J Clin Endocrinol Metab* 1989; **68**: 173–179.

26. Barbieri RL: Hyperandrogenic disorders. *Clin Obstet Gynaecol* 1990; **33**: 640–654.

27. Barth JH, Jenkins M, Belchetz PE: Ovarian hyperthecosis, diabetes and hirsuties in post-menopausal women. *Clin Endocrinol* 1997; **46**: 123–128.

28. Gatee OB, Attia HMA, Salama IA: Hirsutism in the United Arab Emirates: a hospital study. *Postgrad Med J* 1996; **72**: 168–171.

29. Mithal A, Ammini AC, Godbole MM, et al.: Late-onset adrenal hyperplasia in North Indian hirsute women. *Hormon Res* 1988; **30**: 1–4.

30. O'Driscoll JB, Mamtora H, Higginson J, et al.: A prospective study of the prevalence of clear-cut endocrine disorders and polycystic ovaries in 350 patients presenting with hirsutism or androgenic alopecia. *Clin Endocrinol* 1994; **41**: 231–236.

31. Derksen J, Nagesser SK, Meinders AE, Haan HR, Van de Velde CJ: Identification of virilizing adrenal tumours in hirsute women. *N Engl J Med* 1994; **331**: 968–973.

32. King DR, Lack EE: Adrenal cortical carcinoma. A clinical and pathological study of 49 cases. *Cancer* 1979; **44**: 239–244.

33. Woodruff JD, Parmley TH: Virilizing ovarian tumours. In: Mahesh VB, Greenblatt RB (eds.). *Hirsutism and Virilism: Pathogenesis and Management.* London, Wright PSG, 1983: 29–158.

34. Moltz L, Pickartz H, Sörensen R, Schwartz U, Hammerstein J: Ovarian and adrenal vein steroids in seven patients with androgen-secreting ovarian neoplasms: selective catheterisation findings. *Fertil Steril* 1984; **42**: 585–593.

35. Spritzer P, Billaud L, Thalabrd JC, et al.: Cyproterone acetate versus hydrocortisone treatment in late-onset adrenal hyperplasia. *J Clin Endocrinol Metab* 1990; **70**: 642–646.

36. Chetkowski RJ, Defazio J, Shamonki I, Judd HL, Chang RJ: The incidence of late-onset congenital adrenal hyperplasia due to 21-hydroxylase deficiency among hirsute women. *J Clin Endocrinol Metab* 1984; **58**: 595–598.

34

Constitutional hirsutism: the SAHA syndrome

Francisco M Camacho

Introduction

The term 'hirsutism' defines the presence, in women, of hair and vellous hair with male characteristics, in locations that are typical of the male. It is, therefore, a response of the female organism to a greater or abnormal induction of androgens. Hypertrichosis, in contrast, is only an increase in the 'amount' of hair.[1,2]

Hirsutism is related to an increase in androgen levels, which is why it appears after puberty. At puberty, the secondary sexual characteristics develop in men, leading to changes in the voice, palpable muscle mass and the appearance of hair on the moustache, beard, thorax, shoulders, back, arms, thighs, pubic diamond and buttocks. If these changes are seen in women, there is often an endocrinological alteration with an increased secretion of androgens. Nevertheless, it is also possible that the androgen serum levels are normal and that the woman has symptoms of hyperandrogenism,[3] namely, an increase in the concentration of androgens, or an exaggerated clinical response to the androgenetic action.[4] The androgen responsible for the change in the voice and the increase in the muscle mass in women is testosterone, and that responsible for hirsutism and androgenetic alopecia is dihydrotestosterone (DHT).[5] The action of androgens on the hair follicle is discussed by Randall in Chapter 5.

Since the pathogenesis and clinical features of different types of hirsutism were described in two previous chapters (see Chapters 32 and 33), this chapter concentrates on 'constitutional hirsutism'. As the pathology of constitutional hirsutism is entirely dermatological, with symptoms of seborrhea, acne, hirsutism and alopecia present, it has also been called 'dermatological hirsutism' or the SAHA syndrome. A special form of ovarian hirsutism known as HAIRAN (Hyper-Androgenism, Insulin Resistance, Acanthosis Nigricans) syndrome will also be described.

The SAHA syndrome

The name 'SAHA' is the acronym of seborrhea, acne, hirsutism and alopecia, and was introduced by Constantine Orfanos in 1982.[6] As all four symptoms are androgen-dependent, we must consider this syndrome as a 'minor' form of the hyperandrogenism syndrome.[7–9] Previously, constitutional or 'dermatological' hirsutism used to be called 'idiopathic' and 'endogenous' hirsutism but these terms are no longer used, as the origin of the increases in the androgens was unknown at that time. Today the origin of the excess androgens produced in some cases is known, together with the reason why they act as though they were being produced in excess when the levels are normal. In this situation the problem is located in the effector organ, which is why some authors use the term 'peripheral hirsutism'.[10,11]

In a study of 110 Hispanic women with constitutional hirsutism being evaluated for androgen receptor (AR) polymorphisms,[12] an inverse relationship was found between the Ferriman and Gallwey's score[36] and CAG trinucleotide repeat size. These findings and also the results of the study by Sawaya and Shalita[12] confirm that the effects of elevated circulating androgens are a marker of hyperandrogenism. Furthermore, when a group of hyperandrogenic women with elevated androgens was studied, an inverse relationship between size of AR polymorphisms and cutaneous signs of hyperandrogenism was demonstrated. This is further evidence that decreased CAG trinucleotide repeats and elevated androgen levels correlate with increased sensitivity to androgens.

In the different types of SAHA, high plasma androgen levels are only found in certain circumstances. As shown in Table 1, when there is a slight increase in the androgens of **adrenal** origin (simple (DHEA) and sulfated dehydro-epiandrosterone (DHEA-S)), the condition is termed 'persistent adrenarche syndrome', and this may occur in women who are very stressed, thin, who have seborrhea, acne and female androgenetic alopecia (FAGA) although this may be of the male pattern (FAGA.M)), generally central hirsutism, and long inter-menstrual periods with long menstruations. If the androgen excess (δ-4-andrestenedione-A-) arises from the ovaries the condition is known as 'excess ovarian androgen release syndrome', which occurs in young women who are generally obese, with the same skin symptomatology, although the alopecia is always of the female pattern, and the menstruations are short, with short cycles.[14] If a slight increase in prolactin is the only alteration found, the 'SAHA syndrome due to hyperprolactinemia' is diagnosed. Finally, if there seems to be no endocrinological alteration, the condition is known as 'familial hirsutism'.

Familial SAHA

This is also known as 'ethnic hyperandrogenism'.[4] It is characterized by certain signs of hyperandrogenization such as 'facial hirsutism in Southern European women or women from the Mediterranean area' (Figure 1) and is seen within families. Women normally consult the physician because of lateral facial hirsutism and less often, mammary hirsutism. The facial

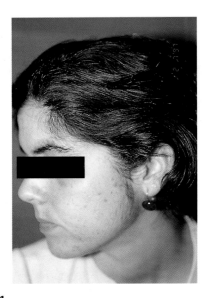

Figure 1

Familial SAHA. Lateral facial hirsutism and slight papulo-pustulous acne can be seen.

hirsutism is accompanied by slight papulopustulous acne, which is located exclusively on the mid-facial area and often accompanied by facial congestion as a result of the increased vascular reactivity.

Although there is usually no hormonal alteration, with biochemical parameters being in the middle levels of normality, biochemical examination should be undertaken.

Ovarian SAHA (excess ovarian androgen release syndrome)

This usually affects young women between the ages of 17 and 20 years. Pustulous or nodulocystic acne with some scars, mammary and lateral facial hirsutism (Figure 2) are seen; sometimes there may also be some central hairiness that does not exceed grade 2, significant seborrhea, and FAGA grade 1. Women are slightly obese or have a tendency to obesity, and they usually have painless, short menstruations and short menstrual cycles.[9]

They may have slightly increased serum A and

Table 1   Constitutional hyperandrogenism.

Familial SAHA
Ovarian SAHA (excess ovarian androgen release syndrome)
Adrenal SAHA (persistent adrenarche syndrome)
Hyperprolactinemic SAHA (pituitary involvement)

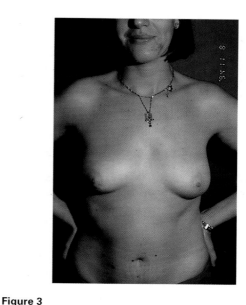

Figure 3

Adrenal SAHA. Slight central hirsutism that is more evident between pubic triangle and the umbilicus, and nodulocystic acne is present.

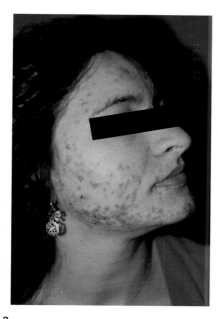

Figure 2

Ovarian SAHA. Lateral facial hirsutism and severe nodulocystic acne with some scarring is shown.

free testosterone (T) levels. Sex hormone binding globulin (SHBG; TeBG) is usually decreased and androstenediol glucuronide is increased. Other biochemical test results are normal, especially that for DHEA-S. The slight increase in testosterone is due to the greater activity of 5-α-reductase.[2]

When mammary hirsutism exceeds grade 2 and the FAGA is grade 2, blood biochemistry should be checked repeatedly to exclude ovarian hyperandrogenism.

Adrenal SAHA (persistent adrenarche syndrome)

This can be compared to an 'adrenal hyperplasia' in which the hydroxylases are present but do not act. As a result, one can see significant seborrhea and nodulocystic acne, with residual scars in the face and on the back. Furthermore, there may be FAGA 1–2 and even FAGA.M 1–2, slight to moderate central and lateral hirsutism (Figure 3), predominantly central, which may join the hair of the pubic triangle with the hair existing on the chin and the central area of the throat, and there is also palmar hyperhidrosis.[9]

In contrast with ovarian SAHA, these patients are usually thin and constantly stressed. Their menstrual cycles are generally longer than 30 days, sometimes skipping a cycle, with menstruations that are generally long, and quite painful on the first day.[2] This fact has been known for quite some time, and it is the reason for the name of this syndrome, which, in 1986, Lucky termed 'exaggerated adrenarche'.[15,16] These are very stressed patients who are working or studying. When the adrenarche is premature, it may be seen in association with a hidradenitis suppurativa.[17]

Biochemically there is an increase in DHEA-S and sometimes also in serum A; prolactin, SHBG, and free testosterone are normal. When there is a certain intensity of the clinical picture, it is useful to request determination of the plasma cortisol level.

Hyperprolactinemic SAHA

The clinical manifestations are the same as those of adrenal SAHA; with the presence of nodulocystic acne and central hirsutism (Figure 4); occasionally however galactorrhea may also be present.

In some cases, the hirsute woman presents with a central and lateral hairiness but most prominent is an oligomenorrhea; this is not usually a reason for consulting the dermatologist, rather the gynecologist. Biochemically, in these women one can see a slight increase in prolactin.

The HAIRAN syndrome

Another special form of hyperandogenism is the HAIRAN syndrome. Although previously considered as a form of familial hyperandrogenism, currently, it is integrated in the type 2 polycystic ovary syndrome (PCOS) as a form of ovarian hyperandrogenism.[18] This syndrome was named HAIRAN because hyperandrogenization (HA) occurs together with insulin resistance (IR) and acanthosis nigricans (AN). Although its relationship, as yet, is not understood, it is present in 2–5% of hirsute patients.[19–21]

The resistance to insulin causes hyperinsulinism, which stimulates the production of ovarian androgens, through the interaction of the insulin receptors and insulin-like growth factor 1 (IGF-1). The insulin receptors are found in the ovaries and it has been shown that IGF-1 stimulates the production of androgens in the ovarian stroma.[4,22] IGF-1 also causes a reduction of SHBG, with which it leads indirectly to hyperandrogenism as there is an excess of free testosterone.[23] The resistance to insulin, as a primary disease, occurs in two forms – types A and B. In both forms, the pathogenic problem is the same; namely, a marked reduction of the binding of insulin to its membrane receptors, causing insulin resistance, resistance to exogenous insulin, and a variable degree of glucose intolerance. Type A is seen in young women, who, in addition to presenting with significant acanthosis nigricans (Figure 5), also have hirsutism, clitorimegaly, accelerated body growth and polycystic ovaries. This is caused either by the decrease in the number of insulin receptors on the cell membrane, or because that, although present in sufficient numbers, they are nonfunctioning.

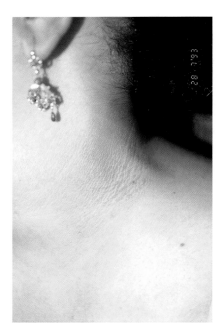

Figure 5

The HAIRAN syndrome. Acanthosis nigricans on the neck.

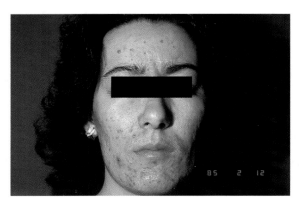

Figure 4

Hyperprolactinemic SAHA. Nodulocystic acne and central hirsutism are seen.

Type B occurs in older women, in whom the acanthosis nigricans is less evident but in whom the alopecia, the arthralgia and the thickening of the salivary glands are common. This is caused by antinuclear antibodies, which bind to the insulin receptors and prevent their function.[24]

Acanthosis nigricans (AN), characterized by cutaneous thickening and hyperpigmentation, is seen in the axillae, the neck (see Figure 5), the inside of the elbow, and the groin, and less frequently in other flexion sites, the umbilical area, and the submammary folds.[25] The AN observed in this syndrome is benign as it does not affect the mucosas, the palms and the soles; moreover, it is not pruriginous, unlike the malignant form. Of all the existing benign forms (e.g. idiopathic, hereditary, drug-induced and endocrine) of this syndrome, in this chapter we are only interested in the endocrine form, specifically that associated with insulin resistance and hyperinsulinemia, a common finding in obese women.

Panidis et al.[26] studied 50 women whom they divided into five groups of ten women each as follows:

(1) With PCOS, abnormal body mass index (BMI), and AN;
(2) With PCOS and an abnormal BMI but without AN;
(3) With PCOS but with a normal BMI and without AN;
(4) With an abnormal BMI but without PCOS;
(5) Normal.

Their conclusions were that insulin resistance is required but not the only factor responsible for acanthosis nigricans in patients with PCO syndrome.

Therefore, the pathogenesis of this syndrome seems clear. The chronic hyperinsulinemia resulting from resistance to insulin stimulates increased androgen secretion by the ovary, and leads to proliferation of the epidermis, which leads to hirsutism, virilization and acanthosis nigricans.[25] An increase in testosterone is now not thought to be the primary metabolic defect of the HAIRAN syndrome. Moreover, it is now known that insulin stimulates the synthesis of DNA in human fibroblasts by binding to the insulin or the IGF-1 receptors contained in fibroblasts and also in keratinocytes. This induces cellular proliferation and results in acanthosis nigricans. In the same way, there have been descriptions of insulin and IGF-1 receptors in the granulosa layer of the ovary, and it is known that this produces testosterone in response to insulin, although which receptor is involved in this stimulation is not yet known.[24]

There have been descriptions of familial cases, with amenorrhea, hirsutism, masculinization, hypertension, hyperinsulinemia, hypertriglyceridemia, and hyperprolactinemia. The suppression of luteinizing hormone (LH) and follicle stimulating hormone (FSH) normalizes the serum androgens but has no effect on the hyperinsulinemia, the hypertriglyceridemia, the hyperprolactinemia, the hypertension, or the acanthosis nigricans. With respect to acanthosis nigricans and trichological alterations, Chuang et al.[27] have published the familial association of acanthosis nigricans with madarosis, indicating that perhaps this is a new entity.

Diagnosis of constitutional hirsutism

Clinical history

Any woman with acne that began between the ages of 16 and 20 years, should have a clinical history taken. Other signs of androgenization should be verified, following defeminizing signs of acne, menstrual alterations, breast atrophy, decreased rugosity of the vaginal columns and sterility, and also following virilizing signs such as hirsutism and also FAGA.M, deepening voice, increased muscle mass, amenorrhea and clitorimegaly.[28]

Every clinical history should include a series of data. Nevertheless, from the prognostic point of view, the most important sign is probably the age of onset of the acne, because if this began after the age of 20 years other causes of hyperandrogenism should be considered. Seborrhea, which will always be present, is a very important parameter when accompanying acne, hirsutism and FAGA, because it suggests significant androgen action.

Hirsutism that begins between the ages of 10 and 20 years and develops slowly, will never be caused by a tumor; however, if it appears suddenly at any age and evolves quickly, and is accompanied by other signs of virilization, the presence of a tumor is indicated.

It is necessary always to ascertain the menstrual history. In ovarian SAHA, menstruations take place every 15–21 days, always fewer than 28 days, and they last 1 or 2 days, while in adrenal or hyperprolactinemic SAHA the menstruations are considerably longer, with cycles of 35–60 days and sometimes more, in other words, some menstrual cycles are skipped. When there are neither present nor previous menstrual alterations, one must consider familial SAHA.[29,30]

The clinical history must also include information about associated diseases such as diabetes, insulin resistance, thyroiditis, other immunological and general disorders, and the possible ingestion of drugs that are able to cause hirsutism.[31]

Clinical examination

This is performed to verify how many of the SAHA signs are present in the patient, and whether or not other androgenization signs exist. In our experience, seborrhea is always present, FAGA present in 20.7%, followed by acne in 10% and hirsutism in 6.15%.[7] Only 21.5% of our patients presented with all four signs of SAHA.[7,9,28,29]

Hirsutism must be evaluated according to Ferriman and Gallwey's score, which we have modified to include only 9 parameters[32] and the alopecia must be assessed according to the FAGA and FAGA.M patterns, which we proposed many years ago.[33]

Of course, if there is insulin resistance and acanthosis nigricans, the hyperandrogenism will not be constitutional but of the ovarian type, making up the HAIRAN syndrome.[34]

Seborrhea measurement using sebumeter is a good method of measurement of androgen action. The FAGA may be measured by trichogram, pull test and pinch sign or Jacquet sign.

Biochemical screening

Six plasma levels are required for diagnosis: free testosterone, DHEA-S, δ-4-androstenedione, SHBG, prolactin and androstenediol glucuronide.[35] In certain cases one can also request FSH, LH, 17-hydroxyprogesterone, ferritin, T4, and antimicrosomal antibodies. In exceptional cases, we will also request cortisol, 11-desoxycortisol, and 17β-estradiol.[2] As to the value of steroid chromatography in 24-hour urine samples, it was shown in 1987 that this has an error margin of 33.3%, so at present there is no sense in requesting this.[7]

In the HAIRAN syndrome, laboratory investigations only reveal increased levels of free testosterone, insulin, and glucose; sometimes there may be an increase in the antibodies against insulin receptors, antinuclear antibodies, gammaglobulins, A1c hemoglobin and cortisol. There may even be leukopenia but the levels of LH, FSH and DHEA-S will be normal.

Other examinations

Other specific examination tests for hyperandrogenism, such as the dexamethasone suppression test, the ACTH stimulation test, computerized axial tomography (CAT), ultrasound, retropneumoperitoneum, and so on are not usually necessary for the assessment of SAHA, although they could be necessary to determine the type of hirsutism.

Diagnostic indicators

As a general guide, patients with familial and ovarian SAHA usually present with papulopustulous acne and, exceptionally, nodulocystic acne on the face (Figure 6) and sometimes a few scattered elements on the chest. Patients with the adrenal and hyperprolactinemic forms of SAHA show nodulocystic acne with residual scars on the face and back (Figures 7 and 8).

With regard to the pattern of alopecia, in ovarian SAHA there will always be FAGA 1–2 (Figure 6), while in adrenal and hyperprolactine-

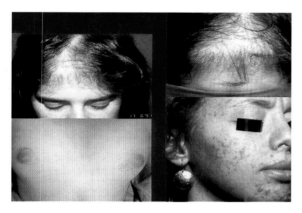

Figure 6

Ovarian SAHA. Nodulocystic acne, FAGA 1 and mammary hirsutism are shown.

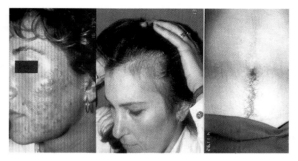

Figure 8

Hyperprolactinemic SAHA. Severe nodulocystic acne, FAGA.M 1 and abdominal hirsutism can be seen.

mic SAHA the FAGA may be of the male pattern (FAGA.M) and reach grade 2[35] (see Figures 7 and 8).

The pattern of hirsutism is assessed according to the Ferriman and Gallwey score.[36] In familial SAHA there is usually facial hirsutism and less frequently, mammary hirsutism; in ovarian SAHA one sees lateral hirsutism, which is more obvious on the mammary and the facial areas (Figure 6); while in adrenal and hyperprolactine-

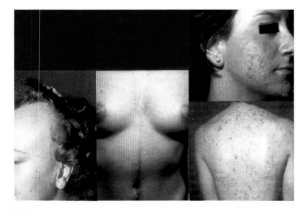

Figure 7

Adrenal SAHA. Nodulocystic acne with scars on the face and back, FAGA.M 1 and central hirsutism are present.

mic SAHA the hirsutism is usually central[2] (Figures 7 and 8). This attempt to define the pattern of hirsutism depending on the type of SAHA is only helpful at the onset as, when the condition has evolved there is usually hairiness both laterally and centrally, although one of these may predominate. For example, in polycystic ovary syndrome there is usually lateral hairiness, while the hairiness of congenital adrenal hyperplasia is usually central. Therefore, for nontumoral SAHA and hirsutism, this may be a valuable diagnostic fact.

Obesity is usually a marker of ovarian SAHA, while in adrenal and hyperprolactinemic SAHA, women are usually thin, nervous and stressed, and frequently have palmar hyperhydrosis.[7]

With regard to menstruation, ovarian SAHA usually coincides with short-cycle menstruations that last several days, while women with adrenal or hyperprolactinemic SAHA usually have long menstruation cycles that may even skip months and that are long-lasting (sometimes lasting more than a week), and very painful initially.[7]

Biochemically, familial SAHA does not show any androgenic alteration. Adrenal SAHA has slightly increased levels of DHEA-S and free testosterone. In ovarian SAHA, there are slightly increased levels of serum A and free testosterone with a decrease in SHBG and an increase in androstenediol glucuronide, while in hyperprolactinemic SAHA, there is a slight increase in prolactin. If the prolactin level is very high, one must examine the pituitary gland.

If all the ovarian or adrenal androgen levels are increased (i.e. DHEA-S, serum A, and free testosterone) it will be necessary to carry out a dexamethasone suppression according to Hatch's scheme,[37] namely 0.5 mg dexamethasone 4 times a day for 7 days. If the suppression is abnormal, an ovarian or an adrenal tumor, polycystic ovary syndrome, or Cushing's syndrome will be present. If the suppression is normal, a prolactinoma or a congenital adrenal hyperplasia, or even a persistent adrenarche syndrome may be present.[9]

References

1. Camacho F: Hipertricosis e hirsutismo. In: Camacho F, Montagna W (eds.). *Tricología. Trichology. Trichologie.* Madrid, Garsi Ed, 1982; 123–138.
2. Camacho F, Sánchez-Pedreño P: Hirsutismo. Concepto, clasificación etiopatogénica y cuadros clínicos. *Monogr Dermatol* 1992; **5**: 342–351.
3. Camacho F: Hirsutism. In: Camacho F, Montagna W (eds.). *Trichology. Diseases of the Pilosebaceus Follicle.* Madrid, Aula Médica Ed, 1997: 265–298.
4. Sperling LC, Heimer WL: Androgen biology as a basis for the diagnosis and treatment of androgenic disorders in women. I. *J Am Acad Dermatol* 1993; **28**: 669–683.
5. Waldstreicher J: The importance of 5α-reductase in dermatology: Clinical Studies With Finasteride. American Academy of Dermatology, New Orleans, February 1995.
6. Orfanos CE: Antiandrógenos en Dermatología. *Arch Arg Dermat* 1982; **32(Suppl 1)**: 51–55.
7. Sánchez-Pedreño P: *Estudio clínico, bioquímico, evolutivo y terapéutico del síndrome SAHA.* Doctoral Thesis. University of Seville, 1987.
8. Hammerstein J: Androgenization in women. Acne, seborrhoea, androgenetic alopecia and hirsutism. Amsterdam. *Excerpta Medica*, 1980.
9. Edwars O, Rock A: Androgen-dependent cutaneous syndromes. In: Rook A, Savin J (eds.). *Recent Advances in Dermatology.* New York, Churchill Livingstone, 1980: 159–183.
10. Glickman SP, Rosenfield RL: Androgen metabolism by isolated hairs from women with idiopathic hirsutism is usually normal. *J Invest Dermatol* 1984; **82**: 62–66.
11. Toscano V, Adamo MV, Caiola S, Foli S, Petrangeli E, Cassilli D, Sciarra F: Is hirsutism an evolving syndrome? *J Endocrinol* 1983; **97**: 379–387.
12. Legro RS, Shahbahrami B, Lobo RA, Kovacs BW: Size polymorphisms of the androgen receptor among female hispanics and correlation with androgenic characteristics. *Obstet Gynecol* 1994; **83**: 701–706.
13. Sawaya ME, Shalita AR: Androgen receptor polymorphisms (CAG repeat lengths) in androgenetic alopecia, hirsutism, and acne. *J Cutan Med Surg* 1998; **3**: 9–15.
14. Bergfeld W, Redmond GP: Hirsutism. *Dermatol Clin* 1987; **5**: 501–507.
15. Lucky AW: Androgens and the skin. Another journey around the cycle. *Arch Dermatol* 1987; **123**: 193–19S.
16. Lucky AW, Rosenfield RL, McGuire J, Rudy S, Helke J: Adrenal androgen hyperresponsiveness to adrenocorticotropin in women with acne and/or hirsutism: adrenal enzyme defects and exaggerated adrenarche. *J Clin Endocrinol Metab* 1986; **62**: 840–848.
17. Levis F, Messenger AG, Wales JKH: Hidradenitis suppurativa as a presenting feature of premature adrenarche. *Br J Dermatol* 1993; **129**: 447–448.
18. Sayag J, Aquilina C: *Hirsutismes. Collection Peau et Phaneres.* Marsella, Solal, 1989.
19. Barbieri RL: Hyperandrogenism, insulin resistance and acanthosis nigricans. 10 years of progress. *J Reprod Med* 1994; **39**: 327–336.
20. Azziz R: The hyperandrogenic-insulin-resistant acanthosis nigricans syndrome: therapeutic response. *Fertil Steril* 1994; **61**: 570–572.
21. Barth JH, Ng LL, Wognarowska F, Dawber RPR: Acanthosis nigricans, insulin resistance and cutaneous virilism. *Br J Dermatol* 1988; **118**: 613–620.
22. Sperling LC, Heimer WL: Androgen biology as a basis for the diagnosis and treatment of androgenic disorders in women. II. *J Am Acad Dermatol* 1993; **28**: 901–916.
23. Aizawa H, Niimura M: Mild insulin resistance during oral glucose tolerance test (OGTT) in women with acne. *J Dermatol* 1996; **23**: 526–529.
24. Esperanza LE, Fenske NA: Hyperandrogenism insulin resistance and acanthosis nigricans (HAIRAN) syndrome: spontaneous remission in a 15-year-old girl. *J Am Acad Dermatol* 1996; **34**: 892–897.
25. Camacho F, Muñoz MA: HAIRAN syndrome. In: Van Neste D, Randall V (eds.). *Hair Research for the Next Millennium.* Amsterdam, Elsevier, 1996: 289–292.
26. Panidis D, Skiadopoulos S, Rousso D, Ioannides D, Panidou E: Association of acanthosis nigricans with insulin resistance in patients with polycystic ovary syndrome. *Br J Dermatol* 1995; **132**: 936–941.
27. Chuang S-D, Jee S-H, Chiu H-C, Chen J-S, Lin J-T: Familial acanthosis nigricans with madarosis. *Br J Dermatol* 1995; **133**: 104–108.

28. Camacho F: SAHA syndrome. In: Camacho F, Montagna W (eds.). *Trichology. Diseases of the Pilosebaceus Follicle.* Madrid, Aula Médica, 1997: 673–690.

29. Camacho F, Sánchez-Pedreño P: Síndrome SAHA. *Piel* 1991; **6**: 272–286.

30. Sánchez-Pedreño P, Camacho F: Acné en el síndrome SAHA. *Monogr Dermatol* 1990; **3**: 76–87.

31. Sotillo I, Jorquera E: Hipertricosis por drogas. *Monogr Dermatol* 1992; **5**: 328–333.

32. Camacho F: Hirsutismo. Diagnóstico y tratamiento. *Monogr Dermatol* 1992; **5**: 352–373.

33. Camacho F, Sánchez-Pedreño P: Alopecia androgenética. *Monogr Dermatol* 1989; **2**: 107–117.

34. Dunaif A, Green G, Phelps RG, Lebwohl M, Futterweit W, Lewy L: Acanthosis nigricans, insulin action, and hyperandrogenism: clinical, histological and biochemical findings. *J Clin Endocrinol Metab* 1991; **73**: 590–595.

35. Camacho F: Alopecias: Androgenética. Areata. Cicatriciales. *Monogr Dermatol* 1993; **6** (núm. extra): 79–104.

36. Ferriman D, Gallwey JD: Clinical assessment of body hair growth in women. *J Clin Endocr Metab* 1961; **21**: 1440–1447.

37. Hatch R, Rosenfield RL, Kim MH, Tredway D: Hirsutism: implications, etiology and management. *Am J Obstetr Gynecol* 1981; **140**: 815–830.

35
Drug treatment of hirsutism

Francisco M Camacho

Introduction

In this chapter the treatment for all types of hirsutisms will be described, particularly the most recent. The classification we shall follow is the same as that for hyperandrogenism (Table 1).

Although contrary to the belief of some dermatologists, gynecologists and endrocrinologists, I believe that the first physician that should see the hirsute woman should be the dermatologist; and that once it is demonstrated that the pathology of the ovaries, adrenal glands or pituitary gland is the most important factor she or he will refer the woman to the corresponding specialist. The dermatologist has the capacity to diagnose peripheral hyperandrogenism, which, as we know from Professor Sciarra's team working in Gainesville,[1] is an evolving syndrome that may modify the hypothalamo-hypophysial-adrenal-ovarian axis, with an adrenal repercussion. The peripheral hyperandrogenism could be a permissive extraovarian factor for polycystic ovary syndrome.

Treatment for peripheral hyperandrogenism is similar to that for organ failure, although the dose will be lower and the treatment shorter in duration. In general, all ovarian pathology, with the exception of tumors, will be treated with estrogens and antiandrogens, the adrenal pathology will be treated using corticosteroids and antiandrogens or estrogens, while problems of hyperprolactinemia will be treated with bromocriptine. Therefore, this chapter will concentrate on the treatment of constitutional hyperandrogenism in detail.

In this chapter the treatment of hirsutism is separated into dermatological therapeutical methods, and extradermatological medical-surgical methods. These are summarized in Table 2 and discussed in the following text.

Table 1 Classification of hyperandrogenism.

Constitutional hyperandrogenism (dermatological)
Familial SAHA
Adrenal SAHA (persistent adrenarche syndrome)
Ovarian SAHA (excess ovarian androgen release syndrome)
Hyperprolactinemic SAHA (pituitary)

Adrenal hyperandrogenism
Congenital adrenal hyperplasia (CAH)
Cushing's syndrome
Tumors

Ovarian hyperandrogenism
Polycystic ovary syndrome
Tumors

Other causes of hyperandrogenism
Hepatic
Pituitary
Iatrogenic
Lack of peripheral conversion of androgens to estrogens
Ectopic androgen production

Dermatological treatment of constitutional hirsutism

It is chiefly patients with 'constitutional hirsutism', previously termed 'idiopathic hirsutism' and also referred to as the 'SAHA syndrome', an acronym of seborrhea, acne, hirsutism and alope-

Table 2 Treatment of hirsutism.

Dermatological treatment
    General therapy
    Topical therapy

Non-dermatological medicosurgical treatment
    Endocrinological treatment
    Gynecological treatment
    Surgical treatment
    Dermatocosmetic measures

cia (see Camacho's Chapter 34) who consult the dermatologist. When patients also present with other symptoms of virilization that would lead us to a diagnosis of ovarian, adrenal, or hypophyseal hirsutism, the dermatologist should refer the woman on to the corresponding specialist.

The treatment of constitutional hyperandrogenism is most interesting for the dermatologist because most women with this syndrome are referred to the dermatologist after visiting the endocrinologist or gynecologist who have diagnosed these women as normal. Their endocrine glands and ovaries are normal but these patients have a peripheral sensitivity, especially in the pilosebaceous follicle in the target organs; they thus develop signs of hyperandrogenism such as seborrea, acne, hirsutism and alopecia – the SAHA syndrome[2–7] (see Chapter 34).

Treatment of familial SAHA

This form is separate from the rest of the SAHAs because of the minimal clinical manifestations and absolutely normal biochemical test results, with plasma levels of androgen not even being close to the upper limits of normality. For this reason a general therapy should not be used, rather, only a local (topical) treatment and a dermatocosmetic treatment should be applied.[6–10] Topical therapy comprises the isolated treatment of symptoms – especially facial hirsutism – which is treated with a local application of 3% spironolactone in a hydroalcohol solution, or 5% in a carbopol gel.[4,8] Also 1–2% canrenone solution, which is the metabolite of spironolactone with similar results,[8] can be also used.

In addition to the application of spironolactone, seborrhea may benefit from a 5% hydroalcoholic progesterone solution associated with 5% propyleneglycol, as the progesterone would block the 5α-reductase. The association of progesterone at doses as low as 0.025% with low doses, 0.05%, of spironolactone also seems very adequate as these complement each other synergistically in reducing the size of the sebaceous glands in the areas in which they are applied.[11]

The fact that this is used locally does not mean that it does not have complications, as contact dermatitis has been described with the use of a 5% spironolactone cream.[12]

Complementary dermatocosmetic treatment may comprise:

(1) Discolouration or bleaching;
(2) Shaving;
(3) Electrolysis; or
(4) Depilation – with tweezers, wax or chemicals.

Complementary dermatocosmetic methods are discussed at the end of this chapter.

Treatment of adrenal SAHA (persistent adrenarche syndrome)

In these patients, local measures include topical spironolactone (3% solution) or its metabolic product, canrenone (1–2% solution). In addition to local measures, adrenal suppression with dexamethasone or prednisone should be instigated. At the same time, the conversion of excess androstenedione and testosterone to dehydrotestosterone (DHT) should be prevented, since, if it reached the cytosol intracellular receptors it would cause pathology. The treatment for this is the use of antiandrogens. To summarize, in adrenal SAHA therapy, glucocorticoids and antiandrogens are used.

With regard to glucocorticosteroid treatment in constitutional hirsutism, for many years we have been using low-dose bedtime prednisone therapy for adrenal suppression. The dose used is 7.5 mg daily for 2 months, reducing this to 5 mg daily and 2.5 mg daily every second month respectively, until 6 months of treatment are completed. In the first 2 months the patient is given 2.5 mg in the morning and 5 mg at night. For the last 7 years (1992–1998) we have treated patients using overnight suppression with low-dose dexamethasone. A dose of 0.5 mg is given each night for 3 months and on alternate nights for another 3 months. These doses of glucocorticoids are enough to reduce the level of dehydroepiandrosterone-sulfate (DHEA-S), androstenedione and testosterone. The only secondary effect is that obese women, which is not normal in the adrenal SAHA, tend to gain a little more weight. If the dexamethasone dose is more than 0.75 mg daily if given for longer cushingoid changes would be seen.[8,13–15]

With regard to antiandrogen therapy, there are seven antiandrogens and 5α-reductase inhibitors available at present: cyproterone acetate; spironolactone; flutamine; finasteride; cimetidine; isotretinoin; and ketoconazole. Our experience with finasteride is limited but as a potent 5α-reductase inhibitor, we consider it to be more useful in the treatment of androgenetic alopecia (for more details see Chapter 13 by Price or Chapter 10 by Randall).

We only use finasteride in cases of SAHA with hirsutism and female androgenetic alopecia (FAGA), and we do not deem cimetidine, isotretinoin and ketoconazole to be useful, at least not in general.[12] The current classification of treatments opposing androgen action is of three types:

Androgenic receptor antagonists (antiandrogens)

For many years we have been using cyproterone acetate. For 4 years (1992–1995), we have been using spironolactone in the treatment of SAHA and hirsutism and flutamine for 3 years. Although some authors stipulate that the effects of cyproterone acetate and spironolactone are similar,[16] we believe that the former is better.

Cyproterone acetate (CA)
Cyproterone acetate acts by suppressing the pituitary-gonadal axis by:

(1) Interfering with the binding of androgens to the androgen receptor of the follicular target organ; and
(2) inhibiting the secretion of FSH and LH due to its progestagen action, which at the same time reduces the ovarian secretion of androgen.[17]

A dose of 50–100 mg a day is recommended from day 5–15 of the menstrual cycle during the 6 months of the period of glucocorticoid suppression.

CA usually causes femininization in the male fetus, and also menstrual alterations in the post-pubertal female, even at doses of 50 mg a day. Therefore it is useful to add 0.050 mg of ethinyl estradiol from day 5–26 of the menstrual cycle,[17,18] or, as we do, to add 0.035 mg from day 1–21, in the first menstrual cycle of treatment.

After 1 week of rest, the women take ethinyl estradiol from day 5–26 of the menstrual cycle.[8,19]

In post-menopausal women with female androgenetic alopecia, and with slight hirsutism, generally on the face, cyproterone acetate can be administered in a dose of 50 mg a day without interruption.

The secondary effects of cyproterone acetate are a decrease of libido, emotional alterations, fatigue, mastodynia, nausea, headaches, depression, elevation of blood pressure and weight increase. CA is completely contraindicated in liver disease. The side-effects are very difficult to see in women taking the doses we administer.[19]

Spironolactone (SL)
The use of SL in the SAHA syndrome with hirsutism and acne at a dose of 50–200 mg a day for at least 6 months, has yielded magnificent results.[20–22] With this dose after 6 months there was a reduction of 40% in the diameter of the facial hair and 83% after 12 months,[8] although better results could be observed after 2 or 3 years of treatment with 100 mg/daily (Figure 1). When the serum androgens were analyzed it was found that SL reduces the concentration of total testosterone and, occasionally, that of DHEA-S.[8]

The antiandrogen effects of SL are related to the selective destruction of cytochrome P_{450} in the gonads and the subsequent decrease of the activity of the different enzymes of steroidogenesis, which depend on the cytochrome P_{450} coenzyme, such as 17α-, 11β- and 21-hydroxylases. The destruction of cytochrome P_{450} is believed to be the result of the degradation of its HEM portions and the apoprotein by a 7α-thiosubstituted metabolite of SL. The peripheral antiandrogenic activity of SL seems to be due to its competition in blocking the intracellular androgen receptors of the follicular target organs, which would therefore block the activation of the hormone response elements in the DNA, preventing gene expression.[8]

Spironolactone causes a series of side-effects in 75–91% of users. These side-effects are generally mild, which means that only a few patients need to abandon the therapy. Among these side-effects, are menstrual irregularities as in an endocrine disorder, decreased libido and an increase in breast size and tension; hypercalcemia and an increase in serum creatinine; sleepiness, headaches, vertigo and even confu-

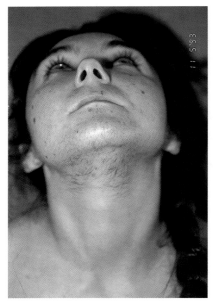

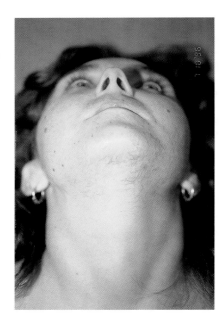

a   b

Figure 1

Adrenal SAHA: **(a)** Central facial hirsutism; **(b)** Same patient as shown in Figure 1a, after 3 years of treatment with 250 mg/day flutamide.

sion; nausea, vomiting, anorexia and diarrhea; and agranulocytosis and eosinophilia.[8,19] As this is a potent antiandrogen, it may also cause feminization of the male fetus which is why it must always be accompanied by contraceptive therapy.[8,23]

The cutaneous side-effects are diverse; namely, pruritus, xerosis, maculopapulous eruptions, urticaria, melasma-type pigmentations, contact dermatitis, erythema annulare centrifugum, vasculitis, erythema multiforme, Raynaud's phenomenon, alopecia, lupus type eruption,[24] and, on two occasions, a lichenoid eruption.[25]

Flutamide

Flutamide is a pure, non-steroidal antiandrogen that lacks any intrinsic progestogenic, estrogenic, corticosteroid or antigonadotropic effect both in vitro and in vivo.[26] When it is administered orally, it metabolizes to hydroxyflutamine, which is an active metabolite that acts by competitive inhibition on the androgen receptor of the target

organs of the pilosebaceous follicle. It has been shown that flutamide causes an inhibition of the activity of adrenal 17,20 desmolase in patients treated for prostate cancer and that it decreases serum DHEA-S levels. This is why it is considered the first choice of antiandrogen in the treatment of cutaneous androgenization syndromes caused by an excessive adrenal production,[26] including adrenal SAHA. We have been using it since 1993 at a dose of 250–375 mg/day for 6 months–2 years,[27,28] finding an improvement in 80% of the patients with complete SAHA (Figure 2), with the improvement being noticeable from the third month. As the risks of fetal malformations with its use during pregnancy are unknown, a tricyclic (estrogen-progestogen) contraceptive should be added. With the low doses we are using, digestive side-effects (which we found in 75% of the patients with doses greater than 500 mg) are usually not seen.[27] Furthermore, the toxic hepatitis that took place in 13% of patients and which required control of the patients every 3 months

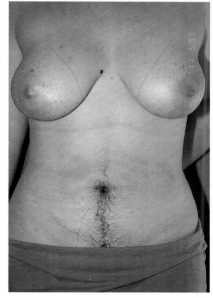

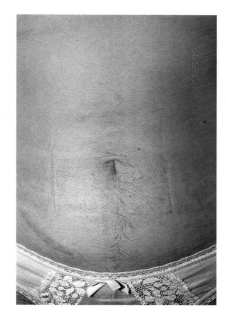

a   b

Figure 2

Adrenal SAHA: **(a)** Central abdominal hirsutism; **(b)** Same patient as shown in Figure 2a, after 2 years of treatment with 250 g/day flutamide.

by means of functional tests did not appear at the lower dosage either. Dodin et al.[29] recommend a maximum dose of 125 mg/day.

We currently recommend this low-dose regime and also insist that it is necessary to use tricyclic contraceptives. The reason for the latter is not only because the possible effects on the fetus are unknown, but also because it has been shown that lower doses reduce the hirsutism and prevent the relapse of hirsutism once the treatment with flutamide is stopped[28] – the reason for this is unknown.

A report of photosensitivity in a male with prostate carcinoma treated with flutamide[30] highlights the need to consider this complication especially in young women who tend to excessive exposure to sunlight in summer.

5α-reductase inhibitors

Before commenting on the 5α-reductase inhibitors it is worth remembering that, at present, two types of 5α-reductase inhibitors are considered according to the two isoenzymes of

5α-reductase. Type 1 has an enzymatic activity at the level of the scalp, sebaceous glands of the face and cutaneous surface of the chest and back, as well as in the liver, adrenals, and kidneys. Type 2 has an enzymatic activity at the level of the beard, skin of the scalp and in the liver. Moreover, in males it acts in the seminal vesicles, the prostate, the epididymis, the testicles and the skin of the scrotum. An example of type 1 inhibitor is known as MK-386, and a type 2 inhibitor is MK-906, the latter being 'finasteride', which is the only one available (Proscar, Propecia). The antiandrogenic effect of isotretinoin is still being discussed.

Finasteride

Finasteride is considered to be a potent inhibitor of the 5α-reductase isoenzyme 2 and is effective both in women to reduce hirsutism, and in men for the treatment of benign prostate hypertrophy[31] and androgenetic alopecia (see Chapter 15 by Price). At a dose of 5 mg/day, the only side-effects observed in men are a decrease in seminal volume, and in less than 4% of patients impotence, an alteration in ejaculation, and a decrease in libido.[32]

This antiandrogen is well absorbed orally and it has a half-life of 6–8 hours; however, its biological half-life is much longer as it depresses serum DHT and androstanediol glucuronide levels for up to 2 weeks after its last administration. Finasteride is excreted in the feces and in the urine.

A dose of 5 mg/day, or 7.5 mg/day, for 3–6 months significantly reduces the serum DHT and decreases the intrafollicular formation of DHT, which is enzymically mediated by 5α-reductase type 2; this is the reason why finasteride should be useful when treating FAGA and facial hirsutism.[33–35] We used finasteride at the dose of 2.5 mg daily in 23 women with facial hirsutism and FAGA, always in association with oral contraceptives. After 2 years of treatment the results were considered to be good, and similar to those for cyproterone acetate.

Although it is well tolerated and safe, finasteride has some side-effects, but these are usually slight – especially in women. As finasteride apparently may cause femininization of the male fetus, it has to be accompanied by anovulatory agents. It does not have any effect on serum lipids or on bone density; nor does it show any drug interactions; however, when used in association with oral contraceptives, there is a marked increase in serum cholesterol levels.[31] It has also been shown that, in hirsute women, there is a slight increase in gonadotropins and testosterone.

Isotretinoin

Although isotretinoin does not appear to have any significant effect on the circulating androgens, it has been shown to decrease the activity of 5α-reductase and thus the production of DHT and its metabolites.[36] We have never used isotretinoin in our establishment for the treatment of constitutional hirsutism; nevertheless, when we used it for nodulocystic acne the seborrhea was decreased similar to the decrease seen with flutamide.

Other antiandrogens

Cimetidine has an 'anecdotal'[15,37] value because, although it acts as a peripheral antiandrogen by inhibiting the binding of DHT to the androgen receptor,[38] its use causes an increase in the androgen secretion through a negative feedback mechanism.[39] Some authors suggest that it could be used in SAHA at a dose of 300 mg five times/day, preferably in association with a contraceptive. The rationale behind this is that it has a blocking effect at the level of receptors in the hair follicle and because of its low incidence of side-effects there has only been one report of a 'fixed exanthema' with its use.[40]

Other antiandrogens of steroid configuration exist, such as 'deoxycorticosterone', 'androstenedione', and 'progesterone'. These may act as competitive inhibitors of the 5α-reductase but have a limited use because of their hormonal effects.

Treatment of ovarian SAHA (excess ovarian androgen release syndrome)

The therapy for ovarian SAHA comprises antiandrogens, and ovarian suppression with contraceptives, always for 2 years, although the beneficial effects begin to be noticeable after 6 months. Antiandrogens were discussed in the treatment of adrenal SAHA so, in this section, we will concentrate on ovarian suppression.

Ovarian suppression

This is achieved by the use of oral contraceptives, and also of antagonists of gonadotropin releasing hormone (GnRH).

Oral contraceptives

Oral contraceptives should not be used in women with headaches, thromboembolic disease, or carcinoma of the breast or the uterus; they are also relatively contraindicated in women with hypertension.

Most products used in contraception contain an estrogen, ethinyl estradiol (EE), and a progestogen, which may be ethinodiol diacetate, norefinodrel, linestranol, norethindrone acetate, norgestrel, desogestrel, or levonorgrestrel. The combination of ethinyl estradiol with norethindrone acetate, norgestrel, and/or levonorgrestrel should be avoided, as these three progestagens have a marked androgenic activity.[41,42]

Our therapeutic standard consists of administering, for a period of 6 months, 100 mg/day of CA from day 5–15 of the menstrual cycle, and 0.035 mg of EE from day 5–26 of the cycle, in other words, for 21 days. The patient would then rest for 1 week before beginning the next therapeutic series. During the remaining 18 months, the patient would take 2 mg of CA and 0.035 mg of EE from post-menstrual day 5–26. It should be pointed out that this last association is only effective in mild SAHA and only as a maintenance therapy; it has no use as primary therapy in the first 6 months.[23,43,44] After 2 years the biochemical tests would be repeated, as some patients require treatment for 3 years or more. Since 1995 our regimen was changed to 125 mg daily of flutamide in all the women who did not have a good response to cyproterone acetate (Figure 3).

The action of EE is based mainly on the fact that it stimulates the production of SHBG, which decreases the amount of free testosterone; it also modifies the binding of DHT to its receptor and, when used for a considerable period of time, the activity of 5α-reductase is decreased. Moreover, at high doses, it also inhibits the secretion of LH.

If the patient does not tolerate oral contraceptives, medroxyprogesterone acetate can be used. It is a synthetic progesterone that is used as an anovulatory agent because it inhibits gonadotropin secretion, especially LH; this consequently reduces the production of testosterone and androstenedione in the ovaries.[45] Its use at 5 mg a day, or twice a day, along with 35 µg of EE during 21 days, with a rest week so that menstruation can occur, is usually very effective in controlling the menstrual cycle. The dose can be increased if there is menorrhage.

In women older than 40 years, the administration of 4 mg of estradiol valerate (EV) orally may be a substitute for EE and, in the case of an oral intolerance to estrogens, 10 mg of EV can be given intramuscularly on days 5 and 15 of the menstrual cycle.[46]

Gonadotropin releasing hormone (GnRH) antagonists

Since 1971, several synthetic analogs of GnRH have been developed; some of them, like nafarelin and leuprolide, have been used successfully in the treatment of hirsutism. This is because they reduce the diameter of the hair shaft and

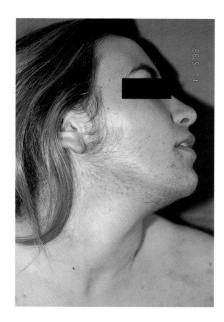

a

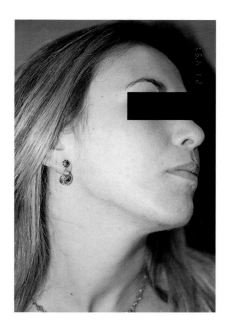

b

Figure 3

Ovarian SAHA: **(a)** Lateral facial hirsutism; **(b)** Same patient as shown in Figure 3a, after 2 years (May 1993–May 1995) with cyproterone acetate with poor results. The later treatment with 125 mg/day of flutamide from 1995–1997 gave excellent results.

the grading on the Ferriman and Gallwey score. Although their use in the SAHA syndrome is not usually considered, we must not forget that this syndrome may resemble ovarian hyperandrogenism, and polycystic ovary syndrome; indeed GnRH antagonists have been shown to be especially useful if the hirsutism is accompanied by seborrhea and acne.[47]

The effects of GnRH antagonists result from a continual stimulation of the pituitary gland, thus reducing luteinizing hormone (LH) and follicle stimulating hormone (FSH) production. The LH reduction in turn leads to a reduction of testosterone produced by the ovary. Its use is limited, however, as its side-effects cause loss of bone matter as a result of estrogenic depletion. As a result, GnRH antagonists are currently administered in association with estrogens and progesterone, and these in turn increase SHBG levels while reducing free testosterone.

In this way, leuprolide, at a dose of 3.75 mg/month given intramuscularly and 0.625 mg/day in conjunction with estrogens and 10 mg of medroxyprogesterone acetate from day 1–12 of the menstrual cycle has shown a significant reduction in hirsutism.[48] Moreover, nafarelin, at an intranasal dose of 400 µg with 1 mg norethindrone and 35 µg of ethinyl estradiol, has also been shown to reduce hirsutism much more than if the nafarelin or the estrogen were used as single therapies.[49]

Although the use of GnRH analogs, such as goserelin causes suppression of testosterone and of the free testosterone index, these compounds do not exert sufficient influence on hair growth or the diameter of the hair for this therapy to be considered effective in the treatment of hirsutism.[50]

More recently, triptorelin, a long-acting GnRH agonist, was introduced for the treatment of hirsutism. A comparative study between CA 2 mg with 0.035 mg of ethinyl estradiol (Diane group), CA 50 mg on days 5–15 of the menstrual cycle and ethinyl estradiol 0.050 mg on days 5–26 each month (CA group), and triptorelin 3.75 mg intramuscularly every 28 days, with the addition of conjugated estrogen 0.625 mg on days 1–21 and medroxyprogesterone acetate 10 mg on days 12–21 (GnRH group), was performed. All women were treated for 1 year with a 1-year follow-up.[51] After 1 year of treatment, hirsutism decreased in all three groups, with greater changes in the

CA and GnRH groups. Following treatment, hirsutism increased rapidly in the Diane and CA groups and more gradually in the GnRH group.

Hyperprolactinemic SAHA

Some cases that resemble adrenal SAHA syndrome have the peculiarity that patients present with premature amenorrhea, and they have hyperprolactinemia. If the hyperprolactinemia is severe, with concomitant amenorrhea, the patient should be treated by the gynecologist. However, if the prolactin levels are not too high and the young woman is not amenorrheic but, as in adrenal SAHA, her menstrual cycles are 2 months or longer, and the predominant feature is the cutaneous one, we can treat her with the corticosteroid doses indicated earlier, together with 2.5–7.5 mg bromocriptine, a dopaminergic agonist, which achieves normalization of the prolactin levels within 3–5 months[52] and thus gonadal function and fertility are also restored in most cases of hyperprolactinemia (Figure 4).

It should also be remembered that CA acts at the level of the pituitary which is why it should be used in cases of hyperprolactinemic SAHA.[8]

Treatment of adrenal hirsutism

Congenital adrenal hyperplasia (CAH) and Cushing's syndrome must be treated with the same drugs as adrenal SAHA but using higher doses. Adrenal hyperplasia is treated with substitutive corticosteroid therapy, regardless of the enzymatic deficiency. Cushing's syndrome benefits from substitution therapy with corticosteroids associated with surgery and/or irradiation.

The best antiandrogen to be used is flutamide at a dose of 250–750 mg daily for 6–9 months, with an improvement of the four dermatological signs after 9 months.[26] Spironolactone (SL) is also used in adrenal hirsutism. The most efficient dose of SL seems to be 200 mg daily since this reduces the diameter of the facial vellus hairs in 83% of patients in 12 months. Cyproterone acetate must also be used at a dose of 100 mg/day from day 5–15 of the menstrual cycle during the 6 months

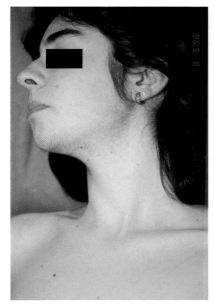

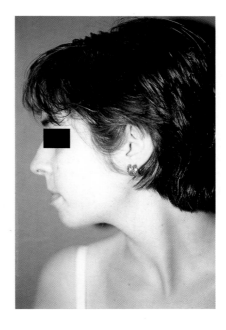

a   b

Figure 4

Hyperprolactinemic SAHA: **(a)** Central and lateral facial hirsutism. **(b)** Same patient as shown in Figure 4a, after 8 months treatment with bromocriptine 5 mg/day.

of the glucocorticoid suppression therapy period. In my opinion, CA has less effect on adrenal hirsutism than flutamide and spironolactone.

Treatment of ovarian hirsutism

Polycystic ovary syndrome (PCOS) must be treated by a gynecologist using higher doses than those used to treat the ovarian SAHA. Nevertheless, there are 'overlap cases' or ovarian SAHA cases that resemble polycystic ovary syndrome as a consequence of the evolving hypothalamo-hypophysial-adrenal-ovarian axis modification. In this situation there may be adrenal repercussions, which must be diagnosed and treated by dermatologists.

Other causes of hyperandrogenism

Treatment of pituitary hirsutism

Cases with high levels of prolactin arising from a pituitary adenoma can be treated by a dermatologist using 2.5–7.5 mg/day bromocriptine, while the patient is referred to the endocrinologist or gynecologist.

Treatment of iatrogenic hirsutism

If the hirsutism is drug-induced, the drug responsible should be eliminated and, on occasion, dermocosmetic measures should be used if the hirsutism has not disappeared after a certain time.

Treatment of other types of hirsutism

It is very rare to find hirsutism of hepatic origin or hirsutism resulting from the lack of peripheral conversion of androgens to estrogens. The specialist would diagnose the main cause of the hyperandrogenism and treat it. Nevertheless, every hirsute woman will benefit from 'losing weight', as this will decrease androgen levels and increase plasma SHBG.[53]

Non-dermatological medicosurgical treatments

These refer to treatment administered by the endocrinologist, gynecologist, or the general surgeon in cases of hirsutism resulting from endocrine or ovarian disorders.

The medical treatment of early- or late-onset congenital adrenal hyperplasias, Cushing's syndrome, and hirsutism caused by pituitary hypofunction, with possible acromegaly gigantism and hyperprolactinemia, will belong to the endocrinologist.

The gynecologist will treat all hirsutism that is accompanied by amenorrhea or significant menstrual disorders, which may lead to infertility. For this reason, it is within their territory to treat polycystic ovary syndrome, ovarian hyperthecosis or polycystic hyperplasia of the ovaries, pseudotumoral tecomatosis, the different ovarian tumors such as arrhenoblastoma, hilus cell, granular cell and Brenner tumors, which are responsible for androgenization, and hyperprolactinemias.

When the hyperprolactinemia is severe, with concomitant amenorrhea, it should be treated by the gynecologist. Bromocriptine may also be effective in slowing down the progression of hirsutism in certain anovulatory states; nevertheless, clomiphene citrate remains the treatment of choice when ovulation induction is desired. Regrettably, clomiphene has no value in the treatment of hirsutism since it is an indirect ovarian stimulator, which can increase the output of ovarian androgens.

General or specialized surgeons can treat the tumor of adrenal or pituitary glands, or other tumors that are capable of producing ectopic androgens.

Complementary dermatocosmetic methods

Currently, the methods of hair removal vary between simple, inexpensive home methods (e.g. depigmentation, shaving, plucking, depilatories) and expensive and potentially time-consuming methods, usually used by physicians and other healthcare professionals (e.g. laser, electrolysis).[54]

Home methods

Discoloration or bleaching

This technique may be useful for fair skinned women although the process must be repeated until acceptable cosmetic results are obtained. Its use by tanned women, however, does not usually have good results as the bleached hair can be more noticeable that it was before the bleaching.

Shaving

This technique is one of the most widely used methods of removing hair from the legs. However, it is not usually accepted as a method of removing facial hair by women. Recently, an electrical system has been introduced. This has a vibrating spiral which pulls out the hairs. Its main disadvantage is the pain it causes as a result of which it cannot be used in the axillar and inguinal areas.

Other mechanical shaving mechanisms such as the use of sand paper and pumice stone are not accepted by most women.

Depilation with tweezers

This is a safe and easy method for eliminating isolated hairs on the eyebrows, chin or periareolar areas. It is, however, painful and difficult to carry out in areas where there are many hairs.

Wax depilation

This is very effective and is the most efficient procedure for the depilation of the upper lip. The intervals between depilations vary from 2–6 weeks with the hair needing to be a minimum length of 1 mm in order for it to adhere to the wax and be pulled out.

Depilation with chemical substances

This is based on the use of substances which reduce the disulfur links of the cortex of the hair shaft, softening the hair shaft. The main ingredient of these products is thioglycolic acid, particularly calcium thioglycolate at a concentration of 2–4%. The high level of alkalis (Ph between 12 and 13) means that in order to prevent irritation these products can only be used on limited areas. The intervals between successive applications should be longer than with the wax method because this depilatory agent not only acts on the cortex of the emerged hair but also reaches the part of the hair which is hidden.[4]

Physician performed methods

Laser

This is the most popular method of hair removal but must be performed by a physician. This method is discussed in chapter 36.

Electrolysis

This is the second most popular method of hair removal. To perform this technique it is necessary to have a machine which produces a galvanic current (galvanic electrolysis) and a high frequency alternate current (thermolysis). This method of electrolysis is called 'blend' and it is the one used at present.[55] The galvanic current produces sodium hydroxide which destroys the bulb, including the papilla, but this is a slow method which requires a minute or more on each hair. In contrast, thermolysis is a quick method which produces heat to destroy the hair in a few seconds. This heat destroys the vellus hair but thick hairs are more problematic making combined use of the two methods necessary.[57] It

is most important that the electrode be placed exactly in the direction of the hair shaft. Once the electric current has passed for 3–5 seconds, the hair can be removed easily with tweezers. The needles destroy the bulb and papilla of anagen hair and coagulate an area which varies between 0.7 and 4 mm underneath the skin surface. A whitish halo around the follicular pore indicates that the current, or the time during which it was applied, was too great and this may leave scars.[58,59] If, after passing the current, there is no white halo but the hair is not easily removed, the procedure will have to be repeated as there was insufficient coagulation. After the procedure, an antiseptic, an emollient, an anti-inflammatory agent or even ice are usually applied for 30 seconds.

There is another form of electrical depilation which is called 'high frequency wave depilation' or 'depilation with electrical tweezers'. The apparatus used has such a low frequency that electronecrosis cannot by produced in the neighbouring tissues. The procedure consists of administering a high frequency wave through tweezers applied to a hair. The hair acts as an electrode and transports the energy to the bulb. This is known as the 'tip effect'.

The main problem with electrolysis is that 15–50% of the hairs treated in this way return.[55,56] 'Cotsarelli's hypothesis of the bulge'[60] explains that only those follicles in telogen or anagen I-II are destroyed definitely; that is to say, those in which the bulge and secondary germ in which the matrix cells of the bulb and the dermal papilla are located are close enough for the electric discharge to cause destruction of both without causing an important peripheral deterioration.

References

1. Toscano V, Adamo MV, Caiola S, et al.: Is hirsutism an evolving syndrome? *J Endocrinol* 1983; 97: 379–387.
2. Camacho F: Hypertricosis and hirsutism. In: Camacho F, Montagna W (eds.). *Tricología. Trichology. Trichologie.* Madrid, Garsi, 1982: 123–138.
3. Camacho F, Sánchez-Pedreño P: Hirsutismo. Concepto clasificación etiopatogénica y cuadros clínicos. *Monogr Dermatol* 1992; 5: 342–351.
4. Camacho F: Hirsutism. In: Camacho F, Montagna

W (eds.). *Trichology. Diseases of the Pilosebaceus Follicle.* Madrid, Aula Médica, 1997; 265–298.

5. Orfanos CE: Antiandrógenos en Dermatología. *Arch Arg Dermatol* 1982; **23(suppl 1)**: 51–55.
6. Sánchez-Pedreño P: *Estudio clínico, bioquímico, evolutivo y terapéutico del síndrome SAHA.* Doctoral Thesis. University of Seville, 1987.
7. Camacho F, Sánchez-Pedreño P: Síndrome SAHA. *Piel* 1991; **6**: 272–286.
8. Camacho F: Hirsutismo. Diagnóstico y tratamiento. *Monogr Dermatol* 1992; **5**: 352–373.
9. Camacho F: SAHA syndrome. In: Camacho F, Montagna W (eds.). *Trichology. Diseases of the Pilosebaceus Follicle.* Madrid, Aula Médica, 1997: 673–690.
10. Sánchez-Pedreño P, Camacho F: Acné en el síndrome SAHA. *Monogr Dermatol* 1990; **3**: 76–87.
11. Matias JR, Malloy VL, Orentreich N: Synergistic antiandrogenic effects of topical combination of 5-alpha-reductase and androgen receptor inhibitors in the hamster sebaceous glands. *J Invest Dermatol* 1988; **91**: 429–433.
12. Vincenzi C, Trevisi P, Farina P, Stinchi C, Tosti A: Facial contact dermatitis due to spironolactone in an antiacne cream. *Contact Dermatitis* 1993; **29**: 277.
13. Hatch R, Rosenfield RL, Kim MH, Tredway D: Hirsutism: implications, etiology and management. *Am J Obstetr Gynecol* 1981; **140**: 815–830.
14. Camacho F, Mazuecos J: Avances en terapéutica dermatológica 1993. *Monogr Dermatol* 1994; **7**: 211–235.
15. Alexandre S: Common baldness in women. *Sem Dermatol* 1985; **4**: 1–3.
16. O'Brien RC, Cooper ME, Murray RML, Seeman E, Thomas AK, Jerums G: Comparison of sequential cyproterone acetate/estrogen versus spironolactone/oral contraceptive in the treatment of hirsutism. *J Clin Endocrinol Metab* 1991; **72**: 1008–1013.
17. Bergfeld W, Redmond GP: Alopecia androgénetica femenina. *Monogr Dermatol* 1989; **2**: 118–126.
18. Ludwig E: Classification of the types of androgenetic alopecia (common baldness). Occurrence in the female sex. *Br J Dermatol* 1977; **97**: 249–254.
19. Camacho F: Alopecias: Androgenética. Areata. Cicatriciales. *Monogr Dermatol* 1993; **6**: 79–104.
20. Verschoore M: Aspects hormonaux de l'acne. *Ann Dermatol Vénéréol* 1987; **114**: 439–454.
21. Frieden IJ, Price VH: Androgenetic alopecia. In: Thiers BH, Dobson RL (eds.). *Pathogenesis of the skin disease.* New York, Churchill Livingstone, 1986: 41–55.
22. Camacho F, Sánchez-Pedreño P: Espironolactona en el tratamiento del síndrome SAHA. *Med Cut ILA* 1993; **21**: 107–114.
23. Neumann F, Schleusener A, Albring M: Pharmacology of antiandrogens. In: Hammerstein J (ed.). *Androgenization in Women. Acne, Seborrhoeae,* *Androgenetic Alopecia and Hirsutism.* Amsterdam, Excerpta Medica, 1980: 147–192.
24. Gupta AK, Knowles SR, Shear NH: Spironolactone associated cutaneous effects: a case report and a review of the literature. *Dermatology* 1994; **189**: 402–405.
25. Schon MP, Tebbe B, Trautmann C, Orfanos CE: Lichenoid drug eruption induced by spironolactone. *Acta Dermatol Venereol (Stockh)* 1994; **74**: 476.
26. Cusan L, Dupont A, Gómez JL, Tremblay RR, Labrie F: Comparison of flutamide and spironolactone in the treatment of hirsutism: a randomized controlled trial. *Fertil Steril* 1994; **61**: 281–287.
27. Martín-Hernández T, Jorquera E, Torres A, Camacho F, Herrera E: Comparación de la eficacia de la flutamida y el acetato de ciproterona en el tratamiento del hirsutismo asociado al síndrome de los ovarios poliquísticos. *Actas Dermosifiliogr* 1995: **86**: 327–334.
28. Camacho F: Tratamiento del hirsutismo. *Piel* 1995; **10**: 550–556.
29. Dodin S, Faure N, Cédrin I: Clinical efficacy and safety of low-dose flutamide alone and combined with an oral contraceptive for the treatment of idiopathic hirsutism. *Clin Endocrinol* 1995; **43**: 575–582.
30. Zabala R, Gardeazabal J, Manzano D, Aguirre A, Zubizarreta J, Tunneu A, Diaz Perez JL: Fotosensibilidad por flutamida. *Actas Dermosifiliogr* 1995; **86**: 323–325.
31. Amichai B, Grunwald MH, Sobel R: 5α-reductase inhibitors – a new hope in dermatology? *Int J Dermatol* 1997; **36**: 182–184.
32. Hughes CL: Hirsutism. In: Olsen E (ed.). *Disorders of Hair Growth. Diagnosis and treatment.* New York, McGraw-Hill, 1994: 337–351.
33. Fruzzetti F, de Lorenzo D, Parrini D: Finasteride (Proscar) reduces hair growth in hirsute women without affecting gonadotropin secretion. *J Clin Endocrinol Metab* 1994; **79**: 831–835.
34. Nguyen QH, Chen T, Wang X, Chen Y, Chien P: Finasteride inhibits 5α-reductase activity in human dermal fibroblasts: prediction of its therapeutic application in androgen-related diseases. *Int J Dermatol* 1995; **34**: 720–724.
35. Faure M, Drapier-Faure E: La prise en charge des hyperandrogénies. *Ann Dermatol Vénéréol* 1998; **125**: 533–540.
36. Sperling LC, Heimer WL: Androgen biology as a basis for the diagnosis and treatment of androgenic disorders in women. I. *J Am Acad Dermatol* 1993; **28**: 669–683.
37. Belchetz PE: Hirsutism. In: Verbow J (ed.). *Talking Points in New Clinical Applications Dermatology.* Lancaster, MTP, 1987: 1–25.
38. Sayag J, Aquilina C: *Hirsutismes.* Collection peau et phaneres. Marsella, Solal, 1989.

39. Hatwall A, Bhatt RP, Agrawal JK, Singh G, Bajpai HS: Spironolactone and cimetidine in treatment of acne. *Acta Derm Venereol (Stockh)* 1988; **68**: 84–87.

40. Inoue A, Teramae H, Hisa T, Taniguchi S, Chanoki M, Hamada T: Fixed drug eruption due to cimetidine. *Acta Derm Venereol (Stockh)* 1995; **75**: 250.

41. Bergfeld WF, Redmond GP: Hirsutism. In: Provost TT, Farmer ER (eds.). *Current Therapy in Dermatology – 2*. Philadelphia, BC Decker, 1988: 110–114.

42. Ehrmann DA, Rosenfield RL: Clinical review 10. An endocrinologic approach to the patient with hirsutism. *J Clin Endocrinol Metab* 1990; **71**: 1–4.

43. Jamin C: Hirsutisme. *Ann Dermatol Vénéréol* 1986; **113**: 723–726.

44. Mortimer CH, Rushton H, James KC: Effective medical treatment for common baldness in women. *Clin Exper Dermatol* 1984; **9**: 342–350.

45. Schmidt JB, Huber J, Spona J: Medroxyprogesterone acetate therapy in hirsutism. *Br J Dermatol* 1985; **113**: 161–165.

46. Hammerstein J: Antiandrogens: clinical aspects. In: Orfanos CE, Happle R (eds.). *Hair and Hair Diseases*. Berlin, Springer-Verlag, 1990: 827–886.

47. Shaw JC: Antiandrogen therapy in dermatology. *Int J Dermatol* 1996; **35**: 770–778.

48. Azziz R, Ochoa TM, Bradley EL, Potter HD, Boots LR: Leuprolide and estrogen versus oral contraceptive pills for the treatment of hirsutism: a prospective randomized study. *J Clin Endocrinol Metab* 1995; **80**: 3406–3411.

49. Heiner JS, Greendale GA, Kawakami AK, Fisher LM, Young D, Judd HL: Comparison of a gonadotropin-releasing hormone agonist and low-dose oral contraceptive given alone or together in the treatment of hirsutism. *J Clin Endocrinol Metab* 1995; **80**: 3412–3418.

50. Rademaker M, Simpson NB, Gudmundsson J, Bonduelle M, Fleming R, Coutts JRT: Effect of the gonadotrophin releasing hormone analogue, goserelin, and oestradiol replacement on sebum excretion rates and hair size in mildly hirsute women. *J Dermatol Treat* 1991; **1**: 289–292.

51. Carmina E, Lobo RA: Gonadotrophin-releasing hormone agonist therapy for hirsutism is as effective as high-dose cyproterone acetate but results in a longer remission. *Hum Reprod* 1997; **12**: 663–666.

52. Peserico A, Ruzza G, Veller Fornasa C, Bertoli P, Cipriani R: Bromocriptine treatment in patients with late-onset acne and idiopathic hyperprolactinemia. *Acta Derm Venereol (Stockh)* 1988; **68**: 83–84.

53. Dunaif A: Hirsutism. In: Lebwohl M (ed.). *Difficult Diagnoses in Dermatology*. New York, Churchill Livingstone, 1988: 375–388.

54. Olsen EA: Methods of hair removal. *J Am Acad Dermatol* 1999; **40**: 143–155.

55. Wagner RF: Physical methods for the management of hirsutism. *Cutis* 1990; **45**: 319–326.

56. Chernosky ME: Electroepilation in hirsutism. Letter to the Editor. *J Am Acad Dermatol* 1987; **17**: 142–143.

57. Richard RN, Meharg GE: Electrolysis: Observations from 13 years and 140 000 hours of experience. *J Am Acad Dermatol* 1995; **33**: 662–666.

58. Kaminsky CA, Kaminsky AR, Rubin J, Iribarren NA: Hirsutismo. In Viglioglia PA, Rubin J (eds.). *Cosmiatría II*. Buenos Aires, AP Panamericana, 1989: 239–250.

59. Moreno JC: Tratamiento físico de la hipertricosis e hirsutismo. Depilación. *Monogr Dermatol* 1992; **5**: 384–388.

60. Sun TT, Cotsarelis G, Lavker RM: Hair follicular stem cells: The bulge-activation hypothesis. *J Invest Dermatol* 1991; **95(Suppl)**: 77S–78S.

36

Laser treatment

Hugh Zachariae and Peter Bjerring

Introduction

In principle, the term 'hirsutism' should be restricted to androgen-dependent hair patterns and the term 'hypertrichosis' to other patterns of excessive hair growth; however, the words are often applied interchangeably and indiscriminately to excessive hair growth of any type in any distribution. This has also been the case in the literature on laser treatment of unwanted hair growth disorders.

All patients experiencing unwanted hair are prone to cosmetic, psychological and social problems, which may lead them to seek medical advice.[1,2] Until recently, drug therapy for hirsutism had been the administration of oestrogens, cyproterone acetate, or spironolactone (reviewed by Camacho in Chapter 35); temporary cosmetic measures included plucking, bleaching, waxing, shaving and depilatory creams, while electrolysis and high-frequency electroepilation have been the only accepted methods for more long-lasting epilation. However, the latter treatments are tedious, may cause pitting[3,4] and, for technical reasons, may be followed by an operator-dependent regrowth of 15–50% of hairs.[5] Recently lasers and filtered flash-lamp systems have been used as a simple and fast technique for optical hair removal in hirsutism and hypertrichosis.[6,7] This treatment will be discussed in relation to the existing non-laser technology.

Techniques for laser hair removal

All forms of laser energy represent different types of light. Laser stands for Light Amplification by the Stimulated Emission of Radiation. Most medical lasers, however, do not employ ionizing radiation and consequently should not be associated with the risks inherent with the high-energy forms of ionizing radiation that are normally used in the management of cancer. Several different lasers (Table 1) have been developed to permit treatment of large areas of unwanted hair with less discomfort and fewer complications than electrolysis and electroepilation. Most of the techniques are based upon the principle of a selective photothermolysis taking

Table 1 Parameters of common lasers used for hair removal.

System name	Source	Wavelength (nm)	Pulse width (ms)	Energy fluence (J/cm)	Beam diameter (mm)	Repetition rate (Hz)
Chromos 694	Ruby, normal mode	694	0.5–1.0	10–25	5	1
EpiLaser	Ruby, normal mode	694	3	10–75	10–12	0.5
Meltemi	Ruby, normal mode	694	0.5	20	2	?
EpiTouch	Ruby, dual mode	694	0.8	5–10	4–6	1.2
SOFTLight	Nd:YAG	1064	10–20	2.5 (1.2)	7	?
EpiTouch 5100	Alexandrite	755	2	25–40	7	5
LightSheer	Diode	800	5–30	15–40	9	?

place in the hair follicle in order to reduce unwanted injury to perifollicular tissue.[6] To accomplish this, light of the right combination of wavelength, energy fluence and pulse duration should be delivered, while the target should be capable of absorbing light of the particular wavelength in an amount of time that is equal to or less than its thermal relaxation time. In order to have an effect on hair growth, precise damage must be applied to the areas of hair follicle germinal cells. Two different techniques have been used:[6] in the first technique, light is absorbed by normal components like melanin keratohyalin; in the second, an exogenous material has been absorbed by the hair or placed in the follicular orifice.

Ruby lasers

Melanin present in the follicular epithelium and papillae acts as a chromophore for the red light at a wavelength of 694 nm delivered by the ruby lasers.[8] A limiting factor for hair removal is that melanin is also found in the epithelial cells of the epidermis, and because of high epidermal absorption in patients with dark-brown or black skin, these patients should not be offered ruby laser depilation. In fair skin the ruby light is transmitted through the epidermis to the dermis, where the light is scattered in all directions by sudden changes of refractory indices of the different anatomical structures. Approximately 15–20% of the ruby light penetrates through the entire dermis. Here it enters the hair follicles at different levels and is absorbed in hair melanin and converted to heat, resulting in selective thermolysis. The treatment technique includes preoperative shaving of the treatment area to prevent long and dark hairs from conducting thermal energy to adjacent skin surfaces, leading to injury.

The Chromos 694 (SLS/Biophile), the Meltemi (NWL), and the EpiLaser (Spectrum Medical) are normal-mode long-pulse ruby lasers, while the EpiTouch (Laser Industries/Sharplan) is a dual-mode ruby laser, that is designed to be operated by the so-called Q-switched mode to emit very short pulses in the nano-second range for treatment of tattoos and benign pigmented lesions and normal long pulses for removal of unwanted

hair. The EpiLaser and the EpiTouch are equipped with cooling devices. The parameters of the different lasers are listed in Table 1.

The results have shown[8-16] that prolonged and even permanent hair loss is possible using ruby lasers (Figure 1). Animal studies[17] and human experience[9] have shown that the hair growth cycle affects hair follicle destruction by ruby laser pulses. Actively growing and pigmented anagen hair follicles have been found to be sensitive to hair removal by normal mode ruby laser exposure, whereas catagen and telogen stage hair follicles seem resistant to the laser irradiation. Selective thermal injury to follicles has been observed histologically, and hair regrowth has been found to be fluence-dependent. In animals exposed during the anagen phase, intermediate fluences induced non-scarring alopecia, whereas high fluences induced scarring alopecia. These findings should be taken into consideration for optimal laser hair removal.

The great variation in clinical results is probably the result of the use of different types of lasers, different laser fluences, different durations of laser pulses, and assessment periods varying from 8 days to 12 months. Grossman et al,[8] using a normal mode ruby laser, found that the pulses produced a fluence-dependent growth

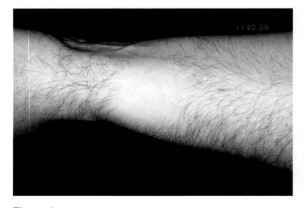

Figure 1

Alopecia induced by a Chromos 694 ruby laser on the lower arm following two treatments with a 1-year interval. The photograph was taken 3 years after the first treatment.

delay of hair follicles and apparently permanent hair removal in some subjects, while McCoy and Evans[16] showed that the dual-mode ruby laser in all cases only switched hairs from anagen to a prolonged catagen phase. Moreover, Walther et al.[18] found no evidence for histological damage to hair follicles, while Bjerring,[19] in a limited preliminary study, demonstrated destruction of hair and hair follicles (Figure 2). (Refer to Table 1 for the differences in physical parameters between the different ruby lasers.) Pulse durations of more than 1 ms and a spot size of more than 5 mm have been recommended for obtaining a long-term effect.[18]

Variations in body region may also play a role. These variations are considerable, with respect to both hair depth and hair growth cycles[20] (Table 2). Figure 3 shows the result of hair removal from one-half of the upper lip 4 weeks after therapy with the Chromos 694 ruby laser. Figure 4 is a photomicrograph showing thermal injury to a dark terminal hair, together with a non-affected vellus hair 2 hours after therapy, while Figure 2 shows the photomicrograph of a destroyed hair and hair follicle approximately 4 months following exposure to ruby laser treatment.

Intervals between treatments should be selected specifically for each anatomical region in order to be able to treat all hairs in the anagen phase. In theory, if hair removal by lasers should be considered permanent, two treatments would be necessary but also sufficient. The possibility of achieving this is illustrated by Figure 1, which shows an area of the lower arm that was treated twice by ruby laser with a 1-year interval. The photograph was taken 3 years after the first treatment. For practical reasons, however, patients should expect at least four treatments. In one

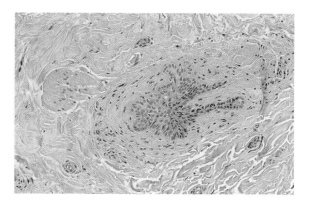

Figure 2

Coagulation, fibrosis and inflammation at hair follicle level. This photograph was taken approximately 4 weeks after ruby laser treatment.

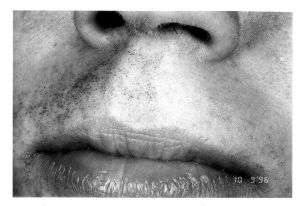

Figure 3

Results of hair removal by ruby laser of one-half of the upper lip. This photograph was taken approximately 4 months after treatment.

Table 2   Hair growth cycle in different body regions.[19]

Body region	Anagen duration (months)	Phase (%)	Telogen duration (months)	Phase (%)
Beard (chin)	12	70	3	30
Moustache	16	65	6	35
Leg	21	20	19	80
Pubic region	8	30	0.5	70
Arm	13	20	13	80
Axilla	4–6	30	3	70

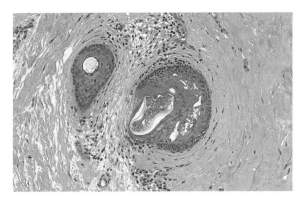

Figure 4

Coagulated brown terminal hair 2 hours after laser treatment. Note the intact vellus hair.

study,[9] where success was defined as greater than 50% hair removal, 59% of patients reported successful results after 90 days or more after the last treatment, and with a success defined as greater than 25% hair removal, successful treatment was raised to 75%. In the same study only a few side-effects were observed; in general, pain was no clinical problem, and no significant scarring was observed. A temporary hypopigmentation was experienced by approximately 10%, but in only one patient did this persist until 90 days following treatment. The discomfort of ruby laser therapy can be diminished by the use of topical anaesthesia. A slight itch, and transient erythema and oedema are not uncommon but usually of little concern to the patients.

The limitations of the use of ruby laser therapy are evident in patients with lightly pigmented hair, whether grey, white, yellow or red. In the study mentioned[9] an overall statistically significant inverse correlation between percentage of grey hair and the patient's report of successful removal of hair was found ($p = 0.003$). When more than 50% grey hairs were present, the success rate dropped from approximately 70% to approximately 40%. It was also observed, that previously electroepilated or tweezers-treated scarred areas needed higher laser energy for successful therapy, probably because of the lower light transmittance through the scar tissue.

The alexandrite laser

Alexandrite laser absorption in melanin is somewhat lower than that of the ruby laser. The claim has been that this should not modify absorption in the hair shafts but that it might give less absorption by darker epidermis. The EpiTouch 5100 (Sharplan/Allendale) pulsed alexandrite laser operates at a wavelength of 755 nm with a 7 mm spot at energy fluences of 25–40 J/cm^2. A 15-month study[21] of 126 patients on a wide range of body sites, operating at a repetition rate of up to 5 Hz and using a transparent gel as epidermal heat sink, resulted in a hair count reduction close to 65% of the pre-treatment value before the second treatment, and lower than 12% 3 months after the last treatment. The intervals between treatments ranged from 4 weeks to $3\frac{1}{2}$ months. The side-effects were transient redness, transient very superficial burns sometimes with blistering and transient slight hypopigmentation. No statements on permanency could be made from this study.

The Q-switched neodymium:ytrium-aluminium-garnet (Nd:YAG) laser

The infrared light at a wavelength of 1064 nm is poorly absorbed by melanin, therefore the Nd:YAG laser known as the SOFTLight (Thermolase Corp) is considered to need another chromophore. In one study, to achieve this a topical mineral oil lotion containing a carbon-based material was massaged into the skin prior to treatment.[22] A wax epilation of the area to be treated has also been recommended prior to the procedure to increase the penetration of the mineral oil–carbon solution.[23] The carbon material located deep within the follicles can then be activated by laser light as in the treatment of tattoos. The particles undergo a rapid temperature increase and produce thermal injury to the germinative cells of the follicle. Besides producing thermal energy kinetic energy is also produced. This leads to a shock wave that propels carbon particles at high speed in many directions within the follicle, resulting in mechanical damage.

Initial results with this laser have demonstrated a high degree of temporary reduction in hair density with minimal and only temporary side-effects such as erythema and oedema. Rare petechiae may persist for up to 5 days. The results, however, do not seem to be permanent, as the delay in regrowth only lasts, on average, from 3–6 months.[22] The hair that regrows is often small in calibre and lighter. The Nd:YAG laser has been tried without adjuvant topical preparation[24] but the studies with this modality are limited.

Diode lasers

Diode lasers (Star Medical), or coherent lasers, using wavelengths of 800 nm with a pulse width of 5–30 ms and an energy per pulse of 15–40 J/cm^2 have recently been introduced for hair removal. On a short-term basis they have been successful but no data on the long-term efficacy are available at present. In a comparison with a ruby laser (3 ms and max. fluence of 50 J/cm^2) the percentage regrowth at 1 month was significantly higher for the diode laser but the efficacy after two treatments was higher for the diode laser.[25]

Laser hair removal based on photodynamic therapy

This technique is only in an early stage of development[26] but deserves a mention since it offers the ability to treat that is independent of skin or hair colour. The photodynamic treatment with topical aminolevulinic acid (ALA), which induces the synthesis of the potent photosensitizer protoporphyrin IX, has for several years been offered for treatment of cutaneous malignancies. Since ALA is more selectively absorbed by hair follicles than by the epidermis, the exposure to red light that activates the photosensitizer may cause the necessary selective cell damage for the destruction of the unwanted hair.

Comparison with non-laser technology

Direct comparisons with electrolysis and electroepilation cannot easily be made at present because of the lack of long-term follow-up of laser therapy. Potential advantages of laser therapy are that many more hairs can be treated per session and that treatment discomfort in general is considered to be less in laser therapy. The latter has been confirmed by the use of a post-treatment questionnaire.[9] When restricting therapy to patients with fair skin, longer-lasting hypopigmentation seems extremely rare after laser therapy and permanent depigmentation is probably absent.[6,9] Hyperpigmentation is common in electroepilation but only rarely reported after laser therapy; firm data are, however, still lacking. The duration of a hyperpigmentation reported by questionnaire[9] was only around 7 days, leading to the view, that the patients had misinterpreted a crust formation as hyperpigmentation. No permanent scarring has been found following laser-assisted hair removal; this is not so after electroepilation. Although scarring in electroepilation has been reduced following the introduction of an isolated needle, which limits heat generation to the base of the follicle,[27] both insulated and non-insulated epilating needles are still in use, and we still find signs of scarring in patients fairly recently electroepilated, when they turn up for laser therapy. It should also be brought to attention, that the correct placement of the insulated needle remains very important as well as the use of appropriate intensities and durations of treatment.

More recently, an intense source of white light from a flashlamp modified by appropriate filtering has been designed for removal of unwanted hair allowing adjustments in pulse duration, pulse delay, wavelength, and energy fluence.[28] Preliminary results seem promising, and so do preliminary comparisons with a 35 J/cm^2, 4 mm spotsize ruby laser.[29] New filtered flashlamp systems are underway.

Conclusions

The use of lasers has assumed an increasingly important role in the treatment of a variety of cutaneous lesions over the past few decades. Lasers, when properly used, often offer clear advantages when compared with older, traditional approaches. They occasionally, however, have created unrealistic expectations. At present, laser treatment of hirsutism and hypertrichosis should be considered a useful method for many patients. The principles of selective photothermolysis of hair and hair follicles have been employed with success to large areas of the skin with minimal discomfort and with low risk of scarring. The present laser therapy usually requires no or only topical analgesia. It is possible to remove some hair permanently with certain lasers, and to induce a prolonged delay in regrowth by switching hairs from anagen to a prolonged catagen phase using others. At present, the largest and longest experience is with the ruby lasers; nevertheless, in these cases more clinical investigations are needed to describe the long-term efficacy of the treatment. Further developments within technology may improve the rate of permanency of laser treatment (as well as of treatment with filtered flashlamps) of unwanted hair.

References

1. Rabinowitz S, Cohen R, Le Roith D: Anxiety and hirsutism. *Psychol Rep* 1983; **53**: 827–833.
2. Sonino N, Fava G, Mani E, et al.: Quality of life of hirsute women. *Postgrad Med J* 1993; **69**: 186–189.
3. Richards R, Meharg G. Electrolysis: observations from 13 years and 140,000 hours of experience. *J Am Acad Dermatol* 1995; **33**: 662–666.
4. Grunnet E, Zachariae H: Hypertrichosis. *Mdskr Prakt Lœgeg* 1980; **58**: 485–492.
5. Wagner R: Physical methods for the management of hirsutism. *Cutis* 1990; **45**: 199–202.
6. Wheeland R: Laser-assisted hair removal. *Dermatol Clin* 1997; **15**: 469–477.
7. Zachariae H: Can the lasers remove hair permanently. *Forum for Nord Derm Ven* 1997; **2**: 13–14.
8. Grossman M, Dierickx C, Farinelli W, et al.: Damage to hair follicles by normal-mode ruby laser pulses. *J Am Acad Dermatol* 1996; **35**: 889–894.
9. Bjerring P, Zachariae H, Lybecker H, Clement M: Evaluation of the free-running ruby laser for hair removal. *Acta Derm Venereol (Stockh)* 1998; **78**: 48–51.
10. Solomon M: Hair removal using the lung-pulsed ruby laser. *Ann Plast Surg* 1998; **41**: 1–6.
11. Sommer S, Render C, Burd R, Sheehan-Dare R: Ruby laser treatment for hirsutism: clinical response and patient tolerance. *Br J Dermatol* 1998; **138**: 1009–1014.
12. Lask G, Elman M, Slatkin M, et al.: Laser-assisted hair removal by selective photothermolysis. Preliminary results. *Dermatol Surg* 1997; **23**: 737–739.
13. William R, Havoonjian H, Isagholian K, et al.: A clinical study of hair removal using the lung-pulsed ruby laser. *Dermatol Surg* 1998; **24**: 837–842.
14. Dierickx C, Grossmann M, Farinelli W, Anderson R: Permanent hair removal by normal-mode ruby laser. *Arch Dermatol* 1998; **134**: 837–842.
15. Vander Kam V, Achauer B: Hair removal with the ruby laser (694 nm). *Plast Surg Nurs* 1997; **17**: 144–145.
16. McCoy S, Evans A: Long pulsed ruby laser for hair removal – a histological analysis. *Austral J Dermatol* 1997; **38**: A329.
17. Lin T, Manuskiatti W, Dierickx C, et al.: Hair growth cycle affects hair follicle destruction by ruby laser pulses. *J Invest Dermatol* 1998; **41**: 1–6.
18. Walther T, Bäumler W, Wenig M, et al.: Selective photothermolysis of hair follicles by normal-mode ruby laser treatment. *Acta Derm Venereol (Stockh)* 1998; **78**: 443–444.
19. Bjerring P: The ruby laser for depilation. *Fifth Congress of the European Academy of Dermatology and Venereology, Lisbon, October, 1996.*
20. Braun-Falco O: Dynamik des normalen und pathologischen Haarwachstum. *Arch Kiln Exp Dermatol* 1966; **227**: 419–452.
21. Finkel B, Eliezri Y, Waldman A, Slatkine M: Pulsed alexandrite laser technology for non-invasive hair removal. *J Clin Laser Med Surg* 1957; **15**: 225–229.
22. Goldberg D, Littler C, Wheeland R: Topical suspension-assisted Q-switched Nd:YAG laser hair removal. *Dermatol Surg* 1997; **23**: 741–745.
23. Nanni C, Alster T: Optimizing treatment parameters for hair removal using a topical carbon-based solution and 1064-nm Q-switched neodymium:YAG laser energy. *Arch Dermatol* 1997; **133**: 1546–1549.
24. Kilmer S, Chotzen V: Q-switched Nd:YAG laser (1064 nm) hair removal without adjuvant topical preparation. *Laser Surg Med* 1997; **9(suppl)**: 31.
25. Dierickx C, Grossman M, Farinelli A, et al.: Comparison between a long pulsed ruby laser and a pulsed infrared laser system for hair removal. *Laser Surg Med* 1998; **10**: 42.

26. Grossman M, Wimberly J, Dwyer P, et al.: PDT for hirsutism. *Laser Surg Med* 1995; **7**: 44.

27. Kobayashi T: Electrosurgery using insulated needles: epilation. *J Dermatol Surg Oncol* 1985; **11**: 993.

28. Gold M, Bell M, Foster T, Street S: Long-term epilation using the EpiLight broad band, intense pulsed light hair removal system. *Dermatol Surg* 1997; **23**: 909–913.

29. Hebel T, Drosner M: Comparison of normal mode ruby laser and epilight for hair removal on the face. *Laser Surg Med* 1998; **10(suppl)**: 57.

Index